COMPREHENSIVE REVIEW OF RESPIRATORY CARE

SECOND EDITION

William V. Wojciechowski, M.S., R.R.T.

Chairman and Associate Professor
Department of Respiratory Care and Cardiopulmonary Sciences
University of South Alabama
Mobile, Alabama

Paula E. Neff, M.S., R.R.T., J.D.

Associate Professor and Director
Department of Respiratory Therapy
Division of Allied Health Sciences
Indiana University Northwest
Gary, Indiana

Adjunct Associate Professor of Respiratory Therapy
Division of Allied Health Sciences
Indiana University School of Medicine

A WILEY MEDICAL PUBLICATION
JOHN WILEY & SONS

New York • Chichester • Brisbane • Toronto • Singapore

PB 922/97986.

Library of Congress Cataloging in Publication Data:

Wojciechowski, William V.
    Comprehensive review of respiratory care.

    (A Wiley medical publication)
    Rev. ed. of: Comprehensive review of respiratory
therapy. c1981.
    Includes bibliographies and index.
    1. Respiratory therapy—Examinations, questions, etc.
I. Neff, Paula E.   II. Wojciechowski, William V.
Comprehensive review of respiratory therapy.
III. Title.   IV. Series.   [DNLM: 1. Respiratory Therapy
—examination questions. WB 18 W847c]

RC735.I5W64   1986   615.8'36'076   86-26644
ISBN 0-471-83090-9 (pbk.)

Printed in the United States of America

10 9 8 7 6 5 4 3 2 1

PREFACE

Because the first edition of this book was used for purposes beyond that originally intended by the authors, this edition has been expanded to meet more completely these multiple needs.

Originally, the first edition was written to assist those persons preparing to sit for the National Board for Respiratory Care (NBRC) written registry examination. However, the first edition was frequently used by (1) students in both technician and therapist programs to assist them in preparation for their course examinations, (2) instructors for providing assistance in formulating course examinations in their respiratory care programs, and (3) persons preparing for the Entry Level Certification Examination and the Advanced Practitioner Examination.

The second edition has been structured using the curriculum content areas listed in the Essentials and Guidelines of an Accredited Educational Program for the Respiratory Care Practitioner recently implemented by the Joint Review Committee for Respiratory Therapy Education (JRCRTE).

These curriculum content areas include the following:

1. Basic Sciences
   a. Cardiopulmonary anatomy and physiology
   b. Chemistry
   c. Mathematics
   d. Microbiology
   e. Pharmacology
   f. Physics
2. Clinical Sciences
   a. Cardiopulmonary diseases
   b. Pediatrics and perinatology
3. Respiratory Care Content Areas
   a. Aerosol therapy
   b. Airway management
   c. Cardiopulmonary assessment
   d. Cardiopulmonary diagnostics and interpretation
   e. Cardiopulmonary monitoring and interpretation
   f. Cardiopulmonary rehabilitation and home care
   g. Chest physiotherapy

    h. Oxygen therapy
    i. Medical gas therapy
    j. Humidity therapy
    k. Hyperinflation therapy
    l. Mechanical ventilation
    m. Pediatrics and perinatology

This edition has been fashioned to meet a variety of educational needs. The question, answer, analysis, and references format has been retained to assist (1) students in respiratory therapy programs (technician and therapist), (2) graduates preparing for credentialing examinations (Entry Level Certification Examination and Advanced Practitioner Examination), and (3) practitioners seeking to review subject matter. This edition is more comprehensive and encompasses the matrices of both national credentialing examinations.

Content areas that have been added include hemodynamic monitoring, home respiratory care, cardiopulmonary rehabilitation, pediatrics, neonatology, chest radiography, and high frequency ventilation. A special mathematics section has been added to assess computational skills pertinent to cardiopulmonary physiology and clinical care. More calculations in a variety of content areas have, likewise, been included.

Furthermore, clinically oriented questions have been included in this revision. This book will be useful to assess knowledge, understanding, and clinical application of the principles and practices associated with respiratory care. The analyses have been expanded to be more instructional and to review more information. More diagrams have been inserted to better illustrate the concepts and practices related to the curriculum content areas.

                                                                                 W.V.W.

ACKNOWLEDGMENTS

Sincere thanks and gratitude are given to Fred Hill, M.A., R.R.T., for his thorough review of the entire manuscript. Deserving of accolades is Deanna Howell for her unrelenting efforts in typing the manuscript. Appreciation also goes to Wendy Hill for the magnificent job that she did on the original illustrations.

W.V.W.

CONTENTS

Section 4. RESPIRATORY CARE CONTENT AREAS ASSESSMENTS
AND ANALYSES   279

Section 5. APPENDIXES   631

SECTION 1

INTRODUCTION

TEXT OBJECTIVES

The objectives of this text are to:

1. Prepare persons for the National Board for Respiratory Care (NBRC) credentialing examinations (Entry Level and Advanced Practitioner).
2. Assist respiratory care students (technician and therapist levels) in preparing for course examinations.
3. Prepare practitioners for legal credentialing (state) examinations.
4. Determine content areas requiring remediation.
5. Present an organized approach to examination preparation.
6. Reinforce learning by providing several cross-references for each question.
7. Clarify theoretical and clinical aspects of cardiopulmonary care via analysis of each question.
8. Provide a self-assessment mechanism for credentialed respiratory care practitioners.
9. Supplement hospital in-service education programs.
10. Assist respiratory care educators in developing evaluation instruments.
11. Assist nurses preparing to sit for the Critical Care Registered Nurses (CCRN) Examination.
12. Provide nursing students and other allied health personnel with the rudiments of respiratory care, fostering an interdisciplinary approach to respiratory care.

EXAMINATION PREPARATION

STUDY HINTS

If you are using this book to prepare for any of the NBRC credentialing examinations, establish a timetable for complete review of the material. The timetable that you establish should be realistic. If you are employed, your timetable should take your work schedule into consideration. Additionally, your timetable should include time required to read and study the question analyses, as well as time needed to read and study appropriate references.

Note: It is *not* necessary to have all the references listed here. Two or three of the standard texts should be sufficient.

A suggested schedule for the completion of this study guide is shown below:

TIME	CONTENT AREA
Week 1	1. Mathematics (25 items); cardiopulmonary anatomy and physiology (100 items)
Week 2	2. Chemistry (50 items); microbiology (35 items); pharmacology (50 items); physics (50 items)
Week 3	3. Cardiopulmonary diseases (50 items); pediatrics and perinatology (50 items)
Week 4	4. Oxygen/gas therapy (50 items); aerosol/humidity therapy (65 items); hyperinflation therapy (45 items); chest physiotherapy (40 items); cardiopulmonary resuscitation (50 items)

Week 5   5. Airway management (50 items); mechanical ventilation (50 items); cardiopul-
             monary evaluation/cardiopulmonary monitoring and interpretation (55 items)

Week 6   6. Cardiopulmonary diagnostics and interpretation (80 items); pediatrics and perina-
             tology (50 items); cardiopulmonary rehabilitation and home care (50 items)

Keep in mind that the NBRC examinations represent a critical stage in your professional career. Successful completion of these examinations is essential to your professional
growth. You owe it to yourself to impose strict measures of self-discipline and to adhere to
your established timetable. Once you begin a test section, you should proceed uninterrupt-
edly to its completion.

Simulate testing conditions as closely as possible. Sit at a desk or table in a well-
lighted, ventilated, quiet area.

The assessments should be taken without specific advance preparation. You should rely
on your educational and experiential background at this point. This policy will provide
you with a baseline from which to begin charting your progress as you work through this
book.

If you are using this book to prepare for course examinations in the content categories
contained here, perform the appropriate assessment(s) in a simulated test-taking environment. Then study the analyses of the questions you answered incorrectly and those that
you may have answered correctly by guessing. Also, refer to some of the references pertaining to the question(s).

TEST-TAKING HINTS

As you work through any of the examinations contained here, occasionally note the time.
Try not to spend more than 1 minute per question.

If you are uncertain as to which response to select after reading the question, attempt to
eliminate responses that may be obviously incorrect. The rationale for this action is to increase your "educated guessing" percentage. For example, if you have five responses from
which to choose and have no idea what the correct response is, your chance of selecting
the correct answer is only 1 in 5, or 20%. If you can realistically eliminate any re-
sponse(s), you automatically increase your percentage to something greater than 20%, depending upon how many responses you can eliminate. Do not leave any questions unan-
swered.

If you encounter any difficult questions or if you guess, somehow mark these questions
so that you can return to them to study the information that they contain.

NBRC CREDENTIALING EXAMINATION FORMAT

INSTRUCTIONS

Two types of test instructions are found on the NBRC examinations. One type describes
how to respond to the multiple-choice and multiple true-false questions. The other type explains how to respond to the situational sets.

Multiple-choice and multiple true-false instructions read as follows:

DIRECTIONS: Each of the questions or incomplete statements below is followed by five sug-gested answers or completions. Select the one which is best in each case and then blacken the corresponding space on the answer sheet.

Situational set instructions read as follows:

DIRECTIONS: Each group of questions below concerns a certain situation. In each case, first study the description of the situation. Then, choose the one best answer to each question follow-ing it and blacken the corresponding space on the answer sheet.

MULTIPLE-CHOICE QUESTIONS

EXAMPLE

Mobile is a(n) ———————.
A. city
B. country
C. state

D. island
E. planet

The one best response is A.

Multiple-choice test items require that you choose the one best response from five plau-sible selections. This style of test item is constructed in such a manner as to present all five choices as plausible responses. You must determine which choice represents the one best response. The phrase *one best response* refers to the choice that, among those present, most accurately completes the stem of the question. The best response may not actually be the precise answer; however, from the five selections available, it represents the best choice.

Read the question carefully and completely. Be mindful of key words, such as

1. Most
2. Not
3. Generally
4. Should
5. Recommend
6. Usually

For example, you might encounter a question worded thus:

IPPB is generally contraindicated when the patient has. . . .

Here *generally* means "under most circumstances." This is not to say that IPPB would never be given to a patient exhibiting any of the contraindications that might be listed. The statement means that IPPB usually would not be given but there may be circumstances that would require its administration despite what is generally considered accepted. Again, read both the stem and the responses carefully and completely.

MULTIPLE TRUE-FALSE QUESTIONS

EXAMPLE

Which statements describe the city of Mobile, Alabama?

    I. It is the state capital.
   II. It is located in the Gulf Coast area.
  III. It is located in the southern region of the state.
  IV. It is the annual site for the American Junior Miss Pageant.
   V. It is the site of the annual Senior Bowl football game.

A. I, II, III, IV, V   D. II, III, IV, V only
B. I, III, IV only   E. I, II, III, IV only
C. III, V only

The correct response is D.

You must select the statements that refer to or describe the stem. The statements range in number from four to five. All the true statements relating to the stem must be selected.

The process of elimination is easier to use with this type of question. For example, referring to the sample question, suppose you were certain that III and IV were true concerning the stem and that I was false but you were uncertain about II. You could automatically eliminate A, B, and E knowing that I was false. Choice C can be eliminated because it does not contain IV, which you know is true. Since no selection is provided using III and IV only, D represents your logical choice.

As you read through the responses available, you should indicate the true responses with some kind of mark (X, T, etc.). You will thus save time by not having to reread selections.

SITUATIONAL SETS

EXAMPLE

Exploration in the Mobile River area began in 1519 when the Spanish Admiral Alonzo Alverez de Piñeda entered and charted the area known as Mobile Bay. The old fort, now known as Fort Morgan, guarding Mobile Bay was first fortified by the Spanish in 1599. Settled in 1711 by the French, the Bay area has had a tradition rich in culture and essential in the affairs of the nation from its formative years to the present.

    Trade and shipping are vital to the economy of the area. More than thirty-five million tons of shipping are handled annually through the Port of Mobile, which is rated among the top ports in the country. More than ten million tons of shipping are carried yearly on the Tombigbee–Black Warrior Waterway with its modern locks and dams. The intracoastal waterway, crossing the southern end of the state, is connected at Mobile Bay with both inland and ocean shipping. Four railroads and four airlines serve the Bay area. Diversified farming, woodland crops, and seafood and fisheries are major factors in the economy of the area. (Taken from *The University of South Alabama Bulletin,* 1979–1980.)

1. Fort Morgan was first fortified by the Spanish in what period of time?

  A. during the Renaissance   D. in 1519
  B. sometime before 1610   E. last Thursday
  C. after 1700

(B is the best response.)

2. Which statement(s) refer(s) to Mobile Bay?

  I. It helps irrigate the diversified farming and woodland crops in the area.
  II. It is responsible for the large trade and shipping industry in the Mobile area.
  III. Ten million tons of shipping are carried yearly through the Bay.
  IV. A major municipal airport is located immediately adjacent to the Bay.
  V. The French were the first people to explore the Mobile Bay area.

  A. II only   D. IV, V only
  B. III, IV only   E. I, II, IV only
  C. II only

  (C is the correct response.)

The scenario should be read carefully and understood completely. The scenario should be reread if the situation described is not clear. After reading the questions, refer to the narrative for information needed to make the correct choice. The example given does not describe a clinical situation. However, it serves to illustrate this type of question.

In the first question (multiple-choice) the exact data presented in the narrative were not asked for in the stem. Instead, a time period was sought; therefore, B (sometime before 1610) represents the one best response.

The second question (multiple true-false) sought much more information than the first. Statement I should not have been chosen because the narrative did not state that Mobile Bay was responsible for irrigation, nor did the narrative imply it. Statement II is the only applicable statement in terms of the stem. Statements III, IV, and V are not true regarding the stem.

All information should be considered, including that which is found in the questions following the narrative. Your responses to previous questions about the situation should be kept in mind as you consider responses to other questions within the same scenario. For example, if four questions are asked within a situational set, you should consider your responses to the previous three questions when pondering the fourth.

HOW TO USE THIS TEXT

CONTENT AREA ASSESSMENTS AND ANALYSES

Complete the 19 individual categories. If you score 70% or better on any of the assessment examinations, you are probably strong in those areas. However, do not fall into the trap of false security that may result from a passing score. You should not ignore that subject matter in your examination preparation. Achieving a passing score simply means that you should not spend the same amount of time on that subject category as you should on one that represents a weak area. You should study all content categories before taking any of the NBRC examinations.

Each assessment section should be systematically approached, that is, first the examination, then the review and study of analyses, and then the review and study of references. Do not study only the questions and their letter answers. Work toward understanding the concepts and principles contained in the questions and analyses. Avoid the common pitfall of preparing for examinations by memorizing or learning previously reviewed test questions. Seek understanding, not rote memorization.

Only you can determine the amount of time that should be spent studying each area. However, be realistic in your approach and adhere to your established timetable. Feel confident that the effort you are expending is beneficial to you.

Upon completing your study in a category identified as being weak, you may elect to take the assessment examination once again.

BASIC SCIENCES

This section is composed of the following content categories

1. Mathematics (25 items)
2. Cardiopulmonary anatomy and physiology (100 items)
3. Chemistry (50 items)
4. Microbiology (35 items)
5. Pharmacology (50 items)
6. Physics (50 items)

The mathematics section is intended to assess basic mathematics skills as they pertain to cardiopulmonary physiology and therapeutic intervention. The other content categories deal with basic science principles, laws, theories, and calculations relevant to the discipline of respiratory care.

MATHEMATICS ASSESSMENT

PURPOSE: The purpose of this 25-item section is to provide the reader with the opportunity to evaluate fundamental mathematics skills. Addition, subtraction, multiplication, division, and certain algebraic and logarithmic operations will be presented in the context of respiratory care practice and cardiopulmonary physiology. Knowledge and understanding of the underlying principles will *not* be evaluated. However, some persons may decide to use this section to evaluate their capabilities of recalling the variety of conversion factors, formulae, etc., needed to solve the problems included in this section. Therefore, the pertinent conversion factors, formulae, etc., are listed in Appendix I for your convenience.

DIRECTIONS: Each of the questions or incomplete statements below is followed by five suggested answers. Select the one which is the best in each case and then blacken the corresponding space on the answer sheet.

1. A weight of 197 lb is equal to _____ kg.

    A. 433.0 kg   D. 89.6 kg
    B. 199.2 kg   E. 50.0 kg
    C. 194.8 kg

2. What is the Fahrenheit equivalent of 38°C?

    A. 249.1°F   D. 70.0°F
    B. 126.0°F   E. 36.4°F
    C. 100.4°F

3. How should 0.0000008 be expressed in proper scientific notation?

    A. 8.00×10^7 D. 8.00×10^8
    B. 8.00×10^{-7} E. 0.08×10^{-5}
    C. 80.0×10^{-8}

4. Perform the operation $\dfrac{10^{-4}}{10^7}$.

   A. 10^{-11} D. 10^3

   B. 10^{-3} E. 10^{-28}

   C. 10^{11}

5. Convert 713 mm Hg to its equivalent in cm H_2O.

   A. 969.7 cm H_2O D. 714.4 cm H_2O

   B. 905.7 cm H_2O E. 711.6 cm H_2O

   C. 524.3 cm H_2O

6. Calculate the relative humidity for a volume of air containing 18 g/m^3 (content) of water at 37°C.

   A. 18%   D. 43%

   B. 37%   E. 125%

   C. 41%

7. Calculate the percent of the forced vital capacity (FVC) exhaled in one second (FEV$_1$) given the following data

   FVC: 6.44 liters
   FEV$_1$: 5.02 liters

   A. 1,144.0%   D. 114.4%

   B. 142.0%   E. 77.9%

   C. 128.2%

8. Determine the amount of oxygen bound to hemoglobin (content) for a patient who has an oxygen saturation of 90% and an oxygen-carrying capacity of 20 vol%.

   A. 18 vol%   D. 170 vol%

   B. 22 vol%   E. 450 vol%

   C. 70 vol%

9. Compute the mean arterial pressure (MAP) for a patient whose blood pressure is 140 mm Hg systolic pressure over 80 mm Hg diastolic pressure (140/80).

   A. 100 mm Hg   D. 140 mm Hg

   B. 120 mm Hg   E. 360 mm Hg

   C. 130 mm Hg

10. Reynold's equation is written as

$$R_N = \frac{velocity \times density \times diameter}{viscosity}$$

Cancel out the units as they would occur during the calculation of Reynold's number (R_N) to determine the unit(s) for that value.

A. $\dfrac{kg}{sec \times cm}$

B. $\dfrac{sec \times cm}{kg}$

C. $\dfrac{kg^2}{sec^2 \times cm^2}$

D. $\dfrac{sec^2 \times cm^2}{kg^2}$

E. R_N has no units.

11. The compliance of the lung (C_L) is 0.2 liter/cm H_2O and the compliance of the chest wall (C_{CW}) is 0.2 liter/cm H_2O. Determine the lung-chest wall or total compliance ($C_{L\text{-}CW}$).

    A. 10 liters/cm H_2O

    B. 0.5 liter/cm H_2O

    C. 0.4 liter/cm H_2O

    D. 0.1 liter/cm H_2O

    E. 0.04 liter/cm H_2O

12. If the driving pressure (ΔP) across a conducting system is 30 cm H_2O and the flowrate ($\dot{V}$) through the system is 10 liters/sec, calculate the resistance (R).

    A. 300 cm H_2O/liter/sec

    B. 30 cm H_2O/liter/sec

    C. 3 cm H_2O/liter/sec

    D. 1 cm H_2O/liter/sec

    E. 0.3 cm H_2O/liter/sec

13. Determine the air-oxygen ratio for an oxygen delivery system operating at 12 lpm and entraining 9 lpm of room air.

    A. 0.30:1

    B. 0.50:1

    C. 0.75:1

    D. 1:0.50

    E. 1:075

14. What is the Celsius equivalent of 86°F?

    A. 30.0°C

    B. 44.4°C

    C. 65.6°C

    D. 97.2°C

    E. 212.4°C

15. $(4.80 \times 10^6) \div (5.30 \times 10^8) =$ _____ .

    A. 1.10×10^{-2}

    B. 1.10×10^{14}

    C. 9.00×10^{-3}

    D. 9.00×10^{14}

    E. 2.54×10^{15}

16. Calculate the inspiratory/expiratory ratio from the information given below:

    Inspiratory time: 2.0 seconds
    Expiratory time: 1.5 seconds

A. 3.5:1   D. 0.75:1

B. 1.3:1   E. 0.2:1

C. 1:3

17. Determine the dead space/tidal volume ratio for a patient who has a dissolved arterial carbon dioxide tension of 40 mm Hg and a mean exhaled carbon dioxide tension of 28 mm Hg.

A. 1.3   D. 0.3

B. 0.7   E. 0.1

C. 0.5

18. Calculate the percent shunt using the classic shunt equation and the data presented below.

The end-pulmonary capillary O_2 content: 24.78 vol%
The arterial O_2 content: 24.36 vol%
The venous O_2 content: 20.86 vol%

A. 8.9%   D. 13.8%

B. 10.7%   E. 15.1%

C. 12.0%

19. log (L × M × N) = _____ .

A. log L − log M − log N   D. $\dfrac{\log L + \log M}{\log N}$

B. log L/log M/log N   E. log L + log M + log N

C. $\dfrac{\log L - \log M}{\log N}$

20. Calculate the amount of water in a volume of air (absolute humidity or content) when the humidity deficit is 15.7 mg/liter and the capacity is 44.0 mg/liter.

A. 3.5 mg/liter   D. 15.7 mg/liter

B. 5.5 mg/liter   E. 28.3 mg/liter

C. 13.3 mg/liter

21. Determine a person's body surface area (BSA) if her cardiac index (C.I.) is 3.4 liters/min/m² and her cardiac output (C.O.) is 6.7 liters/min.

A. 0.50 m²   D. 10.10 m²

B. 1.97 m²   E. 22.78 m²

C. 3.30 m²

Questions 22 and 23 refer to the same data.

22. Obtain the factor relating pressure drop to gas volume for an oxygen cylinder containing 200 cu ft of gas under a filling pressure of 2,200 psig.

A. 2.40 liters/psig   D. 2.87 liters/psig
B. 2.57 liters/psig   E. 3.14 liters/psig
C. 2.63 liters/psig

23. How long will this full oxygen cylinder last if it is the gas source for an oxygen delivery device operating at 15 lpm?

A. 5.8 hours   D. 7.0 hours
B. 6.2 hours   E. 7.6 hours
C. 6.4 hours

24. Find the antilogarithm of 3.8828. (See Appendix II.)

A. 7625   D. 8828
B. 7630   E. 8833
C. 7635

25. What concentration of racemic epinephrine would result if 0.5 cc of 2.25% (W/V) racemic epinephrine was diluted with 5.0 cc of 0.9% (W/V) NaCl?

A. 1.105%   D. 0.250%
B. 0.315%   E. 0.205%
C. 0.286%

ASSESSMENT ANSWER SHEET

DIRECTIONS: Darken the space under the selected answer.

	A	B	C	D	E			A	B	C	D	E
1.	[ ]	[ ]	[ ]	[ ]	[ ]	14.	[ ]	[ ]	[ ]	[ ]	[ ]
2.	[ ]	[ ]	[ ]	[ ]	[ ]	15.	[ ]	[ ]	[ ]	[ ]	[ ]
3.	[ ]	[ ]	[ ]	[ ]	[ ]	16.	[ ]	[ ]	[ ]	[ ]	[ ]
4.	[ ]	[ ]	[ ]	[ ]	[ ]	17.	[ ]	[ ]	[ ]	[ ]	[ ]
5.	[ ]	[ ]	[ ]	[ ]	[ ]	18.	[ ]	[ ]	[ ]	[ ]	[ ]
6.	[ ]	[ ]	[ ]	[ ]	[ ]	19.	[ ]	[ ]	[ ]	[ ]	[ ]
7.	[ ]	[ ]	[ ]	[ ]	[ ]	20.	[ ]	[ ]	[ ]	[ ]	[ ]
8.	[ ]	[ ]	[ ]	[ ]	[ ]	21.	[ ]	[ ]	[ ]	[ ]	[ ]
9.	[ ]	[ ]	[ ]	[ ]	[ ]	22.	[ ]	[ ]	[ ]	[ ]	[ ]
10.	[ ]	[ ]	[ ]	[ ]	[ ]	23.	[ ]	[ ]	[ ]	[ ]	[ ]
11.	[ ]	[ ]	[ ]	[ ]	[ ]	24.	[ ]	[ ]	[ ]	[ ]	[ ]
12.	[ ]	[ ]	[ ]	[ ]	[ ]	25.	[ ]	[ ]	[ ]	[ ]	[ ]
13.	[ ]	[ ]	[ ]	[ ]	[ ]						

MATHEMATICS ANALYSES

Note: The references listed after each analysis are numbered and keyed to the reference list located at the end of this section. The first number indicates the text. The second number indicates the page where information about the question can be found. For example, (1:219,394) means that reference number 1 is to be used and that on pages 219 and 394 information about the question will be found. Frequently, it will be necessary to read beyond the page number indicated to obtain complete information. Therefore, reference to the question will be found either on the page indicated or on subsequent pages.

1. D. Because 1 kilogram (kg) equals 2.2 pounds (lb), the number of pounds given in the problem can be divided by 2.2. The factor 2.2 can be viewed as indicating that there are 2.2 lb per kg (2.2 lb/kg). Therefore,

$$\frac{(197 \text{ lb})}{2.2 \text{ lb/kg}} = 89.6 \text{ kg}$$

   or

$$197 \text{ lb}\left(\frac{1 \text{ kg}}{2.2 \text{ lb}}\right) = 89.6 \text{ kg}$$

   When performing any conversion from the metric system to the English system, or vice versa, it is advisable to express equivalents in the form of a fraction because such expressions are equal to unity (one). For example, because 2.2 lb equal 1 kg, the fraction

$$\frac{1 \text{ kg}}{2.2 \text{ lb}}$$

   equals one (1). Any number multiplied by one does not change in value. Hence

$$197 \text{ lb}\left(\frac{1 \text{ kg}}{2.2 \text{ lb}}\right) = 197 \text{ (1)}$$

   (1:702), (2:29), (4:12)

2. C. By using the formula °F = $(\frac{9}{5})$(°C) + 32, the Fahrenheit equivalent of 38°C can be obtained as follows

$$°F = \left(\frac{9}{5}\right)(38°C) + 32$$
$$°F = (1.8)(38°C) + 32$$
$$°F = 68.4 + 32$$
$$°F = 100.4$$

   (1:702), (2:87–88), (4:9–10)

3. B. To avoid using numbers in a long form, it is useful to be able to express numbers in scientific notation. In addition to allowing easier comprehension of their magnitude, scientific notation provides the additional benefit of expediting mathematical manipulations by simplifying the numbers.

When one expresses a number in proper scientific notation, the whole number should be greater than or equal to 1, but should not exceed 9. For example, expressing the number 8,210 as 82.1×10^2 is not considered proper scientific notation because the whole number (82) exceeds 9. The correct form is 8.21×10^3, where the whole number is greater than 1 but does not exceed 9.

For values less than 1, the same rule applies. For instance, writing the number 0.0749 as 0.749×10^{-1} is incorrect. In proper scientific notation it should be written as 7.49×10^{-2}.

(1:699), (2:2)

4. A. Exponents are algebraically subtracted during division according to the rule

$$\frac{10^x}{10^y} = 10^x \div 10^y = 10^{x-y}$$

Therefore, $\frac{10^{-4}}{10^7} = 10^{-4} \div 10^7 = 10^{-4-(+7)} = 10^{-4-7} = 10^{-11}$

(2:4)

5. A. The factor 1.36 cm H_2O/mm Hg is obtained by dividing the atmospheric pressure in cm H_2O (1,034 cm H_2O = 1 atm) by the atmospheric equivalent in mm Hg (760 mm Hg). For example,

$$\frac{1{,}034 \text{ cm } H_2O}{760 \text{ mm Hg}} = 1.36 \text{ cm } H_2O/\text{mm Hg}$$

Therefore, 713 mm Hg =

$$(713 \text{ mm Hg})(1.36 \text{ cm } H_2O/\text{mm Hg}) = 969.7 \text{ cm } H_2O$$

(1:12–13), (2:116–118), (4:20–21)

6. C. The expression:

$$\text{relative humidity} = \frac{\text{content}}{\text{capacity}} \times 100$$

provides for the calculation of the relative humidity when the content is divided by the capacity and the quotient is multiplied by 100 to express that ratio as a percent. For example,

$$\text{relative humidity} = \frac{18 \text{ g/m}^3}{43.8 \text{ g/m}^3} \times 100$$
$$= 0.41 \times 100$$
$$= 41\%$$

(1:17,337), (2:14–15), (4:21–22)

7. E. The relationship

$$FEV_{T\%} = \frac{FEV_T}{FVC} \times 100$$

is the general equation used to obtain the percent of any of the $FEV_{T}s$ ($FEV_{0.5}$, FEV_1, FEV_2, and FEV_3) expressed as a percentage of the FVC. For example,

$$FEV_{1\%} = \frac{FEV_1}{FVC} \times 100$$

$$= \frac{5.02 \text{ liters}}{6.44 \text{ liters}} \times 100$$

$$= 0.779 \times 100$$

$$= 77.9\%$$

(1:175), (2:15–16), (4:281), (6:232–233), (14:146–147)

8. A. The formula for oxygen saturation (S_{O_2}) is

$$S_{O_2} = \frac{\text{content}}{\text{capacity}} \times 100$$

The relationship can be rearranged to solve for any of the factors in the expression when two of the three factors are known. For example,

$$\frac{(S_{O_2})(\text{capacity})}{100} = \text{content}$$

$$\frac{(90\%)(20 \text{ vol}\%)}{100} = \text{content}$$

$$(0.90)(20 \text{ vol}\%) = 18 \text{ vol}\%$$

(1:203–204), (2:17–18), (4:184), (6:260), (8:78), (9:129), (12:186), (14:69–70), (27:83), (29:125–126), (32:134)

9. A. Insert the values given in the problem into the equation

$$MAP = \frac{\text{systolic pressure} + (2)(\text{diastolic pressure})}{3}$$

$$= \frac{140 \text{ mm Hg} + 2(80 \text{ mm Hg})}{3}$$

$$= \frac{300 \text{ mm Hg}}{3}$$

$$= 100 \text{ mm Hg}$$

(4:231)

10. E. Dimensional analysis of Reynold's equation demonstrates that Reynold's number is a dimensionless value.

$$\text{velocity} = \text{cm/sec}$$

$$\text{density} = \text{kg/cm}^3$$

$$\text{diameter} = \text{cm}$$

$$\text{viscosity} = \frac{\text{kg} \times \text{cm} \times \text{sec}}{\text{sec}^2 \times \text{cm}^2}$$

Therefore,

$$R_N = \dfrac{\dfrac{cm}{sec} \times \dfrac{kg}{cm^3} \times cm}{\dfrac{kg \times cm \times sec}{(sec \times sec) \times (cm \times cm)}}$$

STEP 1: Perform cancellations in the numerator.

$$\dfrac{\cancel{cm}}{sec} \times \dfrac{kg}{cm^3} \times \cancel{cm} = \dfrac{kg}{sec \times cm}$$

STEP 2: Perform cancellations in the denominator.

$$\dfrac{kg \times \cancel{cm} \times \cancel{sec}}{(sec \times \cancel{sec}) \times (\cancel{cm} \times cm)} = \dfrac{kg}{sec \times cm}$$

STEP 3: Place the numerator over the denominator and cancel remaining like units.

$$\dfrac{\dfrac{\cancel{kg}}{\cancel{sec} \times \cancel{cm}}}{\dfrac{\cancel{kg}}{\cancel{sec} \times \cancel{cm}}} = \text{a numerical value with no units}$$

(2:164–165)

11. D. When obtaining the total system compliance (lung-chest wall), the reciprocals of the lung and chest wall compliances are added. For example,

$$\dfrac{1}{C_L} + \dfrac{1}{C_{CW}} = \dfrac{1}{C_{L-CW}}$$

$$\dfrac{1}{0.2 \text{ liter/cm } H_2O} + \dfrac{1}{0.2 \text{ liter/cm } H_2O} = \dfrac{1}{C_{L-CW}}$$

$$5 \text{ cm } H_2O/\text{liter} + 5 \text{ cm } H_2O/\text{liter} = \dfrac{1}{C_{L-CW}}$$

$$10 \text{ cm } H_2O/\text{liter} = \dfrac{1}{C_{L-CW}}$$

$$C_{L-CW} = \dfrac{1}{10 \text{ cm } H_2O/\text{liter}}$$

$$C_{L-CW} = 0.1 \text{ liter/cm } H_2O$$

(1:140–141,183–184), (2:169–170), (3:46–47), (4:27–28,77–80), (6:247–249, 1025), (8:22–26), (29:70–74), (32:22–24)

12. C. Resistance (R) is a function of the driving pressure (ΔP) and the flowrate ($\dot{V}$). The formula for resistance is

$$R = \dfrac{\Delta P}{\dot{V}} = \dfrac{30 \text{ cm } H_2O}{10 \text{ liters/sec}}$$

$$R = 3 \text{ cm } H_2O/\text{liter/sec}$$

(1:145), (2:153–159), (4:30–32), (6:249–251), (8:30–39), (29:30), (32:34)

13. C. The air-oxygen ratio is obtained by placing the flowrate of the entrained air over the oxygen flowrate. For example,

$$\frac{\text{air flowrate}}{\text{oxygen flowrate}} = \frac{9 \text{ liters/min}}{12 \text{ liters/min}} = \frac{0.75}{1} = 0.75\!:\!1$$

(1:472), (2:7–8), (4:377), (5:107), (6:407), (30:18)

14. A. To convert temperatures from the Fahrenheit scale to degrees Celsius, the formula

$$°C = (°F - 32)\frac{5}{9}$$

is used. For example,

$$°C = (86°F - 32)\frac{5}{9}$$

$$= (54)\frac{5}{9}$$

$$= (6)\frac{5}{1}$$

$$= 30.0 °C$$

(1:702), (2:87–88), (4:9–10)

15. C. When dividing numbers containing exponents, the exponents are subtracted and the coefficients are divided. For example, $(4.80 \times 10^6) \div (5.30 \times 10^8)$.

   STEP 1: The coefficient 5.30 is divided into 4.80 and the exponent 10^8 is subtracted from 10^6.

$$\left(\frac{4.80}{5.30}\right) 10^{6-8} = 0.90 \times 10^{-2}$$

   STEP 2: Express 0.90×10^{-2} in proper scientific notation.

$$0.90 \times 10^{-2} = 9.00 \times 10^{-3}$$

(2:2–5)

16. B. Place the inspiratory (I) time over the expiratory (E) time and divide to obtain the I/E ratio, i.e.,

$$\frac{\text{inspiratory time}}{\text{expiratory time}} = \frac{2.0 \text{ seconds}}{1.5 \text{ seconds}} = \frac{1.3}{1.0} = 1.3\!:\!1$$

(2:8), (30:217)

17. D. The Bohr equation is used for determining the dead space/tidal volume (V_D/V_T) ratio. When the dissolved arterial carbon dioxide tension (Pa_{CO_2}) and the mean ex-haled carbon dioxide tension $(P\bar{E}_{CO_2})$ are given, the V_D/V_T can be calculated as follows.

$$\frac{V_D}{V_T} = \frac{Pa_{CO_2} - P\bar{E}_{CO_2}}{Pa_{CO_2}}$$

$$\frac{V_D}{V_T} = \frac{40 \text{ mm Hg} - 28 \text{ mm Hg}}{40 \text{ mm Hg}}$$

$$\frac{V_D}{V_T} = \frac{12 \text{ mm Hg}}{40 \text{ mm Hg}}$$

$$\frac{V_D}{V_T} = 0.30$$

(1:119–120), (2:9–10), (4:226–227), (6:242–243), (8:139), (14:19,163), (27:73,234–235), (29:60,244), (32:64–65)

18. B. The classic shunt equation allows for the calculation of the percent shunt. For example,

$$\frac{\dot{Q}_S}{\dot{Q}_T} = \frac{Cc_{O_2} - Ca_{O_2}}{Cc_{O_2} - C\bar{v}_{O_2}}$$

where

$\dot{Q}_S$ = shunt cardiac output
$\dot{Q}_T$ = total cardiac output
Cc_{O_2} = end-pulmonary capillary O_2 content
Ca_{O_2} = arterial O_2 content
$C\bar{v}_{O_2}$ = venous O_2 content

$$\frac{\dot{Q}_S}{\dot{Q}_T} = \frac{24.78 \text{ vol\%} - 24.36 \text{ vol\%}}{24.78 \text{ vol\%} - 20.86 \text{ vol\%}} \times 100$$

$$= \frac{0.42 \text{ vol\%}}{3.95 \text{ vol\%}} \times 100$$

$$= (0.1071)(100)$$

$$= 10.71\%$$

(2:18–20), (3:318–319,321), (4:217–218), (6:1000), (14:52–55), (27:213–214), (32:110)

19. E. When the logarithms of two or more numbers are to be multiplied add the logarithms.

$$\log (L \times M \times N) = \log L + \log M + \log N$$

(2:38)

20. E. The expression

$$\text{humidity deficit} = \text{capacity} - \text{content}$$

can be re-arranged to solve for the content as follows:

$$\text{content} = \text{capacity} - \text{humidity deficit}$$
$$= 44.0 \text{ mg/liter} - 15.7 \text{ mg/liter}$$
$$= 28.3 \text{ mg/liter}$$

(1:338)

21. B. The formula for determining the cardiac index (C.I.) can be re–arranged to solve for the body surface area (BSA) when the C.I. and the cardiac output (C.O.) are given, i.e.,

$$\text{BSA} = \frac{\text{C.O.}}{\text{C.I.}}$$

$$= \frac{6.7 \text{ liters/min}}{3.4 \text{ liters/min/m}^2}$$

$$= 1.97 \text{ m}^2$$

(3:300), (9:127)

22. B. Insert into the formula the values that are given in the problem.

$$\text{conversion factor} = \frac{(200 \text{ cu-ft})(28.3 \text{ liters/cu-ft})}{2,200 \text{ psig}}$$

$$= \frac{5,660 \text{ liters}}{2,200 \text{ psig}}$$

$$= 2.57 \text{ liters/psig}$$

(1:431), (4:360)

23. B. Insert into the formula the known values and solve for the duration of flow

$$\text{flow duration} = \frac{(2,200 \text{ psig})(2.57 \text{ liters/psig})}{15 \text{ liters/min}}$$

$$= \frac{5,654}{15 \text{ min}^{-1}}$$

$$= 376.9 \text{ minutes}$$

Because 1 hour equals 60 minutes,

$$\text{flow duration} = \frac{376.9 \text{ min}}{60 \text{ min/hr}}$$

$$= 6.2 \text{ hours}$$

(1:432), (4:360), (6:396)

24. C. The following steps will describe how to find the antilogarithm (antilog), i.e., the number. To find the antilog or number, use the reverse process of that for finding the logarithm or exponent (power).

   STEP 1: From the log table (Appendix II) find the range of mantissas within which the desired mantissa (8828) lies, and determine the high-low mantissa difference.

   8831 high mantissa

   −8825 low mantissa

   ──────────────────────

   6 high-low mantissa difference

   STEP 2: From the log table find the range of corresponding numbers within which the desired mantissa lies and determine the high-low number difference.

7640 high number

−7630 low number

10 high-low number difference

STEP 3: Calculate the difference between the desired mantissa and the low mantissa.

8828 desired mantissa

−8825 low mantissa

3 desired-low mantissa difference

STEP 4: Set up the following proportion to solve for X (desired-low number difference).

$$\frac{\text{desired–low mantissa difference}}{\text{high-low mantissa difference}} = \frac{X}{\text{high-low number difference}}$$

$$\frac{3}{6} = \frac{X}{10}$$

$$\frac{(3)(10)}{6} = X$$

$$\frac{30}{6} = X$$

$$5 = X$$

STEP 5: Add X to the lower number to obtain the antilog.

7630 low number

+   5 high-low number difference

7635 antilog

STEP 6: The characteristic of the logarithm determines the position of the decimal point with the number. For example, because the characteristic of the log is 3, the number must contain four digits to the left of the decimal point.* Therefore, the antilog of 3.8828 is 7635.

Exponentially, the expression is

$$10^{3.8838} = 7635$$

Logarithmically, the expression reads

$$\log_{10} 7635 = 3.8838$$

(2:30–38)

25. E. Disregard the concentration of the diluent, i.e., 0.9% (W/V) NaCl. It will *not* enter into the calculations.

STEP 1: Set up the proportion $V_1 C_1 = V_2 C_2$ where

*Review how the characteristic is obtained from Wojciechowski, W., *Respiratory Care Sciences: An Integrated Approach*, John Wiley & Sons, New York, 1985, p. 32.

V_1 = the original volume
C_1 = the original concentration
V_2 = the final volume
C_2 = the final concentration

STEP 2: Determine the value of V_2.

$$V_2 = \text{volume of diluent} + V_1$$
$$= 5.0 \text{ cc} + 0.5 \text{ cc}$$
$$= 5.5 \text{ cc}$$

STEP 3: Insert known values into the proportion and solve for C_2.

$$V_1 C_1 = V_2 C_2$$

where

V_1 = 0.5 cc racemic epinephrine
C_1 = 2.25% (W/V) racemic epinephrine
V_2 = 5.5 cc
C_2 = ?

$$(0.5 \text{ cc})(2.25\%) = (5.5 \text{ cc})(C_2)$$
$$\frac{(0.5 \text{ cc})(2.25\%)}{5.5 \text{ cc}} = C_2$$
$$0.205\% = C_2$$

(1:63–64), (2:11–13), (3:114–115), (4:6–7)

REFERENCES

1. Spearman, C., and Sheldon, R., *Egan's Fundamentals of Respiratory Therapy*, 4th ed., C.V. Mosby, St. Louis, 1982.
2. Wojciechowski, W., *Respiratory Care Sciences: An Integrated Approach*, John Wiley & Sons, New York, 1985.
3. Shapiro. B., Harrison, R., Kacmarek, R., and Cane, R., *Clinical Application of Respiratory Care*, 3rd ed., Year Book Medical Publishers, Chicago, 1985.
4. Kacmarek, R., Mack, C., and Dimas, S., *The Essentials of Respiratory Therapy*, 2nd ed., Year Book Medical Publishers, Chicago, 1985.
5. McPherson, S., *Respiratory Therapy Equipment*, 3rd ed., C.V. Mosby, St. Louis, 1985.
6. Burton, G., and Hodgkin, J., *Respiratory Care: A Guide to Clinical Practice*, 2nd ed., J.B. Lippincott, Philadelphia, 1985.
7. Frownfelter, D., *Chest Physical Therapy and Cardiopulmonary Rehabilitation, An Interdisciplinary Approach*, Year Book Medical Publishers, Chicago, 1978.
8. Cherniack, R., and Cherniack, L., *Respiration in Health and Disease*, 3rd ed., W.B. Saunders, Philadelphia, 1983.
9. Daily, E., and Schroeder, G., *Techniques in Bedside Hemodynamic Monitoring*, 3rd ed., C.V. Mosby, St. Louis, 1985.
10. Des Jardins, R., *Clinical Manifestations of Respiratory Disease*, Year Book Medical Publishers, Chicago, 1984.

11. Mitchell, R., *Synopsis of Clinical Pulmonary Disease*, 3rd ed., C.V. Mosby, St. Louis, 1982.

12. Comroe, J., *Physiology of Respiration*, 3rd ed., Year book Medical Publishers, Chicago, 1974.

13. West, J., *Pulmonary Pathophysiology—The Essentials*, 2nd ed., Williams & Wilkins, Baltimore, 1982.

14. West, J., *Respiratory Physiology—The Essentials*, 3rd ed., Williams & Wilkins, Baltimore, 1985.

15. Martz, K., et al., *Management of the Patient-Ventilator System: A Team Approach*, 2nd ed., C.V. Mosby, St. Louis, 1984.

16. Shoup, C., and McHenry, R., *Laboratory Exercises in Respiratory Therapy*, 2nd ed., C.V. Mosby, St. Louis, 1983.

17. Ruppel, G., *Manual of Pulmonary Function Testing*, 3rd ed., C.V. Mosby, St. Louis, 1982.

18. Appelbaum, E., and Bruce, D., *Tracheal Intubation*, W.B. Saunders, Philadelphia, 1976.

19. Rau, J., *Respiratory Therapy Pharmacology*, 2nd ed., Year Book Medical Publishers, Chicago, 1984.

20. United States Department of Health, Education, and Welfare, Public Health Service, *Isolation Techniques for Use in Hospitals*, 2nd ed., Washington, D.C., 1975.

21. Brooks, S., *Integrated Basic Science*, 4th ed., C.V. Mosby, St. Louis, 1979.

22. Comroe, J., *The Lung*, Year Book Medical Publishers, Inc., Chicago, 1962.

23. Shibel, E., and Moser, K., *Respiratory Emergencies*, 2nd ed., C.V. Mosby, St. Louis, 1982.

24. Tisi, G., *Pulmonary Physiology in Clinical Medicine*, 2nd ed., Williams & Wilkins, Baltimore, 1985.

25. Cherniack, R., *Pulmonary Function Testing*, W.B. Saunders, Philadelphia, 1977.

26. Altose, M., *The Physiological Basis of Pulmonary Function Testing*, Clinical Symposia–CIBA, Vol. 31, No. 2, Summit, New Jersey, 1979.

27. Shapiro, B., Harrison, R., and Walton, J., *Clinical Applications of Arterial Blood Gases*, 3rd ed., Year Book Medical Publishers, Chicago, 1982.

28. West, J., *Ventilation/Blood Flow and Gas Exchange*, 3rd ed., Blackwell Scientific Publications, 1979.

29. Slonim, N., and Hamilton, K., *Respiratory Physiology*, 4th ed., C.V. Mosby, St. Louis, 1981.

30. Rarey, K., and Youtsey, J., *Respiratory Patient Care*, Prentice-Hall, Englewood Cliffs, 1981.

31. Berne, R., and Levy, M., *Physiology*, C.V. Mosby, St. Louis, 1983.

32. Levitzky, M., *Pulmonary Physiology*, 2nd ed., McGraw-Hill, New York, 1986.

33. Wilson, P., Bell, C., and Norton, A., *Rehabilitation of the Heart and Lungs*, SensorMedics, 1980.

34. Clausen, J., and Zarins, L., *Pulmonary Function Testing Guildlines and Controversies*, Academic Press, New York, 1982.

35. Klaus, M., and Fanaroff, A., *Care of the High-Risk Neonate*, 2nd ed., W.B. Saunders, Philadelphia, 1979.

36. Lough, M., et al., *Pediatric Respiratory Therapy*, 3rd ed., Year Book Medical Publishers, Chicago, 1985.

37. Levin, D., et al., *A Practical Guide to Pediatric Intensive Care*, 2nd ed., C.V. Mosby, St. Louis, 1984.

38. O'Ryan, J., and Burns, D., *Pulmonary Rehabilitation from Hospital to Home*, Year Book Medical Publishers, Chicago, 1984.

39. Bell, C., et al., *Home Care and Rehabilitation in Respiratory Medicine*, J.B. Lippincott, Philadelphia, 1984.

40. Wilkins, R., et al., *Clinical Assessment in Respiratory Care*, C.V. Mosby, St. Louis, 1985.

41. Jones, N., and Campbell, E., *Clinical Exercise Testing*, 2nd ed., W.B. Saunders, Philadelphia, 1982.

42. Goldsmith, J., and Karotkin, E., *Assisted Ventilation of the Neonate*, W.B. Saunders, Philadelphia, 1981.

43. Blowers, M., and Sims, R., *How to Read an ECG*, 3rd ed., Medical Economics, New Jersey, 1983.

44. Eubanks, D., and Bone, R., *Comprehensive Respiratory Care*, C.V. Mosby, St. Louis, 1985.

45. Rattenborg, C., *Clinical Use of Mechanical Ventilation*, Year Book Medical Publishers, Chicago, 1981.

46. Witkowski, A.S., *Pulmonary Assessment: A Clinical Guide*, J.B. Lippincott, Philadelphia, 1985.

47. Op't Holt, Timothy B., *Assessment Based Respiratory Care*, John Wiley & Sons, New York, 1986.

CARDIOPULMONARY ANATOMY AND PHYSIOLOGY ASSESSMENT

PURPOSE: This section (100 items) is intended to assess your understanding and comprehension of cardiopulmonary anatomy and physiology. In this section you will be tested on the following content:

1. Cardiovascular anatomy
2. Blood and circulation
3. Hemodynamics
4. Electrical and contractile properties of the heart
5. Respiratory anatomy
6. Mechanics of ventilation
7. Blood gas transport
8. Pulmonary blood flow
9. Regulation of ventilation
10. Ventilation/perfusion ($\dot{V}/\dot{Q}$) relationships
11. Acid-base physiology

DIRECTIONS: Each of the questions or incomplete statements is followed by five suggested answers. Select the one which is the best in each case and then blacken the corresponding space on the answer sheet.

1. As _____, surface tension of the alveolar liquid lining layer _____ . (Assume the presence of a normal amount of pulmonary surfactant.)

    I. inflation pressure increases; decreases

    II. alveolar radius decreases; increases

    III. alveolar diameter increases; increases

    IV. alveolar radius decreases; changes according to airway resistance measurements

A. III only

B. II only

C. I, III only

D. I, II only

E. II, IV only

2. Calculate the V_A of a patient who has a 160-ml V_D, a 550-cc V_T, and a ventilatory rate of 15 breaths/min.

A. 10.65 liters

B. 6.75 liters

C. 5.85 liters

D. 710.00 cc

E. 390.00 cc

3. Calculate the amount of reduced hemoglobin in a patient who has the following clinical data while breathing room air:

Pa_{O_2} 30 torr
Pa_{CO_2} 90 torr
pH 7.25
[Hb] 20 g%
Sa_{O_2} 51%
$S\bar{v}_{O_2}$ 45%

A. 5.0 g%

B. 8.5 g%

C. 10.0 g%

D. 12.0 g%

E. 20.0 g%

4. Which of the following substances function as urine buffers?

I. NH_3

II. $HPO_4^=$

III. $H_2PO_4^-$

IV. HCO_3^-

V. Pr^-

A. II, III, IV, V only

B. I, II, III, IV only

C. II, III, IV only

D. II, IV only

E. I, II, IV only

5. Which statement(s) is(are) true about the steep portion of the oxyhemoglobin dissociation curve?

I. It reflects the unloading of oxygen at the tissue level.

II. Small fluctuations in the P_{O_2} at this point are associated with large changes in oxygen saturation.

III. Shifts in the Hb-O_2 dissociation curve either to the right or left affect the steep portion more than the upper flat portion.

A. II, III only

B. III only

C. I, II only

D. I, II, III

E. I only

6. Calculate the percent shunt of a patient on controlled mechanical ventilation with an $F_{I_{O_2}}$ of 0.60 and a Swan-Ganz catheter in place.

   Given: P_B 760 mm Hg
   Body temperature 37°C
   $P_{A_{CO_2}}$ 40 mm Hg
   P_{H_2O} 47 mm Hg
   $P_{a_{O_2}}$ 150 mm Hg
   $P_{a_{CO_2}}$ 40 mm Hg
   pH 7.35 (arterial)
   [Hb] 15 g%
   $S_{a_{O_2}}$ 100%
   $P_{\bar{v}_{O_2}}$ 30 mm Hg
   $P_{\bar{v}_{CO_2}}$ 45 mm Hg
   pH 7.32 (mixed venous)
   $S_{\bar{v}_{O_2}}$ 75%
   Respiratory quotient 1.0

   A. 21.36%   D. 11.72%
   B. 17.29%   E. 2.57%
   C. 14.18%

7. Calculate a patient's $\dot{Q}_T$ given the following data:

   heart rate: 100 beats/min
   blood pressure: 135/90
   stroke volume: 60 cc

   A. 6.5 liters/min   D. 5.0 liters/min
   B. 6.0 liters/min   E. 4.5 liters/min
   C. 5.5 liters/min

8. A person who hypoventilates would be expected to have a(n) _____ P_{CO_2} in his _____ compared with a person with a normal ventilatory pattern.

   I. decreased; cerebrospinal fluid
   II. decreased; arterial blood
   III. increased; cerebrospinal fluid
   IV. increased; arterial blood
   V. equivalent; cerebrospinal fluid

   A. III, IV only   D. II, III only
   B. I, IV only   E. V only
   C. I, II only

9. Which physiologic alteration(s) would stimulate the peripheral chemoreceptors into sending hyperventilation impulses to the medulla?

   I. a decreased partial pressure of oxygen in arterial blood
   II. an acute rise in dissolved arterial CO_2

III. an acute increase in arterial [H$^+$]

IV. an acute increase in arterial blood pH

A. I only	D. I, II, III only
B. II, III, IV only	E. I, II, III, IV
C. I, II only	

10. Which of the following structures comprise a functional aspect of the mucociliary blanket in the tracheobronchial tree?

    I. goblet cells

   II. submucosal glands

  III. the vagus nerve

  IV. macrophages

A. III, IV only	D. II, III only
B. I, II, III only	E. I, II, III, IV
C. I, III only	

11. Each heme group in the hemoglobin molecule has the potential to combine with _____ oxygen molecule(s).

A. 1	D. 4
B. 2	E. 5
C. 3	

12. Calculate the theoretical maximum Pa$_{O_2}$ that can be achieved by a normal person breathing an F$_{I_{O_2}}$ of 1.0 at 1 atm under normal resting conditions. Assume a $\dot{V}_A/\dot{Q}_C$ of 1.0.

A. 730 mm Hg	D. 673 mm Hg
B. 720 mm Hg	E. 616 mm Hg
C. 713 mm Hg	

13. Which selection best describes the relationship between the Pa$_{O_2}$ and the amount of oxygen dissolved in the arterial blood expressed as *volumes percent?*

A. The two factors are inversely related.

B. Their relationship is sigmoid in nature.

C. No apparent relationship exists.

D. A direct relationship exists between these two factors.

E. The actual relationship is determined by body temperature, which is *not* given; therefore, no interpretation can be made.

14. The law of continuity is manifested in which physiologic situation(s)?

    I. the movement of gases across the alveolar-capillary membrane

   II. the movement of alveolar macrophages in the alveolar liquid lining layer

  III. the flow of blood through pulmonary circulation

  IV. the movement of gas from the trachea to the alveoli during inspiration

A. IV only

B. II only

C. I, III only

D. III, IV only

E. II, IV only

15. Which of the following statements accurately describe the mucociliary blanket?

   I. The cilia are bathed in the sol layer, while their whipping action moves the uppermost gel layer.
   II. The cilia are rigid during their cephalad stroke and become flaccid during their recovery stroke.
   III. Smoke, alcohol, and hypoxemia impair ciliary activity.
   IV. The mucociliary blanket is useful for removing impurities in the inspired air from the lungs.

   A. II, III, IV only

   B. I, II only

   C. III, IV only

   D. II, IV only

   E. I, II, III, IV

16. Persistent fetal circulation may include which of the following anatomic shunts?

   I. umbilical arteries
   II. patent foramen ovale
   III. umbilical vein
   IV. patent ductus venosus
   V. patent ductus arteriosus

   A. II, V only

   B. I, III only

   C. II, IV only

   D. I, III, IV only

   E. II, IV, V only

17. A metabolic alkalosis would be associated with a(n) _____ in _____ .

   I. normal P_{50}; arterial and venous blood
   II. decrease; P_{50}
   III. decrease; Hb-O_2 affinity
   IV. increase; Hb-O_2 affinity
   V. increase; P_{50}

   A. I only

   B. III, V only

   C. IV only

   D. V only

   E. II, IV only

18. Which of the following statements are true about carbonic anhydrase?

   I. It is present only in erythrocytes.
   II. It catalyzes the reaction $CO_2 + H_2O \rightarrow H_2CO_3$.
   III. It is present in kidney tubule cells.
   IV. It facilitates the combination of O_2 to hemoglobin.

A. I, II, IV only
B. I, II only
C. II, III, IV only

D. I, IV only
E. II, III only

19. Which of the following statements are true about the anatomic features of the lungs?

    I. The left lung is divided into two lobes by the horizontal fissure.
    II. The medial surfaces of both lungs are concave.
    III. The right hemidiaphragm is situated higher in the thorax than the left hemidiaphragm.
    IV. The root of the lung enters the lung at the hilum.

    A. I, II, III, IV
    B. II, III, IV only
    C. I, II, IV only

    D. III, IV only
    E. I, II only

20. Calculate the cardiac index given the data below, and then the chart shown in Figure 1.

    systolic pressure: 140 torr
    diastolic pressure: 90 torr
    cardiac rate: 63 beats/min
    stroke volume: 72 ml
    height: 72 in
    weight: 190 lb

    A. 9.12 liters/min/m²
    B. 4.47 liters/min/m²
    C. 2.16 liters/min/m²

    D. 1.92 liters/min/m²
    E. 1.39 liters/min/m²

21. Which of the following CO_2 transport mechanisms carries the majority of the CO_2 from the tissues to the lungs?

    A. reversibly bound to Hb
    B. Pa_{CO_2}
    C. H_2CO_3

    D. bicarbonate
    E. carbamino protein

22. Which of the following mathematical relationships will provide for the computation of the ventilation time constant?

    A. $\Delta P/\Delta V \times \Delta P/\dot{V}$
    B. $\Delta P/\Delta \dot{V} \times \Delta \dot{V}/\Delta P$
    C. $\Delta V/\Delta \dot{V} \times \Delta V/\Delta P$
    D. $\Delta V/\Delta P \times \Delta P/\dot{V}$
    E. $\dot{V}/\Delta P \times V_T/\Delta P$

23. Which structures do *not* branch directly off the aortic arch?

    I. left subclavian artery
    II. brachiocephalic artery

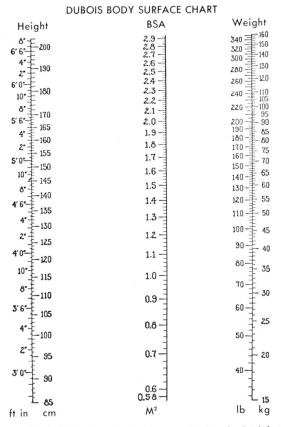

FIGURE 1. Find the patient's height in either feet or centimeters in the left column and the patient's weight in pounds or kilograms in the right column. Connect these two points with a ruler. The BSA is indicated at the point where the ruler crosses the middle column. (From DuBois, E. F., *Basal Metabolism in Health and Disease,* 3rd ed., Lea & Febiger, Philadelphia, 1936.)

III. right common carotid artery

IV. coronary arteries

V. right subclavian artery

A. I, II, IV only

B. I, II only

C. III, IV, V only

D. I, IV only

E. III, V only

24. Which quantitative relationship expresses the Bohr equation?

A. $P_{A_{O_2}} = F_{I_{O_2}}(713) - Pa_{CO_2}\left(F_{I_{O_2}} + \dfrac{1 - F_{I_{O_2}}}{R}\right)$

B. $\dfrac{V_D}{V_T} = \dfrac{Pa_{CO_2} - P\overline{E}_{CO_2}}{Pa_{CO_2}} \times 100$

C. $\dfrac{\dot{Q}s}{\dot{Q}T} = \dfrac{(P_{A_{O_2}} - Pa_{O_2})0.003}{3.5 + (P_{A_{O_2}} - Pa_{O_2})0.003} \times 100$

D. $\dot{V}_A = \dot{V}_D - V_T(f)$

E. $P(A\text{-}a)O_2 = 140 - (Pa_{O_2} + Pa_{CO_2})$

25. If a person hyperventilates, she would be expected to have a(n) _____ P_{CO_2} in the _____ in comparison with a person with a normal ventilatory pattern.

   I. increased; cerebrospinal fluid
   II. increased; arterial blood
   III. decreased; cerebrospinal fluid
   IV. decreased; arterial blood

A. I, II only
B. IV only
C. III, IV only
D. I, IV only
E. II, III only

26. Which structure in fetal circulation has the highest partial pressure of oxygen?

A. ductus arteriosus
B. aorta
C. superior vena cava
D. umbilical arteries
E. umbilical vein

27. Which of the following anatomic features are cartilages located in the larynx?

   I. epiglottis
   II. glottis
   III. cricoid
   IV. thyroid
   V. cuneiform

A. I, III, IV only
B. I, II, III, IV only
C. I, II, V only
D. I, III, IV, V only
E. I, II, III, IV, V

28. Which of the following anatomic terms refer to arterial anastomoses?

   I. palmar arch
   II. plantar arch
   III. circle of Willis
   IV. internal and external carotid arteries

A. I, II, III only
B. I, III, IV only
C. II, IV only
D. I, II only
E. I, II, III, IV

29. Calculate the arterial-venous oxygen content difference at pH 7.20, using Figure 2. This patient has 13 g% Hb, Pa_{O_2} 100 torr, and $P\overline{v}_{O_2}$ 40 torr.

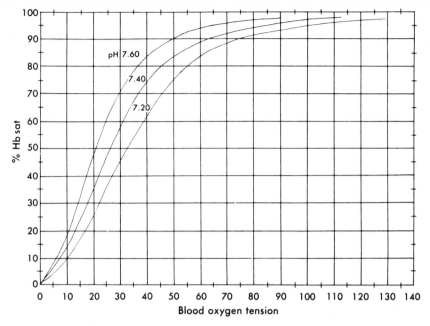

FIGURE 2

A. 5.00 vol%   D. 7.01 vol%

B. 5.75 vol%   E. 7.34 vol%

C. 6.60 vol%

30. A 150-lb (ideal weight) male is receiving mechanically controlled ventilation with a V_T of 500 ml at a rate of 12 breaths/min. Calculate his $\dot{V}_A/\dot{Q}_C$ given the following data:

$\dot{V}_{O_2}$ 240 ml/min
Ca_{O_2} 20 vol%
$C\bar{v}_{O_2}$ 14 vol%

A. 3.33   D. 1.45

B. 2.31   E. 1.05

C. 2.08

31. According to the Fick equation, as the cardiac output _____ , when the $\dot{V}_{O_2}$ remains constant, the $Ca_{O_2} - C\bar{v}_{O_2}$ gradient _____ .

I. increases; increases

II. decreases; decreases

III. increases; decreases

IV. decreases; increases

A. III only   D. III, IV only

B. II only   E. I, II only

C. II, III only

32. Which veins contribute to the normal anatomic shunt?

    I. azygos
    II. bronchial
    III. Thebesian
    IV. saphenous

    A. I, II, III, IV   D. I, III only
    B. I, II, IV only   E. I, II, III only
    C. II, III only

33. Calculate the amount of deoxygenated hemoglobin present in a patient with the following clinical features and diagnostic data:

    Pa_{O_2} 55 torr; Pa_{CO_2} 61 torr; pH 7.33
    $F_{I_{O_2}}$ 0.24
    Sa_{O_2} 84%; $S\bar{v}_{O_2}$ 70%
    [Hb] 19 g%

    A. 8.74 g%   D. 3.45 g%
    B. 5.70 g%   E. 2.66 g%
    C. 4.37 g%

34. Figure 3 illustrates the distribution of pulmonary blood flow in the normal upright lung. The abscissa indicates the different lung regions, and the ordinate represents the amount of pulmonary blood flow. Which of the following graphs (Figures 4 through 8) might represent the distribution of blood flow if there was a decrease in pulmonary artery pressure?

    A. A   D. D
    B. B   E. E
    C. C

35. Which of the following statements characterize sinus bradycardia?

    I. regular rhythm
    II. normal QRS interval
    III. a longer interval between ventricular repolarization and atrial depolarization
    IV. a normal PR interval

    A. II, III only   D. I, II, IV only
    B. I, III, IV only   E. I, II, III, IV
    C. II, III, IV only

36. Calculate the dead space volume to tidal volume ratio for a patient having an end-tidal carbon dioxide tension of 44 torr and mean exhaled carbon dioxide tension of 33 mm Hg.

    A. 11%   D. 25%
    B. 13%   E. 75%
    C. 21%

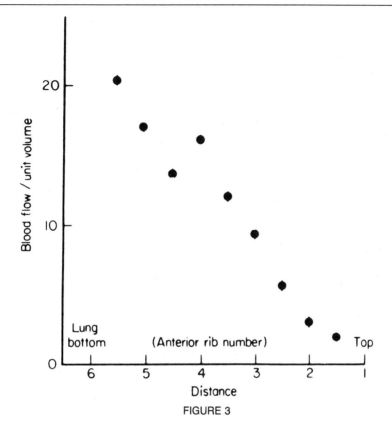

FIGURE 3

A.

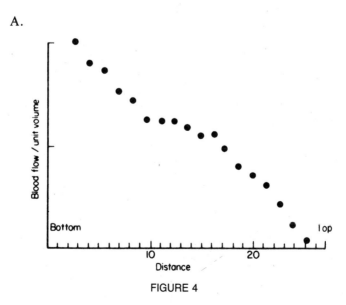

FIGURE 4

B.

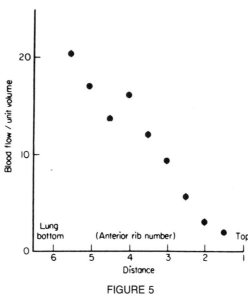

FIGURE 5

C.

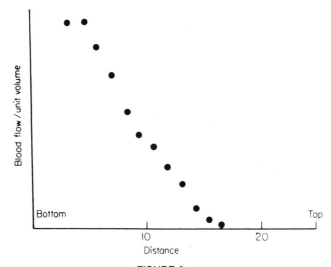

FIGURE 6

D.

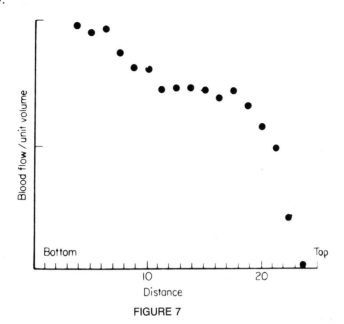

FIGURE 7

E.

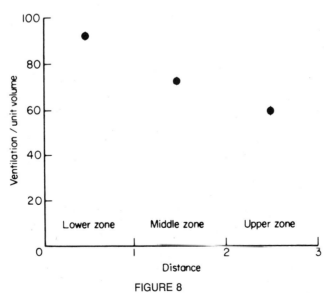

FIGURE 8

37. The valve between the right atrium and right ventricle is called the _____ valve.

   I. tricuspid
   II. bicuspid
   III. mitral
   IV. semilunar
   V. aortic

   A. II, III only   D. II only
   B. II, V only   E. I only
   C. III only

38. The systemic arterial circulation to the tracheobronchial tree down to the respiratory bronchioles occurs via the _____ .

   A. bronchial circulation   D. pulmonary arteries
   B. thoracic aorta   E. pulmonary capillaries
   C. pleural circulation

39. Which of the following statements describes the situation associated with normal, resting exhalation?

   A. Intrapulmonic pressure is negative.
   B. The diaphragm descends.
   C. Pressure in the intrapleural space is below that of the atmosphere.
   D. Intra-alveolar pressure is less than atmospheric.
   E. Transairway pressure is subatmospheric.

40. Which group of specialized cells is considered to be the heart's pacemaker?

   A. AV node   D. SA node
   B. bundle of His   E. Purkinje fibers
   C. cardiac sphincters

41. From which bone do the superior and middle turbinates arise?

   A. ethmoid   D. sphenoid
   B. vomer   E. frontal
   C. palatine

42. Calculate the percent shunt on a patient having the following clinical data, assuming normal ambient conditions.

   Pa_{O_2} 287 torr
   Pa_{CO_2} 38 torr
   pH 7.42
   Sa_{O_2} 100%
   $P\bar{v}_{O_2}$ 40 torr
   $P\bar{v}_{CO_2}$ 46 torr
   $S\bar{v}_{O_2}$ 70%

Body temperature 37° Respiratory quotient = normal
F_{IO_2} 1.0
[Hb] 14g%

A. 20.11%   D. 15.49%
B. 19.39%   E. 13.38%
C. 17.27%

43. Which physiologic factors are responsible for fluid leaving the pulmonary vaculature?

    A. pulmonary capillary hydrostatic pressure and interstitial osmotic pressure
    B. pulmonary capillary oncotic pressure and interstitial fluid hydrostatic pressure
    C. intra-alveolar pressure and pulmonary vascular osmotic pressure
    D. interstitial fluid osmotic pressure and pulmonary capillary osmotic pressure
    E. pulmonary capillary hydrostatic pressure and interstitial fluid hydrostatic pressure

44. What molecule is illustrated in Figure 9?

    A. pyrrole   D. porphyrin
    B. heme   E. hemoglobin
    C. globin

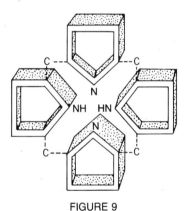

FIGURE 9

45. How many grams of water will be provided by the respiratory mucosa to the inspired air having a relative humidity of 10% at body temperature over a 2-hour period. This individual has a tidal volume of 500 cc and a ventilatory rate of 14 breaths/min.

    A. 84.00 g   D. 33.11 g
    B. 42.00 g   E. 16.59 g
    C. 39.50 g

46. What event is taking place along the muscle fiber shown in Figure 10?

    A. repolarization   D. absolute refractory period
    B. depolarization   E. resting potential
    C. relative refractory period

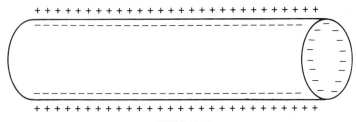

FIGURE 10

47. Extracellular fluid is comprised of which of the following compartments?

   I. interstitial fluid
   II. intravascular fluid
   III. intracellular fluid
   IV. extravascular fluid

   A. I, II only
   B. III, IV only
   C. II, III only

   D. I, IV only
   E. I, II, IV only

48. Which of the following statements accurately compares or contrasts renal system compensation and respiratory system compensation?

   I. Renal compensation can be readily observed.
   II. Respiratory compensation is rapid and complete.
   III. Renal compensation eventually reaches a point of completeness.
   IV. A metabolic alkalosis is rarely compensated by a respiratory acidosis with a Pa_{CO_2} beyond 50 torr.

   A. I, III, IV only
   B. I, III only
   C. II, III only

   D. III, IV only
   E. I, IV only

49. Which of the following factors influence the Hb-O_2 affinity?

   I. Pa_{CO_2}
   II. pH
   III. 2,3-DPG
   IV. temperature

   A. I, II, III, IV
   B. I, II, III only
   C. I, II, IV only

   D. II, III, IV only
   E. II, IV only

50. Which protein is most responsible for the presence of the oncotic pressure present in circulation?

A. globulin   D. fibrinogen
B. hemoglobin   E. albumin
C. prothrombin

51. Calculate the glomerular filtration pressure given the data below:

   glomerular capillary hydrostatic pressure: 65 torr
   colloid osmotic pressure: 33 torr
   cortical interstitial fluid hydrostatic pressure: 3 torr
   Bowman's capsule hydrostatic pressure: 17 torr
   pulmonary capillary wedge pressure: 12 torr

   A. 32 torr   D. 3 torr
   B. 15 torr   E. 0 torr
   C. 12 torr

52. Which of the following statements most accurately describes the normal ventilation/ perfusion relationship between the bases and apices?

   A. The bases are better ventilated than perfused.
   B. The lung apices are better perfused than ventilated.
   C. The apices are more perfused than the bases.
   D. The apices are better ventilated than perfused.
   E. Both the bases and apices are equally ventilated and perfused.

53. Which of the following conditions would cause someone to hyperventilate via peripheral chemoreceptor stimulation?

    I. methemoglobinemia
   II. polycythemia
   III. a sea-level resident ascending to an altitude of 10,000 ft
   IV. cyanide poisoning
    V. carbon monoxide poisoning

   A. I, III, IV only   D. II, V only
   B. I, II, III, IV only   E. I, II, III, IV, V
   C. III, IV only

54. What is the normal systolic pressure range for the right ventricle?

   A. 5 to 10 torr   D. 50 to 60 torr
   B. 15 to 25 torr   E. 110 to 120 torr
   C. 35 to 45 torr

55. Which blood component can be classified as a colloid?

   A. HCO_3^- D. white blood cells
   B. Na^+ E. albumin
   C. red blood cells

56. Which of the following depictions (Figures 11 through 15) most accurately represents intracellular fluid?

A. A   D. D

B. B   E. E

C. C

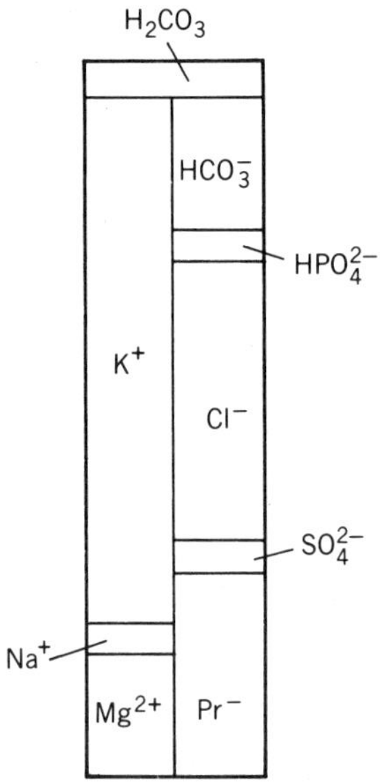

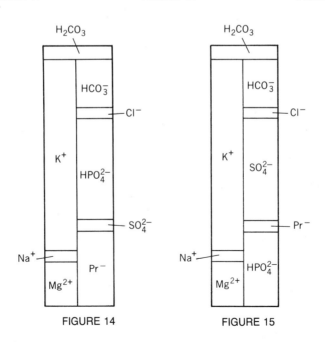

FIGURE 11 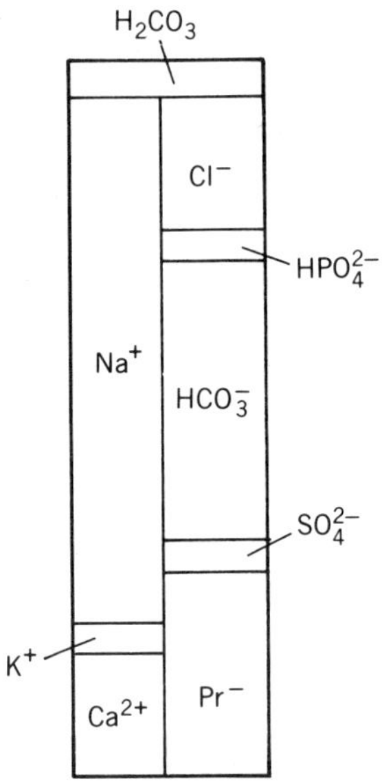   FIGURE 12 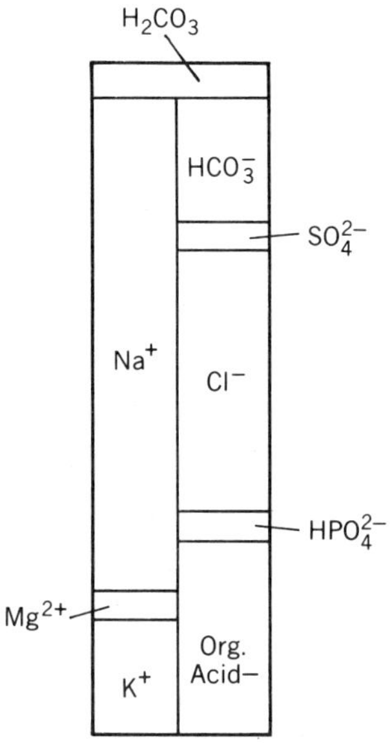   FIGURE 13

FIGURE 14   FIGURE 15

57. Which statements accurately compare and/or contrast bronchi (generations 1 to 9) and bronchioles (generations 10 to 15)?

    I. Generations 1 to 9 have smooth muscle, whereas generations 10 to 15 do *not*.
    II. The bronchioles posses *no* cartilage, whereas the bronchi do.
    III. Both structures have mucous glands.
    IV. Both are composed of pseudostratified ciliated columnar epithelium.

    A. I, II, III, IV
    B. II, III only
    C. I, III only
    D. II, III, IV only
    E. I, II, IV only

58. Carbaminohemoglobin can be best described as _____ .

    A. carbon monoxide combined with hemoglobin
    B. carbon dioxide combined with hemoglobin
    C. another name for CO_2 compounds in the erythrocytes
    D. CO_2 released from hemoglobin
    E. CO_2 combined with protein compounds

59. Which of the following statements are true about gas activity at the alveolar level?

    I. The molecules are under the influence of the pressure gradient that initiated the inspiration.
    II. O_2 diffuses faster than CO_2 within the alveoli.
    III. The addition of H_2O vapor from the respiratory tract reduces the P_{O_2} from 149 mm Hg in tracheal air to an alveolar P_{O_2} of approximately 100 mm Hg.
    IV. Gases move in rapid, random motion known as Brownian movement.
    V. CO_2 diffuses across the alveolar-capillary membrane 19 times faster than O_2.

    A. I, III, IV, V only
    B. II, III, IV, V only
    C. II, IV, V only
    D. I, III, IV only
    E. IV, V only

60. Which of the following anatomic features are components of an acinus?

    I. alveolar sacs
    II. vallecula
    III. respiratory bronchioles
    IV. channels of Lambert
    V. alveolar macrophages

    A. I, III, IV, V only
    B. I, III, V only
    C. II, IV only
    D. I, II, III only
    E. I, III only

61. Which of the following statements are true concerning the renal regulation of H^+ ion concentration?

I. The $[H^+]$ is principally regulated by the kidney by either increasing or decreasing extracellular HCO_3^-.

II. H^+ ion secretion varies inversely with the Pa_{CO_2}.

III. For every H^+ ion secreted, one HCO_3^- ion is filtered to form a weak acid and to maintain ionic neutrality.

IV. H^+ ion secretion is optimum up to a tubular fluid pH of 4.50.

A. I, IV only   D. II, III, IV only
B. I, III, IV only   E. I, II, III, IV
C. I, II, III only

62. Which statement most closely describes the Valsalva maneuver?

A. air voluntarily forced against a closed epiglottis
B. a reduction in the mean intrathoracic pressure accompanied by an increased cardiac output
C. an elevated mean intrathoracic pressure accompanied by a reduced venous return
D. a voluntary abdominal muscle contraction causing decreased intrathoracic pressure
E. a voluntary breathing maneuver similar to that performed when one sips liquid through a straw

63. Anatomic dead space is best described as ———————— .

A. physiologic dead space minus alveolar dead space
B. alveoli receiving ventilation but no perfusion
C. alveolar dead space minus physiologic dead space
D. intrapulmonary shunting
E. fast alveoli

64. Which of the following statements are true about the hemoglobin molecule?

I. Unsaturated hemoglobin is a more effective buffer than oxygenated hemoglobin.

II. The amount of hemoglobin present influences the amount of dissolved O_2 in the blood.

III. One mole of oxygen (32 g) will combine with 66,700 g of hemoglobin.

IV. One hemoglobin molecule can maximally accommodate four oxygen molecules.

A. I, IV only   D. II, IV only
B. II, III, IV only   E. I, III, IV, V only
C. I, IV, V only

65. Which blood vessels supply arterial blood to the left ventricle?

I. marginal artery

II. posterior descending branch of the right coronary artery

III. anterior descending branch of the left coronary artery

IV. circumflex artery

A. I, II, III only
B. II, III only
C. III, IV only

D. I, III only
E. II, III, IV only

66. Which of the following substances is secreted by the juxtaglomerular apparatus?

A. renin
B. aldosterone
C. angiotensin I

D. antidiuretic hormone
E. angiotensin II

67. What is the local response to a regional increase in alveolar dead space ventilation?

A. Alveolar CO_2 tension increases.
B. The alveolar partial pressure of CO_2 decreases.
C. Blood HCO_3^- concentration increases.
D. The partial pressure of alveolar oxygen decreases.
E. Shunting increases.

68. How many cervical vertebrae are normally present?

A. 12
B. 7
C. 6

D. 5
E. 4

69. Which type of cell exhibits the function of producing pulmonary surfactant?

A. globlet cells
B. sebaceous gland cells
C. type I alveolar cells

D. type II alveolar cells
E. synovial cells

70. Which of the following statements are true about Figure 16?
   I. The transpulmonary pressure gradient in the lung bases is greater than that in the apices.
   II. The transpulmonary pressure gradient differences cause alveoli in the bases to contain a greater volume at FRC than the apical alveoli.

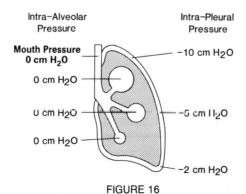

FIGURE 16

III. When compared with the apices, any given inspiratory ΔP in the bases is accompanied by a greater ΔV.

IV. The elastance is greater in the apices than in the bases of the upright, normal lung.

A. I, III, IV only
B. II, IV only
C. III, IV only
D. I, III only
E. II, III only

71. If the distance from lung apex to lung base is 30 cm, and, if the main pulmonary artery trunk is approximately midway between the apex and the base in an erect person, calculate the minimum pressure needed for apical perfusion to occur during right ventricular diastole.

A. 10 mm Hg
B. 11 mm Hg
C. 12 mm Hg
D. 13 mm Hg
E. 22 mm Hg

72. Calculate a patient's $\dot{V}A$ given the following data:

heart rate: 100 beats/min
blood pressure: 140/85
stroke volume: 50 cc
$\dot{V}A/\dot{Q}C$: 0.6:1.0

A. 0.012 liter/min
B. 0.6 liter/min
C. 30.0 ml/sec
D. 3.0 liters/min
E. 12.0 liters/min

73. Why is fluoroscopy generally *not* used for Swan-Ganz catheter insertion?

I. The prolonged exposure to radiation during catheter insertion would destroy myocardial tissue.

II. The catheter has flow-directed capabilities provided by the inflatable balloon at the catheter tip.

III. Each cardiac chamber and associated vessels generate characteristic pressure waveforms allowing for the discernment of the catheter position.

IV. The catheter is *not* radiopaque; consequently, fluoroscopy would *not* be useful.

A. IV only
B. I, II, III only
C. II, III only
D. I, III only
E. I, II only

74. Which of the following statements are true about low $\dot{V}A/\dot{Q}C$ units.

I. Arterial blood gas values, i.e., P_{O_2} and P_{CO_2}, tend to be altered more by low $\dot{V}A/\dot{Q}C$ units than by high $\dot{V}A/\dot{Q}C$.

II. Low $\dot{V}A/\dot{Q}C$ units can be described as either shunting or shunt effect.

III. Low $\dot{V}A/\dot{Q}C$ units are equivalent to alveolar dead space.

IV. Low $\dot{V}A/\dot{Q}C$ units can result in hypoxemia in the presence of normocapnia.

A. I, III, IV only
B. III, IV only
C. I, II only

D. II, IV only
E. I, II, IV only

75. The normal amount of CO_2 dissolved in arterial blood is _____ vol%.

A. 0.37
B. 1.20
C. 2.06

D. 2.68
E. 53.53

76. What would be the O_2 content (amount of O_2 bound to Hb) in the venule leading away from the two alveoli in the following illustration? (Assume that these alveoli belong to a person who is normal except for the partially obstructed alveolus shown in Figure 17.)

A. 33.56 vol%
B. 16.79 vol%
C. 14.07 vol%

D. 19.49 vol%
E. 5.42 vol%

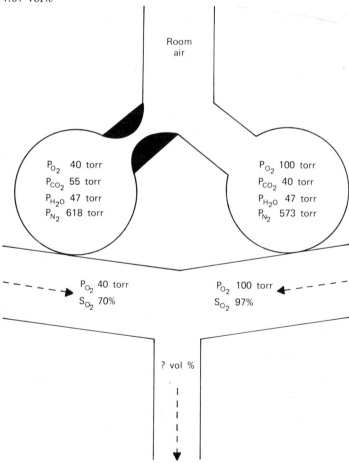

FIGURE 17

77. Calculate the $P(A-a)O_2$ given the following data:

    Pa_{O_2}: 325 mm Hg
    Pa_{CO_2}: 45 mm Hg
    pH: 7.34
    $[HCO_3^-]$: 24 mEq/liter
    Sa_{O_2}: 100%
    P_B: 760 mm Hg
    P_{H_2O}: 47 mm Hg
    R: normal
    F_{IO_2}: 1.0

    A. 429 mm Hg   D. 339 mm Hg
    B. 388 mm Hg   E. 317 mm Hg
    C. 348 mm Hg

78. Which nerve innervates the diaphragm?

    A. phrenic   D. thoracic
    B. vagus   E. glossopharyngeal
    C. trigeminal

79. Determine the mean arterial blood pressure given the data below.

    systolic: 110 torr
    diastolic: 80 torr
    oncotic pressure: 25 torr
    barometric pressure: 760 torr

    A. 135 torr   D. 80 torr
    B. 95 torr   E. 72 torr
    C. 90 torr

80. Calculate the mean exhaled P_{CO_2} based on the data below for a 200-lb (ideal body weight) person.

    tidal volume: 650 cc
    arterial P_{CO_2}: 45 torr

    A. 59 torr   D. 31 torr
    B. 46 torr   E. 38 torr
    C. 40 torr

81. Which statements are true concerning Figure 18?

    I. As the F_{ICO_2} increases, minute ventilation increases.
    II. The graph shown above is sigmoid shaped.
    III. The greatest response for increased breathing occurs between F_{ICO_2} 0.01 and 0.04.
    IV. At an F_{ICO_2} of around 0.10, minute ventilation begins to decrease.

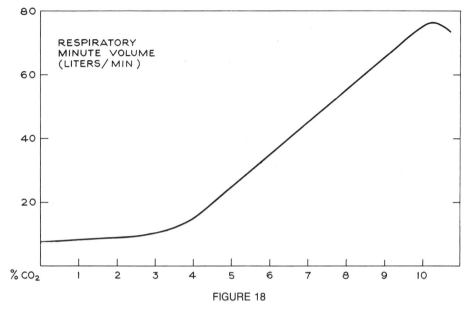

FIGURE 18

A. II, III only   D. I, II only
B. I, III, IV only   E. I, IV only
C. II, IV only

82. To compensate for an increased $\dot{V}E$, which of the following parameters could be increased to maintain a constant Pa_{CO_2}?

    I. $\dot{V}E$
   II. V_T
  III. ventilatory rate
  IV. V_A

A. I, II, III, IV   D. I, IV only
B. I, II, III only   E. I, II, IV only
C. II, III only

83. Which of the following physiologic events would accentuate intrapulmonary shunting?

    I. increased oxygen consumption
   II. increased tidal volume
  III. decreased cardiac output
  IV. increased cardiac contractility

A. I, II only   D. II, III only
B. II, IV only   E. I, III only
C. I, IV only

84. Which nerve innervates the carotid bodies?

    A. vagus   D. phrenic
    B. glossopharyngeal   E. trigeminal
    C. recurrent laryngeal

85. Identify letter C in the pressure tracings shown in Figure 19?

    A. central venous pressure   D. pulmonary artery pressure
    B. right ventricular pressure   E. pulmonary capillary wedge pressur
    C. left atrial pressue

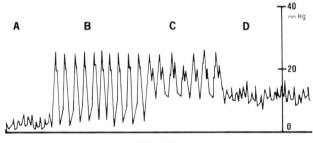

FIGURE 19

Questions 86, 87, and 88 refer to Figures 20 and 21.

86. Based on the data shown in Figure 20, determine the resultant Sa_{O_2} when blood from alveolus I mixes with blood from alveolus II.

    A. 100.0%   D. 70.7%
    B. 97.5%   E. 50.1%
    C. 83.8%

87. Based on the resultant Sa_{O_2}, what will be the accompanying Pa_{O_2} when blood from alveolus I mixes with blood from alveolus II?

    A. >100 torr   D. 38 torr
    B. 100 torr   E. 26 torr
    C. 52 torr

88. What would be the expected PA_{O_2} and PA_{CO_2} in alveolus I in Figure 20? (Assume room air breathing.)

    A. PA_{O_2} 40 torr; PA_{CO_2} 46 torr
    B. PA_{O_2} 100 torr; PA_{CO_2} 40 torr
    C. PA_{O_2} 140 torr; PA_{CO_2} 0 torr
    D. PA_{O_2} 159 torr; PA_{CO_2} 0 torr
    E. PA_{O_2} 60 torr; PA_{CO_2} 55 torr

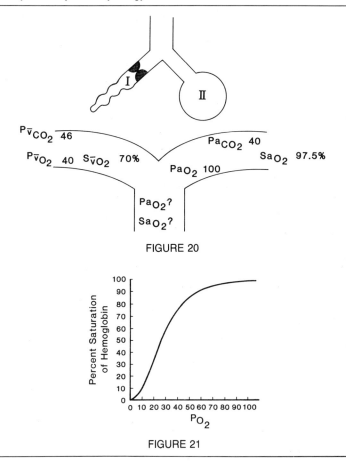

FIGURE 20

FIGURE 21

89. Calculate the net filtration pressure from the information given Figure 22

    CHP = capillary hydrostatic pressure
    IHP = interstitial hydrostatic pressure
    COP = colloid osmotic pressure
    IOP = interstitial osmotic pressure

    A. 1 mm Hg   D. 12 mm Hg
    B. 6 mm Hg   E. 30 mm Hg
    C. 10 mm Hg

90. When the pH of plasma is 7.40, urine pH is approximately _____.

    A. 7.40   D. 3.60
    B. 6.00   E. 2.00
    C. 4.50

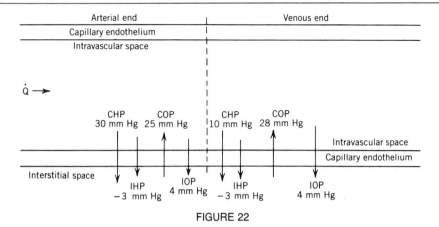

FIGURE 22

91. Which of the following statements are true concerning the control of extracellular fluid osmolality?

   I. When extracellular fluid osmolality increases, the pituitary gland is stimulated to release antidiuretic hormone.

   II. Extracellular sodium ion concentration almost entirely determines extracellular osmolality.

   III. When extracellular osmolality increases, both sodium ions and water are reabsorbed.

   IV. The juxtaglomerular apparatus senses changes in extracellular osmolality and influences aldosterone secretion accordingly.

   A. I, IV only   D. II, III, IV only
   B. II, IV only   E. I, II, III, IV
   C. I, II, III only

92. Calculate the amount of oxygen combined to hemoglobin in a patient having 13 g% Hb and an arterial oxygen saturation of 86%.

   A. 20.10 vol%   D. 14.98 vol%
   B. 17.42 vol%   E. 13.64 vol%
   C. 15.32 vol%

93. The hyperventilation that is associated with diabetic acidosis is caused by which physiologic mechanism?

   A. The peripheral chemoreceptors are stimulated by the low Pa_{O_2}.
   B. The central chemoreceptors are stimulated by the increased Pa_{CO_2}.
   C. The peripheral chemoreceptors respond to the increased arterial $[H^+]$.
   D. The central chemoreceptors respond to the increased CSF $[H^+]$.
   E. The cerebral cortex sends a greater number of impulses to medullary inspiratory center.

94. As the left ventricle fails as a pump, which pressure measurements would reflect the severity of that failure?

    I. central venous pressure
    II. pulmonary artery systolic pressure
    III. left ventricular end-diastolic pressure
    IV. pulmonary capillary wedge pressure

    A. III, IV only
    B. II, III only
    C. II, IV only
    D. I, II only
    E. I, II, III, IV

95. Which statement(s) best describe(s) the purpose of central venous pressure (CVP) monitoring?

    I. It reflects left ventricular activity.
    II. It reflects right ventricular activity.
    III. CVP monitors left atrial emptying pressure.
    IV. CVP represents the pressure in the venous system as blood returns to the heart.

    A. I only
    B. III, IV only
    C. I, III only
    D. II only
    E. II, IV only

96. Calculate the $\dot{Q}_T$ given the information below.

    tissue oxygen consumption: 230 ml/min
    ABGs: Pa_{O_2} 95 torr
    Pa_{CO_2} 45 torr
    pH 7.42
    Sa_{O_2} 94%
    mixed venous blood gases: $P\bar{v}_{O_2}$ 40 torr
    $P\bar{v}_{CO_2}$ 49 torr
    pH 7.33
    $S\bar{v}_{O_2}$ 70%
    hemoglobin concentration: 16 g%

    A. 5.23 liters/min
    B. 5.00 liters/min
    C. 4.81 liters/min
    D. 4.52 liters/min
    E. 4.33 liters/min

97. A person having an acute nonrespiratory alkalosis would be expected to have a(n) _____ CSF pH and a(n) _____ arterial blood pH.

    A. increased; increased
    B. increased; decreased
    C. decreased; increased
    D. decreased; decreased
    E. normal; increased

98. The peripheral chemoreceptors would send hyperventilatory signals to the respiratory center in the brain in response to which acid-base disturbance(s)?

    I. respiratory acidosis
    II. metabolic acidosis
    III. respiratory alkalosis
    IV. metabolic alkalosis

A. I, II, III, IV
B. III, IV only
C. II, IV only

D. I, II only
E. II only

99. During the initial phase of a normal tidal inspiration, the Pa_{CO_2} ———————— and the Pa_{O_2} ———————— .

A. decreases; increases
B. decreases; decreases
C. increases; decreases

D. increases; increases
E. remains constant; increases

100. Which lung zone(s) most likely reflect(s) the ideal $\dot{V}_A/\dot{Q}_C$ ratio range?

A. middle
B. upper
C. lower

D. middle and lower
E. upper, middle, and lower

ASSESSMENT ANSWER SHEET

DIRECTIONS: Darken the space under the selected answer.

	A	B	C	D	E		A	B	C	D	E
1.	[ ]	[ ]	[ ]	[ ]	[ ]	28.	[ ]	[ ]	[ ]	[ ]	[ ]
2.	[ ]	[ ]	[ ]	[ ]	[ ]	29.	[ ]	[ ]	[ ]	[ ]	[ ]
3.	[ ]	[ ]	[ ]	[ ]	[ ]	30.	[ ]	[ ]	[ ]	[ ]	[ ]
4.	[ ]	[ ]	[ ]	[ ]	[ ]	31.	[ ]	[ ]	[ ]	[ ]	[ ]
5.	[ ]	[ ]	[ ]	[ ]	[ ]	32.	[ ]	[ ]	[ ]	[ ]	[ ]
6.	[ ]	[ ]	[ ]	[ ]	[ ]	33.	[ ]	[ ]	[ ]	[ ]	[ ]
7.	[ ]	[ ]	[ ]	[ ]	[ ]	34.	[ ]	[ ]	[ ]	[ ]	[ ]
8.	[ ]	[ ]	[ ]	[ ]	[ ]	35.	[ ]	[ ]	[ ]	[ ]	[ ]
9.	[ ]	[ ]	[ ]	[ ]	[ ]	36.	[ ]	[ ]	[ ]	[ ]	[ ]
10.	[ ]	[ ]	[ ]	[ ]	[ ]	37.	[ ]	[ ]	[ ]	[ ]	[ ]
11.	[ ]	[ ]	[ ]	[ ]	[ ]	38.	[ ]	[ ]	[ ]	[ ]	[ ]
12.	[ ]	[ ]	[ ]	[ ]	[ ]	39.	[ ]	[ ]	[ ]	[ ]	[ ]
13.	[ ]	[ ]	[ ]	[ ]	[ ]	40.	[ ]	[ ]	[ ]	[ ]	[ ]
14.	[ ]	[ ]	[ ]	[ ]	[ ]	41.	[ ]	[ ]	[ ]	[ ]	[ ]
15.	[ ]	[ ]	[ ]	[ ]	[ ]	42.	[ ]	[ ]	[ ]	[ ]	[ ]
16.	[ ]	[ ]	[ ]	[ ]	[ ]	43.	[ ]	[ ]	[ ]	[ ]	[ ]
17.	[ ]	[ ]	[ ]	[ ]	[ ]	44.	[ ]	[ ]	[ ]	[ ]	[ ]
18.	[ ]	[ ]	[ ]	[ ]	[ ]	45.	[ ]	[ ]	[ ]	[ ]	[ ]
19.	[ ]	[ ]	[ ]	[ ]	[ ]	46.	[ ]	[ ]	[ ]	[ ]	[ ]
20.	[ ]	[ ]	[ ]	[ ]	[ ]	47.	[ ]	[ ]	[ ]	[ ]	[ ]
21.	[ ]	[ ]	[ ]	[ ]	[ ]	48.	[ ]	[ ]	[ ]	[ ]	[ ]
22.	[ ]	[ ]	[ ]	[ ]	[ ]	49.	[ ]	[ ]	[ ]	[ ]	[ ]
23.	[ ]	[ ]	[ ]	[ ]	[ ]	50.	[ ]	[ ]	[ ]	[ ]	[ ]
24.	[ ]	[ ]	[ ]	[ ]	[ ]	51.	[ ]	[ ]	[ ]	[ ]	[ ]
25.	[ ]	[ ]	[ ]	[ ]	[ ]	52.	[ ]	[ ]	[ ]	[ ]	[ ]
26.	[ ]	[ ]	[ ]	[ ]	[ ]	53.	[ ]	[ ]	[ ]	[ ]	[ ]
27.	[ ]	[ ]	[ ]	[ ]	[ ]	54.	[ ]	[ ]	[ ]	[ ]	[ ]

	A	B	C	D	E		A	B	C	D	E
55.	[ ]	[ ]	[ ]	[ ]	[ ]	83.	[ ]	[ ]	[ ]	[ ]	[ ]
56.	[ ]	[ ]	[ ]	[ ]	[ ]	84.	[ ]	[ ]	[ ]	[ ]	[ ]
57.	[ ]	[ ]	[ ]	[ ]	[ ]	85.	[ ]	[ ]	[ ]	[ ]	[ ]
58.	[ ]	[ ]	[ ]	[ ]	[ ]	86.	[ ]	[ ]	[ ]	[ ]	[ ]
59.	[ ]	[ ]	[ ]	[ ]	[ ]	87.	[ ]	[ ]	[ ]	[ ]	[ ]
60.	[ ]	[ ]	[ ]	[ ]	[ ]	88.	[ ]	[ ]	[ ]	[ ]	[ ]
71.	[ ]	[ ]	[ ]	[ ]	[ ]	89.	[ ]	[ ]	[ ]	[ ]	[ ]
72.	[ ]	[ ]	[ ]	[ ]	[ ]	90.	[ ]	[ ]	[ ]	[ ]	[ ]
73.	[ ]	[ ]	[ ]	[ ]	[ ]	91.	[ ]	[ ]	[ ]	[ ]	[ ]
74.	[ ]	[ ]	[ ]	[ ]	[ ]	92.	[ ]	[ ]	[ ]	[ ]	[ ]
75.	[ ]	[ ]	[ ]	[ ]	[ ]	93.	[ ]	[ ]	[ ]	[ ]	[ ]
76.	[ ]	[ ]	[ ]	[ ]	[ ]	94.	[ ]	[ ]	[ ]	[ ]	[ ]
77.	[ ]	[ ]	[ ]	[ ]	[ ]	95.	[ ]	[ ]	[ ]	[ ]	[ ]
78.	[ ]	[ ]	[ ]	[ ]	[ ]	96.	[ ]	[ ]	[ ]	[ ]	[ ]
79.	[ ]	[ ]	[ ]	[ ]	[ ]	97.	[ ]	[ ]	[ ]	[ ]	[ ]
80.	[ ]	[ ]	[ ]	[ ]	[ ]	98.	[ ]	[ ]	[ ]	[ ]	[ ]
81.	[ ]	[ ]	[ ]	[ ]	[ ]	99.	[ ]	[ ]	[ ]	[ ]	[ ]
82.	[ ]	[ ]	[ ]	[ ]	[ ]	100.	[ ]	[ ]	[ ]	[ ]	[ ]

CARDIOPULMONARY ANATOMY AND PHYSIOLOGY ANALYSES

Note: The references listed after each analysis are numbered and keyed to the reference list located at the end of this section. The first number indicates the text. The second number indicates the page on which information about the question will be found. For example, (1:219,384) means that reference number 1 is to be used and that on pages 219 and 394 information about the question will be found. Frequently, it will be necessary to read beyond the page number indicated to obtain complete information. Therefore, reference to the question will be found either on the page indicated or on subsequent pages.

1. A. Under normal physiologic conditions the alveoli do not behave in accordance with the law of LaPlace, which states that pressure (dynes/cm^2) within the sphere is inversely related to the radius (cm) and directly related to the surface tension (dynes/cm) at the air-liquid interface. Quantitatively, the law of LaPlace is written

$$P = \frac{2\ ST}{r}$$

   where,

$$P = \text{distending pressure (dynes/cm}^2)$$
$$ST = \text{surface tension (dynes/cm)}$$
$$r = \text{radius (cm)}$$

   According to the law of LaPlace, the surface tension increases as the radius decreases. Conversely, it also states that the surface tension decreases as the radius increases.

   Because of the presence of pulmonary surfactant, surface tension inside the alveoli decreases as the alveolar radius decreases (exhalation). The decreased surface tension at this point in the ventilatory cycle reduces the work of breathing as less pressure is needed to inflate the alveoli.

   During inspiration the surface tension of the alveolar lining layer increases as surfactant becomes less concentrated and alveolar radius increases.
   (1:134–140), (2:174–176,232–234), (3:20,34–35), (4:28–29,134), (6:226,706), (8:21–22), (12:105), (14:90–94,166).

2. E. The formula used here is

$$V_T - V_D = V_A$$

   where

$$V_T = \text{tidal volume (cc)}$$
$$V_D = \text{dead space volume (cc)}$$
$$V_A = \text{alveolar volume (cc)}$$

   Therefore,

$$550\ cc - 160\ cc = 390\ cc$$

   V_A should *not* be confused with $\dot{V}_A$ which is the product of $V_A \times f$.
   (1:116), (2:151), (8:50–51), (14:15)

3. C. Cyanosis will appear if a person has 5.0 g% (5.0 g/dl) or more of unsaturated Hb in total circulation (arterial and venous). The degree of unsaturation can be calculated as follows:

STEP 1: Calculate the percentage of unsaturated arterial hemoglobin.

$$\frac{100\%}{- 51\% \ Sa_{O_2}}$$

49% unsaturated arterial Hb

STEP 2: Determine the percentage of unsaturated venous hemoglobin.

$$\frac{100\%}{- 45\% \ S\bar{v}_{O_2}}$$

55% unsaturated venous Hb

STEP 3: Compute the amount of reduced hemoglobin in arterial blood. 20 g% Hb × 0.49 = 9.8 g% reduced Hb (arterial)

STEP 4: Obtain the amount of reduced hemoglobin in venous blood.

20 g% Hb × 0.55 = 11.0 g% reduced Hb (venous)

STEP 5: Calculate the amount of reduced hemoglobin in total circulation (average of that in arterial and venous blood).

$$\frac{9.8 \ g\% + 11.0 \ g\%}{2} = \frac{20.8 \ g\%}{2}$$

$$= 10.4 \ g\% \text{ reduced Hb in total circulation.}$$

Because the amount of total unsaturated (reduced) Hb in this example is greater than 5.0 g%, this person will display cyanosis.
(1:281–282), (8:184)

4. E. The three major buffers found in the urine are NH_3, $HPO_4^=$, and HCO_3^-.
(4:162–165), (27:96–97)

5. D. The steep portion of the Hb-O_2 dissociation curve reflects the unloading of oxygen to the tissues (internal respiration); the flat portion of the curve reflects the binding of oxygen to hemoglobin at the lung level (external respiration).

At the steep portion of the curve, small changes in P_{O_2} are associated with large fluctuations in saturation. Conversely, large fluctuations in P_{O_2} are associated with small changes in oxygen saturation on the flat portion of the curve.

For example, in Figure 23 a P_{O_2} decrease of 20 torr (from 100 torr to 80 torr) on the flat portion of the curve is associated with a fall in S_{O_2} of only about 3.5% (i.e., an S_{O_2} of 97.5% at a P_{O_2} of 100 torr compared with an S_{O_2} of 94.0% at a P_{O_2} of 80 torr). The same drop in P_{O_2} (20 torr) on the steep portion of the curve produces a decrease in the S_{O_2} of approximately 26% i.e., an S_{O_2} of 83% at a P_{O_2} of 50 torr compared with an S_{O_2} of 57% at a P_{O_2} of 30 torr).

Factors such as pH, temperature, P_{CO_2}, and 2,3-DPG influence the steep aspect of the curve more than the flat portion.
(1:205–210), (2:242–246), (3:169–171), (4:185–187), (6:260–261), (8:78–80), (12:186–191)

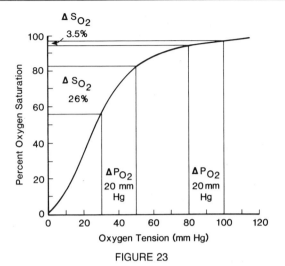

FIGURE 23

6. D. STEP 1: Use the clinical shunt equation.

$$\frac{\dot{Q}s}{\dot{Q}T} = \frac{(P_{AO_2} - P_{aO_2})0.003}{(P_{AO_2} - P_{aO_2})0.003 + (C_{aO_2} - C\bar{v}_{O_2})} \times 100$$

STEP 2: Calculate the arterial O_2 content.

$$\begin{aligned}
C_{aO_2} &= \text{dissolved arterial } O_2 + \text{combined arterial } O_2 \\
&= (150 \text{ torr} \times 0.003) + (1.00 \times 15g\% \text{ Hb} \times 1.34) \\
&= 20.55 \text{ vol}\%
\end{aligned}$$

STEP 3: Calculate the venous O_2 content.

$$\begin{aligned}
C\bar{v}_{O_2} &= \text{dissolved venous } O_2 + \text{combined venous } O_2 \\
&= (30 \text{ torr} \times 0.003) + (0.75 \times 15 \text{ g}\% \text{ Hb} \times 1.34) \\
&= 15.17 \text{ vol}\%
\end{aligned}$$

STEP 4: Use the alveolar air equation to compute the P_{AO_2}.

$$P_{AO_2} = (P_B - P_{H_2O})F_{IO_2} - P_{ACO_2}*\left(F_{IO_2} + \frac{1 - F_{IO_2}}{R}\right)$$

Because R = 1.0,

$$\left(F_{IO_2} + \frac{1 - F_{IO_2}}{R}\right) = \left(0.6 + \frac{1 - 0.6}{1}\right) = 1.0$$

Therefore,

$$P_{AO_2} = (760 \text{ torr} - 47 \text{ torr}) 0.6 - 40 \text{ torr}(1.0) = 388 \text{ torr}$$

*The P_{aCO_2} can substitute for the P_{ACO_2} in the alveolar air equation because equilibration across the alveolar-capillary membrane is assumed.

STEP 5: Insert values in the clinical shunt equation.

$$\frac{\dot{Q}s}{\dot{Q}T} = \frac{(388 \text{ torr} - 150 \text{ torr})0.003}{(388 \text{ torr} - 150 \text{ torr})0.003 + (20.55 \text{ vol\%} - 15.17 \text{ vol\%})} \times 100$$

$$\frac{\dot{Q}s}{\dot{Q}s} = 11.72\%$$

Alternatively, the classic shunt equation (below) can sometimes be used.

$$\frac{\dot{Q}s}{\dot{Q}T} = \frac{Cc_{O_2} - Ca_{O_2}}{Cc_{O_2} - C\bar{v}_{O_2}} \times 100$$

where

$\dot{Q}s$ = that portion of the cardiac output that does *not* exchange with alveolar air

$\dot{Q}T$ = total cardiac output

Cc_{O_2} = total end-pulmonary capillary oxygen content

Ca_{O_2} = total arterial oxygen content

$C\bar{v}_{O_2}$ = total venous oxygen content

If the alveolar-arterial oxygen tension difference, that is, $(P_{A_{O_2}} - P_{a_{O_2}}) \times (0.003)$, is equal to the $Cc_{O_2} - Ca_{O_2}$ gradient, the expression $Cc_{O_2} - C\bar{v}_{O_2}$ in the clinical shunt equation can be replaced by $(P_{A_{O_2}} - P_{a_{O_2}}) \times (0.003) + (Ca_{O_2} - C\bar{v}_{O_2})$. Additionally, if the hemoglobin in the arterial blood is 100% saturated, then the expression $Cc_{O_2} - Ca_{O_2}$ in the clinical shunt equation can be replaced by the alveolar-arterial oxygen tension difference, that is $(P_{A_{O_2}} - P_{a_{O_2}}) \times (0.003)$.
(2:18–22), (3:318–326), (4:217–219), (13:30,32), (14:52–55), (17:185–186), (27:213–215)

7. B. The cardiac output ($\dot{Q}T$) is the product of the heart rate and the stroke volume.

heart rate $\times$ stroke volume = cardiac output
100 beats/min $\times$ 0.06 liter = 6.0 liters/min

(8-111)

8. A. As a person hypoventilates, the amount of CO_2 dissolved in arterial blood increases. Subsequently, the amount of CO_2 in the CSF will also increase because CO_2 passively moves across the blood-brain barrier into the CSF. For a given metabolic rate, the Pa_{CO_2} and $P_{CSF_{CO_2}}$ are inversely related to the ventilatory rate.
(1:222–227), (3:29), (4:92–93), (6:229,230), (10:134), (12:59), (14:116–118)

9. D. The peripheral chemoreceptors are essentially the oxygen (Pa_{O_2}) sensors in the blood. However, hyperventilation occurs when arterial blood acutely high in carbon dioxide or acutely high in H^+ ions flows through the carotid and aortic bodies.
(1:222–227), (3:29–30), (4:91–92), (6:229,230), (7:43), (8:97,102–103), (10:33), (12:38,57,68), (14:118–119)

10. B. Goblet cells are interspersed among the pseudostratified ciliated columnar epithelium cells. The goblet cells maintain the efficacy of the mucociliary layer along with secretions of the submucosal glands. The submucosal glands are located beneath the respiratory mucosal layer.

The vagus nerve, when stimulated, causes increased mucous gland and goblet cell activity.

(3:13–15), (4:40–42), (6:372–374), (8:148), (13:140)

11. A. The hemoglobin molecule contains four nonprotein heme groups and one protein globin portion. Each heme group is normally capable of chemically and reversibly combining with one oxygen molecule. Therefore, the entire hemoglobin molecule has the ability to combine with four oxygen molecules.

Note the simplified depiction of the hemoglobin molecule below:

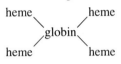

(1:203), (2:239,240–241), (4:183–184), (27:19–23)

12. D. Theoretically, all the perfusion would come into contact with all the ventilation. Gas exchange would be perfect throughout these perfect lungs. An $F_{I_{O_2}}$ of 1.0 would result in the washout of all the nitrogen. The only gases that would remain in the lungs along with the oxygen would be CO_2 and water vapor (P_{H_2O}).

$$
\begin{array}{ll}
 & 760 \text{ torr } P_B \\
- & 47 \text{ torr } P_{H_2O} \\
\hline
 & 713 \text{ torr corrected } P_B \\
- & 40 \text{ torr } P_{CO_2} \\
\hline
 & 673 \text{ torr } P_{O_2} \text{ (theoretical maximum)}
\end{array}
$$

(1:123), (2:127–132)

13. D. A direct relationship exists between the $P_{a_{O_2}}$ and the amount of oxygen dissolved in the arterial blood expressed as vol%. Both measurements represent the same parameter; however, each is expressed in a different unit.

The $P_{a_{O_2}}$ is usually expressed as mm Hg, torr, or kPa. It can also be expressed as vol% by multiplying the unit mm Hg or torr by the conversion factor 0.003 vol%/mm Hg. For example, a $P_{a_{O_2}}$ of 100 mm Hg can be converted to vol% as follows

$$100 \ \cancel{mm \ Hg} \times 0.003 \ vol\%/\cancel{mm \ Hg} = 0.3 \ vol\%$$

Therefore, as the $P_{a_{O_2}}$ increases, the amount of oxygen dissoved in the arterial blood, expressed as vol%, also increases. The converse is also true. Note Figure 24.

(1:202), (2:39), (12:184–185)

14. D. The law of continuity, based on the law of conservation of matter, explains the relationship between the cross-sectional area of a tube through which a fluid is flowing and the velocity of the flowing fluid. In quantitative terms the product of

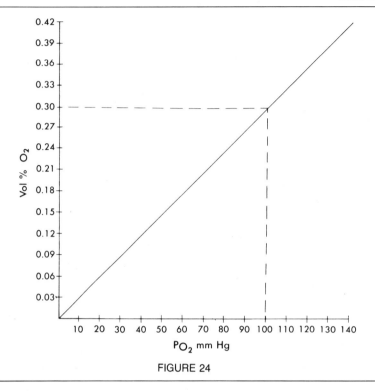

FIGURE 24

the cross-sectional area times the velocity for a given flowrate is constant. Therefore, the two factors, cross-sectional area and velocity, are inversely related; that is, as the cross-sectional area decreases for a given flowrate, the velocity of the flowing gas increases and vice versa.

The continuity equation can be shown as

$$A \times v = k$$

where

        A = the cross-sectional area of the tubes
a   v = the velocity of the flowing fluid
        k = a constant

or as

$$A_1 \times v_1 = A_2 \times v_2$$

which indicates that the product of the cross-sectional area and the velocity at any two points in the conducting system are the same for a constant flowrate.

As blood travels from the pulmonary artery (Figure 25), it encounters an increased cross-sectional area upon entering and traversing the pulmonary capillary bed. The physiologic advantages of this situation are to reduce blood velocity as it passes near ventilated alveoli, allowing more time for gas exchange, and to provide an increased surface area for gas exchange.

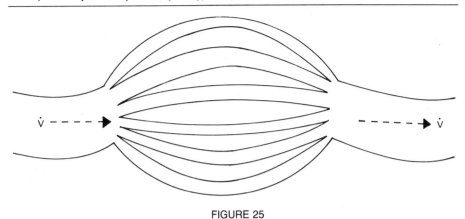

FIGURE 25

As inspired gas moves from the trachea (generation 0) to the alveoli, 23 generations of airways are encountered. This system of dichotomous branching results in
an increased cross-sectional area with each branching. Gas velocity is reduced to
Brownian movement in the alveoli, as a consequence. The physiologic advantage
of this arrangement is to allow gas molecules to move through small airways (≤ 2
mm diameter) into the alveoli for gas exchange.

(2:133–138), (4:29), (12:36–38))

15. E. Portions of the respiratory mucosa are lined by pseudostratified ciliated columnar
epithelium and ciliated cuboidal epithelium. These cellular structures house goblet
cells that secrete mucus. In addition, the submucosal glands contribute to the fluid
layer that bathes the cilia. The fluid layer has a watery component in which the
cilia are totally immersed. The gel layer atop the watery component functions as a
trap for foreign particles and prevents the desiccation of the layer below.

The cilia move in a cephalad (toward the head) direction. They are so efficient
that no retrograde motion occurs during their recovery stroke. They are rigid when
they whip forward and become flaccid when they recover. Certain noxious chemicals and environmental factors impair ciliary activity, for example, tobacco
smoke, alcohol, and hypoxemia.

(1:352–353,455), (3:13–15), (4:40–42), (8:147–149), (12:222), (14:10)

16. A. Persistent fetal circulation may be characterized by a patent foramen ovale
(communication between the two atria) and/or a patent ductus arteriosus
(communication between the pulmonary artery and the aorta). Such a condition
results from a high pulmonary vascular resistance, which is aggravated by progressive hypoxemia resulting from this significant right-to-left shunting.

(4:167–170), (8:118–123), (12:241)

17. E. The normal P_{50} value is 27 mm Hg. This value represents the oxygen tension at
which 50% of the hemoglobin in circulation is combined with oxygen under the
following conditions: Pa_{CO_2} 40 mm Hg, pH 7.40, and a normal body temperature
(37°C).

Inspection of the Hb-O_2 dissociation curve (Figure 26) shows that as the curve
shifts to the left ($\downarrow$ [H$^+$]; $\uparrow$ pH; $\downarrow$ Pa_{CO_2}; $\downarrow$ temperature; $\downarrow$ 2,3-DPG), the release

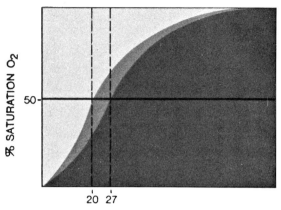

PARTIAL PRESSURE O$_2$

FIGURE 26

of oxygen to the tissues is hindered (↑ Hb-O$_2$ affinity). At the same time, the P$_{50}$ value decreases. When the curve shifts to the left, a lower partial pressure of oxygen is needed to saturate 50% of the hemoglobin in circulation.

(1:208–209), (3:170–171), (4:186–187), (6:261–262), (7:53–54), (12:183–191), (14:72), (27:84–86)

18. E. Carbonic anhydrase is not found only in the red blood cells. It is also found in the kidney tubule cells. Carbonic anhydrase catalyzes the reaction between CO$_2$ and H$_2$O. In the presence of carbonic anhydrase, the hydration of carbon dioxide occurs 13,000 times faster.

(1:213), (4:161), (6:276), (12:208), (14:72)

19. B. The medial surface of both lungs display concavity, to accommodate mediastinal structures, such as the great veins and arteries, and the heart.

The right hemidiaphragm is situated higher than that on the left in order to accommodate the liver beneath.

The root of the lung (pulmonary artery, pulmonary veins, lymph vessels, nerves, and mainstem bronchi) enters the lung at the lung's hilum.

(4:63), (6:217–218)

20. C. The cardiac index (C.I.) provides a more specific measurement of the cardiac status than does the cardiac output (C.O.). It is obtained by dividing the C.O. by the body surface area (BSA) expressed in square meters (m^2).

$$C.I. = \frac{C.O.}{BSA}$$

STEP 1: Calculate the cardiac output (C.O.).

$$
\begin{aligned}
C.O. &= \text{stroke volume} \times \text{heart rate} \\
&= 72 \text{ ml/beat} \times 63 \text{ beats/min} \\
&= 4.54 \text{ lpm}
\end{aligned}
$$

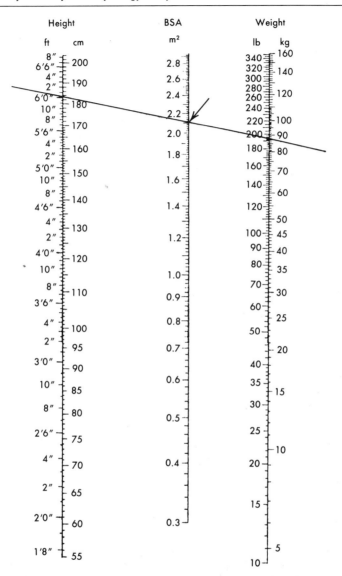

FIGURE 27. Find the patient's height in either feet or centimeters in the left column and the patient's weight in pounds or kilograms in the right column. Connect these two points with a ruler. The BSA is indicated at the point where the ruler crosses the middle column. (From DuBois, E.F., *Basal Metabolism in Health and Disease*, 3rd ed., Lea & Febiger, Philadelphia, 1936.)

STEP 2: Obtain the BSA from the Dubois Body Surface Chart in Figure 27. The BSA has been found to be 2.10 m².

STEP 3: Calculate the cardiac index (C.I.).

$$\text{C.I.} = \frac{4.54 \text{ liters/min}}{2.10 \text{ m}^2} = 2.16 \text{ liters/min/m}^2$$

The normal range for the C.I. is 2.50 to 4.00 liters/min/m^2.
(9:127,287)

21. D. Carbon dioxide is primarily transported in blood as HCO_3^-. The majority of this HCO_3^- is formed in the red blood cells (RBC). Carbon dioxide is involved in a number of reactions in the RBC. (1) Some CO_2 physically dissolves in erythrocyte water as P_{CO_2}; (2) a portion of CO_2 reversibly combines with the globin portion of the Hb molecules; and (3) the majority of the CO_2 is hydrated in the presence of carbonic anhydrase (C.A.). This reaction is

$$CO_2 + H_2O \xrightarrow{C.A.} H_2CO_3 \longrightarrow H^+ + HCO_3^-$$

In the RBC this reaction is favored to the right at the tissue level because (1) C.A. catalyzes the reaction 13,000 times; (2) unsaturated Hb buffers the H^+ ions produced by this reaction; and (3) the HCO_3^- ions passively diffuse out of the RBC in exchange for Cl^- ions (Hamburger phenomenon or chloride shift).
(1:213–216), (2:79–80), (4:189–191), (6:274–275), (8:81–84), (12:207–210)

22. D. The amount of time required to fill a lung unit with air can be calculated by multiplying the resistance times compliance characteristics of the lungs.

$$\text{Resistance} \times \text{compliance} = \text{time constant}$$
$$\cancel{cm\ H_2O}/\text{liter/sec} \times \text{liters}/\cancel{cm\ H_2O} = \#\ \text{of sec}$$

(3.82, (4:34–51), (8:36–38,56), (14:109,155,157)

23. C. The right common carotid artery and the coronary arteries do not branch directly off the aortic arch; the brachiocephalic, left subclavian, and left common carotid arteries do. The right subclavian and right common carotid arteries both arise later from the brachiocephalic.
(21:286)

24. B. The equation for calculating the VD/VT ratio is derived from the Bohr equation. The technically correct equation is

$$\frac{V_D}{V_T} = \frac{\dot{V}_E(F_{A_{CO_2}} - F\overline{E}_{CO_2})}{F_{A_{CO_2}}}$$

where

$$V_D = \text{anatomic dead space}$$
$$V_T = \text{tidal volume}$$
$$\dot{V}_E = \text{minute ventilation } (V_T \times f)$$
$$F_{A_{CO_2}} = \text{fraction of alveolar carbon dioxide}$$
$$F\overline{E}_{CO_2} = \text{fraction of mean exhaled carbon dioxide}$$

However, clinically, the equation conveniently becomes

$$\frac{V_D}{V_T} = \frac{(Pa_{CO_2} - P\overline{E}_{CO_2})}{Pa_{CO_2}}$$

where

$$Pa_{CO_2} = \text{arterial carbon dioxide tension}$$
$$P\overline{E}_{CO_2} = \text{mean exhaled carbon dioxide tension}$$

(1:119–120), (2:9–10), (6:242), (8:402), (14:20,162)

25. C. Hyperventilation will result in a decreased Pa_{CO_2} and a respiratory alkalosis. At the same time, because carbon dioxide is passively permeable across the blood–brain barrier, cerebrospinal fluid carbon dioxide tension will also fall.
    (1:222–227,233–234), (3:92), (4:29), (10:134), (12:59), (14:116)

26. E. The umbilical vein transports arterial blood from the placenta to the fetus. The umbilical vein normally carries oxygenated blood. The umbilical arteries carry fetal venous blood to the placenta for gas exchange.
    (4:167–169), (8:11,119), (14:140)

27. D. The larynx is composed of nine cartilages. These cartilages include the thyroid and cricoid cartilages, the epiglottis, the arytenoids (1 pair), and the cuneiform (1 pair) and corniculate (1 pair) cartilages. The glottis is simply the opening between the vocal cords.
    (3:7–8), (4:50)

28. A. The palmar arch, the plantar arch, and the circle of Willis are arterial anastomoses. The palmar arch is the union of the radial and ulnar arteries in the palm of the hand. The planter arch is the joining of the dorsalis pedis and plantar arteries in the sole of the foot. The circle of Willis is formed by the anterior and posterior communicating arteries, the anterior and posterior cerebral arteries, and the internal carotid arteries.
    (21:290–291)

29. B. At 100 torr Pa_{O_2} the corresponding Sa_{O_2} at pH 7.20 would be approximately 94% or 0.94. The $S\overline{v}_{O_2}$ at pH 7.20 and $P\overline{v}_{O_2}$ 40 torr would be about 62% or 0.62.

    STEP 1: Convert the Pa_{O_2} to vol%.

    $$Pa_{O_2} \times 0.003 \text{ vol\%/torr} = \text{vol\%}$$
    $$100 \text{ torr} \times 0.003 \text{ vol\%/torr} = 0.3 \text{ vol\%}$$

    STEP 2: Calculate the amount of O_2 combined to hemoglobin (arterial).

    $$Sa_{O_2} \times [Hb] \times 1.34 \text{ ml } O_2/g \text{ Hb} = O_2 \text{ combined to Hb (vol\%)}$$
    $$0.94 \times 13 \text{ g\%} \times 1.34 \text{ ml } O_2/g \text{ Hb} = 16.37 \text{ vol\%}$$

    STEP 3: Calculate the arterial O_2 content.

    $$\text{combined arterial} + \text{dissolved arterial} = \text{arterial } O_2 \text{ content}$$
    $$16.37 \text{ vol\%} + 0.3 \text{ vol\%} = 16.67 \text{ vol\%}$$

    STEP 4: Convert the $P\overline{v}_{O_2}$ to vol%.

    $$P\overline{v}_{O_2} \times 0.003 \text{ vol\%/torr} = \text{volumes \%}$$
    $$40 \text{ torr} \times 0.003 \text{ vol\%/torr} = 0.12 \text{ vol\%}$$

STEP 5: Calculate the amount of O_2 combined to hemoglobin (venous).

$$S\bar{v}_{O_2} \times [Hb] \times 1.34 \text{ ml } O_2/g \text{ Hb} = O_2 \text{ combined to Hb (vol\%)}$$
$$0.62 \times 13g\% \times 1.34 \text{ ml } O_2/g \text{ Hb} = 10.80 \text{ vol\%}$$

STEP 6: Calculate the venous O_2 content.

$$\text{combined venous} + \text{dissolved venous} = \text{venous } O_2 \text{ content}$$
$$10.80 \text{ vol\%} + 0.12 \text{ vol\%} = 10.92 \text{ vol\%}$$

STEP 7: Calculate the arterial-venous difference.

$$\text{arterial } O_2 \text{ content} - \text{venous } O_2 \text{ content} = \text{a-v difference}$$
$$16.67 \text{ vol\%} - 10.92 \text{ vol\%} = 5.75 \text{ vol\%}$$

(1:207–208), (2:20,22), (4:509–510)

30. E. The first four steps will provide for the calculation of the alveolar minute ventilation ($\dot{V}_A$):

STEP 1: Approximately, 1 lb of ideal body weight equals 1 cc of anatomic dead space.

150 lb of ideal body weight = 150 cc of anatomic dead space.

STEP 2: Calculate the minute dead space ventilation ($\dot{V}_D$):

$$V_D \times f = \dot{V}_D$$
$$150 \text{ cc} \times 12 \text{ breaths/min} = 1{,}800 \text{ cc/min}$$

STEP 3: Calculate the minute ventilation ($\dot{V}_E$):

$$V_T \times f = \dot{V}_E$$
$$500 \text{ cc} \times 12 \text{ breaths/min} = 6{,}000 \text{ cc/min}$$

STEP 4: Calculate the alveolar minute ventilation ($\dot{V}_A$):

$$\dot{V}_E - \dot{V}_D = \dot{V}_A$$
$$6{,}000 \text{ cc/min} - 1{,}800 \text{ cc/min} = 4{,}200 \text{ cc/min}$$

The cardiac output can be determined by using the Fick equation

$$\dot{Q}_T = \frac{\dot{V}_{O_2}}{Ca_{O_2} - C\bar{v}_{O_2}}$$

where

$$\dot{Q}_T = \text{cardiac output}$$
$$\dot{V}_{O_2} = \text{oxygen consumption}$$
$$Ca_{O_2} = \text{arterial } O_2 \text{ content}$$
$$C\bar{v}_{O_2} = \text{venous } O_2 \text{ content}$$

(Recall that $Ca_{O_2} - C\bar{v}_{O_2}$ is the a-v oxygen content difference expressed in vol%.)

STEP 5: Insert the known values into the Fick equation to calculate the cardiac output ($\dot{Q}_T$).

$$\dot{Q}_T = \frac{240 \text{ ml/min}}{20 \text{ vol\%} - 14 \text{ vol\%}}$$

$$= \frac{240 \text{ cc/min}}{\left(\dfrac{20 \text{ cc } O_2}{100 \text{ cc blood}}\right) - \left(\dfrac{14 \text{ cc } O_2}{100 \text{ cc blood}}\right)}$$

$$= \frac{240 \text{ cc/min}}{\left(\dfrac{6 \text{ cc } O_2}{100 \text{ cc blood}}\right)}$$

$$= 4{,}000 \text{ cc/min, or } 4.0 \text{ liters/min.}$$

STEP 6: Calculate the $\dot{V}_A/\dot{Q}_C$ ratio.

$$\frac{\dot{V}_A}{\dot{Q}_C} = \frac{4{,}200 \text{ cc/min}}{4{,}000 \text{ cc/min}}$$

$$= 1.05$$

(1:308), (3:315–316), (4:236)

31. D. The Fick equation is as follows:

$$\dot{Q}_T = \frac{\dot{V}_{O_2}}{Ca_{O_2} - C\bar{v}_{O_2}}$$

where

$$\dot{Q}_T = \text{cardiac output}$$
$$\dot{V}_{O_2} = \text{oxygen consumption}$$
$$Ca_{O_2} = \text{arterial oxygen content}$$
$$C\bar{v}_{O_2} = \text{venous oxygen content}$$

In the equation, if the $\dot{V}_{O_2}$ is constant, $\dot{Q}_T$ and $Ca_{O_2} - C\bar{v}_{O_2}$ (arterial − venous oxygen content difference) are inversely related. Therefore, if the $\dot{Q}_T$ increases, the $Ca_{O_2} - C\bar{v}_{O_2}$ (a-v difference) decreases. The converse is also true.
(2:10–11,41), (3:315–316), (4:236), (9:128), (14:39,164), (17:185)

32. C. The normal anatomic shunt (2.5%) results from (1) a small portion of bronchial venous blood draining into the pulmonary veins, (2) a small amount of coronary venous blood depositing directly into the right atrium via the Thebesian veins, and (3) a small amount of blood from the pleural veins entering the arterial blood. Therefore, the bronchial, Thebesian, and pleurel veins account for the normal anatomic shunt.
(1:204), (3:60), (4:214), (6:265), (8:322,324)

33. C. STEP 1: Determine the degree of unsaturation in both the arterial and venous blood.

a) arterial unsaturation

$$\begin{array}{r} 100\% \text{ total saturation} \\ - \ 84\% \ Sa_{O_2} \\ \hline 16\% \text{ Hb unsaturated} \end{array}$$

b) venous unsaturation

$$100\% \text{ total saturation}$$
$$\underline{-\ 70\% \text{ S}\bar{v}_{O_2}}$$
$$30\% \text{ Hb unsaturated}$$

STEP 2: Determine the amount of Hb unsaturated in both arterial and venous blood.

   a) hemoglobin unsaturated in arterial blood

$$19 \text{ g}\% \text{ Hb} \times 0.16 = 3.04 \text{ g}\% \text{ of Hb unsaturated}$$

   b) hemoglobin unsaturated in venous blood

$$19 \text{ g}\% \text{ Hb} \times 0.30 = 5.70 \text{ g}\% \text{ of Hb unsaturated}$$

STEP 3: Calculate the amount of Hb unsaturated in total circulation.

$$\frac{3.04 \text{ g}\% + 5.70 \text{ g}\%}{2} = 4.37 \text{ g}\%$$

Note: Cyanosis is exhibited when there is 5.00 g% or more of unsaturated Hb in total circulation.

(1:281–282), (8:184)

34. C. The normal distribution of pulmonary blood flow from base to apex changes when the pulmonary artery pressure (PAP) decreases. When a decrease in PAP occurs, less than normal blood flow reaches the apices. The slope of the graph becomes steeper when compared with a normal PAP. Pulmonary venous pressure was kept low in both instances (Figures 28 and 29).

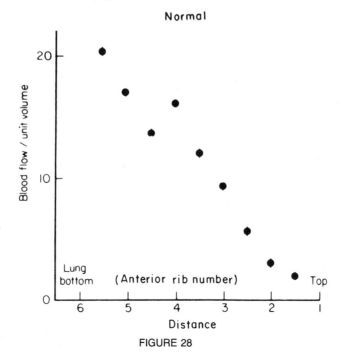

FIGURE 28

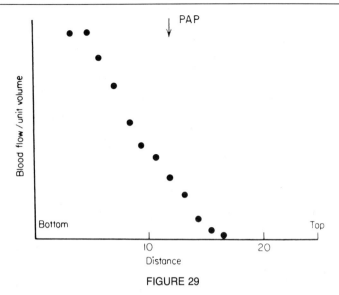

FIGURE 29

When pulmonary venous pressure (PVP) is increased (Figure 30), pulmonary blood distribution becomes more uniform in the bases and middle zone. Also, more blood flow will enter the apices.

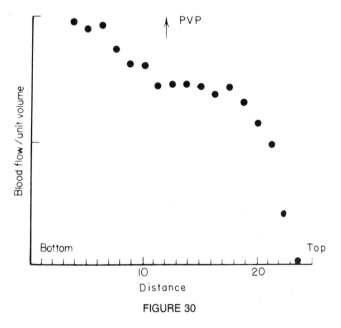

FIGURE 30

The foregoing information refers to normal subjects standing upright. (3:54–56), (8:62–68), (12:145–146), (14:40–43), (28:18–22).

35. E. Sinus bradycardia (Figure 31) has the following ECG characteristics:

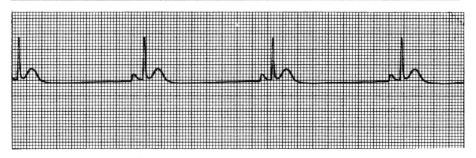

FIGURE 31

1. regular rhythm (distance between QRS complexes is equal)
2. normal QRS complex
3. rate is less than 60 beats per minute
4. P waves precede each QRS complex
5. normal and constant PR interval

Sinus bradycardia is a common finding in the early period of an acute myocardial infarction (AMI), especially on the inferior surface of the myocardium. An AMI may decrease the cardiac output, and lead to congestive heart failure.

(30:368)

36. D. The equation

$$V_D/V_T = \frac{Pa_{CO_2} - P\overline{E}_{CO_2}}{Pa_{CO_2}}$$

where

V_D = dead space ventilation (cc)
V_T = tidal volume (cc)
Pa_{CO_2} = arterial carbon dioxide tension (mm Hg); end-tidal CO_2 tension can be used also
$P\overline{E}_{CO_2}$ = mean exhaled carbon dioxide tension (mm Hg)

allows for the calculation of the dead space to tidal volume ratio. The end-tidal carbon dioxide tension can substitute for the Pa_{CO_2} because the end-tidal P_{CO_2} is from the alveolar air and actually is the PA_{CO_2}. The Pa_{CO_2} and PA_{CO_2} are considered to be in equilibrium.

end-tidal P_{CO_2} = 44 mm Hg
mean exhaled P_{CO_2} = 35 mm Hg

$$\frac{44 \text{ mm Hg} - 33 \text{ mm Hg}}{44 \text{ mm Hg}} = 0.25$$

or $100 \times 0.25 = 25\%$

(2:9–10), (4:225 × 226), (6:242–243), (14:19,163), (27:73,234–235)

37. E. The tricuspid valve between the right atrium and right ventricle opens during atrial contraction and closes during ventricular contraction.

(3:284–285), (4:108,112–113)

38. A. The bronchial artery, which branches off the thoracic aorta, supplies arterial blood to the entire tracheobronchial tree down to, but not including, the respiratory bronchioles. The respiratory bronchioles, alveolar ducts, and alveolar sacs (alveoli) receive their blood supply from the pulmonary arterial circulation.

(1:104–106), (12:3), (24:9–10)

39. C. Because the rib cage has a natural tendency to expand (bow out), and the lungs are inclined to collapse, a subatmospheric (negative pressure) environment is normally maintained in the intrapleural (intrathoracic) space throughout quiet breathing (inhalation and exhalation). Normally, the only time the intrapleural pressure rises above atmospheric pressure is during a rapid or forceful exhalation.

(1:129–132), (3:31–34), (4:72–76), (8:14–18), (12:99–102), (24:97–98)

40. D. The sinoatrial (SA) node is located in the right posterior atrial wall, immediately below the opening of the superior vena cava. This specialized group of nervous tissue is called the heart's pacemaker. It emits electric impulses that radiate across the heart structure 60 to 100 times/min.

(1:244), (4:256,258)

41. A. The ethmoid bone (lightest of the cranial bones) forms part of the cranial floor and the upper portion of the nasal cavity. The superior and middle turbinates (conchae) are processes fo the ethmoid bone. The inferior turbinates are separate bones.

(21:223–227)

42. D. The following steps are used to calculate the percent shunt:

STEP 1: Use the alveolar air equation.*

$$P_{AO_2} = F_{IO_2}(P_B - P_{H_2O}) - P_{ACO_2}\left(F_{IO_2} + \frac{1 - F_{IO_2}}{R}\right)$$

$$= 1.0(760 \text{ torr} - 47 \text{ torr}) - 38 \text{ torr}\left(1.0 + \frac{1 - 1.0}{0.8}\right)$$

$$= 675 \text{ torr}$$

STEP 2: Calculate the amount of O_2 combined to hemoglobin (arterial).

$$C_{aO_2} = S_{aO_2} \times [Hb] \times 1.34 \text{ ml } O_2/\text{g Hb}$$

$$- 1.0 \times 14 \text{ g\% Hb} \times 1.34 \text{ ml } O_2/\text{g Hb}$$

$$= 18.76 \text{ vol\%}$$

*In the alveolar air equation the P_{aCO_2} can substitute for the P_{ACO_2} because equilibration across the alveolar-capillary membrane is assumed.

STEP 3: Convert the Pa_{O_2} to its equivalent in vol%.

$$\text{arterial dissolved vol\%} = Pa_{O_2} \times 0.003 \text{ vol\%/torr}$$
$$= 287 \text{ torr} \times 0.003 \text{ vol\%/torr}$$
$$= 0.86 \text{ vol\%}$$

STEP 4: Calculate the amount of O_2 combined to hemoglobin (venous).

$$C\bar{v}_{O_2} = S\bar{v}_{O_2} \times [\text{Hb}] \times 1.34 \text{ ml } O_2/\text{g Hb}$$
$$= 0.70 \times 14 \text{ g\% Hb} \times 1.34 \text{ ml } O_2/\text{g Hb}$$
$$= 13.13 \text{ vol\%}$$

STEP 5: Convert the $P\bar{v}_{O_2}$ to its equivalent in vol%.

$$\text{venous dissolved vol\%} = P\bar{v}_{O_2} \times 0.003 \text{ vol\%/torr}$$
$$= 46 \text{ torr} \times 0.003 \text{ vol\%/torr}$$
$$= 0.14 \text{ vol\%}$$

STEP 6: Calculate the arterial oxygen content.

$$\text{arterial } O_2 \text{ content} = \text{combined } O_2 + \text{dissolved } O_2$$
$$= 18.76 \text{ vol\%} + 0.86 \text{ vol\%}$$
$$= 19.62 \text{ vol\%}$$

STEP 7: Calculate the venous oxygen content.

$$\text{venous } O_2 \text{ content} = \text{combined } O_2 + \text{dissolved } O_2$$
$$= 13.13 \text{ vol\%} + 0.14 \text{ vol\%}$$
$$= 13.27 \text{ vol\%}$$

STEP 8: Use the clinical shunt equation.

$$\frac{\dot{Q}_S}{\dot{Q}_T} = \frac{(PA_{O_2} - Pa_{O_2})0.003}{(PA_{O_2} - Pa_{O_2})0.003 + (Ca_{O_2} - C\bar{v}_{O_2})} \times 100$$
$$= \frac{(675 \text{ torr} - 287 \text{ torr})0.003}{(675 \text{ torr} - 287 \text{ torr})0.003 + (19.62 \text{ vol\%} - 13.27 \text{ vol\%})} \times 100$$
$$= 15.49\%$$

(2:20–22), (3:318–319,321), (4:217–219), (17:76–77,186), (27:215)

43. A. Pulmonary capillary hydrostatic pressure pushes fluid out of pulmonary circulation. It is in direct opposition to the protein osmotic (oncotic) pressure in the blood. Outside the vasculature, interstitial fluid hydrostatic pressure pushes fluid back into circulation, whereas interstitial fluid osmotic pressure pulls fluid out of circulation. The pulmonary lymphatic vessels transport the fluid, which does not reenter the pulmonary circulation, and deposit this fluid into general circulation at the junction of the left subclavian and internal jugular veins.

(2:182–190), (3:469), (4:157,244–247), (12:147–148), (14:44–46)

44. D. A porphyrin ring is comprised of four pyrrole molecules cyclically held together by four methylene bridges. Figure 32 shows the component structure of the por-

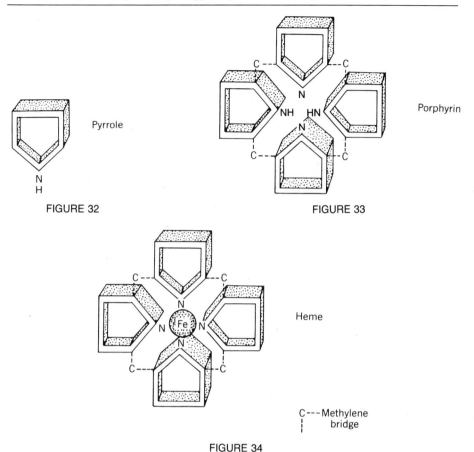

Pyrrole

FIGURE 32

Porphyrin

FIGURE 33

Heme

C --- Methylene
　　　bridge

FIGURE 34

phyrin ring. Figure 33 depicts a porphyrin ring bound together by four methylene bridges. Figure 34 illustrates a heme structure having an iron (Fe^{+2}) center. (2:238–241), (4:183–184), (27:19–21)

45. D. STEP 1: Calculate the minute ventilation ($\dot{V}E$).

$$V_T \times f = \dot{V}_E$$
$$500 \text{ cc} \times 14 \text{ breaths/min} = 7,000 \text{ cc/min}$$
$$= 7.0 \text{ liters/min}$$

STEP 2: Calculate the hourly ventilation.

$$\dot{V}_E \times 60 \text{ min/hr} = \text{liters/hr}$$
$$7.0 \text{ liters/min} \times 60 \text{ min/hr} = 420 \text{ liters/hr}$$

STEP 3: Determine the ventilation over a 2-hour period.

$$\text{hourly ventilation} \times 2 \text{ hr} = \text{ventilation over 2 hr}$$
$$420 \text{ liters/hr} \times 2 \text{ hr} = 840 \text{ liters/2 hr}$$

STEP 4: Determine the absolute humidity (content). The maximum weight of water in air at 37°C (body temperature) is 43.8 g/m³ (43.8 g/1000 liters), or 43.8 mg/liter.

$$\frac{\text{content}}{\text{capacity}} \times 100 = \% \text{ relative humidity}$$

$$\begin{array}{r} 43.8 \text{ g/m}^3 \\ \times\ 10\% \text{ relative humidity} \\ \hline 4.38 \text{ g/m}^3 \text{ absolute humidity} \end{array}$$

STEP 5: Calculate the humidity deficit.

$$\text{capacity} - \text{content} = \text{humidity deficit}$$
$$43.80 \text{ g/1000 liters} - 4.38 \text{ g/1000 liters} = 39.42 \text{ g/1000 liters}$$

STEP 6: Determine the amount of H_2O rendered by the respiratory mucosa per liter of gas.

$$\frac{39.42 \text{ g}}{1000 \text{ liters}} = 0.3942 \text{ g/liter}$$

STEP 7: Calculate the amount of H_2O rendered by the respiratory mucosa in 2 hours.

$$0.3942 \text{ g/liter} \times 840 \text{ liters/2 hr} = 33.11 \text{ g/2 hr}$$

(1:17–18,336–338), (2:14–15), (4:21–22)

46. E. Figure 35 depicts a resting potential.

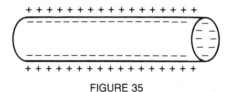

FIGURE 35

During a wave of depolarization (Figure 36) the membrane becomes more permeable to sodium (Na^+) and an influx of positive charges traverse the membrane realigning the order of charges along the surface of the membrane.

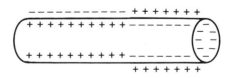

Wave of depolarization

FIGURE 36

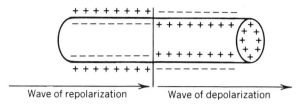

Wave of repolarization   Wave of depolarization

FIGURE 37

Immediately following the wave of depolarization is a wave of repolarization (Figure 37).

(1:247–248), (4:260)

47. A. Extracellular (outside the cell) fluid includes the following fluid compartments

   1. interstitial fluid—the fluid immediately outside the cell
   2. intravascular fluid—the fluid (blood) confined within the vasculature

   Extravascular fluid refers to fluid outside the vasculature and includes interstitial fluid and intracellular fluid.

   (4:241–242)

48. B. Renal compensation is slow in becoming clinically recognizable; however, the kidneys generally completely compensate for primary respiratory problems. In cases of CO_2 retention, the kidneys will respond by retaining more HCO_3^- and by excreting more H^+. It is not uncommon to observe HCO_3^- values in the high 30s in order to return the pH to within its normal range in the face of chronic hypercapnia.

   Similarly, when chronic hyperventilation causes hypocapnia, the renal compensatory mechanism responds by excreting more HCO_3^- and by retaining more H^+, thus bringing the arterial pH to a near-normal value.

   During a primary metabolic alkalosis, the ventilatory rate slows very quickly causing CO_2 retention in an attempt to elevate the blood pH. In this acid-base disorder the Pa_{CO_2} rarely exceeds 50 mm Hg because higher CO_2 levels can induce CO_2 narcosis. Hypoxemia can be a complication of the alveolar hypoventilation.

   (3:101,246), (4:95,204–210), (8:84–92)

49. A. Each of the four factors listed (Pa_{CO_2}, pH, 2,3-DPG, and temperature) influences Hb-O_2 affinity. Those that cause a rightward shift in the Hb-O_2 dissociation curve are: ↑ Pa_{CO_2}; ↓ pH; ↑ 2,3-DPG; ↑ temperature. Those causing a leftward shift in the Hb-O_2 curve are: ↓ Pa_{CO_2}; ↑ pH; ↓ 2,3-DPG; ↓ temperature.

   (1:207–210), (2:243), (3:82–83), (4:187), (8:78–79)

50. E. The proteins within the vasculature that are responsible for the oncotic (colloid osmotic, protein osmotic) pressure are albumin, globulin, and fibrinogen. Albumin, having the highest concentration in plasma, is the greatest contributor toward the oncotic pressure.

   (2:181–182), (4:242)

51. B. Starling's law of the capillaries can be used to describe the filtration of blood in the kidneys at the glomerulus. Fluid (blood) in the glomerular capillary tuft is filtered into Bowman's capsule. However, hydrostatic pressure in the glomerulus overcomes the hydrostatic pressure in Bowman's capsule and the colloid osmotic pressure of the blood itself to filter across the glomerular membrane.

$$\begin{matrix} \text{glomerular filtration} \\ \text{pressure} \end{matrix} = \begin{matrix} \text{glomerular capillary} \\ \text{hydrostatic pressure} \end{matrix} - \left(\begin{matrix} \text{colloid osmotic} \\ \text{pressure} \end{matrix} + \begin{matrix} \text{Bowman's} \\ \text{capsule} \\ \text{hydrostate} \\ \text{pressure} \end{matrix} \right)$$

$$= 65 \text{ torr} - (33 \text{ torr} + 17 \text{ torr})$$
$$= 15 \text{ torr}$$

(2:177–190), (4:157)

52. D. Both pulmonary perfusion and ventilation are influenced by gravity. In a normal, erect person the perfusion in the lung bases exceeds the ventilation in that area. In the apices, however, ventilation exceeds perfusion.
(3:54–56), (4:83–85), (6:227–228), (8:48–68), (12:142,171,177–178)

53. C. Any situation that causes a reduced blood supply to the aortic and carotid bodies (peripheral chemoreceptors) results in an increase in ventilation. For example, ascending to a higher altitude (hypoxic hypoxia), and cyanide poisoning (histotoxic hypoxia).

Certain conditions that do not reduce the Pa_{O_2} will not stimulate the peripheral chemoreceptors to emit hyperventilatory signals to the medulla. These include methemoglobinemia (Fe^{+3} instead of Fe^{+2} in the center of the heme structure), and CO poisoning (CO binds 210 times stronger to Hb than does O_2).

In cyanide poisoning oxygen transport in the blood can be normal (Pa_{O_2} 100 mm Hg and Sa_{O_2} 97.5%). However, the tissues, including the peripheral chemoreceptors, are unable to use the oxygen because of the presence of hydrocyanic acid in the cells. Therefore, regardless of a normal Pa_{O_2}, the peripheral chemoreceptors would send hyperventilatory signals to the medulla.

In the case of ascending to a higher altitude, fewer oxygen molecules diffuse across the alveolar–capillary membrane. Hence, the Pa_{O_2} decreases and the peripheral chemoreceptors are stimulated.
(1:208,224,232), (3:29–30,535), (4:91,140,303,332–333,370–371), (6:216,229, 262–263,044), (8:97,80,365)

54. B. The systolic pressure ranges of the right and left ventricles of the heart are approximately 15 to 25 torr and 90 to 140 torr, respectively.
(1:261–263), (4:125), (6:227), (9:283)

55. E. Colloids are solutes having a diameter in the range of 1 μ to 100 μ. They also have a large molecular weight. Crystalloids (true solutes) have a diameter less than 1 μ.

The protein molecules (albumin, globulin, fibrinogen) are classified as collids. Electrolytes (K^+, Cl^-, Na^+, etc.) are classified as crystalloids.
(2:181), (4:244), (6:880–881)

56. D. The intracellular fluid compartment comprises approximately 60% of the total body fluids. Intracellular fluid has the following components

CONSTITUENTS	m Osmol/L of H_2O
sodium (Na^+)	10
potassium (K^+)	141
calcium (Ca^{+2})	0
magnesium (Mg^{+2})	31
chlorine (Cl^-)	4
bicarbonate (HCO_3^-)	10
monophosphate (HPO_4^-)	11
diphosphate ($H_2PO_4^{-2}$)	11
sulfate (SO_4^{-2})	1
protein	4

(4:243), (31:827)

57. B. Generations 1 to 9 are composed of pseudostratified ciliated *columnar* epithelium, whereas generations 10 to 15 have ciliated *cuboidal* epithelium. Cartilage is absent beginning around generation 10. Goblet cells and submucosal glands begin to diminish at this point also.
(4:54–57), (6:222)

58. B. Carbaminohemoglobin is formed by the combination of carbon dioxide and hemoglobin. More specifically, the reaction can be shown as

$$Hb \cdot NH_2 + CO_2 \rightleftharpoons Hb \cdot NH \cdot COOH$$

Carboxyhemoglobin results from the reaction between carbon monoxide and hemoglobin.
(1:213), (2:244), (4:188,190,332), (8:82–83)

59. C. Once gas molecules reach the alveolar level, they are no longer under the influence of the pressure gradient originally responsible for gas flow in that direction. The law of continuity is effective in reducing gas velocity through the branchings at each airway generation. When the inspired gas reaches the alveoli, it moves via its own kinetic energy ($\frac{1}{2} Dv^2$), that is, rapid, random movement (Brownian motion).

The movement of gases *inside* (*within*) the alveoli is explained by the following relationship described by Graham's law of diffusion of a gas within a gas:

$$\frac{r_{O_2}}{r_{CO_2}} = \frac{\sqrt{CO_2 \text{ molecular weight}}}{\sqrt{O_2 \text{ molecular weight}}} = \frac{\sqrt{44}}{\sqrt{32}} = \frac{6.66}{5.66} = 1.17$$

O_2 is a lighter molecule; consequently, it will move faster within the gaseous medium inside the alveoli.

The movement of gases *across* the alveolar-capillary membrane is described by the following relationship, stated again by Graham, explaining the diffusion of gases in a liquid medium:

$$\frac{r_{CO_2}}{r_{O_2}} = \frac{(CO_2 \text{ solubility coefficient})(\sqrt{O_2 \text{ molecular weight}})}{(O_2 \text{ solubility coefficient})(\sqrt{CO_2 \text{ molecular weight}})}$$

$$= \frac{(0.510)(5.66)}{(0.023)(6.66)}$$

$$= \frac{19}{1}$$

CO_2 is much more soluble across lipid membranes than O_2; hence CO_2 is faster than O_2 moving across the alveolar-capillary membrane.

The P_{O_2} change from 149 torr in the trachea to 100 torr in the alveoli is caused by the mixing with alveolar air and the oxygen uptake by the pulmonary circulation. (1:196–198), (2:67–69,127–132,136), (4:25–26), (27:8–9), (29:21,26–27), (32:120–121)

60. E. The following anatomic structures compose an acinus: respiratory bronchioles, alveolar ducts, alveolar sacs, and alveoli. (6:223), (29:38–39), (32:10)

61. A. Extracellular fluid hydrogen ion concentration is related to both ventilatory (volatile acid) and renal (nonvolatile acids) function. Extracellular fluid hydrogen ion concentration is influenced by the amount of dissolved carbon dioxide in the arterial blood (Pa_{CO_2}), and by either reabsorption or excretion of HCO_3^- ions. Hydrogen ion secretion is directly related to the Pa_{CO_2}. For each H^+ ion secreted, one HCO_3^- ion is reabsorbed.

The secretion of H^+ ions is optimum up to a urine pH of 4.50. When arterial pH is 7.40, urine pH is about 6.10. (4:161–162), (17:96), (31:882–885)

62. C. The Valsalva maneuver performed during defecation and childbirth consists of forcing intrapulmonic air against a closed glottis along with diaphragmatic elevation and abdominal muscle contraction. Both intrathoracic and intraabdominal pressures markedly increase. Venous return is reduced; however, left ventricular output is generally not reduced because an adequate volume of blood resides in the pulmonary vasculature.

The Valsalva maneuver is voluntary and is sustained briefly for a few seconds at a time. (4:47), (6:220)

63. A. Physiologic dead space includes all the anatomic and alveolar dead space. Therefore, deducting the alveolar dead space from the physiologic dead space leaves the anatomic dead space. (1:116–118), (2:9–10,151), (3:59–60), (4:224–225), (6:242), (8:48–50)

64. C. The term *reduced hemoglobin* is a misnomer. The binding of oxygen to hemoglobin does not involve oxidation (loss of electrons). Consequently, the release of oxygen by hemoglobin to the tissues does not involve reduction (gain of electrons). A more appropriate term is either *unsaturated* or *deoxygenated*

hemoglobin. The term *reduced Hb* will remain in use, but one should be aware of the actual meaning of the expression.

Unsaturated Hb is a more effective buffer than saturated Hb. At the tissue level, $KHbO_2$ (saturated Hb) releases oxygen, which enters the tissues. Unsaturated Hb combines with CO_2 (attaches to globin). At the same time, the following reaction:

$$CO_2 + H_2O \xrightarrow{\text{C.A.}^*} H_2CO_3 \longrightarrow H^+ + HCO_3^-$$

within the RBC elevates the H^+. The unsaturated Hb, having a higher H^+ binding capacity than $KHbO_2$, effectively buffers the H^+ ions. The reaction in the RBC at the tissues is

$$K^+ + HbO_2^- + H^+ + HCO_3^- \longrightarrow K^+ + HCO_3^- + HHb + O_2$$

Each one of the four heme groups on the Hb molecule can bind one oxygen molecule, that is, a total of four oxygen molecules per Hb molecule.

(1:203), (2:238–246), (4:183–185), (12:183–195), (29:125–127), (32:148)

65. E. The left coronary artery branches into the anterior descending artery and the circumflex artery. The anterior descending artery provides blood flow to both ventricles. The circumflex artery supplies the left atrium and left ventricle.

The right coronary artery branches into the posterior descending artery and the marginal artery. The posterior descending artery serves both ventricles, and the marginal artery provides blood supply to the right atrium and right ventricle.

(31:596–597)

66. A. The juxtaglomerular apparatus illustrated in Figure 38 is located in the kidney and is formed by the direct physical contact between the distal convoluted tubule and the afferent arteriole within each nephron.

When renal perfusion pressure decreases, the juxtaglomerular apparatus secretes renin, which, in turn, begins a series of biochemical reactions ultimately producing the potent vasoconstrictor, angiotensin II. The alpha-adrenergic activity of angiotensin II tends to restore renal perfusion pressure.

Additionally, angiotensin II stimulates the adrenal glands to secrete aldosterone which causes the reabsorption of sodium and water. The consequence of this activity is to expand the fluid volume to similarly restore perfusion pressure.

(4:161), (31:830)

67. B. Alveolar dead space represents alveoli that are ventilated but not perfused. The structures do not participate in gas exchange. The gas composition of such alveolar units should closely approximate that of tracheal air.

The predominant source of alveolar CO_2 is the person's metabolic functions (atmospheric CO_2 is 0.04% of 760 torr, or 0.3 torr). If blood flow to certain alveolar units is prevented, P_{ACO_2} levels will decrease in those regions.

(1:306), (12:13,178–180), (14:2,16–19, 41)

**CA: Carbonic anhydrase is an enzyme catalyst for the CO_2 hydration reaction.

Proximal convoluted tubule

Afferent arteriole

Capillary loop

Juxtaglomerular apparatus

Distal convoluted tubule

Macula densa

Bowman's capsule

Efferent arteriole

Mesangium cell

Bowman's space

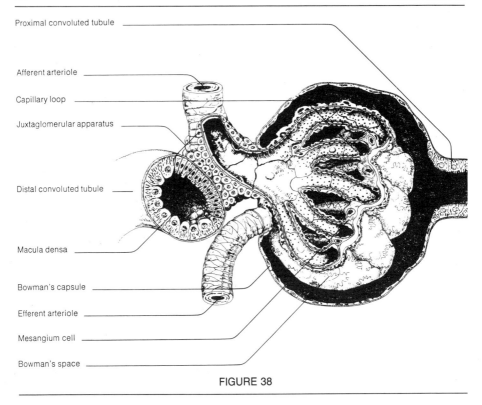

FIGURE 38

68. B. There are 7 cervical, 12 thoracic, and 5 lumbar vertebrae. The adult sacrum is formed by the unification of 5 sacral vertebrae, and the adult coccyx results from the merging of 4 coccygeal vertebrae.
(21:223)

69. D. Pulmonary surfactant reduces the surface tension of the fluid that lines the alveolar epithelium. This substance, a phospholipid, is produced by type II alveolar cells.

As the alveoli expand during inspiration, their surface area increases. As inspiration proceeds, the pulmonary surfactant is spread thin throughout each gas exchange unit. Therefore, as alveolar radius increases, surface tension increases. Conversely, as alveolar radius decreases, surface tension forces decrease because the same amount of pulmonary surfactant is confined to a smaller space.

Consequently, the direct relationship between alveolar radius and surface tension forces in the presence of pulmonary surfactant prevents alveolar collapse during exhalation and limits lung expansion during inhalation.
(1:134–140), (2:232–234), (3:18,20), (4:29), (6:224,226), (8:19–21), (12:110–114), (13:94), (14:46,90–95)

70. C. The transpulmonary pressure gradient (intra-alveolar pressure minus intrapleural pressure) varies across the tracheobronchial tree. At FRC, that gradient is greater in the apices than it is in the bases. Therefore, at FRC, the apical alveoli are more

distended than the basal alveoli. This is one of the reasons why gas on inspiration goes preferentially to the basal segments, and why over the course of time, the bases experience a greater minute ventilation ($\dot{V}E$) than the apices.

Because elastance (E) is the reciprocal of compliance (C),

$$C = \frac{\Delta V}{\Delta P} = \frac{\text{liter}}{\text{cm H}_2\text{O}}$$

$$E = \frac{\Delta P}{\Delta V} = \frac{\text{cm H}_2\text{O}}{\text{liter}}$$

$$C = \frac{1}{E} \quad \text{and} \quad E = \frac{1}{C}$$

The pulmonary elastance is greater in the apices than in the bases of an upright, normal lung.

(2:169–172), (3:34,46,56,335), (4:27–28,72–73), (6:247–248), (12:127)

71. C. Assuming that the pulmonary artery enters the lung midway between the apex and base (Figure 39), the blood would have to move against gravity a distance of 15 cm. A vertical distance of 15 cm is equivalent to a pressure of 15 cm H_2O. 15 cm H_2O can be converted to mm Hg as follows:

$$\frac{1 \text{ atm in cm H}_2\text{O}}{1 \text{ atm in mm Hg}} = \frac{1{,}034 \text{ cm H}_2\text{O}}{760 \text{ mm Hg}} = 1.36 \text{ cm H}_2\text{O/mm Hg}$$

$$\frac{15 \text{ cm } H_2O}{1.36 \text{ cm } H_2O/\text{mm Hg}} = 11 \text{ mm Hg}$$

The vertical distance of 15 cm on the pressure 15 cm H_2O is equal to 11 mm Hg. This indicates that gravity is exerting a pressure of 11 mm Hg against apical perfusion. Therefore, to achieve a flow of blood in the apices, a pressure greater than 11 mm Hg would be required. From the choices listed in the question the *minimum* pressure that will produce a flow is 12 mm Hg. Therefore, a diastolic pres-

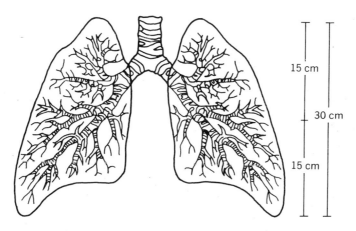

15 cm

30 cm

15 cm

FIGURE 39

sure of 12 mm Hg would provide blood flow to the apices during that portion of the cardiac cycle.

(3:54–56), (4:83–85), (28:15)

72. D. $\dot{V}_A$ = alveolar minute ventilation
                                 $\dot{Q}_C$ = pulmonary capillary minute perfusion

$$\frac{\dot{V}_A}{\dot{Q}_C} \quad \frac{\text{alveolar minute ventilation}}{\text{pulmonary capillary minute perfusion}}$$

STEP 1: Calculate the cardiac output ($\dot{Q}_T$) according to the following formula:

$$\text{heart rate} \times \text{stroke volume} = \dot{Q}_T$$
$$100 \text{ beats/min.} \times 0.05 \text{ liter} = 5 \text{ liters/min}$$

It is assumed here that normal physiology prevails. Therefore, right ventricular output will equal left ventricular output. Because the right ventricle's output enters the pulmonary vasculature, $\dot{Q}_C$ will also be 5.0 liters/min.

STEP 2: Set up a proportion.

$$\frac{0.6}{1} = \frac{\dot{V}_A}{\dot{Q}_C}$$
$$\frac{0.6}{1} = \frac{x}{5}$$
$$\frac{(0.6)(5)}{1} = 3 \text{ liters/min.}$$

(4:192–193), (29:109–120), (32:104)

73. C. Swan-Ganz catheter insertion does not require fluoroscopy because the catheter has flow-directed capabilities (balloon tip), and because each catheter position displays a characteristic waveform as shown in Figure 40.

                  RA = right atrium pressure
                  RV = right ventricle pressure
                  PA = pulmonary artery pressure
              PCW = pulmonary capillary wedge pressure

(9:76–77,98)

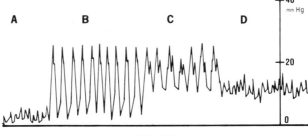

FIGURE 40

74. E. Low $\dot{V}A/\dot{Q}C$ units alter arterial blood gas values more than high $\dot{V}A/\dot{Q}C$ units because more blood volume is involved in conjuction with low $\dot{V}A/\dot{Q}C$ units, as perfusion exceeds ventilation. Low $\dot{V}A/\dot{Q}C$ units that are correctable by oxygen therapy are termed shunt effect because on room air they do not completely arterialize the venous blood flowing past them. Hypoxemia and normocapnia can co-exist in the presence of low $\dot{V}A/\dot{Q}C$ units if enough high $\dot{V}A/\dot{Q}C$ units compensate. In such cases high $\dot{V}A/\dot{Q}C$ units can compensate for the increased CO_2 but cannot correct for the hypoxemia.

(1:298–302), (8:66–71), (12:173–179), (29:109–120)

75. D. The amount of carbon dioxide physically dissolved in the arterial blood (Pa_{CO_2}) is ordinarily expressed as mm Hg or torr. However, mm Hg and torr can be converted to vol% in a two-step fashion.

STEP 1: Change the normal Pa_{CO_2} of 40 mm Hg to mEq/liter (mmol/liter).

$$40 \text{ mm Hg} \times 0.03 \text{ mEq/liter/mm Hg} = 1.20 \text{ mEq/liter}$$

STEP 2: Convert 1.20 mEq of CO_2/liter to vol%.

$$1.20 \text{ mEq/liter} \times 2.23 \text{ vol\%/mEq/liter} = 2.68 \text{ vol\%}$$

(1:216,219–220), (2:64–67), (4:191–192)

76. B. The O_2 content represents only the amount of oxygen combined with hemoglobin. Total arterial O_2 content refers to the sum of the combined oxygen and the dissolved oxygen.

STEP 1: Calculate the O_2 content leaving the unobstructed alveolus.

$$0.97 \times 15 \text{ g\% Hb} \times 1.34 \text{ ml } O_2/\text{g Hb} = 19.50 \text{ vol\%}$$

STEP 2: Calculate the O_2 content leaving the partially obstructed alveolus.

$$0.70 \times 15 \text{ g\% Hb} \times 1.34 \text{ ml } O_2/\text{g Hb} = 14.07 \text{ vol\%}$$

STEP 3: Determine the overall (average) O_2 content in the pulmonary venule leading away from these two alveoli.

$$\begin{array}{r} 19.50 \text{ vol\%} \\ + \ 14.07 \text{ vol\%} \\ \hline 33.57 \text{ vol\%} \end{array}$$

$$\frac{33.57 \text{ vol\%}}{2} = 16.79 \text{ vol\%}$$

(1:203–206), (2:17–18), (3:193), (4:185)

77. D. STEP 1: Determine the PA_{O_2} using the alveoler air equation.

$$PA_{O_2} = (PB - P_{H_2O})FI_{O_2} - PA_{CO_2}\left(FI_{O_2} + \frac{1 - FI_{O_2}}{R}\right)^*$$

*The Pa_{CO_2} may substitute for the PA_{CO_2} because compelete equilibration across the alveolar capillary membrane is assumed.

$$= (760 \text{ mm Hg} - 47 \text{ mm Hg})1.0 - 45 \text{ mm Hg}\left(1 + \frac{1-1}{0.8}\right)^*$$
$$= 713 \text{ mm Hg} - 45 \text{ mm Hg}$$
$$= 664 \text{ mm Hg}$$

STEP 2: Calculate the $P(A\text{-}a)O_2$,

$$P(A\text{-}a)O_2 = 664 \text{ mm Hg} - 325 \text{ mm Hg}$$
$$= 339 \text{ mm Hg}$$

(1:198–201,303,717), (2:19,22), (17:182), (27:210), (30:224), (32:72)

78. A. The phrenic nerve, which originates at C-3, C-4, and C-5, is one of the major branches of the cervical plexus. The phrenic nerve innervates the musculature of the diaphragm.
   (1:121), (3:27), (4:68), (6:220), (8:10), (29:67), (32:17,169)

79. C. The formula for determining the mean arterial pressure (MAP) is shown below.

$$MAP = \frac{\text{systolic pressure} + 2 \text{ (diastolic pressure)}}{3}$$
$$= \frac{110 \text{ torr} + 2 \text{ (80 torr)}}{3}$$
$$= \frac{270 \text{ torr}}{3}$$
$$= 90 \text{ torr}$$

(4:231), (9:102)

80. D. The Bohr equation shown below can be used to determine the mean exhaled carbon dioxide tension ($P\overline{E}_{CO_2}$).

$$\frac{V_D}{V_T} = \frac{Pa_{CO_2} - P\overline{E}_{CO_2}}{Pa_{CO_2}}$$

STEP 1: The dead space volume (V_D) can be estimated according to the guideline that 1 cc of ideal body weight approximates the V_D. For example, a person with an ideal body weight of 200 1b has a V_D of approximately 200 cc.

STEP 2: Insert the known values and calculate the $P\overline{E}_{CO_2}$.

$$\frac{200 \text{ cc}}{650 \text{ cc}} = \frac{45 \text{ torr} - P\overline{E}_{CO_2}}{45 \text{ torr}}$$
$$0.31 \text{ (45 torr)} = 45 \text{ torr} - P\overline{E}_{CO_2}$$
$$P\overline{E}_{CO_2} = 45 \text{ torr} - 13.95 \text{ torr}$$
$$P\overline{E}_{CO_2} = 31 \text{ torr}$$

(1:119–120), (2:9–10), (4:226–227,464), (8:49), (27:73,234–235), (29:60,244)

---

*Whenever the F_{IO_2} is 1.0, the factor $[F_{IO_2} + (1 - F_{IO_2})/R]$ will be unity.

81. **E.** The graph plots the $CO_2\%$ on the x axis and the minute volume on the y axis. According to the data plotted, minute volume increases slightly from a $CO_2\%$ of 1% to 4%. (F_{ICO_2} of 0.01 to 0.04). However, from a $CO_2\%$ of 4% to 10% (F_{ICO_2} of 0.04 to 0.10) the minute volume shows essentially a linear increase. At about 10% CO_2 (F_{ICO_2} 0.10) the minute ventilation begins to fall. This point represents the onset of CO_2 narcosis.
    (12:55–56), (29:169)

82. **A.** To compensate for an increased $\dot{V}D$, one would need to increase his tidal volume (VT) and/or ventilatory rate (f) to maintain an adequate $\dot{V}A$. By increasing either or both the VT or f, the $\dot{V}E$ would increase.

    $$VT(f) = \dot{V}E$$
    $$\dot{V}A + \dot{V}D = \dot{V}E$$

    where

    $$\dot{V}A = \text{alveolar minute ventilation } [VA(f)]$$
    $$\dot{V}D = \text{dead space minute ventilation } [VD(f)]$$
    $$\dot{V}E = \text{minute ventilation } [VT(f)]$$

    (1:118–119), (2:151), (4:225), (8:101–102), (29:63)

83. **E.** Both a decreased cardiac output (stroke volume × heart rate) and an increased oxygen consumption ($\dot{V}_{O_2}$) tend to make a shunt worse. A decreased cardiac output ($\dot{Q}T$) impacts adversely on a shunt because less blood per unit time is sent to the lungs for oxygenation and less blood per unit time is also pumped out to the tissues. If the tissues become more metabolically active, thus increasing their oxygen demands, any degree of shunt present becomes intensified. The Fick equation can be used for showing this relationship.

    $$\dot{Q}T = \frac{\dot{V}_{O_2}}{Ca_{O_2} - C\bar{v}_{O_2}}$$

    where

    $$\dot{Q}T = \text{cardiac ouput (liters/min)}$$
    $$\dot{V}_{O_2} = \text{oxygen consumption (liters/min)}$$
    $$Ca_{O_2} = \text{arterial oxygen content (vol\%)}$$
    $$C\bar{v}_{O_2} = \text{venous oxygen content (vol\%)}$$

    The $Ca_{O_2} - C\bar{v}_{O_2}$ is the arterial-venous oxygen content difference.
    (3:313–317,322–324), (4:217,236–237), (27:211–213,215–219), (29:99–101, 125)

84. **B.** The IX cranial nerve, i.e., the glossopharyngeal nerve, innervates the carotid bodies. The X cranial nerve (vagus nerve) innervates the aortic bodies.
    (4:90), (8:97)

85. **D.** The diagram depicts the characteristic waveforms that should be observed during the insertion of a Swan-Ganz catheter in a person.

waveform A = right atrium pressure
waveform B = right ventricle pressure
waveform C = pulmonary artery pressure
waveform D = pulmonary capillary wedge pressure

(9:98), (*Pressure Monitoring Instruments for Critical Care*, Spacelabs, Figure 35, page 5-2)

86. C. The saturation of the blood resulting from blood from alveolus I mixing with blood from alveolus II can be determined as follows

$$70.0\% \ S_{O_2} \text{ of blood from alveolus I}$$
$$+ \quad 97.5\% \ S_{O_2} \text{ of blood from alveolus II}$$
$$167.5\%$$

$$\frac{167.5\%}{2} = 83.8\% \ S_{O_2} \text{ of mixture}$$

(1:301), (3:192), (4:376)

87. C. The Pa_{O_2} of blood having an oxygen saturation of 83.7% will be approximately 52 torr. This value can be obtained from the oxyhemoglobin dissociation curve shown in Figure 41.

(1:205–210), (3:168–171), (4:185–186), (8:78–79), (29:125–128)

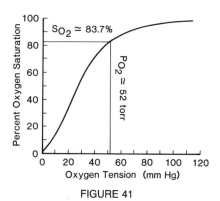

FIGURE 41

88. A. The gases in the obstructed alveolus would eventually equilibrate with the venous blood. Therefore, the $P_{A_{O_2}}$ would ultimately be 40 torr and the $P_{A_{CO_2}}$ would be 46 torr.

(1:306–307), (3:193–196), (14:58), (28:36)

89. D. The diagram depicts the four pressures that determine the magnitude and direction of fluid movement across the systemic capillary endothelium.

On the arterial end of the systemic capillary the following pressures enhance the movement of fluid out of circulation, i.e., filtration:

1. CHP: capillary hydrostatic pressure
2. IHP: interstitial hydrostatic pressure (subatmospheric)*
3. IOP: interstitial osmotic pressure

Quantitatively, this value is

$$\begin{array}{l}
\text{30 mm Hg CHP} \\
\text{3 mm Hg IHP} \\
\underline{\text{4 mm Hg IOP}} \\
\text{37 mm Hg total pressure tending to push fluid out of circulation}
\end{array}$$

The colloid osmotic pressure acts against the factors that favor filtration. Therefore, the net filtration pressure can be determined by subtracting the colloid osmotic pressure from the sum of the pressures that favor filtration.

$$\begin{array}{l}
\text{37 mm Hg (favoring filtration)} \\
\underline{-25 \text{ mm Hg (opposing filtration)}} \\
\text{12 mm Hg net filtration pressure}
\end{array}$$

(2:186–193), (3:469–478), (4:157,244–247), (13:113), (14:45,164), (32:100–101)

90. B. When arterial blood pH is 7.40, urine pH is approximately 6.00. Urine pH generally ranges between 4.50 to 8.00.
    (4:154), (32:163–165)

91. C. Extracellular fluid osmolality is predominately controlled by osmoreceptors in the hypothalamus. When the osmolality increases (excess Na^+), the osmoreceptors increase their rate of impulse discharge and cause more antidiuretic hormone (ADH) to be secreted by the posterior pituitary gland. When extracellular osmolality decreases (decreased Na^+), the osmoreceptors cause less ADH to be secreted.

    Increased ADH increases the permeability to water of both the distal convoluted tubule and collecting duct of the nephron. More water is retained and the osmolality of the extracellular fluid returns to normal. Less ADH in circulation results in more H_2O excretion.

    Because sodium is the most abundant cation in the extracellular fluid compartment, it essentially determines extracellular fluid osmolality.

    Aldosterone is secreted by the adrenal cortex in response to the activity of the juxtaglomerular apparatus. The juxtaglomerular apparatus senses renal perfusion pressure and controls the renin-angiotensin system accordingly.
    (3:160–161), (31:633,830,1003–1008), (32:214)

92. D. The amount of oxygen bound to hemoglobin (content) can be determined according to the following steps:

*The subatmospheric IHP is acting in the same direction as the other filtration pressures (CHP and IOP). Therefore, despite the negative value of the IHP, it is added as a positive number to the CHP and IOP.

STEP 1: Rearrange the formula to solve for content.

$$\frac{content}{capacity} \times 100 = saturation$$

$$content = saturation \times capacity$$

STEP 2: Insert values and calculate content.

$$content = 0.86(1.34 \text{ ml } O_2/g \text{ Hb} \times 13 \text{ g\% Hb})$$
$$= 0.86 \ (17.42 \text{ vol\%})$$
$$= 14.98 \text{ vol\%}$$

(1:203–204), (2:17–18), (3:185), (8:78), (14:70), (32:133–134)

93. C. Diabetic ketoacidosis is associated with an acute rise in nonvolatile acids causing an acute decrease in the arterial blood pH ($\uparrow H^+$). The peripheral chemoreceptors (aortic and carotid bodies) respond immediately to this sudden increase in H^+ by sending hyperventilatory signals to the medulla.

   The ventilatory response then is to increase minute ventilation ($\dot{V}_E$) to blow off the volatile acid, H_2CO_3, in the form of CO_2. This compensatory mechanism falls far short of correcting the metabolic acidosis.

   (1:224–226,234–236), (3:91–92,209), (27:245), (29:140,171), (32:161,183, 185–186)

94. A. A four-lumen Swam-Ganz catheter provides a means for measuring pulmonary artery pressure (PAP), pulmonary capillary wedge pressure (PCWP), central venous pressure (CVP), and cardiac output via thermodilution.

   Both the left ventricular end-diastolic pressure (LVEDP) and the PCWP reflect the severity of left ventricular failure.

   Normal mean PCWP ranges from 6 to 12 mm Hg. When the left ventricle fails as a pump, back pressure will be exerted from the left ventricle into the left atrium. This pressure will be manifested as an elevated PCWP.

   The PCWP is frequently used to monitor left ventricular preload. Left ventricular preload is represented by the LVEDP, which reflects the volume of blood present in the left ventricle immediately before ventricular systole. As the left ventricle fails, the preload increases as reflected by an increased LVEDP. At the end of diastole the mitral valve is still open. At this time, pressure created by the blood volume in the left ventricle equilibrates with that in the left atrium, pulmonary veins, and pulmonary capillaries. It is at this point in the cardiac cycle that the pulmonary artery diastolic pressure correlates well with the LVEDP.

   Pulmonary artery pressure (PAP) during systole reflects right ventricular function; during diastole it assesses pulmonary artery resistance. Essentially, the central venous pressure (CVP) reflects right atrial pressure, which, in turn, is influenced by right ventricular function.

   (1:270–273), (3:301–304), (4:231–235), (6:943–944), (9:66–67,193)

95. E. The central venous pressure (CVP) monitor essentially measures pressure changes in the right ventricle. The pressure changes are also reflected to the right atrium. Additionally, the CVP reflects blood volume and venous return.

   (1:270), (3:301), (4:231), (6:943)

96. E. The Fick equation can be used to calculate the cardiac output ($\dot{Q}_T$). The following steps provide for this calculation.

STEP 1: Determine the arterial O_2 content (Ca_{O_2}).
    a) 95 torr $\times$ 0.003 vol%/torr = 0.29 vol%
    b) 0.94(16g% Hb $\times$ 1.34 ml O_2/g Hb) = 20.15 vol%
    c) 0.29 vol% + 20.15 vol% = 20.44 vol%

STEP 2: Determine the venous O_2 content ($C\bar{v}_{O_2}$).
    a) 40 torr $\times$ 0.003 vol%/torr = 0.12 vol%
    b) 0.70(16g% Hb $\times$ 1.34 ml O_2/g Hb) = 15.01 vol%
    c) 0.12 vol% + 15.01 vol% = 15.13 vol%

STEP 3: Obtain the arterial-venous oxygen content difference ($Ca_{O_2} - C\bar{v}_{O_2}$).

$$\begin{array}{r} 20.44 \text{ vol\% arterial } O_2 \text{ content} \\ -15.13 \text{ vol\% venous } O_2 \text{ content} \\ \hline 5.31 \text{ vol\% a-v difference} \end{array}$$

STEP 4: Use the Fick equation and insert the known values.

$$\dot{Q}_T = \frac{\dot{V}_{O_2}}{Ca_{O_2} - C\bar{v}_{O_2}}$$

$$= \frac{230 \text{ ml/min}}{5.31 \text{ vol\%}}$$

$$= \frac{230 \text{ ml/min}}{\dfrac{5.31 \text{ ml/}O_2}{100 \text{ cc blood}}}$$

$$= 4.33 \text{ liters/min}$$

(3:315–316), (4:236–237), (9:127–128), (14:38), (29:99–100)

97. C. A person having an acute nonrespiratory (metabolic) alkalosis would be expected to have a decreased CSF pH and an increased arterial blood pH. During a metabolic alkalosis the HCO_3^- level increases; the respiratory system compensates via hypoventilation. As the person hypoventilates, the dissolved arterial $CO_2(Pa_{CO_2})$ increases. Because the blood-brain barrier is diffusible to CO_2, the CSF P_{CO_2} also increases. The elevated CSF P_{CO_2} causes the CSF H^+ concentration to also increase, thereby lowering the CSF pH.
(1:224–227,236–237), (4:91,92,94,205), (32:162–163)

98. D. An acute rise in Pa_{CO_2} or drop in pH can result in peripheral chemoreceptor stimulation and hyperventilation. The increased arterial $[H^+]$ during a metabolic acidosis stimulates the peripheral chemoreceptors to send hyperventilatory signals to the medulla.
(1:224–227), (3:29–30), (4:91–92), (14:116–119), (29:169–171), (32:162–163)

99. C. The lungs do not completely empty during exhalation. The gas that previously occupied the alveoli (CO_2-rich and O_2-poor) now occupies the anatomic dead space areas of the lungs. At the same time, CO_2 continues to leave pulmonary circulation and enters the alveoli.

The ensuing inspiration is characterized by an initial (brief) increase in Pa_{CO_2} and decrease in Pa_{O_2} because the previous alveolar gas (CO_2-rich and O_2-poor) enters the alveoli first. As inspiration continues, fresh air (O_2-rich and CO_2-poor) eventually raises the Pa_{O_2} and decreases the Pa_{CO_2}.

(12:12)

100. A. Because of the influence of gravity, the lung bases receive more pulmonary blood flow than ventilation, and the lung apices receive more ventilation than perfusion. As a consequence, the middle areas of the lungs (normal, standing upright subject) receive relatively equal amounts of perfusion and ventilation. (3:55–56), (4:82–85), (8:62–63), (12:177–178), (29:111–112), (32:103)

References

1. Spearman, C., and Sheldon, R., *Egan's Fundamentals of Respiratory Therapy,* 4th ed., C. V. Mosby, St. Louis, 1982.
2. Wojciechowski, W., *Respiratory Care Sciences: An Integrated Approach,* John Wiley & Sons, New York, 1985.
3. Shapiro, B., Harrison, R., Kacmarek, R., and Cane, R., *Clinical Application of Respiratory Care,* 3rd ed., Year Book Medical Publishers, Chicago, 1985.
4. Kacmarek, R., Mack, C., and Dimas, S., *The Essentials of Respiratory Therapy,* 2nd ed., Year Book Medical Publishers, Chicago, 1985.
5. McPherson, S., *Respiratory Therapy Equipment,* 3rd ed., C. V. Mosby, St. Louis, 1985.
6. Burton, G., and Hodgkin, J., *Respiratory Care: A Guide to Clinical Practice,* 2nd ed., J. B. Lippincott, Philadelphia, 1985.
7. Frownfelter, D., *Chest Physical Therapy and Cardiopulmonary Rehabilitation, An Interdisciplinary Approach,* Year Book Medical Publishers, Chicago, 1978.
8. Cherniack, R., and Cherniack, L., *Respiration in Health and Disease,* 3rd ed., W. B. Saunders, Philadelphia, 1983.
9. Daily, E., and Schroeder, G., *Techniques in Bedside Hemodynamic Monitoring,* 3rd ed., C. V. Mosby, St. Louis, 1985.
10. Des Jardins, R., *Clinical Manifestations of Respiratory Disease,* Year Book Medical Publishers, Chicago, 1984.
11. Mitchell, R., *Synopsis of Clinical Pulmonary Disease,* 3rd ed., C. V. Mosby, St. Louis, 1982.
12. Comroe, J., *Physiology of Respiration,* 3rd ed., Year Book Medical Publishers, Chicago, 1974.
13. West, J., *Pulmonary Pathophysiology—The Essentials,* 2nd ed., Williams & Wilkins Baltimore, 1982.
14. West, J., *Respiratory Physiology—The Essentials,* 3rd ed., Williams & Wilkins, Baltimore, 1985.
15. Martz, K., et al., *Management of the Patient-Ventilator System: A Team Approach,* 2nd ed., C. V. Mosby, St. Louis, 1984.
16. Shoup, C., and McHenry, R., *Laboratory Exercises in Respiratory Therapy,* 2nd ed., C. V. Mosby, St. Louis, 1983.
17. Ruppel, G., *Manual of Pulmonary Function Testing,* 3rd ed., C. V. Mosby, St. Louis, 1982.
18. Appelbaum, E., and Bruce, D., *Tracheal Intubation,* W. B. Saunders, Philadelphia, 1976.
19. Rau, J., *Respiratory Therapy Pharmacology,* 2nd ed., Year Book Medical Publishers, Chicago, 1984.

20. United States Department of Health, Education, and Welfare, Public Health Service, *Isolation Techniques for Use in Hospitals,* 2nd ed., Washington, D.C., 1975.
21. Brooks, S., *Integrated Basic Science,* 4th ed., C. V. Mosby, St. Louis 1979.
22. Comroe, J., *The Lung,* Year Book Medical Publishers, Chicago, 1962.
23. Shibel, E., and Moser, K., *Respiratory Emergencies,* 2nd ed., C. V. Mosby, St. Louis, 1982.
24. Tisi, G., *Pulmonary Physiology in Clinical Medicine,* 2nd ed., Williams & Wilkins, Baltimore, 1985.
25. Cherniack, R., *Pulmonary Function Testing,* W. B. Saunders, Philadelphia, 1977.
26. Altose, M., *The Physiological Basis of Pulmonary Function Testing,* Clinical Symposia-CIBA, Vol. 31, No. 2, Summit, New Jersey, 1979.
27. Shapiro, B., Harrison, R., and Walton, J., *Clinical Application of Arterial Blood Gases,* 3rd ed., Year Book Medical Publishers, Chicago, 1982.
28. West, J., *Ventilation/Blood Flow and Gas Exchange,* 3rd ed., Blackwell Scientific Publications, 1979.
29. Slonim, N., and Hamilton, K., *Respiratory Physiology,* 4th ed., C. V. Mosby, St. Louis, 1981.
30. Rarey, K., and Youtsey, J., *Respiratory Patient Care,* Prentice-Hall, Englewood Cliffs, 1981.
31. Berne, R., and Levy, M., *Physiology,* C. V. Mosby, St. Louis, 1983.
32. Levitzky, M., *Pulmonary Physiology,* 2nd ed., McGraw-Hill, New York, 1986.
33. Wilson, P., Bell, C., and Norton, A., *Rehabilitation of the Heart and Lungs,* SensorMedics, 1980.
34. Clausen, J., and Zarins, L., *Pulmonary Function Testing Guidlines and Controversies,* Academic Press, New York, 1982.
35. Klaus, M., and Fanaroff, A., *Care of the High-Risk Neonate,* 2nd ed., W. B. Saunders, Philadelphia, 1979.
36. Lough, M., et al., *Pediatric Respiratory Therapy,* 3rd ed., Year Book Medical Publishers, Chicago, 1985.
37. Levin, D., et al., *A Practical Guide to Pediatric Intensive Care,* 2nd ed., C. V. Mosby, St. Louis, 1984.
38. O'Ryan, J., and Burns, D., *Pulmonary Rehabilitation from Hospital to Home,* Year Book Medical Publishers, Chicago, 1984.
39. Bell, C., et al., *Home Care and Rehabilitation in Respiratory Medicine,* J. B. Lippincott, Philadelphia, 1984.
40. Wilkins, R., et al., *Clinical Assessment in Respiratory Care,* C. V. Mosby, St. Louis, 1985.
41. Jones, N., and Campbell, E., *Clinical Exercise Testing,* 2nd ed., W. B. Saunders, Philadelphia, 1982.
42. Goldsmith, J., and Karotkin, E., *Assisted Ventilation of the Neonate,* W. B. Saunders, Philadelphia, 1981.
43. Blowers, M., and Sims, R., *How to Read an ECG,* 3rd ed., Medical Economics, New Jersey, 1983.
44. Eubanks, D., and Bone, R., *Comprehensive Respiratory Care,* C. V. Mosby, St. Louis, 1985.
45. Rattenborg, C., *Clinical Use of Mechanical Ventilation,* Year Book Medical Publishers, Chicago, 1981.
46. Witkowski, Arthur S., *Pulmonary Assessment: A Clinical Guide,* J. B. Lippincott, Philadelphia, 1985.
47. Op't Holt, Timothy B., *Assessment Based Respiratory Care,* John Wiley & Sons, New York, 1986.

CHEMISTRY ASSESSMENT

PURPOSE: The purpose of this 50-item section is to assess your knowledge and comprehension of a variety of chemistry principles as they relate to the practice of respiratory care and cardiopulmonary physiology. You will be questioned on such concepts as osmosis, diffusion, chemical laws, electrochemistry, and acid-base chemistry. Mathematical problems pertaining to chemical laws, electrochemistry, solution concentrations, temperature conversions, and acid-base chemistry also have been included.

DIRECTIONS: Each of the questions or incomplete statements is followed by five suggested answers. Select the one which is the best in each case and then blacken the corresponding space on the answer sheet.

1. As the pH of a solution _____ , the number of nanomoles of hydrogen ions per liter of solution _____ .

   I. increases; increases
   II. increases; decreases
   III. decreases; decreases
   IV. decreases; increases

   A. I, III only
   B. II, IV only
   C. I only

   D. III only
   E. II only

2. Predict the events that would occur in Figure 42. (Assume the membrane to be permeable to all species present.)

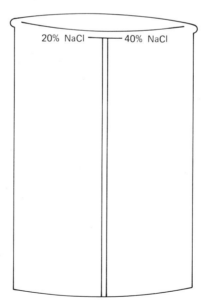

FIGURE 42

I. Na^+ ions, Cl^- ions, and H_2O molecules move in all directions through the solution, collide with each other and with the membrane.

II. Initially, more Na^+ ions and Cl^- ions leave the 20% compartment and enter the 40% compartment.

III. Net diffusion of NaCl occurs from the solution where NaCl concentration is initially greater into the one where its concentration is initially less.

IV. The fluid volume of the 20% NaCl compartment will decrease, whereas that of the 40% NaCl compartment will increase.

V. The movement of NaCl and H_2O occurs simultaneously but in opposite directions.

A. I, II, III, V only
B. I, II, IV, V only
C. II, IV, V only

D. I, III, V only
E. III, IV only

3. Which aqueous solutions would make strong electrolyte solutions?

I. H_2O
II. H_2CO_3
III. HCl
IV. NaOH
V. acetic acid

A. I, II, III, V only
B. III, IV only
C. II, III, IV only

D. IV, V only
E. I, IV, V only

4. Calculate the pH of a blood sample when the combined CO_2 is 21 mmol/liter and the dissolved CO_2 is 25 mm Hg.

A. 6.10
B. 7.37
C. 7.46

D. 7.55
E. 7.59

5. Which statements accurately describe the compound NaCl?

I. The compound forms by having the Na atom transfer two of its electrons to the Cl atom.

II. When NaCl is placed in water, it undergoes ionization.

III. NaCl has a molecular weight of 58.5 amu.

IV. A solution of aqueous NaCl can be classified as an electrolyte solution.

A. I, II, III, IV
B. III, IV only
C. I, II, IV only

D. II, III, IV only
E. I, II, III only

6. A solution having a pH 7.40 is considered to be a(n) _____ solution according to the overall chemical pH scale.

A. alkaline
B. acidic
C. neutral

D. isotonic
E. hypotonic

7. A substance formed from the reaction of elements via the transferring of electrons is termed a(n) _____ .

A. electrovalent compound
B. ionic bond
C. covalent compound

D. covalent-ionic compound
E. valence compound

8. A hypothetical atom having an atomic weight of 20 amu, and having 15 electrons situated around its nucleus will have an atomic number of _____ .

A. 35
B. 20
C. 15

D. 10
E. 5

9. Which of the following materials are the basic constituents of an electrochemical cell?

I. electrolyte solution
II. cathode
III. anode
IV. ammeter

A. I, II, III, IV
B. I, II, III only
C. I, IV only

D. II, III only
E. III, IV only

10. Which formula(s) and/or equation(s) correctly define pH?

I. $-\log_{10}[H^+]$
II. $\text{antilog}^{10}[H^+]$
III. $\log_{10} \dfrac{1}{[H^+]}$
IV. $[H^+][OH^-] = K$

A. I, II, III only
B. II, III, IV only
C. I, III, IV only

D. II, IV only
E. I, III only

11. Separation of a crystalloid from a colloid by means of a semipermeable membrane is called _____ .

A. osmosis
B. dialysis
C. filtration

D. diffusion
E. diapedesis

12. The outermost orbit of any atom has a maximum of _____ electrons.

A. 2   D. 8
B. 4   E. 10
C. 6

13. Which substance is a cation?

A. Al^{+++} D. HCl
B. OH^- E. NH_3
C. H_2O

14. Which factors influence the rate of a chemical reaction?

   I. concentration of products
   II. catalysis
   III. temperature
   IV. concentration of reactants

A. I, II, III, IV   D. I, II, III only
B. I, IV only   E. II, III, IV only
C. II, III only

15. What is the normality of a 2.0 M H_2SO_4 solution?

A. 0.2 N D. 3.0 N
B. 1.0 N E. 4.0 N
C. 2.0 N

16. Which statement is true about the van der Waals forces?

A. They oppose the kinetic action of gas molecules.
B. They tend to cause the heavier molecules to fall out of suspension.
C. They have a tendency to cause the gas molecules to coalesce and form a liquid.
D. They cause gas molecules to repel one another, thus allowing the gas to occupy a large volume.
E. They have no effect on the interaction of molecules.

17. One mole of oxygen at STP would weigh _____ .

A. 6.023×10^{23} g   D. 32 g
B. 8 g   E. 64 g
C. 16 g

18. How many moles of hemoglobin are represented by 133,400 g Hb?

A. 124.00 moles   D. 2.00 moles
B. 22.40 moles   E. 1.34 moles
C. 18.60 moles

19. One mole of carbon dioxide will occupy how many liters at STP?

A. 44.00 liters   D. 1.96 liters

B. 32.00 liters   E. 1.52 liters

C. 22.40 liters

20. What is the Kelvin equivalent of $-8°F$?

A. 226.6°K   D. 295.0°K

B. 240.8°K   E. 319.4°K

C. 251.0°K

21. The tendency of a substance to undergo either reduction or oxidation reactions is indicated by the _____ of that substance.

A. valence   D. atomic weight

B. oxidation potential   E. electromotive force

C. molecular weight

22. How many electrons can maximally reside in principal energy level 2?

A. 2   D. 32

B. 8   E. 50

C. 18

23. Convert a Pa_{O_2} of 83 torr to its equivalent in vol%.

A. 0.25 vol%   D. 1.39 vol%

B. 0.83 vol%   E. 2.49 vol%

C. 1.34 vol%

24. Calculate the total carbon dioxide given the following information.

HCO_3^-: 24 mEq/liter
Pa_{CO_2}: 40 torr

A. 64.0 mEq/liter   D. 34.4 mEq/liter

B. 53.0 mEq/liter   E. 25.2 mEq/liter

C. 42.4 mEq/liter

25. Which gases exist as diatomic molecules?

I. oxygen

II. helium

III. nitrogen

IV. chlorine

A. I, II, III, IV   D. I, III, IV only

B. I, III only   E. I, II, IV only

C. II, IV only

26. The aluminum atom has three electrons in its outermost shell (i.e., principal energy level 3). How many protons does an aluminum atom have?

A. 16   D. 9
B. 13   E. 3
C. 10

27. The specific gravity of nitrous oxide is _____ . (N = 14 amu; 0 = amu.)

    A. 1.11   D. 1.96
    B. 1.33   E. 2.31
    C. 1.51

28. Which statement most accurately describes molarity?

    A. It is defined as the number of moles of solvent per liter of solution.
    B. Molarity equals the number of gram-equivalents per 10^3 cc of solvent.
    C. Molarity is defined as the number of moles of solute per 1,000 cc of solution.
    D. It is defined as the number of gram-equivalents of solute per liter of solution.
    E. Molarity equals the number of moles of solvent per liter of solute.

29. Convert 53.5 vol% of CO_2 to mmol/liter.

    A. 18.8 mmol/liter   D. 40.9 mmol/liter
    B. 24.0 mmol/liter   E. 53.5 mmol/liter
    C. 31.5 mmol/liter

30. Calculate the relative rates of diffusion of the gases carbon dioxide and oxygen across the alveolar-capillary membrane. Assume body temperature to be 37°C.

    oxygen: density 1.43 g/liter
                   solubility coefficient 0.023
    carbon dioxide: density 1.96 g/liter
                   solubility coefficient 0.510

    A. $r_{CO_2} = 0.117\, r_{O_2}$ D. $r_{CO_2} = 14.7\, r_{O_2}$
    B. $r_{CO_2} = 2.54\, r_{O_2}$ E. $r_{CO_2} = 19.0\, r_{O_2}$
    C. $r_{CO_2} = 8.63\, r_{O_2}$

31. Calculate the normality of a liter solution containing 100 g of $Al_2(SO_4)_3$.

    A. 3.25 N   D. 1.11 N
    B. 2.35 N   E. 0.89 N
    C. 1.75 N

32. Each individual suborbital within a shell, or energy level, can maximally hold _____ electrons.

    A. 1   D. 4
    B. 2   E. 8
    C. 3

33. Calculate the voltage of a galvanic cell analyzer having a silver cathode and a lead anode. (See Appendix V.)

A. 0.55 volt   D. 0.93 volt
B. 0.67 volt   E. 1.00 volt
C. 0.75 volt

34. Which law states that the amount of gas that dissolves in a liquid is directly propor-
    tional to the pressure of the gas above the liquid and is inversely proportional to the
    temperature?

    A. Pascal's law   D. Stoke's law
    B. Graham's law   E. Starling's law
    C. Henry's law

35. Calculate the density of cyclopropane $(CH_2)_3$. (C = 12 amu; H = 1 amu.)

    A. 1.45 g/liter   D. 1.96 g/liter
    B. 1.74 g/liter   E. 2.03 g/liter
    C. 1.87 g/liter

36. What law is the basis for the Henderson-Hasselbalch equation?

    A. law of conservation of energy   D. Newton's second law of thermodynamics
    B. law of mass action   E. law of conservation of momentum
    C. law of conservation of matter

37. Which statement best describes Avogadro's law?

    A. When the temperature of a gas is constant, the volume and pressure are inversely
       proportional.
    B. Equal volumes of gases under the same conditions or temperature and pressure
       contain the same number of molecules.
    C. As the partial pressure of a gas above a liquid is increased, more gas will dissolve
       in that liquid.
    D. When a liquid is in a confined space, the pressure will be distributed equally
       throughout the system if a force is applied to a point in the system.
    E. When the volume of gas is constant, the pressure and temperature are directly re-
       lated.

38. Which properties refer to carbon dioxide gas at normal atmospheric conditions?

     I. colorless
    II. odorless
   III. a density of 1.43 g/liter
    IV. a specific gravity of 1.52

    A. I, II, III, IV   D. I, III, IV only
    B. I, II, IV only   E. II, III only
    C. I, II, III only

39. Calculate the HCO_3^- at pH 7.46 and Pa_{CO_2} 26 mm Hg.

A. 27.8 mmol/liter

B. 24.0 mmol/liter

C. 17.9 mmol/liter

D. 15.7 mmol/liter

E. 14.1 mmol/liter

40. What is the oxidation potential of the zinc anode in an electrochemical cell that contains a copper cathode and has a total voltage of 1.10 volts? (See Appendix V.)

A. 0.76 volt

B. 0.55 volt

C. 0.47 volt

D. 0.36 volt

E. 0.13 volt

41. Determine the density of 0.00654 liter of a substance weighing 89 g.

A. 5.8 g/ml

B. 13.6 g/ml

C. 14.0 g/ml

D. 15.1 g/ml

E. 16.2 g/ml

42. Calculate the specific gravity of oxygen.

A. 2.01

B. 1.43

C. 1.11

D. 0.93

E. 0.75

43. Determine the Pa_{CO_2} when the pH is 7.24 and the HCO_3^- is 26 mmol/liter. (See Appendix II.)

A. 74 mm Hg

B. 70 mm Hg

C. 63 mm Hg

D. 58 mm Hg

E. 28 mm Hg

44. Calculate the relative rates of diffusion of the gases O_2 and CO_2 *within* an alveolus. The molecular weight of O_2 is 32 and that for CO_2 is 44.

A. $r_{O_2} = 0.05\ r_{CO_2}$

B. $r_{O_2} = 0.50\ r_{CO_2}$

C. $r_{O_2} = 0.75\ r_{CO_2}$

D. $r_{O_2} = 1.08\ r_{CO_2}$

E. $r_{O_2} = 1.17\ r_{CO_2}$

45. Convert a Pa_{CO_2} of 55 torr to mEq of CO_2 per liter.

A. 0.17 mEq/liter

B. 0.98 mEq/liter

C. 1.42 mEq/liter

D. 1.65 mEq/liter

E. 1.89 mEq/liter

46. A pH of 7.20 is equivalent to how many nanomoles of hydrogen ions per liter of solution? (See Appendix II.)

A. 63 nanomoles/liter

B. 57 nanomoles/liter

C. 44 nanomoles/liter

D. 37 nanomoles/liter

E. 33 nanomoles/liter

47. What is the Fahrenheit equivalent of 210°K?

    A. −81.4°F

    B. 87.8°F

    C. 98.6°F

    D. 127.5°F

    E. 145.4°F

48. Which of the following statements are true concerning an electrochemical cell?

    I. The cathode is the electrode at which oxidation takes place.

    II. In the electrolyte solution the cations migrate to the cathode.

    III. A voltmeter senses the electron flow through the wires.

    IV. An electric current results from the oxidation-reduction reactions occurring in the cell.

    A. I, II, III only

    B. II, IV only

    C. III, IV only

    D. I, II only

    E. I, II, III, IV

49. What is the pH of a solution that contains 7.85×10^{-7} mole/liter?

    A. 7.85

    B. 7.77

    C. 7.21

    D. 6.54

    E. 6.10

50. Convert 1.2 mmol CO_2/liter to vol%.

    A. 2.68 vol%

    B. 10.42 vol%

    C. 24.00 vol%

    D. 47.61 vol%

    E. 53.50 vol%

ASSESSMENT ANSWER SHEET

DIRECTIONS: Darken the space under the selected answer.

	A	B	C	D	E		A	B	C	D	E
1.	[ ]	[ ]	[ ]	[ ]	[ ]	26.	[ ]	[ ]	[ ]	[ ]	[ ]
2.	[ ]	[ ]	[ ]	[ ]	[ ]	27.	[ ]	[ ]	[ ]	[ ]	[ ]
3.	[ ]	[ ]	[ ]	[ ]	[ ]	28.	[ ]	[ ]	[ ]	[ ]	[ ]
4.	[ ]	[ ]	[ ]	[ ]	[ ]	29.	[ ]	[ ]	[ ]	[ ]	[ ]
5.	[ ]	[ ]	[ ]	[ ]	[ ]	30.	[ ]	[ ]	[ ]	[ ]	[ ]
6.	[ ]	[ ]	[ ]	[ ]	[ ]	31.	[ ]	[ ]	[ ]	[ ]	[ ]
7.	[ ]	[ ]	[ ]	[ ]	[ ]	32.	[ ]	[ ]	[ ]	[ ]	[ ]
8.	[ ]	[ ]	[ ]	[ ]	[ ]	33.	[ ]	[ ]	[ ]	[ ]	[ ]
9.	[ ]	[ ]	[ ]	[ ]	[ ]	34.	[ ]	[ ]	[ ]	[ ]	[ ]
10.	[ ]	[ ]	[ ]	[ ]	[ ]	35.	[ ]	[ ]	[ ]	[ ]	[ ]
11.	[ ]	[ ]	[ ]	[ ]	[·]	36.	[ ]	[ ]	[ ]	[ ]	[ ]
12.	[ ]	[ ]	[ ]	[ ]	[ ]	37.	[ ]	[ ]	[ ]	[ ]	[ ]
13.	[ ]	[ ]	[ ]	[ ]	[ ]	38.	[ ]	[ ]	[ ]	[ ]	[ ]
14.	[ ]	[ ]	[ ]	[ ]	[ ]	39.	[ ]	[ ]	[ ]	[ ]	[ ]
15.	[ ]	[ ]	[ ]	[ ]	[ ]	40.	[ ]	[ ]	[ ]	[ ]	[ ]
16.	[ ]	[ ]	[ ]	[ ]	[ ]	41.	[ ]	[ ]	[ ]	[ ]	[ ]
17.	[ ]	[ ]	[ ]	[ ]	[ ]	42.	[ ]	[ ]	[ ]	[ ]	[ ]
18.	[ ]	[ ]	[ ]	[ ]	[ ]	43.	[ ]	[ ]	[ ]	[ ]	[ ]
19.	[ ]	[ ]	[ ]	[ ]	[ ]	44.	[ ]	[ ]	[ ]	[ ]	[ ]
20.	[ ]	[ ]	[ ]	[ ]	[ ]	45.	[ ]	[ ]	[ ]	[ ]	[ ]
21.	[ ]	[ ]	[ ]	[ ]	[ ]	46.	[ ]	[ ]	[ ]	[ ]	[ ]
22.	[ ]	[ ]	[ ]	[ ]	[ ]	47.	[ ]	[ ]	[ ]	[ ]	[ ]
23.	[ ]	[ ]	[ ]	[ ]	[ ]	48.	[ ]	[ ]	[ ]	[ ]	[ ]
24.	[ ]	[ ]	[ ]	[ ]	[ ]	49.	[ ]	[ ]	[ ]	[ ]	[ ]
25.	[ ]	[ ]	[ ]	[ ]	[ ]	50.	[ ]	[ ]	[ ]	[ ]	[ ]

CHEMISTRY ANALYSES

Note: The references listed after each analysis are numbered and keyed to the reference list located at the end of this section. The first number indicates the text. The second number indicates the page where information about the question will be found. For example, (1:219,384) means that reference number 1 is to be used and that on pages 219 and 384 information about the question will be found. Frequently, it will be necessary to read beyond the page number indicated to obtain complete information. Therefore, reference to the question will be found either on the page indicated or on subsequent pages.

1. B. To avoid using pH units (logarithmic expressions) when determining the hydrogen ion concentration of a solution, the unit *nanomoles* is sometimes used. The Greek prefix "nano" represents one one-billionth or 10^{-9}. The unit nanomole, therefore, indicates one one-billionth of a mole or 10^{-9} mole.

    As pH increases, the number of nanomoles of hydrogen ions per liter of solution decreases. The converse is also true. Note Table 1 below.

    (2:74–75), (4:10–11)

2. D. Figure 42 depicts two NaCl solutions of different concentrations separated by a membrane diffusible to H_2O molecules, Na^+ ions, Cl^- ions, and NaCl molecules. In time, equilibrium between the two compartments will occur. In the meantime, however, H_2O molecules will experience a net diffusion from the 20% solution to the 40% solution. Similarly, net diffusion of Na^+ ions, Cl^- ions, and NaCl molecules will occur in the opposite direction. Because the membrane is permeable to all species present, no volume change will occur in either compartment. Molecules of gases and liquids move randomly in all directions; however, net diffusion will take place from the area of higher concentration to that of lower concentration until equilibrium is reached.

    (2:177–178), (4:10,25)

3. B. Compounds that break down into their ionic species when placed in an aqueous solution can be electrolyte solutions. The degree to which a compound will pro-

TABLE 1

pH	nanomoles/liter	pH	nanomoles/liter
7.52	30	7.37	43
7.50	32	7.36	44
7.45	35	7.35	45
7.44	36	7.34	46
7.43	37	7.33	47
7.42	38	7.32	48
7.41	39	7.31	49
7.40	40	7.30	50
7.39	41	7.26	55
7.38	42	7.25	56

duce ions will determine how strong or weak an electrolyte solution it will become. Covalent compounds that produce ions are said to dissociate. Ionic compounds producing ions ionize. HCl and NaOH are strong electrolytes.
(1:64–71), (2:61–62,89), (4:3–4,194)

4. D. The pH, HCO_3^-, or Pa_{CO_2} can be calculated using the Henderson-Hasselbalch equation when any two of those three variables are given.

STEP 1: Set up the Henderson-Hasselbalch equation.

$$pH = 6.10 + \log \frac{HCO_3^-}{(P_{CO_2})(0.03)}$$

STEP 2: Insert known values and calculate the pH.

$$pH = 6.10 + \log\left[\frac{21 \text{ mmol/liter}}{(25 \text{ mmHg})(0.03 \text{ mmol/liter/mm Hg})}\right]$$
$$= 6.10 + \log\left[\frac{21 \text{ mmol/liter}}{0.75 \text{ mmol/liter}}\right]$$
$$= 6.10 + \log 28$$
$$= 6.10 + 1.45$$
$$= 7.55$$

(1:218–219,220–221), (2:81–83), (4:196–197), (6:278)

5. D.   Na = 23 amu
                             Cl = 35.5 amu
Molecular weight of NaCl = 58.5

NaCl ionizes to a large degree when placed in an aqueous solution. Therefore, it is a strong electrolyte.
(1:68–69,76), (2:56,177–179), (4:3)

6. A. The pH scale ranges from 0 to 14. A pH of 7 is considered neutral. A pH less than 7 is acidic, whereas a pH greater than 7 is alkaline. A pH of 7.40 is alkaline.
(1:78–79), (2:72–74), (4:10–11)

7. A. Elements that combine to form another substance via the transferring of electrons produce an electrovalent or ionic compound. The compounds are held together by an electrovalent or ionic bond.
(1:46–47), (2:61), (4:3)

8. C. An atom is electrostatically neutral. It contains equal numbers of protons and electrons.

Atomic weight = number of protons + number of neutrons

Because an atom, which is electrostatically neutral, is under consideration here, the electrons will equal the protons. Therefore, this hypothetical atom contains 15 protons.
(1:39–40), (2:54), (4:1)

9. A. An electrochemical cell has the following basic constituents: (1) a cathode, (2) an anode, (3) an electrolyte solution, and (4) a current meter (ammeter). Figure 43 illustrates these components in relation to each other.

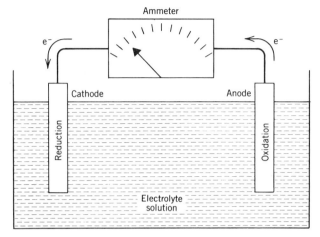

FIGURE 43

10. E. pH can be expressed mathematically as

   1. The negative log (to base 10) of the hydrogen ion concentration. $pH = -\log_{10}[H^+]$
   2. The log (to base 10) of the reciprocal of the hydrogen ion concentration: $pH = \log_{10}\dfrac{1}{[H^+]}$

   (1:79), (2:72–74), (4:10–11), (17:74–75)

11. B. The diffusion of crystalloids across a semipermeable membrane that prevents the passage of colloids is called dialysis. The capillary endothelium resembles such a membrane.
   (21:75–76,381–382)

12. D. The rule of eight is the tendency of elements to arrange their electrons in such a manner as to end up with eight electrons in the outermost shell. The outermost shell of any atom will hold no more than eight electrons.
   (1:43), (2:61)

13. A. An atom that loses electrons becomes an ion, more specifically, a cation, and undergoes oxidation. Any atom that gains electrons will have an excess of electrons (negative charges). Such an ion is called an anion (e.g., Cl⁻). Atoms that gain electrons are reduced.
   (1:46), (2:61), (4:1)

14. A. The following factors influence the rate of a chemical reaction:

1. concentration of products
2. concentration of reactants
3. catalysis
4. temperature

For example, the reversible reaction

$$CO_2 + H_2O \rightleftharpoons H_2CO_3 \rightleftharpoons H^+ + HCO_3^-$$

is favored to the right in the red blood cells at the tissue level because the catalyst carbonic anhydrase increases the rate to 13,000 times that of the same reaction in the plasma, which lacks this enzyme. At the same time, the HCO_3^- that forms at the tissue level from the dissociation of H_2CO_3 is removed from the red blood cell during the chloride shift. Additionally, deoxygenated hemoglobin buffers the H^+ ions produced as H_2CO_3 dissociates. All three of these activities cause the rate of the hydration of CO_2 to proceed rapidly to the right.
(2:79–80)

15. E. 1. $Normality = \dfrac{\text{number of gram-equivalents}}{\text{liter of solution}}$

2. $\dfrac{\text{Molecular weight}}{\text{Valence}} = \text{weight of 1 g-equivalent}$

3. $H_2SO_4 = 98$ amu (molecular weight)
H_2SO_4 valence $= 2$

4. $\dfrac{98 \text{ amu}}{2} = 49$ weight of 1 g-equivalent of H_2SO_4

5. 1 mole of $H_2SO_4 = 98$ g
A 2.0 M H_2SO_4 solution contains 196 g of H_2SO_4 in 1 liter of solution.

6. 196 g $H_2SO_4 = 4$ g-equivalents

7. $\dfrac{4 \text{ g-equivalents}}{1 \text{ liter}} = 4.0 \, N$

(1:50–55,60–61), (2:70–72), (4:7–9)

16. A. The kinetic theory of matter states that gas molecules are attracted to each other by weak forces. This attraction among the molecules is called van der Waals, or London, forces. Because gas molecules are greatly separated and travel at a high velocity, the van der Waals forces in a gas weaken. However, if the temperature decreases, the kinetic energy of the gas molecules decreases and the van der Waals forces increase.
(1:29), (2:116,159), (4:16)

17. D. The quantity of a substance, the weight of which in grams is numerically equal to its molecular weight in atomic mass units (amu), is called a mole, or a gram-molecular weight. For example, 1 mole of oxygen equals 32 g. Oxygen is a diatomic molecule having a molecular weight of 32 amu.
(1:6–7), (2:67–70), (4:18)

18. D. Hemoglobin has a molecular weight of 66,700 amu.* Since,

$$\frac{\text{Number of grams}}{\text{Molecular weight}} = \text{number of moles}$$

therefore,

$$\frac{133,400 \text{ g}}{66,700 \text{ amu}} = 2 \text{ moles of Hb}$$

(1:203), (4:184)

19. C. Based on Avogadro's work, 1 mole (gram molecular weight) of any ideal gas under standard conditions (0°C; 760 torr) will occupy a volume of 22.4 liters.
(1:6–7), (2:132–133), (4:18–19), (6:1017)

20. C. °C = 5/9(°F − 32)
      = 5/9(−8° − 32)
      = 5/9(−40°)
      = −22°
  °K = °C + 273
      = −22° + 273
      = 251°

(1:4), (2:87–88), (4:25), (6:379–380)

21. B. The oxidation potential indicates the tendency of a substance to undergo either reduction or oxidation reactions. Oxidation potentials are obtained by comparing an electrode made of a given substance, for example, gold, lead, etc., to a hydrogen electrode that serves as the standard electrode. The voltage of the battery (cell) is indicated by a voltmeter. The voltage and direction of the current represent the substance's tendency to undergo either reduction or oxidation.
(2:94–96), (4:11)

22. B. The number of electrons that can maximally reside in any of the principal energy levels of an atom can be determined by the formula $2(n^2)$, where n is the numerical value of the principal energy level. For example,

PRINCIPAL ENERGY LEVEL	FORMULA	MAXIMUM NUMBER OF ELECTRONS
1	$2(1^2)$	2
2	$2(2^2)$	8
3	$2(3^2)$	18
4	$2(4^2)$	32
etc.	etc.	etc.

(1:43), (2:56)

*Physiologically, one gram molecular weight of hemoglobin (66,700) can combine with 4 moles of oxygen.

23. A. The conversion factor for changing mm Hg or torr to vol% is derived as follows:
STEP 1: The solubility coefficient of oxygen is divided by 760 mm Hg.

$$\frac{0.023 \text{ ml } O_2/\text{ml plasma}}{P_{O_2} \text{ 760 mm Hg}} = 0.00003 \text{ ml } O_2/\text{ml plasma/mm Hg}$$

STEP 2: Convert the unit *ml O_2/ml plasma/mm Hg* to *vol%/mm Hg*.

0.00003 ml O_2/ml plasma/mm Hg × 100 ml plasma
= 0.003 ml O_2/100 ml plasma/mm Hg

OR

0.003 ml O_2/100 ml plasma/mm Hg = 0.003 vol%/mm Hg

Therefore, the formula used to change any P_{O_2} expressed in mm Hg or torr to vol% is shown as follows:

P_{O_2} × 0.003 vol%/mm Hg = vol%
83 torr × 0.003 vol%/torr = 0.25 vol%

(1:201–202), (2:63–64), (4:183)

24. E. Total carbon dioxide is the sum of the combined CO_2 and the dissolved CO_2. The combined CO_2 refers to the CO_2 carried as HCO_3^- in the plasma, and the dissolved CO_2 is the partial pressure of CO_2 in the plasma (Pa_{CO_2}). Total CO_2 is expressed in millimoles/liter or milliequivalents/liter.* The dissolved CO_2 usually needs to be converted from torr or mm Hg to mmol/liter or mEq/liter. This conversion is accomplished by multiplying any P_{CO_2} (torr or mm Hg) by 0.03 mmol/liter/torr P_{CO_2}.
STEP 1: Change torr (P_{CO_2}) to mmol/liter.

P_{CO_2} × 0.03 mmol/liter/torr
40 torr × 0.03 mmol/liter/torr = 1.2 mmol/liter or 1.2 mEq/liter

STEP 2: Add the combined CO_2 to the dissolved CO_2.

HCO_3^- + P_{CO_2} = total CO_2
24 mEq/liter + 1.2 mEq/liter = 25.2 mEq/liter

(1:215–216,219), (2:64–67), (4:191–192)

25. D. Oxygen (O_2), nitrogen (N_2), and chlorine (Cl_2) are all diatomic molecules; that is, they consist of two atoms.
(2:54), (13:53,55,60)

26. B. The aluminum atom has a total of 13 electrons. They are positioned about its nucleus as follows:

1 orbit, *s* suborbital = 2 electrons
2 orbit, *s* suborbital = 2 electrons
2 orbit, *p* suborbital = 6 electrons

*In this example the units millimoles of CO_2/liter (mmol/liter) and milliequivalents of CO_2/liter (mEq/liter) are equal, and can be used interchangeably.

3 orbit, *s* suborbital = 2 electrons

3 orbit, *p* suborbital = 1 electrons

An atom is electrostatically neutral; therefore, it contains the same number of protons and electrons. Aluminum has 13 protons. Keep in mind that an ion has an imbalance of charged particles. A cation has more protons than electrons; an anion has more electrons than protons.

(1:39–49), (2:54, *Periodic Table*), (4:1–2)

27. C. The density of any gas can be obtained by dividing the gram molecular weight of the gas by the volume occupied by 1 mole of that gas under standard conditions. Gas density can be calculated as follows:

$$\text{Density} = \frac{\text{gram molecular weight}}{22.4 \text{ liters}}$$

Nitrous oxide's molecular weight = 44 amu

$$\text{Density} = \frac{44 \text{ g}}{22.4 \text{ liters}} = 1.96 \text{ g/liter}$$

Calculation of specific gravity for a gas:

$$\frac{\text{Density of the gas}}{\text{Density of the standard}} = \text{specific gravity}$$

The standard used for gases is the density of air 1.29 g/liter.

$$\frac{1.96 \text{ g/liter}}{1.29 \text{ g/liter}} = 1.51$$

(1:7–8), (2:87), (4:19)

28. C. Molarity is defined as the number of moles of solute per liter of solution. The formula for molarity (*M*) is

$$M = \frac{\text{moles}}{\text{liter}}$$

A mole is the quantity of a substance whose weight in grams is numerically the same as the molecular weight in atomic mass units. The weight in grams can be converted into moles by using the following relationship.

$$\frac{\text{Number of grams}}{\text{Molecular weight}} = \text{number of moles}$$

(1:60), (2:69–70)

29. A. The amount of CO_2 expressed as vol% can be converted to millimoles of CO_2/liter (mmol/liter) as follows:

STEP 1: Use the quantitative expression that relates volumes percent (vol%) to mmol/liter.

$$mmol/liter = \frac{vol\%}{2.23 \ vol\%/mmol/liter}$$

STEP 2: Insert the values.

$$mmol/liter = \frac{53.5 \ \cancel{vol\%}}{2.23 \ \cancel{vol\%}/mmol/liter}$$
$$= 24.0 \ mmol/liter$$

(1:221), (2:65–66)

30. E. According to Graham's law of diffusion the relative rates of the diffusion of gases across the alveolar-capillary membrane can be quantified as follows:

$$\frac{r_1}{r_2} = \frac{(\sqrt{D_2})(Cs_1)}{(\sqrt{D_1})(Cs_2)}$$

where

r = rate of gas diffusion
D = gas density (molecular weights can also be used)
Cs = solubility coefficient of the gas

STEP 1: Set up the relationship in terms of carbon dioixde and oxygen.

$$\frac{r_{CO_2}}{r_{O_2}} = \frac{(\sqrt{D_{O_2}})(Cs_{CO_2})}{(\sqrt{D_{CO_2}})(Cs_{O_2})}$$

STEP 2: Insert values and calculate the relative rates of diffusion.

$$\frac{r_{CO_2}}{r_{O_2}} = \frac{(\sqrt{1.43 \ g/L})(0.510)}{(\sqrt{1.96 \ g/L})(0.023)}$$
$$= \frac{(1.195)(0.510)}{(1.400)(0.023)}$$
$$= \frac{0.609}{0.032}$$
$$r_{CO_2} = 19 \ r_{O_2}$$

Note: Oxygen is 1.17 times more diffusible than carbon dioxide when the rates of diffusion of these two gases are compared within a gaseous medium.

$$\frac{r_{O_2}}{r_{CO_2}} = \frac{\sqrt{D_{CO_2}}}{\sqrt{D_{O_2}}} = \frac{1.400}{1.195} = 1.17$$

(1:196–197), (2:67–69), (4:26–27)

31. C. STEP 1: Calculate the gram molecular weight of $Al_2(SO_4)_3$.

$$Al = 27 \text{ g}$$
$$S = 32 \text{ g}$$
gram atomic weights of constituent atoms of
$$O = 16 \text{ g}$$
$Al_2(SO_4)_3$

$$(2 \times 27 \text{ g}) + (3 \times 32 \text{ g}) + (12 \times 16 \text{ g}) = 342 \text{ g}$$

STEP 2: Calculate the weight of 1 gram-equivalent of $Al_2(SO_4)_3$.

$$(342\text{g/mole})\left(\frac{1 \text{ mole}}{6 \text{ Eq*}}\right) = 57 \text{ g/Eq}$$

1 gram-equivalent of $Al_2(SO_4)_3$ weighs 57 g.

STEP 3: Determine the number of gram equivalents of $Al_2(SO_4)_3$ present in 100 grams of $Al_2(SO_4)_3$.

$$\frac{100 \text{ g}}{57\text{g/Eq}} = 1.75 \text{ Eq}$$

STEP 4: Calculate the normality.

$$N = \frac{Eq}{\text{liter}}$$

where,

$$N = \text{normality}$$
$$Eq = \text{number of gram equivalents}$$
$$N = \frac{1.75 \text{ Eq}}{1 \text{ liter}}$$
$$= 1.75 \text{ } N$$

(1:60–61), (2:70–72)

32. B. For example, the *s* suborbital can maximally contain two electrons. Likewise, each *p* suborbital can maximally contain two electrons. The same holds true for the *d* and *f* suborbitals.

(1:40–44), (2:54–60)

33. D. The voltage for the galvanic cell pictured in Figure 44 can be calculated according to the following equation:

$$E° = E°_{oxidation} + E°_{reduction}$$
$$E° = E°_{Pb;Pb^{+2}} + E°_{Ag^{+1};Ag}$$
$$= 0.13 \text{ volt} + 0.80 \text{ volt}$$
$$= 0.93 \text{ volt}$$

(2:91–92,94–96)

---

*Because $Al_2(SO_4)_3$ would ionize as follows $Al_2(SO_4)_3 \rightleftharpoons 2 \text{ } Al^{+3} + 3 \text{ } SO_4^{-2}$, the gram molecular weight is divided by 6.

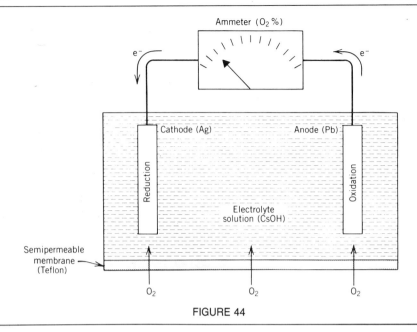

FIGURE 44

34. C. Henry's law states that the amount of gas that dissolves in a liquid is directly proportional to the partial pressure of the gas above the surface of the liquid and inversely proportional to the temperature.

(1:196), (2:63), (4:26), (6:411), (14:163)

35. C. The molecular weight of cyclopropane $(CH_2)_3$ is 42 amu.

$$\text{Gas density} = \frac{\text{gram molecular weight}}{22.4 \text{ liters}}$$

$$\frac{42 \text{ g}}{22.4 \text{ liters}} = 1.87 \text{ g/liter}$$

(1:7–8), (2:87), (4:18–19)

36. B. When two or more chemical substances react, one or more substances different from the reacting species will from. As an example, consider the reaction

$$A + B \longrightarrow C + D$$

where substances A and B chemically react to form the products C and D. It has been experimentally found that a definite relationship exists between the speed, or rate, of the reaction and the concentration of the reacting species. The law of mass action describes this relationship. The rate of a chemical reaction is proportional to the concentration of the reactants.

$$K = \frac{[\text{products}]}{[\text{reactants}]}$$

Basically, the Henderson-Hasselbalch equation is

$$K = \frac{[H^+][HCO_3^-]}{[H_2CO_3]}$$

This expression is based on the reversible reaction

$$CO_2 + H_2O \rightleftarrows H^+ + HCO_3^- \rightleftarrows H_2CO_3$$

Quantitatively, the Henderson-Hasselbalch equation is

$$pH = 6.10 + \log \frac{[HCO_3^-]}{[(P_{CO_2})(0.03)]}$$

(1:217–219), (2:77–85), (4:196–197), (6:278), (14:77–78,166)

37. B. Avogadro's law states that equal volumes of all gases at the same temperature and pressure contain the same number of molecules. Expanding this concept, a gram molecular weight of any compound at STP contains 6.023×10^{23} molecules. (1:6), (2:132–133), (4:18), (6:1017)

38. B. Carbon dioxide gas is colorless and odorless at normal atmospheric conditions. It has a molecular weight of 44 amu. Its density is calculated as follows:

$$\frac{44 \text{ g}}{22.4 \text{ liters}} = 1.96 \text{ g/liter}$$

Using air as the standard, CO_2 has a specific gravity of

$$\frac{1.96 \text{ g/liter}}{1.29 \text{ g/liter}} = 1.52$$

(6:342)

39. C. When any two of the following three factors—pH, HCO_3^-, and P_{CO_2}—are given, the third can be calculated using the Henderson-Hasselbalch equation.
STEP 1: Set up the Henderson-Hasselbalch equation.

$$pH = 6.10 + \log \frac{[HCO_3^-]}{[(P_{CO_2})(0.03)]}$$

STEP 2: Insert known values.

$$7.46 = 6.10 + \log \frac{[HCO_3^-]}{[(26 \text{ mm Hg})(0.03 \text{ mmol/liter/mm Hg})]}$$

STEP 3: Simplify the equation.

$$7.46 - 6.10 = \log \frac{[HCO_3^-]}{0.78 \text{ mmol/liter}}$$

$$1.36 = \log \frac{[HCO_3^-]}{0.78 \text{ mmol/liter}}$$

STEP 4: Determine the antilog of the pH and calculate the $[HCO_3^-]$.

$$\text{antilog } 1.36 = \frac{[HCO_3^-]}{0.78 \text{ mmol/liter}}$$

$$22.9 = \frac{[HCO_3^-]}{0.78 \text{ mmol/liter}}$$

$$[HCO_3^-] = 22.9 \times 0.78 \text{ mmol/liter}$$

$$[HCO_3^-] = 17.9 \text{ mmol/liter}$$

(2:81–84), (3:196–198)

40. A. The question refers to the electrochemical cell illustrated in Figure 45. The following equation is used.

$$E° = E°_{oxidation} + E°_{reduction}$$

where

$E°$ = total voltage of the electrochemical cell (volts)
$E°_{oxidation}$ = total voltage at the anode (volts)
$E°_{reduction}$ = total voltage at the cathode (volts)

$$1.10 \text{ volts} = 0.76 \text{ volt} + E°_{Cu^{+2};Cu}$$

$$E°_{Cu^{+2};Cu} = 1.10 \text{ volts} - 0.76 \text{ volt}$$

$$= 0.34 \text{ volt}$$

(2:94–96)

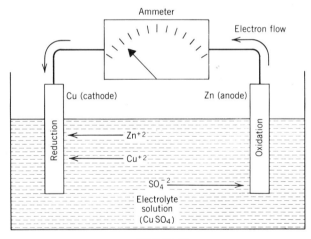

FIGURE 45

41. B. STEP 1: Convert 0.00654 liter to milliliters.

$$0.00654 \text{ liter}\left(\frac{1000 \text{ ml}}{1 \text{ liter}}\right) = 6.54 \text{ ml}$$

STEP 2: Use the formula for calculating density.

$$D = \frac{mass}{volume}$$

$$= \frac{89 \text{ g}}{6.54 \text{ ml}}$$

$$= 13.6 \text{ g/ml}$$

Note: This substance happens to be mercury (Hg).
(2:85–86), (4:20)

42. C. The specific gravity of any gas is determined by comparing the density of the gas to the density of air, which is the standard for gases. The density of air is 1.29 g/liter. The specific gravity of O_2 is determined as follows:

$$\frac{1.43 \text{ g/liter}}{1.29 \text{ g/liter}} = 1.11$$

(1:7–8), (2:87), (4:19)

43. C. STEP 1: Set up the Henderson-Hasselbalch equation.

$$pH = 6.10 + \log \frac{[HCO_3^-]}{[(P_{CO_2})(0.03)]}$$

STEP 2: Insert known values.

$$7.24 = 6.10 + \log\left[\frac{26 \text{ mmol/liter}}{(P_{CO_2})(0.03 \text{ mmol/liter/torr})}\right]$$

STEP 3: Simplify the equation.

$$7.24 - 6.10 = \log\left[\frac{26 \text{ mmol/liter}}{(P_{CO_2})(0.03 \text{ mmol/liter/torr})}\right]$$

$$1.14 = \log 26 - \log[(P_{CO_2})(0.03)]$$

$$1.14 = 1.42 - \log[(P_{CO_2})(0.03)]$$

$$\log[(P_{CO_2})(0.03)] = 1.42 - 1.14$$

$$\log[(P_{CO_2})(0.03)] = 0.28$$

STEP 4: Find the antilogarithm of 0.28 and calculate the P_{CO_2}.

$$(P_{CO_2})(0.03) = \text{antilog } 0.28$$

$$(P_{CO_2})(0.03) = 1.90$$

$$P_{CO_2} = \frac{1.90}{0.03}$$

$$P_{CO_2} = 63 \text{ torr}$$

(1:221–222), (2:81–85)

44. E. According to Graham's law of diffusion for a gas *within* a gas, the lighter

molecules will diffuse faster than the heavier ones. This condition can be quantified as follows:

$$r_1\sqrt{\text{mol wt}_1} = r_2\sqrt{\text{mol wt}_2}$$

where

mol wt = molecular weight of the gas (gas density,
i.e., mass/volume, can also be used)

r = rate of diffusion

$$r_{O_2}\sqrt{32} = r_{CO_2}\sqrt{44}$$

$$\frac{r_{O_2}}{r_{CO_2}} = \frac{\sqrt{44}}{\sqrt{32}}$$

$$\frac{r_{O_2}}{r_{CO_2}} = \frac{6.633}{5.657}$$

$$r_{O_2} = 1.17\ r_{CO_2}$$

Note: When the rates of diffusion of these two gases are compared *across* the alveolar-capillary membrane, CO_2 is 19 times more diffusible than O_2. See question 30.

(2:67–69)

45. D. By using the conversion factor 0.03 mEq/liter/torr*, any P_{CO_2} (mm Hg or torr) can be expressed in mEq/liter. For example,

$$P_{CO_2} \times 0.03\ \text{mEq/liter/torr} = \text{mEq/liter}$$

55 t̶o̶r̶r̶ $\times$ 0.03 mEq/liter/t̶o̶r̶r̶ = 1.65 mEq/liter

(1:219–220), (2:66), (4:192,200), (8:84–85)

46. A. STEP 1: Set up the equation for converting pH to nanomoles/liter.

nanomoles/liter = antilog (9 − pH)

STEP 2: Insert known values.

nanomoles/liter = antilog (9 − 7.20)
= antilog 1.80
= 63 nanomoles/liter

(2:74–76), (4:11)

47. E. STEP 1: Convert 210°K to Celsius.

°K = °C + 273
°C = °K − 273
= 210°K − 273
= −63°C

---

*For the derivation of this factor consult either Spearman, C., and Shelden, R., *Egan's Fundamentals of Respiratory Therapy,* 4th ed., C. V. Mosby, St. Louis, 1982, pages 219–220 or Wojciechowski, W., *Respiratory Care Sciences: An Integrated Approach,* John Wiley & Sons, New York, 1985, 64–66

STEP 2: Convert 63°C to °F.

$$°F = \frac{9}{5}°C + 32$$

$$= \frac{9}{5}(-63°C) + 32$$

$$= -81.4°F$$

(1:3–4), (2:87–88), (4:9–10), (6:379–380)

48. B. In an electrochemical cell reduction (gain of electrons) occurs at the cathode, and oxidation (loss of electrons) occurs at the anode. The electric current (flow of electrons) moves through the wire from the anode to the cathode, and in the electrolyte solution the cations move to the cathode and the anions migrate to the anode.

An ammeter senses the current that results from the oxidation-reduction reactions occurring in the cell.

(2:89–91)

49. E. The mathematical expressions allowing for the calculation of pH include

1. $pH = \log \dfrac{1}{[H^+]}$
2. $pH = -\log [H^+]$

STEP 1: Insert the value given for the $[H^+]$.

$$pH = -\log(7.85 \times 10^{-7})$$

STEP 2: Calculate the pH.

$$pH = -\log 7.85 + (-\log 10^{-7})$$
$$= .8949 + (\log 10^7)$$
$$= -.8949 + 7$$
$$= 6.10$$

(1:219), (2:72–74), (4:10–11)

50. A. STEP 1: Set up the relationship between vol% and mmol/liter.

$$vol\% = (mmol/liter)(2.23 \ vol\%/mmol/liter)$$

STEP 2: Insert known values.

$$vol\% = (1.2 \ \cancel{mmol/liter})(2.23 \ vol\%/\cancel{mmol/liter})$$
$$= 2.68 \ vol\%$$

(1:216,221), (2:65–67)

REFERENCES

1. Spearman, C., and Sheldon, R., *Egan's Fundamentals of Respiratory Therapy*, 4th ed., C.V. Mosby, St. Louis, 1982.

2. Wojciechowski, W., *Respiratory Care Sciences: An Integrated Approach,* John Wiley & Sons, New York, 1985.

3. Shapiro, B., Harrison, R., Kacmarek, R., and Cane, R., *Clinical Application of Respiratory Care,* 3rd ed., Year Book Medical Publishers, Chicago, 1985.

.4. Kacmarek, R., Mack, C., and Dimas, S., *The Essentials of Respiratory Therapy,* 2nd ed., Year Book Medical Publishers, Chicago, 1985.

5. McPherson, S., *Respiratory Therapy Equipment,* 3rd ed., C.V. Mosby, St. Louis, 1985.

6. Burton, G., and Hodgkin, J., *Respiratory Care: A Guide to Clinical Practice,* 2nd ed., J.B. Lippincott, Philadelphia, 1985.

7. Frownfelter, D., *Chest Physical Therapy and Cardiopulmonary Rehabilitation, An Interdisciplinary Approach,* Year Book Medical Publishers, Chicago, 1978.

8. Cherniack, R., and Cherniack, L., *Respiration in Health and Disease,* 3rd ed., W. B. Saunders, Philadelphia, 1983.

9. Daily, E., and Schroeder, G., *Techniques in Bedside Hemodynamic Monitoring,* 3rd ed., C.V. Mosby, St. Louis, 1985.

10. Des Jardins, R., *Clinical Manifestations of Respiratory Disease,* Year Book Medical Publishers, Chicago, 1984.

11. Mitchell, R., *Synopsis of Clinical Pulmonary Disease,* 3rd ed., C.V. Mosby, St. Louis, 1982.

12. Comroe, J., *Physiology of Respiration,* 3rd ed., Year Book Medical Publishers, Chicago, 1974.

13. West, J., *Pulmonary Pathophysiology—The Essentials,* 2nd ed., Williams & Wilkins, Baltimore, 1982.

14. West, J., *Respiratory Physiology—The Essentials,* 3rd ed., Williams & Wilkins, Baltimore, 1985.

15. Martz, K., et al., *Management of the Patient-Ventilator System: A Team Approach,* 2nd ed., C.V. Mosby, St. Louis, 1984.

16. Shoup, C., and McHenry, R., *Laboratory Exercises in Respiratory Therapy,* 2nd ed., C.V. Mosby, St. Louis, 1983.

17. Ruppel, G., *Manual of Pulmonary Function Testing,* 3rd ed., C.V. Mosby, St. Louis, 1982.

18. Appelbaum, E., and Bruce, D., *Tracheal Intubation,* W.B. Saunders, Philadelphia, 1976.

19. Rau, J., *Respiratory Therapy Pharmacology,* 2nd ed., Year Book Medical Publishers, Chicago, 1984.

20. United States Department of Health, Education, and Welfare, Public Health Service, *Isolation Techniques for Use in Hospitals,* 2nd ed., Washington, D.C., 1975.

21. Brooks, S., *Integrated Basic Science,* 4th ed., C.V. Mosby, St. Louis, 1979.

22. Comroe, J., *The Lung,* Year Book Medical Publishers, Chicago, 1962.

23. Shibel, E., and Moser, K., *Respiratory Emergencies,* 2nd ed., C.V. Mosby, St. Louis, 1982.

24. Tisi, G., *Pulmonary Physiology in Clinical Medicine,* 2nd ed., Williams & Wilkins, Baltimore, 1985.

25. Cherniack, R., *Pulmonary Function Testing,* W. B. Saunders, Philadelphia, 1977.

26. Altose, M., *The Physiological Basis of Pulmonary Function Testing,* Clinical Symposia-CIBA, Vol. 31, No. 2, Summit, New Jersey, 1979.

27. Shapiro, B., Harrison, R., and Walton, J., *Clinical Application of Arterial Blood Gases,* 3rd ed., Year Book Medical Publishers, Chicago, 1982.

28. West, J., *Ventilation/Blood Flow and Gas Exchange,* 3rd ed., Blackwell Scientific Publications, 1979.

29. Slonim, N., and Hamilton, K., *Respiratory Physiology,* 4th ed., C.V. Mosby, St. Louis, 1981.

30. Rarey, K., and Youtsey, J., *Respiratory Patient Care,* Prentice-Hall, Englewood Cliffs, 1981.

31. Berne, R., and Levy, M., *Physiology,* C.V. Mosby, St. Louis, 1983.

32. Levitzky, M., *Pulmonary Physiology,* 2nd ed., McGraw-Hill, New York, 1986.

33. Wilson, P., Bell, C., and Norton, A., *Rehabilitation of the Heart and Lungs,* SensorMedics, 1980.

34. Clausen, J., and Zarins, L., *Pulmonary Function Testing Guildlines and Controversies,* Academic Press, New York, 1982.

35. Klaus, M., and Fanaroff, A., *Care of the High-Risk Neonate,* 2nd ed., W. B. Saunders, Philadelphia, 1979.

36. Lough, M., et al., *Pediatric Respiratory Therapy,* 3rd ed., Year Book Medical Publishers, Chicago, 1985.

37. Levin, D., et at., *A Practical Guide to Pediatric Intensive Care,* 2nd ed., C.V. Mosby, St. Louis, 1984.

38. O'Ryan, J., and Burns, D., *Pulmonary Rehabilitation from Hospital to Home,* Year Book Medical Publishers, Chicago, 1984.

39. Bell, C., et al., *Home Care and Rehabilitation in Respiratory Medicine,* J.B. Lippincott, Philadelphia, 1984.

40. Wilkins, R., et al., *Clinical Assessment in Respiratory Care,* C.V. Mosby, St. Louis, 1985.

41. Jones, N., and Campbell, E., *Clinical Exercise Testing,* 2nd ed., W.B. Saunders, Philadelphia, 1982.

42. Goldsmith, J., and Karotkin, E., *Assisted Ventilation of the Neonate,* W.B. Saunders, Philadelphia, 1981.

43. Blowers, M., and Sims, R., *How to Read an ECG,* 3rd ed., Medical Economics, Inc., New Jersey, 1983.

44. Eubanks, D., and Bone, R., *Comprehensive Respiratory Care,* C.V. Mosby, St. Louis, 1985.

45. Rattenborg, C., *Clinical Use of Mechanical Ventilation,* Year Book Medical Publishers, Chicago, 1981.

46. Witkowski, A. S., *Pulmonary Assessment: A Clinical Guide,* J.B. Lippincott, Philadelphia, 1985.

47. Op't Holt, Timothy B., *Assessment Based Respiratory Care,* John Wiley & Sons, New York, 1986.

MICROBIOLOGY ASSESSMENT

PURPOSE: The purpose of this 35-item assessment is to provide you with the opportunity to determine the extent of your understanding and knowledge of basic microbiology principles. This section includes questions pertaining to normal inhabitants of the respiratory tract, bacterial and viral ultrastructures, bacterial morphology and staining characteristics, bacterial growth requirements, and fungal characteristics.

DIRECTIONS: Each of the questions or incomplete statements is followed by five suggested answers. Select the one which is the best in each case and then blacken the corresponding space on the answer sheet.

1. Which of the following types of microbes will colonize bacterial culture media?

   I. anaerobic bacteria

   II. viruses

   III. rickettsiae

   IV. aerobic bacteria

A. I, IV only   D. I, III, IV only
B. II, IV only   E. I, II only
C. II, III only

2. Which of the following microorganisms are spore forming?

   I. *Pseudomonas aeruginosa*
   II. *Bacillus anthracis*
   III. *Clostridium perfringens*
   IV. *Mycobacterium tuberculosis*

   A. I, II, III, IV   D. II, III only
   B. I, II, III only   E. I, II only
   C. III, IV only

3. Chemical agents that inhibit bacterial growth are termed _____ .

   A. germicidal   D. aseptic
   B. bactericidal   E. bacteriostatic
   C. sporicidal

4. Which cellular organization has the simplest cells?

   A. prokaryote   D. protists
   B. mesokaryote   E. eukaryote
   C. monokaryote

5. Which of the following microorganisms are considered normal inhabitants of the respiratory tract?

   I. *Actinomyces israelii*
   II. *Pseudomonas aeruginosa*
   III. *Neisseria meningitidis*
   IV. *Staphylococcus aureus*
   V. *Escherichia coli*

   A. I, II, III only   D. II, IV, V only
   B. I, III only   E. I, II, V only
   C. I, III, IV only

6. What name is given to microorganisms that live off dead organic matter?

   A. autotroph   D. virus
   B. saprophyte   E. heterotroph
   C. parasite

7. Identify point *B* on the bacterial growth curve shown in Figure 46.

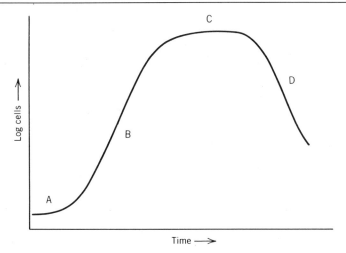

FIGURE 46

A. lag phase   D. stationary phase
B. logarithmic phase   E. acclimatization phase
C. death phase

8. An intracellular parasite characterized by a lack of independent metabolism and by the ability to reproduce only within living cells is called a _____ .

A. fungus   D. bacterium
B. virus   E. yeast cell
C. spore

9. What are the two characteristic morphologies of fungi?

A. yeasts and molds   D. spores and molds
B. hyphae and mycelia   E. yeasts and spores
C. hyphae and molds

10. Which method(s) of reproduction is(are) characteristic of bacteria?

   I. parthenogenesis
  II. simple division
 III. binary fission
  IV. missionary fusion
   V. conjugation

A. I only   D. II, III, V only
B. III, V only   E. I, III only
C. II, IV only

11. What term refers to a microorganism that causes disease in a debilitated host?

    A. opportunist   D. parasite
    B. pathogen   E. virulent
    C. endotoxin

12. The living together of microorganisms in which one member gains from the association while the other one is unaffected is called _____ .

    A. exploitation   D. mutualism
    B. marriage   E. commensalism
    C. antibiosis

13. Comma-shaped bacteria are termed _____ .

    A. coccobacillary   D. spirochetes
    B. streptobacillary   E. punctual
    C. vibrios

14. Bacteria that are classified as acid-fast retain what color during the staining procedure?

    A. violet   D. blue
    B. orange   E. red
    C. green

15. The pathogenic capability of microorganisms is described by which term?

    A. pathogenicity   D. pestilence
    B. virulence   E. opportunism
    C. pathognomonic

16. Which of the following substances are the most lethal to the humam organism?

    A. endotoxins   D. digoxins
    B. exotoxins   E. pyrotoxins
    C. enterotoxins

17. A bacterial cell that remains dormant until environmental conditions improve is called a _____ .

    A. fungus   D. virus
    B. macrophage   E. spore
    C. bacteriophage

18. Which of the following statements are true concerning nutritional growth requirements of bacteria?

    I. Bacteria generally require similar growth media.
    II. Carbon requirements for bacterial growth are usually provided by glucose or some other carbohydrate.

III. Some microorganisms require vitamins and amino acids

IV. Some bacteria can be cultured only in animals.

A. I, IV only

B. II, III only

C. II, III, IV only

D. II, IV only

E. I, II, III only

19. Which type(s) of microorganism(s) is(are) poisoned by the presence of oxygen in the environment?

I. obligate aerobes

II. obligate anaerobes

III. facultative anaerobes

A. I, III only

B. I only

C. II only

D. III only

E. II, III only

20. Which of the following components are characteristic of the prototype bacterium?

A. slime layer, cytoplasm, nucleoplasm

B. cell wall, slime layer, appendages

C. cell envelope, cytoplasm, appendages

D. cell wall, cytoplasm, nucleoplasm

E. protoplast, cytoplasm, spheroplast

21. Which statement best describes vector transmission of microorganisms?

A. physical transfer between a susceptible host and an infected person

B. transmission that occurs by the dissemination of droplet nuclei

C. the transfer between contaminated inanimate objects and a susceptible host

D. a carrier that transmits microorganisms from an infected person to a susceptible host

E. environmental conditions, such as wind, carrying infection to a susceptible host

22. The Ziehl-Neelsen's staining procedure will identify which microorganism?

A. *Staphylococcus aureus*

B. *Klebsiella pneumoniae*

C. *Pseudomonas aeruginosa*

D. *Escherichia coli*

E. *Mycobacterium tuberculosis*

23. Following a Gram stain procedure, gram-positive bacteria appear _____, and gram-negative bacteria appear _____ .

A. blue; red

B. pink; red

C. purple; violet

D. red; blue

E. red; violet

24. Which microorganism(s) is(are) classified as anaerobes?

I. *Clostridium tetani*

II. *Mycobacterium tuberculosis*

III. *Proteus vulgaris*
IV. *Corynebacterium diphtheriae*

A. II only
B. III only
C. I only
D. II, III only
E. II, III, IV only

25. Which of the following microorganisms are fungi?

  I. *Candida albicans*
  II. *Mycoplasma hominis*
  III. *Aspergillus fumigatus*
  IV. *Proteus vulgaris*

A. I, II, III only
B. I, III only
C. II, III only
D. I, IV only
E. III, IV only

26. Which microorganism(s) is(are) classified as bacteria?

  I. spirochetes
  II. streptococci
  III. rickettsiae
  IV. protozoa

A. I, II only
B. I, II, III only
C. II only
D. III only
E. I, III, IV only

27. Microorganisms that grow best at normal body temperature are called
_____ .

A. mesophiles
B. pyrogens
C. thermogens
D. temperobes
E. climaphiles

28. Bacteria that appear as irregular clusters when microscopically viewed are called
_____ .

A. diplococci
B. staphylococci
C. streptococci
D. mirococci
E. spirilla

29. Which of the following microorganisms is acid-fast?

A. *Hemophilus influenzae*
B. *Aspergillus fumigatus*
C. *Diplococcus pneumoniae*
D. *Mycobacterium tuberculosis*
E. *Clostridium perfringens*

30. Bacteria that assume various shapes are described as _____ .

A. polynuclear
B. multiprotoplasmic
C. pleolithic
D. pleomorphic
E. multicellular

31. Which of the following substances is used as the counterstain dye in the Gram stain procedure?

A. carbol-fuschin
B. crystal violet
C. safranin
D. methyl blue
E. acid-alcohol

32. What term describes the metabolically active form of a bacterium?

A. parasitic
B. dormant
C. endospore
D. spore
E. vegetative

33. Which of the following microorganisms are classified as lower protists?

I. rickettsiae
II. fungi
III. protozoa
IV. bacteria

A. I, II, III, IV
B. I, II, IV only
C. II, III only
D. I, II, III only
E. I, IV only

34. Which microorganism(s) only reproduce(s) within living cells?

I. rickettsiae
II. viruses
III. chlamydiae
IV. fungi

A. I, II, III only
B. II, IV only
C. III, IV only
D. II only
E. I, III only

35. Which microorganism has a nucleic acid core encapsulated by protein?

A. virus
B. spore
C. vegetative bacterium
D. protozoan
E. spheroplast

ASSESSMENT ANSWER SHEET

DIRECTIONS: Darken the space under the selected answer.

	A	B	C	D	E		A	B	C	D	E
1.	[ ]	[ ]	[ ]	[ ]	[ ]	19.	[ ]	[ ]	[ ]	[ ]	[ ]
2.	[ ]	[ ]	[ ]	[ ]	[ ]	20.	[ ]	[ ]	[ ]	[ ]	[ ]
3.	[ ]	[ ]	[ ]	[ ]	[ ]	21.	[ ]	[ ]	[ ]	[ ]	[ ]
4.	[ ]	[ ]	[ ]	[ ]	[ ]	22.	[ ]	[ ]	[ ]	[ ]	[ ]
5.	[ ]	[ ]	[ ]	[ ]	[ ]	23.	[ ]	[ ]	[ ]	[ ]	[ ]
6.	[ ]	[ ]	[ ]	[ ]	[ ]	24.	[ ]	[ ]	[ ]	[ ]	[ ]
7.	[ ]	[ ]	[ ]	[ ]	[ ]	25.	[ ]	[ ]	[ ]	[ ]	[ ]
8.	[ ]	[ ]	[ ]	[ ]	[ ]	26.	[ ]	[ ]	[ ]	[ ]	[ ]
9.	[ ]	[ ]	[ ]	[ ]	[ ]	27.	[ ]	[ ]	[ ]	[ ]	[ ]
10.	[ ]	[ ]	[ ]	[ ]	[ ]	28.	[ ]	[ ]	[ ]	[ ]	[ ]
11.	[ ]	[ ]	[ ]	[ ]	[ ]	29.	[ ]	[ ]	[ ]	[ ]	[ ]
12.	[ ]	[ ]	[ ]	[ ]	[ ]	30.	[ ]	[ ]	[ ]	[ ]	[ ]
13.	[ ]	[ ]	[ ]	[ ]	[ ]	31.	[ ]	[ ]	[ ]	[ ]	[ ]
14.	[ ]	[ ]	[ ]	[ ]	[ ]	32.	[ ]	[ ]	[ ]	[ ]	[ ]
15.	[ ]	[ ]	[ ]	[ ]	[ ]	33.	[ ]	[ ]	[ ]	[ ]	[ ]
16.	[ ]	[ ]	[ ]	[ ]	[ ]	34.	[ ]	[ ]	[ ]	[ ]	[ ]
17.	[ ]	[ ]	[ ]	[ ]	[ ]	35.	[ ]	[ ]	[ ]	[ ]	[ ]
18.	[ ]	[ ]	[ ]	[ ]	[ ]						

MICROBIOLOGY ANALYSES

Note: The references listed after each analysis are numbered and keyed to the reference list located at the end of this section. The first number indicates the text. The second number indicates the page where information about the question can be found. For example, (1:219,384) means that reference number 1 is to be used and that on pages 219 and 384 information about the question will be found. Frequently, it will be necessary to read beyond the page number indicated to obtain complete information. Therefore, reference to the question will be found either on the page indicated or on subsequent pages.

1. D. Anaerobic, aerobic bacteria, and rickettsiae will colonize bacterial culture media. Viruses are *not* bacteria; therefore, they will not colonize on bacterial media.
   (2:277–280), (6:422–423)

2. D. Both *Bacillus* and *Clostridium* are spore-forming genera.
   (2:276–277), (4:564)

3. E. Chemical agents that inhibit bacterial growth or multiplication are termed bacteriostatic. Bactericidal agents destroy bacteria.
   (4:580), (30:382)

4. A. Procaryotes (lower protists) include bacteria and algae. This category of the kingdom Protista consists of microorganisms lacking cellular organelles, such as a nucleus and mitochondria. Eucaryotes (higher protists), such as protozoa and fungi, have highly organized cellular structure and function.
   (2:268–269), (4:558), (6:417–419)

5. C. *Actinomyces israelii* (fungus), *Neisseria meningitidis* (gram-positive, aerobe), and *Staphylococcus aureus* (gram-positive, aerobe) are microorganisms that are normal residents of the respiratory flora.
   Pseudomonas aeruginosa is a gram-negative, aerobic bacterium found in the soil and water. It is a frequent inhabitant of respiratory care equipment, especially those containing water reservoirs. *Escherichia coli* is also a gram-negative, aerobic bacterium. It, however, is a normal resident of the gastrointestinal tract, sometimes invading the respiratory tract and producing a necrotizing pneumonia.
   (2:287,288–289), (4:569–573)

6. B. Saprophytes live off dead organic matter. Parasites live off living organic matter. Saprophytes and parasites are categorized under the general term heterotrophs, i.e., organisms living off organic matter. Autotrophs live off inorganic matter which they can synthesize into organic material.
   (4:563)

7. B. The various phases on a bacterial growth curve are identified on Figure 47.
   - A = *lag phase:* metabolic priorities are being arranged to synthesize proteins, lipids, and carbohydrates; a critical mass is generated to support cellular division

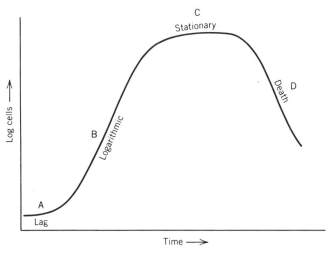

FIGURE 47

B = *logarithmic (exponential) phase:* total mass increases proportionately to the total viable cell number

C = *stationary phase:* depletion of nutrients limits cellular growth and division, and toxic by-products cause cellular death; cellular division equals cellular death

D = *death phase:* cellular death exceeds cellular growth and division.

(2:280–281), (4:562–563)

8. B. Viruses are infectious agents that reproduce only inside living cells. They are obligate intracellular parasites.
(2:292–295), (4:576–577), (6:423)

9. A. Ordinarily, fungi exist either as molds or yeasts. Molds grow from spores that germinate to form long tubular projections called *hyphae*. Numerous hyphae intertwine to form a fungal mass called a *mycelium*. Yeasts are unicellular, microscopic forms that reproduce by forming buds.

Most fungi are monomorphic, i.e., they exist as either molds or yeasts. Few fungi display dimorphism wherein both mold and yeast phases can be demonstrated in one species.
(2:291–292), (4:577–578), (6:420–421)

10. B. Bacterial cells generally divide by binary fission; that is, one cell grows into a two-cell configuration, then separation into two distinct cells occurs. Some bacterial species do, however, reproduce via conjugation (sexually).
(4:562)

11. A. A microorganism that causes disease in a debilitated host is called an opportunist. Pathogens refer to microorganisms that cause disease in a normal host.
(2:290), (4:565), (6:334)

12. E. The living together of two microorganisms in which there is benefit to one but no effect on the other is called *commensalism*. *Mutualism* refers to the living together of two microorganisms wherein both benefit from the association. *Antibiosis* is the living together of two microorganisms that is harmful to one or both.
(4:563), (6:416)

13. C. Morphologically, bacterial species are categorized as follows

1. comma-shaped: vibrios
2. round: cocci
3. cylindrical or rod-shaped: bacilli
4. spindle-shaped: fusiform
5. spiral-shaped: spirochete or spirillum

(2:269–270), (4:564–565), (6:421–422)

14. E. During the acid-fast (Ziehl-Neelsen) staining procedure, bacteria are first stained red with carbol-fuschin. Acid-fast microorganisms retain the red stain after being treated with a solution of acid-alcohol and a methyl blue counterstain. Blue-stained bacteria are not acid-fast.
(2:271), (4:565), (6:424–425)

15. B. Pathogenic microorganisms (disease-causing to normal hosts) are often described in terms of their degree of pathogenicity, known as *virulence*. The potential ability of a microorganism to cause disease is called its *pathogenicity*.
(2:290), (4:566), (6:426)

16. B. Exotoxins are produced by diphtheroids, *Clostridium tetani,* and *Clostridium botulinum*. These exotoxins are the most lethal to humans. *Endotoxins,* generally produced by gram-negative bacteria, are injurious toxins, but they are not as lethally potent as exotoxins.
(2:273,290), (4:566), (6:426)

17. E. Spore-forming bacteria, e.g., *Clostridium* species and *Bacillus anthracis,* are triggered to form spores when nutritional needs become depleted or when adverse conditions occur in the environment. The spore is a dormant form that is resistant to lethal effects of a variety of physical and chemical agents. Upon restoration of favorable environmental conditions, the spore germinates into a single vegetative cell capable of normal growth and cell division.
(2:276–277), (4:564)

18. C. Bacteria have varied nutritional growth requirements. Some require *minimal synthetic media,* i.e., a carbon source (glucose or some other carbohydrate) and inorganic salts. Others need *rich media,* i.e, a complex mixture of organic material (extracts of animal heart, brain, etc.) and inorganic salts. Some bacteria require special supplements such as metal chelating agents, vitamins, and amino acids, known as growth factors. A few bacteria (*Treponema pallidum* and *Mycobacterium leprae*) can be cultured only in animals.
(2:275–278), (4:562), (6:425–426)

19. C. Microorganisms classified as obligate aerobes require the presence of oxygen in their environment for survival. Obligate anaerobes must live in the absence of oxygen; otherwise, they will not survive. Facultative anaerobes have the capability of adjusting to an aerobic environment.
(2:278–279), (4:562), (6:419)

20. C. The typical bacterium has three distinct regions (1) cell envelope, (2) cytoplasm, and (3) appendages. The cell envelope can be either a *capsule* (large quantities of mucilagenous material), a *slime layer* (not a detectable amount of mucilagenous material), a *cell wall,* or a *cell membrane.* The cytoplasm contains various structures, e.g., *plasmids,* and *mesosomes.* Appendages can be either *flagella* or *pili* (sex pilus or common pilus).
(2:271–275), (4:558–562)

21. D. Transmission of infection by arthropods (e.g., insects, crustaceans) is vector transmission of disease. The vector itself may be infected, or it may be a mechanical carrier of the disease.
(21:147)

22. E. The Ziehl-Neelsen's staining procedure identifies microorganisms that are acid-fast, i.e., they retain the red stain from carbol-fuschin after rinsing with an acid-alcohol solution. Examples of microorganisms identified by this method include *Mycobacterium tuberculosis, Mycobacterium leprae,* and *Nocardia.*
(2:270–271), (4:565), (6:424–425)

23. A. The Gram stain procedure is used to identify bacteria that are gram-negative and gram-positive. During the staining procedure crystal violet dye stains the bacteria blue. Alcohol, a decolorizing agent, is then applied. After the decolorization step, a counterstain (red dye safranin) is applied. The bacteria that remain blue are gram-positive; those that stain red are gram-negative.
(2:270–271), (4:564–566), (6:424)

24. C. The bacteria *Clostridium tetani* (causes tetanus) are obligate anaerobes, i.e., they require an environment deprived of oxygen. Other members of the genus *Clostridium* that are anaerobes include *Clostridium botulinum* (causes botulism) and *Clostridium perfringens* (causes gas gangrene).
(2:279), (4:562,568)

25. B. *Candida albicans,* a resident of the normal respiratory flora, and *Aspergillus fumigatus* are fungi.
(2:291), (4:575,577,578), (6:420–421)

26. B. Rickettsiae are closely related to viruses because they survive only within living cells; however, they are classified as bacteria. Protozoa are single-celled animal

microorganisms. Spirochetes are bacteria resembling protozoa. They are spiral shaped and motile. Streptococci are gram-positive bacteria appearing in chains. (2:268,276), (4:564,570,576), (6:419–422)

27. A. Organisms optimally growing within the temperature range of 30°C to 45°C are called *mesophiles*. Some organisms grow best in cold temperatures. These organisms are called *psychrophiles*. *Thermophiles,* on the other hand, experience optimum growth between 55°C and 75°C.
(6:419)

28. B. Some genera of bacteria do not separate completely after cell division. As a result, varying spatial arrangements of cells occur depending on the species. Bacteria that divide in a single plane to their axis and develop into chains are called *strep*. For example, cocci that divide in this manner are referred to as *diplococci* if they occur in pairs, or *streptococci* if they occur as three or more. Organisms that divide in more that one plane to their axis develop into clusters. An example of organisms that divide in this manner are coccus-shaped bacteria called *staphylococci* (*staph* = grape-like clusters). Figure 48 depicts various types and spatial arrangements occurring among bacteria.
(2:270), (6:421)

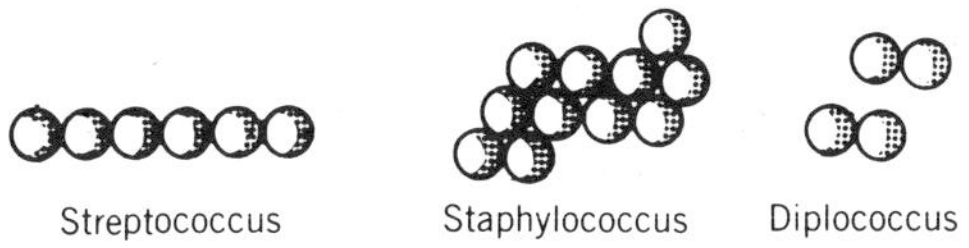

Streptococcus   Staphylococcus   Diplococcus

FIGURE 48

29. D. *Mycobacterium tuberculosis* is a species of rod-shaped bacteria that does not stain easily. However, once stained, it resists decolorization by acid or alcohol. Therefore, members of the species *Mycobacterium tuberculosis* are called "acid-fast" bacilli.
(2:271), (4:565), (6:424–425), (8:302)

30. D. The ability of an organism to assume two or more different forms is termed *pleomorphism*.
(13:125)

31. C. After the microorganisms are exposed to the crystal violet dye, they are washed with acid-alcohol, a decolorizing agent. Then, the counter-stain safranin (red dye) is applied to the microorganisms. Those that retain the blue stain are gram-positive; those that take on the red counterstain are gram-negative.
(2:271), (4:565), (4:424–425)

32. E. The vegetative state of a bacterium represents the metabolically active form of that microorganism.
(4:566)

33. E.

<pre>
                          ─── PROTISTA ───
                        ╱   ╲
HIGHER PROTISTS ───────   ─────── LOWER PROTISTS
protozoa   bacteria
fungi   rickettsiae
slime molds   mycoplasmas
algae   blue-green algae
</pre>

(2:268), (4:558), (6:419)

34. A. Rickettsiae, chlamydiae, and viruses are intracellular parasites, i.e., they only reproduce inside living cells.
(2:276), (4:576), (6:422–423)

35. A. Viruses are particles of protein and nucleic acids occasionally associated with lipids and carbohydrates. The protein forms a coat, or *capsid,* around a nucleic acid core. The nucleic acid can be either deoxyribonucleic acid (DNA) or ribonucleic acid (RNA), but not both.
(2:292), (4:576), (6:418–419,423)

REFERENCES

1. Spearman, C., and Sheldon, R., *Egan's Fundamentals of Respiratory Therapy,* 4th ed., C.V. Mosby, St. Louis, 1982.
2. Wojciechowski, W., *Respiratory Care Sciences: An Integrated Approach,* John Wiley & Sons, New York, 1985.
3. Shapiro, B., Harrison, R., Kacmarek, R., and Cane, R., *Clinical Application of Respiratory Care,* 3rd ed., Year Book Medical Publishers, Chicago, 1985.
4. Kacmarek, R., Mack, C., and Dimas, S., *The Essentials of Respiratory Therapy,* 2nd ed., Year Book Medical Publishers, Chicago, 1985.
5. McPherson, S., *Respiratory Therapy Equipment,* 3rd ed., C.V. Mosby, St. Louis, 1985.
6. Burton, G., and Hodgkin, J., *Respiratory Care: A Guide to Clinical Practice,* 2nd ed., J.B. Lippincott, Philadelphia, 1985.
7. Frownfelter, D., *Chest Physical Therapy and Cardiopulmonary Rehabilitation, An Interdisciplinary Approach,* Year Book Medical Publishers, Chicago, 1978.
8. Cherniack, R., and Cherniack, L., *Respiration in Health and Disease,* 3rd ed., W. B. Saunders, Philadelphia, 1983.
9. Daily, E., and Schroeder, G., *Techniques in Bedside Hemodynamic Monitoring,* 3rd ed., C.V. Mosby, St. Louis, 1985.
10. Des Jardins, R., *Clinical Manifestations of Respiratory Disease,* Year Book Medical Publishers, Chicago, 1984.
11. Mitchell, R., *Synopsis of Clinical Pulmonary Disease,* 3rd ed., C.V. Mosby, St. Louis, 1982.
12. Comroe, J., *Physiology of Respiration,* 3rd ed., Year Book Medical Publishers, Chicago, 1974.
13. West, J., *Pulmonary Pathophysiology—The Essentials,* 2nd ed., Williams & Wilkins, Baltimore, 1982.
14. West, J., *Respiratory Physiology—The Essentials,* 3rd ed., Williams & Wilkins, Baltimore, 1985.

15. Martz, K., et al., *Management of the Patient-Ventilator System: A Team Approach,* 2nd ed., C.V. Mosby, St. Louis, 1984.
16. Shoup, C., and McHenry, R., *Laboratory Exercises in Respiratory Therapy,* 2nd ed., C.V. Mosby, St. Louis, 1983.
17. Ruppel, G., *Manual of Pulmonary Function Testing,* 3rd ed., C.V. Mosby, St. Louis, 1982.
18. Appelbaum, E., and Bruce, D., *Tracheal Intubation,* W. B. Saunders, Philadelphia, 1976.
19. Rau, J., *Respiratory Therapy Pharmacology,* 2nd ed., Year Book Medical Publishers, Chicago, 1984.
20. United States Department of Health, Education, and Welfare, Public Health Service, *Isolation Techniques for Use in Hospitals,* 2nd ed., Washington, D.C., 1975.
21. Brooks, S., *Integrated Basic Science,* 4th ed., C.V. Mosby, St. Louis, 1979.
22. Comroe, J., *The Lung,* Year Book Medical Publishers, Chicago, 1962.
23. Shibel, E., and Moser, K., *Respiratory Emergencies,* 2nd ed., C.V. Mosby, St. Louis, 1982.
24. Tisi, G., *Pulmonary Physiology in Clinical Medicine,* 2nd ed., Williams & Wilkins, Baltimore, 1985.
25. Cherniack, R., *Pulmonary Function Testing,* W. B. Saunders, Philadelphia, 1977.
26. Altose, M., *The Physiological Basis of Pulmonary Function Testing,* Clinical Symposia-CIBA, Vol. 31, No. 2, Summit, New Jersey, 1979.
27. Shapiro, B., Harrison, R., and Walton, J., *Clinical Application of Arterial Blood Gases,* 3rd ed., Year Book Medical Publishers, Chicago, 1982.
28. West, J., *Ventilation/Blood Flow and Gas Exchange,* 3rd ed., Blackwell Scientific Publications, 1979.
29. Slonim, N., and Hamilton, K., *Respiratory Physiology,* 4th ed., C.V. Mosby, St. Louis, 1981.
30. Rarey, K., and Youtsey, J., *Respiratory Patient Care,* Prentice-Hall, Englewood Cliffs, 1981.
31. Berne, R., and Levy, M., *Physiology,* The C.V. Mosby, St. Louis, 1983.
32. Levitzky, M., *Pulmonary Physiology,* 2nd ed., McGraw-Hill, New York, 1986.
33. Wilson, P., Bell, C., and Norton, A., *Rehabilitation of the Heart and Lungs,* SensorMedics, 1980.
34. Clausen, J., and Zarins, L., *Pulmonary Function Testing Guidlines and Controversies,* Academic Press, New York, 1982.
35. Klaus, M., and Fanaroff, A., *Care of the High-Risk Neonate,* 2nd ed., W. B. Saunders, Philadelphia, 1979.
36. Lough, M., et al., *Pediatric Respiratory Therapy,* 3rd ed., Year Book Medical Publishers, Chicago, 1985.
37. Levin, D., et al., *A Practical Guide to Pediatric Intensive Care,* 2nd ed., C.V. Mosby, St. Louis, 1984.
38. O'Ryan, J., and Burns, D., *Pulmonary Rehabilitation from Hospital to Home,* Year Book Medical Publishers, Chicago, 1984.
39. Bell, C., et al., *Home Care and Rehabilitation in Respiratory Medicine,* J. B. Lippincott, Philadelphia, 1984.
40. Wilkins, R., et al., *Clinical Assessment in Respiratory Care,* C.V. Mosby, St. Louis, 1985.
41. Jones, N., and Campbell, E., *Clinical Exercise Testing,* 2nd ed., W. B. Saunders, Philadelphia, 1982.
42. Goldsmith, J., and Karotkin, E., *Assisted Ventilation of the Neonate,* W. B. Saunders, Philadelphia, 1981.
43. Blowers, M., and Sims, R., *How to Read an ECG,* 3rd ed., Medical Economics, New Jersey, 1983.
44. Eubanks, D., and Bone, R., *Comprehensive Respiratory Care,* C.V. Mosby, St. Louis, 1985.

45. Rattenborg, C., *Clinical Use of Mechanical Ventilation,* Year Book Medical Publishers, Chicago, 1981.
46. Witkowski, A. S., *Pulmonary Assessment: A Clinical Guide,* J.B. Lippincott, Philadelphia, 1985.
47. Op't Holt, Timothy B., *Assessment Based Respiratory Care,* John Wiley & Sons, New York, 1986.

PHARMACOLOGY ASSESSMENT

This 50-item section is intended to evaluate your understanding and comprehension of a variety of pharmacologic principles. Included in this assessment are questions pertaining to (1) basic pharmacology, (2) receptor theory, (3) neurologic anatomy and physiology, (4) drug dilution problems, and (5) medications (bronchodilators, corticosteroids, diuretics, etc.).

DIRECTIONS: Each of the questions or incomplete statements is followed by five suggested answers. Select the one which is the best in each case and then blacken the corresponding space on the answer sheet.

1. The term that refers to the time it takes for a drug to be inactivated by or excreted from the body is ——————— .

   A. absorption
   B. threshold level
   C. tolerance

   D. half-life
   E. accumulation

2. Which of the following medications are considered mucokinetic agents?

   I. sodium bicarbonate
   II. 10% saline solution
   III. acetylcysteine
   IV. SSKI

   A. I, II, III, IV
   B. I, II only
   C. I, II, III only

   D. I, III, IV only
   E. I, III only

3. Which of the following terms describes the dosage of a medication that would be lethal to 50% of a population?

   A. ED_{50}
   B. LD_{50}
   C. TI

   D. dose response
   E. adverse reaction

4. How much 20% Mucomyst should be added to 1.0 ml of 0.9% saline to obtain a 13% solution?

A. 0.53 cc   D. 2.85 cc
B. 1.53 cc   E. 16 cc
C. 1.86 cc

5. Which of the following medications are categorized as nondepolarizing neuromuscular blocking agents?

   I. pancuronium
  II. succinylcholine
 III. gallamine
 IV. *d*-Tubocurarine

A. I, II, III, IV
B. II, III, only
C. I, IV only
D. I, III, IV only
E. I, II, III only

6. The therapeutic potential of prostaglandin E (PGE) is its ability to produce

_____ .

A. diuresis   D. pulmonary vasoconstriction
B. positive inotropism   E. bronchodilatation
C. negative chronotropism

7. Which of the following diuretics cause diuresis by inhibiting NaCl transport in the ascending limb of the loop of Henle?

   I. ethacrynic acid
  II. Diuril
 III. Lasix
 IV. mannitol

A. II, IV only   D. III, IV only
B. I, II, III only   E. I, II only
C. I, III only

8. Which diuretic(s) is(are) classified as (a) carbonic anhydrase inhibitor(s)?

   I. mannitol
  II. spironolactone
 III. acetazolamide
 IV. chlorathiazide

A. I, II only   D. II, III only
B. IV only   E. III only
C. III, IV only

9. Which drug is the principal chemical mediator at the majority of the postganglionic neuroeffector junctions along the sympathetic nervous system?

   A. acetylcholine
   B. norepinephrine
   C. anticholinesterase
   D. amine oxidase
   E. doxapram

10. How else can a 1:200 drug solution be expressed?

    A. 0.05%
    B. 0.5%
    C. 1.0%
    D. 1 g/10 cc
    E. 1 ml/200 g

11. Which of the following drugs are classified as sympathomimetic agents?

    I. epinephrine
    II. ephedrine
    III. isoetharine hydrochloride
    IV. isoproterenol hydrochloride
    V. atropine

    A. I, II, III, IV, V
    B. II, III, IV only
    C. I, III, IV, V only
    D. I, II, III, IV only
    E. II, V only

12. Which of the following medications are known for their fungicidal activity?

    I. polymyxin B
    II. amphotericin B
    III. nystatin
    IV. griseofulvin

    A. II, III, IV only
    B. I, II only
    C. I, III, IV only
    D. III, IV only
    E. II, III only

13. Which of the following medications do *not* stimulate alpha-adrenergic receptor sites?

    I. albuterol
    II. terbutaline sulfate
    III. norepinephrine
    IV. epinephrine

    A. I, II, IV only
    B. III, IV only
    C. I, II only
    D. II, IV only
    E. I, III only

14. Which statement(s) accurately describe(s) pharmacologic conditions that influence intracellular levels of cyclic $3'5'$-AMP in bronchial smooth muscle cells?

I. Methylxanthines inhibit the release of guanylate cyclase, thereby decreasing cyclic 3'5'-GMP levels.

II. Alpha-adrenergic drugs inhibit phosphodiesterase activity, thus increasing cyclic 3'5'-AMP levels.

III. Beta-adrenergic drugs increase the release of adenylate cyclase, hence producing greater amounts of cycle 3'5'-AMP.

IV. Stimulation of cholinergic receptors increases guanylate cyclase levels, which, in turn, increases cyclic 3'5'-GMP levels.

A. III, IV only
B. I only
C. II, III, IV only
D. I, II, III only
E. IV only

15. How many milligrams are there in 3 cc of a 10% Mucomyst W/V solution?

A. 3 mg
B. 5 mg
C. 30 mg
D. 300 mg
E. 3,000 mg

16. Which enzyme(s) is(are) responsible for the inactivation of norepinephrine?

I. catechol-o-methyl transferase
II. carbonic anhydrase
III. phosphodiesterase
IV. monoamine oxidase

A. I, IV only
B. I only
C. III only
D. II, IV only
E. II, III, IV only

17. Which of the following medications can be used to reverse the action of morphine?

I. meperdine
II. naloxone
III. methadone
IV. levallorphan

A. I, III only
B. II, IV only
C. I, II only
D. III, IV only
E. II, III only

18. Potential side effects from long-term use of dexamethasone include

I. hirsutism
II. redistribution of body fat
III. hypertension
IV. inactivation of circulating antibodies

A. I, II, IV only

B. II, III, IV only

C. II, III only

D. I, III only

E. I, II, III, IV

19. Which of the following antibiotics exhibit their antimicrobial activity via inhibition of protein synthesis?

   I. streptomycin

  II. chloramphenicol

 III. tobramycin

 IV. erythromycin

A. I, III, IV only

B. II, III only

C. I, IV only

D. I, II only

E. I, II, III, IV

20. Which of the following microorganisms can become penicillin-resistant?

   I. *Pseudomonas aeruginosa*

  II. *Escherichia coli*

 III. *Mycobacterium tuberculosis*

 IV. *Bacillus anthracis*

A. I, IV only

B. II, III only

C. II, III, IV only

D. I, II only

E. I, II, III, IV

21. At which site(s) is(are) muscarinic effects demonstrated?

   I. parasympathetic neuroeffector site

  II. parasympathetic ganglionic synapse

 III. sympathetic ganglionic synapse

 IV. sympathetic neuroeffector site

A. I, II only

B. III, IV only

C. I only

D. IV only

E. II, III, IV only

22. What term describes the influence of two drugs of similar action administered together eliciting a response greater than the sum of the two drugs' individual effects?

A. synergism

B. potentiation

C. cumulation

D. additive

E. antagonism

23. If 2 ml of solute are added to 98 ml of solvent, what percent solution would result?

A. 0.002%

B. 0.02%

C. 0.2%

D. 2.0%

E. 20.0%

24. Which anatomic area of a nerve cell receives the transmitted nerve impulse?

A. axon
B. dendrite
C. perikaryon

D. bouton
E. nodes of Ranvier

25. Sympathetic neurons arise from which area(s) of the spinal cord and /or brain?

I. sacral
II. thoracic
III. brain stem
IV. lumbar
V. midbrain

A. II only
B. I, II, IV only
C. II, IV only

D. I, III, V only
E. II, III, IV only

26. Which enzyme(s) inactivate(s) the neurotransmitter acetylcholine?

I. anticholinesterase
II. monoamine oxidase
III. cholinesterase
IV. phosphodiesterase

A. III only
B. II, III only
C. I, III only

D. II, IV only
E. I only

27. If Mucomyst is ordered for an asthmatic patient, what other medication(s) should be concomitantly administered? (The mode of delivery is nebulization.)

I. Neo-Synephrine
II. cromolyn sodium
III. an antihistamine
IV. isoproterenol hydrochloride
V. any medication having a predominently beta-1 effect

A. I, II only
B. IV, V only
C. II, III only

D. III only
E. IV only

28. Which of the following statements are true concerning racemic epinephrine?

I. It is commercially available in a 1:100 solution.
II. Its beta-2 effect is similar in magnitude to that of Isuprel.
III. It is used as a topical vasoconstrictor.
IV. Its standard dosage is 0.5 ml diluted in 4.0 ml of normal saline.

A. III, IV only

B. II, III only

C. I, III, IV only

D. I, II only

E. I, II, III, IV

29. Sympathomimetic amines may be useful nasal decongestants because _____ .

    A. they may elicit an alpha-adrenergic response
    B. they produce vasodilatation to the nasal mucosa
    C. they inhibit the release of SRS-A
    D. they are able to reduce cardiac output
    E. they stimulate both beta-1 and beta-2 receptors

30. You have been asked to give an aerosol treatment with 10 cc of 1:200 Isuprel. How many milligrams of Isuprel would you be administering to the patient?

    A. 0.05 mg

    B. 0.20 mg

    C. 0.50 mg

    D. 20.00 mg

    E. 50.00 mg

31. Which of the following activities are the result of sympathetic system receptor stimulation?

    I. bronchodilatation
    II. tachycardia
    III. tachypnea
    IV. vasoconstriction

    A. I, II, III, IV

    B. II, III only

    C. I, II only

    D. I, II, IV only

    E. III, IV only

32. If you were asked to administer 4.0 cc of 10% Mucomyst W/V and all that is available is 20% Mucomyst W/V, how much of the 20% solution would be use to give the same dose?

    A. 0.4 cc

    B. 0.2 cc

    C. 2.0 mg

    D. 2.0 cc

    E. 20.0 mg

33. A medication that increases the force of contractility of the myocardium is said to display _____ .

    A. positive chronotropism

    B. positive inotropism

    C. positive contractility

    D. positive depolarization

    E. positive automaticity

34. Which of the following routes of drug administration exemplify the parenteral route?

    I. inhalation

    II. intramuscular

    III. rectal

    IV. oral

    V. intravenous

A. II, V only   D. I, IV only

B. III, IV only   E. I, II, V only

C. I, III, IV only

35. A 5.5% solution with a total weight of 100 g contains how many grams of solute and how many grams of solvent?

    A. 94.5 g of solvent; 5.5 g of solute

    B. 45.0 g of solvent; 55.0 g of solute

    C. 55.0 g of solvent; 45.0 g of solute

    D. 44.5 g of solvent; 55.5 g of solute

    E. 12.0 g of solvent; 88.0 g of solute

36. What is the acceptable dosage for administering 1:100 solution of isoproterenol hydrochloride via nebulization?

    A. 1.0 cc to 3.0 cc in 4 cc of normal saline

    B. 0.25 cc to 0.5 cc in 4 cc of normal saline

    C. 3.5 cc to 4.0 cc in 5 cc of normal saline

    D. 0.5 cc to 1.5 cc in 4 cc of normal saline

    E. 1.0 cc to 1.5 cc in 4 cc of normal saline

37. Which of the following medications *may* be useful in treating acute bronchospasm?

    I. metaproterenol sulfate

    II. Proventil

    III. Intal

    IV. atropine

A. I, II, III, IV   D. I, IV only

B. II, III only   E. I, III only

C. I, II, IV only

38. Which of the following medications are classified as cardiac beta-blocking agents?

    I. metaprolol

    II. butorphanol

    III. propranolol

    IV. levorphanol

A. I, II, IV only   D. II, III only

B. II, IV only   E. I, II, III, IV

C. I, III only

39. The term used to describe a drug's name belonging to one manufacturer only is the
    _____ .

    A. generic name   D. code name
    B. brand name   E. official name
    C. chemical name

40. The log-dose response curve illustrated in Figure 49 demonstrates the
    _____ of drug A compared with drug B.

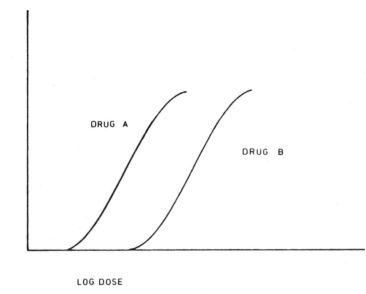

FIGURE 49

    A. therapeutic index   D. compatibility
    B. efficacy   E. potency
    C. affinity

41. Which of the following situations will increase the level of intracellular 3'5'-
    guanosine monophosphate (cyclic GMP) in bronchial smooth muscle cells?

    I. beta-2 stimulation
    II. phosphodiesterase inhibition
    III. cholinergic stimulation
    IV. alpha-stimulation

    A. I, II only   D. III, IV only
    B. II, IV only   E. II, III, IV only
    C. I, III only

42. Which of the following substances are considered mediators released during mast cell
    degranulation?

   I. slow-reacting substance of anaphylaxis

   II. immuglobulin E

   III. heparin

   IV. eosinophilic chemotactic factor of anaphylaxis

A. II, III only

B. I, III, IV only

C. I, IV only

D. I, II, IV only

E. I, II, III, IV

43. How many micrograms are there in 3.0 mg?

A. 0.3 μg

B. 3.0 μg

C. 30.0 μg

D. 300.0 μg

E. 3,000.0 μg

44. The study of the flow and deformation of matter is called _____ .

A. mucokinetics

B. mucology

C. rheology

D. viscosity

E. kinetics

45. How many milliters of diluent must be added to 10 ml of a 20% W/V solution of Mucomyst to make a 10% W/V solution of acetylcysteine?

A. 30 cc

B. 20 cc

C. 15 cc

D. 10 cc

E. 5 cc

46. Which of the following effects are attributed to xanthine administration?

   I. diuresis

   II. bronchodilatation

   III. cardiac stimulation

   IV. central nervous system stimulation

A. I, II, III, IV

B. II, III only

C. I, IV only

D. II, III, IV only

E. I, II, III only

47. Which of the following medications purportedly have *minimal* beta-1 stimulation?

   I. Ventolin

   II. Alupent

   III. Bricanyl

   IV. Bronkosol

A. II, III only

B. I, IV only

C. II, III, IV only

D. I, III only

E. I, II, III, IV

48. What is the primary purpose for nebulizing ethyl alcohol?

    A. to provide topical analgesia
    B. to induce analgesia via systemic absorption
    C. to lyse disulfide bonds in mucus
    D. to reduce the surface tension of the frothy secretions of pulmonary edema
    E. to alleviate respiratory mucosal edema

49. You are asked to administer 700 mg of solu-cortef (cortisol sodium succinate) via aerosolization. You have a 6-cc vial containing 1 g/ml. What volume of the solution must be drawn up to administer the prescribed amount?

    A. 0.7 cc   D. 5.2 cc
    B. 1.4 cc   E. 6.0 cc
    C. 4.2 cc

50. Which of the following responses are considered parasympathetic?

    I. bronchoconstriction
    II. negative inotropism
    III. positive chronotropism
    IV. systemic vasodilatation

    A. I, II, III, IV   D. I, II only
    B. II, III only   E. I, II, IV only
    C. I, IV only

ASSESSMENT ANSWER SHEET

DIRECTIONS: Darken the space under the selected answer.

	A	B	C	D	E		A	B	C	D	E
1.	[ ]	[ ]	[ ]	[ ]	[ ]	26.	[ ]	[ ]	[ ]	[ ]	[ ]
2.	[ ]	[ ]	[ ]	[ ]	[ ]	27.	[ ]	[ ]	[ ]	[ ]	[ ]
3.	[ ]	[ ]	[ ]	[ ]	[ ]	28.	[ ]	[ ]	[ ]	[ ]	[ ]
4.	[ ]	[ ]	[ ]	[ ]	[ ]	29.	[ ]	[ ]	[ ]	[ ]	[ ]
5.	[ ]	[ ]	[ ]	[ ]	[ ]	30.	[ ]	[ ]	[ ]	[ ]	[ ]
6.	[ ]	[ ]	[ ]	[ ]	[ ]	31.	[ ]	[ ]	[ ]	[ ]	[ ]
7.	[ ]	[ ]	[ ]	[ ]	[ ]	32.	[ ]	[ ]	[ ]	[ ]	[ ]
8.	[ ]	[ ]	[ ]	[ ]	[ ]	33.	[ ]	[ ]	[ ]	[ ]	[ ]
9.	[ ]	[ ]	[ ]	[ ]	[ ]	34.	[ ]	[ ]	[ ]	[ ]	[ ]
10.	[ ]	[ ]	[ ]	[ ]	[ ]	35.	[ ]	[ ]	[ ]	[ ]	[ ]
11.	[ ]	[ ]	[ ]	[ ]	[ ]	36.	[ ]	[ ]	[ ]	[ ]	[ ]
12.	[ ]	[ ]	[ ]	[ ]	[ ]	37.	[ ]	[ ]	[ ]	[ ]	[ ]
13.	[ ]	[ ]	[ ]	[ ]	[ ]	38.	[ ]	[ ]	[ ]	[ ]	[ ]
14.	[ ]	[ ]	[ ]	[ ]	[ ]	39.	[ ]	[ ]	[ ]	[ ]	[ ]
15.	[ ]	[ ]	[ ]	[ ]	[ ]	40.	[ ]	[ ]	[ ]	[ ]	[ ]
16.	[ ]	[ ]	[ ]	[ ]	[ ]	41.	[ ]	[ ]	[ ]	[ ]	[ ]
17.	[ ]	[ ]	[ ]	[ ]	[ ]	42.	[ ]	[ ]	[ ]	[ ]	[ ]
18.	[ ]	[ ]	[ ]	[ ]	[ ]	43.	[ ]	[ ]	[ ]	[ ]	[ ]
19.	[ ]	[ ]	[ ]	[ ]	[ ]	44.	[ ]	[ ]	[ ]	[ ]	[ ]
20.	[ ]	[ ]	[ ]	[ ]	[ ]	45.	[ ]	[ ]	[ ]	[ ]	[ ]
21.	[ ]	[ ]	[ ]	[ ]	[ ]	46.	[ ]	[ ]	[ ]	[ ]	[ ]
22.	[ ]	[ ]	[ ]	[ ]	[ ]	47.	[ ]	[ ]	[ ]	[ ]	[ ]
23.	[ ]	[ ]	[ ]	[ ]	[ ]	48.	[ ]	[ ]	[ ]	[ ]	[ ]
24.	[ ]	[ ]	[ ]	[ ]	[ ]	49.	[ ]	[ ]	[ ]	[ ]	[ ]
25.	[ ]	[ ]	[ ]	[ ]	[ ]	50.	[ ]	[ ]	[ ]	[ ]	[ ]

PHARMACOLOGY ANALYSES

Note: The references listed after each analysis are numbered and keyed to the reference list located at the end of this section. The first number indicates the text. The second number indicates the page where information about the question will be found. For example, (1:219,384) means that reference number 1 is to be used and that on pages 219 and 384 information about the question will be found. Frequently, it will be necessary to read beyond the page number indicated to obtain complete information. Therefore, reference to the question will be found either on the page indicated or on subsequent pages.

1. D. The term *half-life* refers to the length of time it takes for half the dosage of a medication to be metabolically broken down and inactivated by the body, or excreted from the body by the renal system.
   (1:383), (19:28)

2. A. Mucokinetic agents can be classified as either inhalational or noninhalational.

INHALATIONAL	NONINHALATIONAL
Sodium bicarbonate	SSKI (potassium iodide)
Normal saline (0.9% NaCl)	Salt (NaCl, NH_4Cl, etc.)
Hypotonic saline (0.45% NaCl)	Terpin hydrate
Hypertonic saline (1.8 to 15% NaCl)	Guaifenesin
Water	Syrup of ipecac
Acetylcysteine (Mucomyst)	
Proteolytic enzymes (DNA, trypsin, streptokinase)	
Alcohol	

   (1:411–415), (3:121), (4:531), (6:459–466), (19:122,129), (30:92–95)

3. B. The designation LD_{50} refers to the medication dose that would be lethal to 50% of a population. The term ED_{50} represents the dosage that would be therapeutically effective for 50% of the population. The therapeutic index (TI) is the ratio of lethal dose to 50% of the population (LD_{50}) to the effective dose to 50% of the population (ED_{50}). Quantitatively,

$$TI = \frac{LD_{50}}{ED_{50}}$$

A low TI value indicates that the lethal and therapeutic dosages are similar, therefore, the medication places the patient at a greater risk for adverse reactions or toxicity.
(4:527), (19:28)

4. C. STEP 1: Disregard the 0.9% W/V NaCl (the diluent) because it will not be considered in the calculation.
   STEP 2: Determine the symbols to use for V_1 and V_2.

1. V_1 can be represented by X.
2. V_2 can be represented by $X + 1$ because V_2 will be the sum of V_1 (which is X) and 1.0 ml of diluent.

STEP 3: Set up a proportion.

$$V_1C_1 = V_2C_2$$

where

V_1 = original volume
C_1 = original concentration
V_2 = new volume
C_2 = new concentration

STEP 4: Insert known values into the proportion and solve for X.

$$V_1C_1 = V_2C_2$$

where

$V_1 = X$
$C_1 = 20\%$
$V_2 = X + 1$
$C_2 = 13\%$
$(X)(20\%) = (X + 1)(13\%)$
$20X = 13X + 13$
$7X = 13$
$X = 1.86$ ml

Alternatively, V_1 can be represented by $X - 1$, and V_2 by X. The calculation would then be as follows

$$(X - 1)(20\%) = (X)(13\%)$$
$$20X - 20 = 13X$$
$$7X = 20$$
$$X = 2.86 \text{ ml}$$

In this case, because $V_2 = X$, you must subtract the 1.0 ml of diluent from V_2 to obtain the original volume of Mucomyst. Therefore,

$$X - 1.0 \text{ ml} = V_1$$
$$2.86 \text{ ml} - 1.0 \text{ ml} = 1.86 \text{ ml}$$

(1:63–64), (2:11–12), (4:6–7), (19:39), (30:109–111)

5. D. Pancuronium bromide (Pavulon), gallamine triethiodide (Flaxedil), and tubocurarine chloride (*d*-Turbocurarine) are classified as nondepolarizing neuromuscular blocking agents, or competitive blockers. These medications paralyze muscles by competing for acetylcholine at the receptor sites at the neuromuscular junction.

Succinylcholine chloride (Anectine) is a depolarizing neuromuscular blocking agent. Depolarization of the muscle membrane occurs, thus preventing muscle stimulation. The postsynaptic membrane is held in a refractory state.

(1:615–616), (4:543–544), (19:200–208), (30:102–104)

6. E. The potential benefit of prostaglandin E (PGE) is its ability to produce bronchodilatation. The mode of action of this drug occurs via direct activity on smooth muscle cells. PGE causes the release of adenylate cyclase, which, in turn, results in
an increased level of intracellular cyclic 3′,5′-adenosine monophosphate (AMP).
Increased intracellular levels of cyclic 3′,5′-AMP promote bronchial smooth muscle relaxation.

(1:408), (6:482), (19:274–280), (30:85)

7. C. Both ethacrynic acid (Edecrin) and furosemide (Lasix) are diuretics (loop diuretics) that act on the ascending limb of the loop of Henle. They cause the inhibition
of NaCl transport at that site on the nephron. The administration of either of these
two drugs can induce a metabolic alkalosis caused by excessive chloride loss or
hypochloremia.

Diuril (chlorothiazide) is a thiazide diuretic. Thiazide diuretics act on the proximal
convoluted tubule inhibiting sodium reabsorption. A metabolic alkalosis can be
induced, as potassium depletion (hypokalemia) also occurs.

Mannitol (Osmitrol) is an osmotic diuretic which prevents the reabsorption of certain substances filtered at the glomerulus.

(4:547–549), (6:277–278), (19:269–271), (30:100)

8. E. Acetazolamide (Diamox) is classified as a carbonic anhydrase inhibitor. Its mechanism of action is to inhibit the activity of the enzyme carbonic anhydrase (CA).
Carbonic anhydrase catalyzes (accelerates) the hydration of carbon dioxide according to the following reaction.

$$CO_2 + H_2O \xrightarrow{\quad CA \quad} H_2CO_3 \longrightarrow H^+ + HCO_3^-$$

By inhibiting carbonic anhydrase in the kidney cells, acetazolamide ultimately
prevents the reaction between H^+ and HCO_3^- in the filtrate. As a result, sodium
and water reabsorption are inhibited. Figure 50 illustrates the interaction among
H^+ secretion, HCO_3^- reabsorption, and the influence of carbonic anhydrase on the
reaction between water and carbon dioxide.

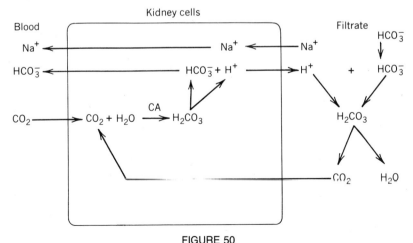

FIGURE 50

(4:163,548), (19:268,269–270)

9. B. Norepinephrine is the mediator or neurotransmitter at the postganglionic neuroeffector junction sites along the sympathetic nervous system. Acetylcholine is the neurotransmitter at (1) the preganglionic synapse along the parasympathetic nervous system, (2) the postganglionic neuroeffector junction along the parasympathetic nervous system, and (3) the preganglionic synapse along the sympathetic nervous system.
   (1:389–391), (4:149–151), (6:275), (19:51–61)

10. B. A 1:200 solution is a ratio solution comprised of 1 g of solute dissolved in 200 ml of solvent. Therefore, it is a weight/volume (W/V) solution.
   Even though this type of solution is not a true percent solution, it can be expressed as a percent. For example, a 1:200 solution represents 1 g/200 ml or

   $$\frac{1}{200} \times 100 = 0.5\%$$

   (1:59), (2:11–13,16), (3:114–115), (4:5), (6:489), (19:43), (30:109–110)

11. D. Pharmacologic agents that stimulate the sympathetic nervous system are classified broadly as sympathomimetics. More specifically, sympathomimetics may be classified according to their receptor activity, such as alpha, beta-1, and beta-2. Epinephrine, ephedrine, isoproterenol hydrochloride, and isoetharine hydrochloride are sympathomimetic agents. Atropine is classified as a parasympatholytic because it blocks the effects of the parasympathetic nervous system. It is also described as an anticholinergic bronchodilator.
   (1:400–402), (4:542), (6:482–483), (19:251), (30:80–81)

12. A. Amphotericin B, nystatin, and griseofulvin are antifungal (fungicidal) agents. Amphotericin B disrupts membrane integrity by binding to sterols. Unfortunately, mammalian cells also contain sterols. Therefore, amphotericin B is highly toxic. Nystatin is a topical antifugal agent. Griseofulvin inhibits nucleic acid synthesis within the fungus.
   (2:287,292), (6:484), (19:192–193)

13. C. The following medications do not stimulate alpha-adrenergic receptor sites.

GENERIC NAME	TRADE NAME
Isoproterenol hydrochloride	Isuprel
Isoetharine hydrochloride	Bronkosol
Metaproterenol sulfate	Alupent, Metaprel
Albuterol	Ventolin, Proventil
Terbutaline sulfate	Bricanyl, Brethine

   The medications primarily elicit bronchodilatation via beta-2 stimulation. They have varying beta-1 influences.
   Both epinephrine and norepinephrine stimulate alpha-adrenergic receptors. Norepinephrine is primarily an alpha-agonist, whereas epinephrine stimulates the alpha, beta-1, and beta-2 receptors more or less equally.
   (1:391,394–399), (3:119), (4:534,536–538), (6:467), (19:66), (30:86–91)

14. A. Proceeding counterclockwise in Figure 51, beta-2 adrenergic agonists (1) are useful for restoring bronchial smooth muscle tone, because they stimulate the activation of adenylate cyclase, thereby increasing bronchial smooth muscle levels of
cyclic AMP and promote bronchodilatation.

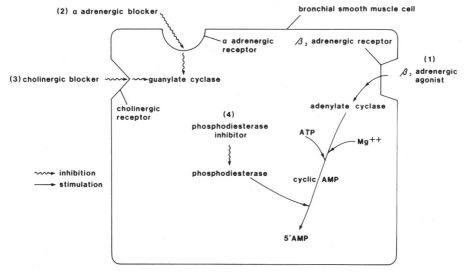

FIGURE 51

Because guanylate cyclase catalyzes the production of cyclic GMP, the cyclic nu-
cleotide thought to be responsible for bronchospasm, its inhibition by pharmacologic agents decreases cyclic GMP levels and promotes bronchodilatation (2).
Therefore, alpha-adrenergic blockers are presumably effective in decreasing intracellular cyclic GMP levels. Likewise, medications that block cholinergic receptor
sites (3) inhibit the activity of guanylate cyclase, lessening cyclic GMP levels and
eliciting bronchial smooth muscle relaxation. Additionally, medications that directly inhibit the action of phosphodiesterase (4), the enzyme responsible for the
degradation of cyclic AMP to 5'-AMP, facilitate the reversal of bronchospasm.
Their utility manifests itself in reducing the degradation or inactivation of cyclic
AMP to 5'-AMP.
(2:255–260), (4:534), (6:466–469), (19:170–181), (30:84–85)

15. D. A 10% Mucomyst W/V solution contains 10 g of solute in 100 ml or cc of solution.

STEP 1: Express the concentration as a fraction of the solute divided by the total
solution.

$$10\% \ \text{W/V} = \frac{10 \ \text{g}}{100 \ \text{ml}}$$

$$= \frac{10,000 \ \text{mg}}{100 \ \text{ml}}$$

STEP 2: Set up a proportion.

$$\frac{3 \text{ cc}}{100 \text{ cc}} = \frac{X}{10,000 \text{ mg}}$$

$$30,000 \text{ mg} = 100 \, X$$

$$\frac{30,000 \text{ mg}}{100} = X$$

$$300 \text{ mg} = X$$

Therefore, a 10% Mucomyst W/V solution contains 300 mg of solute.

(1:63–64), (2:11–13,16), (3:114–115), (4:6–7), (6:489), (19:45–47), (30:109–110)

16. A. The enzymes catechol-o-methyl transferase (COMT) and monoamine oxidase (MAO) are responsible for inactivating the neurotransmitter norepinephrine at the neuroeffector junction along the sympathetic nervous system. The inactivation of norepinephrine at the neuroeffector junction marks the termination of the impulse. During this time the smooth muscle repolarizes in preparation for subsequent impulses. COMT and MAO also act in the liver to catabolize the by-products formed during synaptic inactivation of norepinephrine.
(1:391), (4:145), (19:61–62)

17. B. Analgesics are medications administered for pain relief. Analgesics relieve pain without affecting consciousness. Narcotic analgesics relieve pain by inducing insensibility, sleep, and stupor. Morphine is a narcotic analgesic. Narcotic antagonists are administered to reverse the effects of narcotics. Narcotic antagonists include naloxone (Narcan), levallorphan (Lorfan), and nalorphine (Nalline). Meperdine (Demerol) and methadone (Dolophine) are narcotic analgesics also.
(4:549–551), (19:228–229), (30:108)

18. E. Dexamethasone (Decadron) is a steroid. Long-term use of steroids is associated with the following side effects:

1. Cushing's syndrome (moon face, buffalo hump, redistribution of body fat, hirsutism—abnormal hair growth, muscle wasting)
2. hypertension
3. impaired immunologic system
4. excessive glucose formation
5. osteoporesis—calcium depletion from bones
6. adrenal gland suppression
(1:404–406), (4:546–547), (19:162–163,165), (30:96)

19. E. Antibiotics are chemotherapeutic agents capable of inhibiting the growth of or killing other microorganisms by interfering with a particular step in metabolic sequence, or by altering a structural component necessary for a microorganism's survival. Mechanisms of action of some antibiotics include (1) inhibition of protein synthesis—streptomycin, chloramphenicol, tobramycin, and erythromycin, (2) inhibition of cell wall synthesis—penicillins, cephalosporins, (3) dis-

ruption of cell membrane function—polymyxins, and (4) inhibition of nucleic acid synthesis.

(2:285–287), (4:553–554), (19:183–184), (30:97–99)

20. E. Bacterial resistance to penicillin can be achieved by certain bacteria. This resistance is accomplished by the ability of those bacteria to produce the enzyme *penicillinase*. Bacteria that are capable of producing penicillinase include *Pseudomonas aeruginosa, Escherichia coli, Mycobacterium tuberculosis,* and *Bacillus anthracis.*

(19:187)

21. C. Muscarinic effects (lacrimation, salivation, mucus production, decreased heart rate, vasodilatation, and decreased blood pressure) are elicited by the stimulation of the parasympathetic neuroeffector sites. Nicotinic effects (vasoconstriction, increased blood pressure, and increased heart rate) result from the stimulation of both sympathetic and parasympathetic ganglionic sites, as well as from stimulation of skeletal muscle receptor sites.

(1:391), (19:54–55)

22. B. When the response of two concurrently administered medications is greater than the sum of the two individual responses, the term potentiation is used (2 + 2 = 6). Synergism refers to the enhancing effect that one drug can have on another while producing a total effect greater than that of each drug itself. One drug is inactive on a receptor, while the other is active. The presence of the two causes a greater effect than the active drug along (0 + 3 = 5).

(1:384), (19:27), (30:76)

23. D. The type of solution presented is a volume/volume (V/V) solution.

STEP 1: Use the formula

$$\frac{\text{volume of solute}}{\text{volume of solution}} \times 100 = \% \text{ solution}$$

STEP 2: Determine the volume of the solute and the solution.

1. solute: given in the problem as 2 ml
2. solution: obtained by adding the volume of the solute (2 ml) and the solvent (98 ml)

$$2 \text{ ml} + 98 \text{ ml} = 100 \text{ ml of solution}$$

STEP 3: Insert the known values into the formula and calculate the percent solution.

$$\frac{2 \text{ ml}}{100 \text{ ml}} \times 100 = \% \text{ solution}$$

$$0.02 \times 100 = 2.0\% \text{ solution}$$

(1:59), (2:11–13,16), (3:114–115), (4:6–7), (6:489), (19:44,47)

24. B. The cell body of a nerve cell receives impulses from the dendrites. After passing through the perikaryon (the cell body), the impulses move toward the axon.
(4:142), (13:386)

25. C. The sympathetic neurons arise from the thoracolumbar regions, whereas the parasympathetic neurons originate from the craniosacral regions.
(1:389), (4:149–150), (19:56), (30:83)

26. A. The enzyme cholinesterase inactivates the mediator acetylcholine at both the sympathetic and parasympathetic ganglionic synapses, and at the parasympathetic neuroeffector junction. The enzymes catechol-o-methyl transferase (COMT) and monoamine oxidase (MAO) metabolize the neurotransmitter norepinephrine at the sympathetic neuroeffector junction.
(1:391), (4:151), (19:57–58,61–62), (30:82)

27. E. One of the side effects of Mucomyst is bronchospasm. Therefore, a medication that predominantly stimulates beta-2 receptors should be concomitantly administered, to produce bronchodilatation.
(1:412), (3:121), (4:531), (6:462), (30:92–93)

28. A. Racemic epinephrine is an effective vasoconstrictor. It has a weak beta-1 effect and a moderate beta-2 influence. Its beta-2 stimulation is not great enough to warrant its use to relieve bronchospasm. The standard dosage is 0.5 ml of 2.25% racemic epinephrine diluted with 4.0 ml of normal saline.
(1:398), (3:12), (4:536), (19:85–86)

29. A. The drugs that stimulate alpha-adrenergic receptors, for example, Neo-Synephrine (phenylephrine), produce mucosal vasoconstriction.
(1:386), (3:120), (4:537), (19:139), (30:83–84)

30. E. A 1:200 Isuprel solution is a weight/volume (W/V) solution.
STEP 1: Use the formula

$$\frac{\text{grams}}{100 \text{ ml}} \times 100 = \% \text{ solution}$$

STEP 2: A 1:200 Isuprel solution can be expressed as 1 g/200 ml, or 1,000 mg/ 200 ml.
STEP 3: Set up a proportion and solve for X.

$$\frac{10 \text{ ml}}{200 \text{ ml}} = \frac{X}{1,000 \text{ mg}}$$
$$(0.05)(1,000 \text{ mg}) = X$$
$$X = 50 \text{ mg}$$

(1:59), (2:11–13,16), (3:114–115), (4:6–7), (6:489), (19:45–47), (30:109–110)

31. D. The sympathetic nervous system receptor can be stimulated to produce alpha (α) and beta (β) responses. Beta receptors are classified as beta-1 (stimulate the

heart—increased heart rate and increased myocardial contractility) and beta-2 (bronchodilatation and vasodilatation). Alpha-receptors essentially produce vaso-constriction.

(1:391–392), (3:115–116), (4:533–534), (6:469), (19:66), (30:83–84)

32. D. STEP 1: Use the formula $V_1C_1 = V_2C_2$ where

$$V_1 = \text{original volume}$$
$$C_1 = \text{original concentration}$$
$$V_2 = \text{new volume}$$
$$C_2 = \text{new concentration}$$

STEP 2: Insert the known values and solve for V_2.

$$V_1 = 4.0 \text{ cc}$$
$$C_1 = 10\%$$
$$V_2 = X$$
$$C_2 = 20\%$$
$$(4.0 \text{ cc})(10\%) = (X)(20\%)$$
$$\frac{X}{4.0 \text{ cc}} = \frac{10\%}{20\%}$$
$$X = (4.0 \text{ cc})(0.5)$$
$$X = 2.0 \text{ cc}$$

(1:63–64), (2:11–13,16), (3:114–115), (4:6–7), (6:489), (19:40–42,47)

33. B. Medications, such as digitoxin and digoxin, increase the force of myocardial con-tractility. The ability to elicit this response is termed *positive inotropism*. Drugs that have the opposite effect are said to exhibit *negative inotropism*.

Medications that increase the rate of depolarization of the sinoatrial (S-A) node display *positive chronotropism* because they increase the heart rate. Agents that decrease the rate of S-A node depolarization display *negative chronotropism* be-cause they decrease the heart rate.

(3:286,308), (4:135,256,555), (19:247), (30:104–105)

34. A. Medications that are injected directly into body fluids are said to be administered parenterally (either intramuscularly or intravenously).

(19:8), (30:78)

35. A. The type of solution presented here is a weight/weight (W/W) variety. Therefore, the percentage of solute represents the number of grams in 100 g of the solution.

STEP 1: Use the formula

$$\frac{\text{grams}}{100 \text{ g}} \times 100 = \% \text{ solution}$$

STEP 2: Rearrange the formula to solve for the number of grams of solute in a 5.5% (W/W) solution.

$$\text{grams} = 100 \text{ g}\left(\frac{\text{percentage}}{100}\right)$$

$$X = 100 \text{ g}\left(\frac{5.5\%}{100}\right)$$

$$X = (100 \text{ g})(0.055)$$

$$X = 5.5 \text{ g of solute}$$

STEP 3: Subtract the amount of solute from the total weight of the solution to obtain the weight of the solvent.

$$
\begin{array}{r}
100.0 \text{ g solution} \\
- \quad 5.5 \text{ g solute} \\
\hline
94.5 \text{ g solvent}
\end{array}
$$

(1:59), (2:11–13,16), (3:114–115), (4:6–7), (6:489), (19:42,47)

36. B. The acceptable dosage for the administration of a 1:100 isoproterenol solution is 0.25 cc to 0.5 cc with 4 cc normal saline. Administration of a 1:200 solution should be limited to between 0.5 cc and 1.0 cc with 4 cc normal saline.
(3:119), (4:536), (6:472), (19:86)

37. C. A variety of medications are useful in the treatment of acute bronchospasm. Methylxanthines, for example, aminophylline, are useful because they have strong beta-2 and diuretic effects. The beta-2 stimulation promotes bronchodilatation via phosphodiesterase inhibition within the bronchial smooth muscle cell. The diuresis may somewhat reduce the respiratory mucosal edema associated with bronchospasm. Beta-adrenergic agonists, such as albuterol (Ventolin and Proventil) and metaproterenol sulfate, cause relaxation of bronchial smooth muscle by stimulating beta-2 receptor sites there. Atropine, which is an anticholinergic bronchodilator, may be useful in aerosolized form in the treatment of acute bronchospasm. Sch 1000, also an anticholinergic agent, produces significant bronchodilatation, but it is not available in the United States.

Intal (cromolyn sodium) has prophylactic use in the control of some forms of asthma. It is not beneficial in reversing bronchospasm. Cromolyn sodium prevents mediator (histamine, SRS-A, ECF-A, etc.) release from mast cells.
(1:394,407–408), (2:255–260), (4:310–312), (6:466–469), (8:278–282), (19:153,170), (30:86–91,108–109)

38. C. Cardiac beta-blocking agents decrease the heart rate, prolong impulse conduction time through the atrioventricular (A-V) node, and reduce myocardial contractile force. Medications that elicit these responses include propranolol (Inderal), metaprolol (Lopressor), nadolol (Corgard), and pindolol (Visken). These medications are useful in reducing the work of the myocardium (negative inotropism and negative chronotropism), thereby decreasing the heart's oxygen demands. Caution must be taken with patients who also receive beta-2 adrenergic agonists because cardiac beta-blocking agents block such bronchodilatation effects.

The medications butorphanol (Stadol) and levorphanol (Levo-Dromoran) are narcotic analgesics. These medications are administered to alleviate pain.
(1:394), (4:129,137,543,550), (19:229,250,256)

39. B. The *generic* name is the universal name approved by the FDA and available for all manufacturers. The *trade* name, or *brand* name, is the name of a drug used by a certain manufacturer and restricted for use to that manufacturer. The *chemical* name of a medication refers to the chemical or molecular structure of the drug. The name registered with the United States Pharmacopeia (USP) is termed the *official* name. The generic name is frequently the same as the official name. The *code* name is the name given to an experimental drug by the manufacturer. SCH-100 is the code name for ipratropium bromide.

DESCRIPTIVE TERM	NAME OF MEDICATION
Generic name	Isoproterenol hydrochloride
Trade (*brand*) name	Isuprel (by Winthrop Laboratories), Norisodrine (by Abbott Laboratories)
Chemical name	3,4-Dyhydroxy-[isopropylamino]-benzyl alcohol hydrochloride
Official name	Isoproterenol hydrochloride

(4:528–529), (19:3–4), (30:75)

40. E. The term *potency* refers to the relationship between the degree (strong or weak) of a drug's biologic activity and the dose administered. The log-dose response curve (Figure 49) illustrates that drug A is more potent than drug B. The curve plots the percent response to the drug on the y axis and the dose of the drug on the x axis. Therefore, the closer the curve is to the y axis, the more potent the drug. (4:527,529)

41. D. The following situations will lead to an increased level of intracellular cyclic GMP in bronchial smooth muscles. Alpha-adrenergic stimulation activates the release of the enzyme guanylate cyclase at the surface of bronchial smooth muscle cells. This enzyme catalyzes the conversion of guanosine triphosphate (GTP) to cyclic GMP. Cholinergic (parasympathetic) stimulation of receptors on the surface of bronchial smooth muscle cells also activates guanylate cyclase, thereby causing increased levels of cyclic GMP.

Beta-2 adrenergic stimulation activates the release of adenylate cyclase at the surface of bronchial smooth muscle cells. This enzyme catalyzes the conversion of adenosine triphosphate (ATP) to cyclic AMP (3′,5′-adenosine monophosphate). Phosphodiesterase inhibition by methylxanthine (aminophylline) administration also elevates cyclic AMP levels within the bronchial smooth muscle cells. (1:393–395), (2:255–260), (4:534), (6:466–468), (19:93), (30:84–85)

42. B. When antigen-antibody reactions on the surface of mast cells cause mast cell degranulation, a number of chemical mediators that cause bronchospasm are released. These mediators include the following substances: histamine, eosinophilic chemotactic factor of anaphylaxis (ECF-A), heparin, slow-reacting substance of anaphylaxis (SRS-A), kinins, prostaglandins, and serotonin. The prophylactic administration of cromolyn sodium (Intal) is useful in preventing mast cell degranulation and subsequent mediator release and bronchoconstriction. (2:257–260), (3:122), (6:292–293), (8:279–280), (19:170)

43. E.

$$1 \text{ g} = 1{,}000 \text{ mg or } 10^3 \text{ mg}$$
$$1 \text{ g} = 1{,}000{,}000 \text{ } \mu\text{g or } 10^6 \text{ } \mu\text{g}$$

Therefore,

$$1 \text{ mg} = 10^3 \text{ } \mu\text{g}$$

and

$$3 \text{ mg} = 3 \times 10^3 \text{ } \mu\text{g or } 3{,}000 \text{ } \mu\text{g}$$

(1:702), (4:12), (6:489), (19:36)

44. C. Rheology is the study of the flow and deformation of matter. Viscosity and elasticity are properties of matter that influence the flow and deformation of matter. (3:83), (6:371), (19:125)

45. D. Mucomyst is the trade (brand) name for acetylcysteine (generic name).
STEP 1: Use the formula $V_1C_1 = V_2C_2$
where,

$$V_1 = \text{original volume}$$
$$C_1 = \text{original concentration}$$
$$V_2 = \text{new volume}$$
$$C_2 = \text{new concentration}$$

STEP 2: Set up a proportion using the known values and solve for V_2.

$$V_1 = 10 \text{ cc}$$
$$C_1 = 20\% \text{ Mucomyst W/V}$$
$$V_2 = (X + 10 \text{ cc})$$
$$C_2 = 10\% \text{ Mucomyst W/V}$$
$$V_1C_1 = V_2C_2 \quad \text{or} \quad \frac{V_1C_1}{C_2} = V_2$$

$$(10 \text{ cc})(20\%) = (10\%)(X + 10 \text{ cc})$$
$$200 \text{ cc} = 10X + 100 \text{ cc}$$
$$100 \text{ cc} = 10X$$
$$\frac{100 \text{ cc}}{10} = X$$
$$10 \text{ cc} = X$$

Therefore, 10 cc of diluent must be added to 10 cc of a 20% Mucomyst W/V solution to produce a 10% Mucomyst W/V solution.
(1:63–64), (2:11–13,16), (4:6–7), (6:489), (19:42,47), (30:109)

46. A. Xanthine administration is associated with a variety of physiologic effects. These include central nervous system stimulation, bronchodilatation, diuresis, and skeletal muscle stimulation. Theophylline is the most frequently prescribed xanthine. (1:402–404), (2:260), (4:540), (6:475–478), (19:103–108)

47. E. The following beta-adrenergic agonists are said to have minimum beta-1 (+ inotropic and + chronotropic) effects: Ventolin (albuterol), Alupent (metaproterenol sulfate), Bricanyl (terbutaline sulfate), and Bronkosol (isoetharine).

    (1:394–400), (3:118–119), (4:535–538), (6:470), (19:88–90), (30:87,91)

48. D. Ethyl alcohol (ethanol), a wetting agent, is nebulized for the primary purpose of lowering the surface tension of tracheobronchial secretions. The usual dosage is 5 ml to 15 ml of 30% to 50% of ethyl alcohol. It is mainly used in the treatment of lowering the surface tension of the frothy secretions associated with pulmonary edema. Its clinical use is infrequent.

    (1:413–414), (3:121), (4:533), (6:463), (19:137–138), (30:95)

49. A. STEP 1: Disregard the 6-cc vial. It will *not* enter into the calculation.

    STEP 2: Convert 1 g/ml to milligrams per cubic centimeter (mg/cc).

    $$1 \text{ g} = 1,000 \text{ mg}$$
    $$1 \text{ ml} = 1 \text{ cc}$$
    $$1 \text{ g/ml} = 1,000 \text{ mg/cc}$$

    STEP 3: Set up a proportion.

    $$\frac{1,000 \text{ mg}}{700 \text{ mg}} = \frac{1 \text{ cc}}{X}$$
    $$(1,000)(X) = (700)(1 \text{ cc})$$
    $$X = \frac{700 \text{ cc}}{1,000}$$
    $$X = 0.7 \text{ cc}$$

    0.7 cc of solution needs to be drawn up from the 6-cc vial in order to administer 700 mg of solu-cortef.

    (1:59,63–64), (2:11–12), (3:114–115), (4:6–7), (6:489), (19:42,44,47), (30:109–110)

50. E. Stimulation of the parasympathetic nervous system results in the following responses: bronchoconstriction, pulmonary vasodilatation, vagal stimulation (increased bronchial secretions), negative inotropism (decreased myocardial contractility), negative chronotropism (decreased heart rate), and systemic vasodilatation.

    (1:389,392–393), (3:116–117), (4:152–153), (19:68)

REFERENCES

1. Spearman, C., and Sheldon, R., *Egan's Fundamentals of Respiratory Therapy,* 4th ed., C.V. Mosby, St. Louis, 1982.

2. Wojciechowski, W., *Respiratory Care Sciences: An Integrated Approach,* John Wiley & Sons, New York, 1985.

3. Shapiro, B., Harrison, R., Kacmarek, R., and Cane, R., *Clinical Application of Respiratory Care,* 3rd ed., Year Book Medical Publishers, Chicago, 1985.

4. Kacmarek, R., Mack, C., and Dimas, S., *The Essentials of Respiratory Therapy*, 2nd ed., Year Book Medical Publishers, Chicago, 1985.

5. McPherson, S., *Respiratory Therapy Equipment,* 3rd ed., C.V. Mosby, St. Louis, 1985.

6. Burton, G., and Hodgkin, J., *Respiratory Care: A Guide to Clinical Practice,* 2nd ed., J.B. Lippincott, Philadelphia, 1985.

7. Frownfelter, D., *Chest Physical Therapy and Cardiopulmonary Rehabilitation, An Interdisciplinary Approach,* Year Book Medical Publishers, Chicago, 1978.

8. Cherniack, R., and Cherniack, L., *Respiration in Health and Disease,* 3rd ed., W.B. Saunders, Philadelphia, 1983.

9. Daily, E., and Schroeder, G., *Techniques in Bedside Hemodynamic Monitoring,* 3rd ed., C.V. Mosby, St. Louis, 1985.

10. Des Jardins, R., *Clinical Manifestations of Respiratory Disease,* Year Book Medical Publishers, Chicago, 1984.

11. Mitchell, R., *Synopsis of Clinical Pulmonary Disease,* 3rd ed., C.V. Mosby, St. Louis, 1982.

12. Comroe, J., *Physiology of Respiration,* 3rd ed., Year Book Medical Publishers, Chicago, 1974.

13. West, J., *Pulmonary Pathophysiology—The Essentials,* 2nd ed., Williams & Wilkins, Baltimore, 1982.

14. West, J., *Respiratory Physiology—The Essentials,* 3rd ed., Williams & Wilkins, Baltimore, 1985.

15. Martz, K., et al., *Management of the Patient-Ventilator System: A Team Approach,* 2nd ed., C.V. Mosby, St. Louis, 1984.

16. Shoup, C., and McHenry, R., *Laboratory Exercises in Respiratory Therapy,* 2nd ed., C.V. Mosby, St. Louis, 1983.

17. Ruppel, G., *Manual of Pulmonary Function Testing,* 3rd ed., C.V. Mosby, St. Louis, 1982.

18. Appelbaum, E., and Bruce, D., *Tracheal Intubation,* W.B. Saunders, Philadelphia, 1976.

19. Rau, J., *Respiratory Therapy Pharmacology,* 2nd ed., Year Book Medical Publishers, Chicago, 1984.

20. United States Department of Health, Education, and Welfare, Public Health Service, *Isolation Techniques for Use in Hospitals,* 2nd ed., Washington, D.C., 1975.

21. Brooks, S., *Integrated Basic Science,* 4th ed., C.V. Mosby, St. Louis, 1979.

22. Comroe, J., *The Lung,* Year Book Medical Publishers, Chicago, 1962.

23. Shibel, E., and Moser, K., *Respiratory Emergencies,* 2nd ed., C.V. Mosby, St. Louis, 1982.

24. Tisi, G., *Pulmonary Physiology in Clinical Medicine,* 2nd ed., Williams & Wilkins, Baltimore, 1985.

25. Cherniack, R., *Pulmonary Function Testing,* W.B. Saunders, Philadelphia, 1977.

26. Altose, M., *The Physiological Basis of Pulmonary Function Testing,* Clinical Symposia-CIBA, Vol. 31, No. 2, Summit, New Jersey, 1979.

27. Shapiro, B., Harrison, R., and Walton, J., *Clinical Application of Arterial Blood Gases,* 3rd ed., Year Book Medical Publishers, Chicago, 1982.

28. West, J., *Ventilation/Blood Flow and Gas Exchange,* 3rd ed., Blackwell Scientific Publications, 1979.

29. Slonim, N., and Hamilton, K., *Respiratory Physiology,* 4th ed., C.V. Mosby, St. Louis, 1981.

30. Rarey, K., and Youtsey, J., *Respiratory Patient Care,* Prentice-Hall, Englewood Cliffs, 1981.

31. Berne, R., and Levy, M., *Physiology,* C.V. Mosby, St. Louis, 1983.

32. Levitzky, M., *Pulmonary Physiology,* 2nd ed., McGraw-Hill, New York, 1986.

33. Wilson, P., Bell, C., and Norton, A., *Rehabilitation of the Heart and Lungs,* SensorMedics, 1980.

34. Clausen, J., and Zarins, L., *Pulmonary Function Testing Guildlines and Controversies,* Academic Press, New York, 1982.

35. Klaus, M., and Fanaroff, A., *Care of the High-Risk Neonate,* 2nd ed., W.B. Saunders, Philadelphia, 1979.

36. Lough, M., et al., *Pediatric Respiratory Therapy,* 3rd ed., Year Book Medical Publishers, Chicago, 1985.
37. Levin, D., et al., *A Practical Guide to Pediatric Intensive Care,* 2nd ed., C.V. Mosby, St. Louis, 1984.
38. O'Ryan, J., and Burns, D., *Pulmonary Rehabilitation from Hospital to Home,* Year Book Medical Publishers, Chicago, 1984.
39. Bell, C., et al., *Home Care and Rehabilitation in Respiratory Medicine,* J.B. Lippincott, Philadelphia, 1984.
40. Wilkins, R., et al., *Clinical Assessment in Respiratory Care,* C.V. Mosby, St. Louis, 1985.
41. Jones, N., and Campbell, E., *Clinical Exercise Testing,* 2nd ed., W.B. Saunders, Philadelphia, 1982.
42. Goldsmith, J., and Karotkin, E., *Assisted Ventilation of the Neonate,* W.B. Saunders, Philadelphia, 1981.
43. Blowers, M., and Sims, R., *How to Read an ECG,* 3rd ed., Medical Economics, Inc., New Jersey, 1983.
44. Eubanks, D., and Bone, R., *Comprehensive Respiratory Care,* C.V. Mosby, St. Louis, 1985.
45. Rattenborg, C., *Clinical Use of Mechanical Ventilation,* Year Book Medical Publishers, Chicago, 1981.
46. Witkowski, A.S., *Pulmonary Assessment: A Clinical Guide,* J.B. Lippincott, Philadelphia, 1985.
47. Op't Holt, Timothy B., *Assessment Based Respiratory Care,* John Wiley & Sons, New York, 1986.

PHYSICS ASSESSMENT

PURPOSE: The purpose of this 50-item section is to evaluate your knowledge and understanding of physics concepts as they relate to respiratory care equipment, therapeutic intervention, and cardiopulmonary physiology. The physics principles included here for you to apply include resistance, compliance, fluid dynamics, flow patterns, and physical laws. Numerous mathematical problems are also provided in the areas of the gas laws, pressure and temperature conversions, air entrainment, filtration, and reabsorption.

DIRECTIONS: Each of the questions or incomplete statements is followed by five suggested answers. Select the one which is the best in each and then blacken the corresponding space on the answer sheet.

1. Which formula will allow for the calculation of the unknown resistance in the Wheatstone bridge shown in Figure 52 when the galvanometer reads zero?

   A. $R_1R_x = R_2R_3$

   B. $R_xR_2 = R_1R_3$

   C. $R_3R_x = R_2R_1$

   D. $\dfrac{R_3R_2}{R_1} = R_x$

   E. $\dfrac{R_1R_2}{R_3} = R_x$

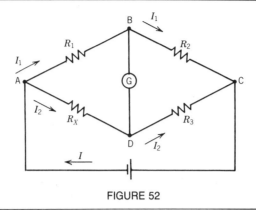

FIGURE 52

Questions 2 and 3 refer to Figure 53.

2. Calculate each resistance encountered as the fluid flows through the tube illustrated in Figure 53.

	ΔP	$\dot{V}$
R_1 (resistance$_1$)	4 torr	2 liters/sec
R_2 (resistance$_2$)	5 torr	2 liters/sec
R_3 (resistance$_3$)	6 torr	2 liters/sec

A. R_1 8.0 torr/liter/sec; R_2 10.0 torr/liter/sec; R_3 12.0 torr/liter/sec
B. R_1 7.5 torr/liter/sec; R_2 7.5 torr/liter/sec; R_3 7.5 torr/liter/sec
C. R_1 2.0 torr/liter/sec; R_2 2.5 torr/liter/sec; R_3 3.0 torr/liter/sec
D. R_1 1.0 torr/liter/sec; R_2 2.0 torr/liter/sec; R_3 3.0 torr/liter/sec
E. R_1 0.5 torr/liter/sec; R_2 0.4 torr/liter/sec; R_3 0.3 torr/liter/sec

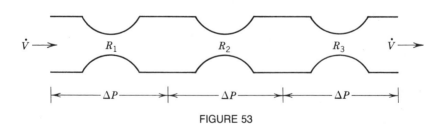

FIGURE 53

3. Determine the total resistance of the system in Figure 53.

A. 30.0 torr/liter/sec   D. 6.0 torr/liter/sec
B. 22.5 torr/liter/sec   E. 1.2 torr/liter/sec
C. 7.5 torr/liter/sec

4. Which statement(s) accurately describe(s) laminar flow?

   I. Eddy currents predominate as a fluid moves through a conduction system.
  II. Laminar flow is dependent upon gas viscosity.
 III. As a gas flows in laminar fashion through a tube of constant radius, the velocity of the molecules is uniform.
  IV. Laminar flow has a parabolically shaped velocity profile.
   V. It normally predominates throughout oral and nasal cavities during resting, spontaneous breathing.

A. I only

B. I, II, V only

C. II, IV only

D. III, V only

E. I, III, V only

5. What is the Fahrenheit equivalent for 30°C?

A. 22°F

B. 27°F

C. 54°F

D. 67°F

E. 86°F

6. Determine the FI_{O_2} of the following gas mixture:

   P_B 760 mm Hg
   P_{O_2} 100 mm Hg
   P_{CO_2} 40 mm Hg
   P_{N_2} 573 mm Hg
   P_{H_2O} 47 mm Hg

A. 1.00

B. 0.18

C. 0.16

D. 0.14

E. 0.13

7. Which of the following mathematical relationships represents spontaneous ventilatory efforts against a closed glottis?

A. $V_1 P_2 = V_2 P_1$

B. $\dfrac{V_1}{V_2} = \dfrac{P_2}{P_1}$

C. $P_a + \frac{1}{2} D v_a^2 = P_b + \frac{1}{2} D v_b^2$

D. $P_T = P_1 + P_2 + P_3 + \cdots P_n$

E. $\eta = \dfrac{\Delta P \pi L}{8 \dot{V} r^4}$

8. Convert 40 mm Hg to kPa.

A. 5.3 kPa

B. 6.1 kPa

C. 7.5 kPa

D. 19.0 kPa

E. 300.0 kPa

9. Find the gas correction factor for a volume of saturated gas collected at 755 mm Hg and at 26°C (ATPS) to a gas saturated at 760 mm Hg and at body temperature (BTPS). (See Appendix III.)

A. 1.000

B. 1.028

C. 1.043

D. 1.061

E. 1.097

10. Based on Reynold's equation which of the following factors contribute to the development of laminar flow?

    I. decreased flowrate
    II. increased gas viscosity
    III. decreased gas velocity
    IV. decreased gas density

    A. I, II, III, IV   D. I, III only
    B. II, III, IV only   E. I, II, III only
    C. II, IV only

Questions 11 and 12 refer to the same patient.

11. A subject with an intra-esophageal balloon in place exhibits an intrapleural pressure of -4 cm H_2O at a resting end-expiratory position. The pressure manometer indicates an intrapleural pressure of -6.5 cm H_2O after the subject inhales 500 cc of air. Calculate this person's pulmonary compliance.

    A. 47.61 liters/cm H_2O D. 0.10 liter/cm H_2O
    B. 5.25 liters/cm H_2O E. 0.05 liter/cm H_2O
    C. 0.20 liter/cm H_2O

12. Calculate the value for pulmonary elastance using the data in the previous question.

    A. 20 liters/cm H_2O D. 0.19 liter/cm H_2O
    B. 10 liters/cm H_2O E. 0.02 liter/cm H_2O
    C. 5 liters/cm H_2O

13. Which statement best describes Pascal's principle?

    A. The weight of liquid displaced equals the buoyant force on a floating or submerged object.
    B. Whenever the pressure in a confined liquid increases or decreases at any point, the pressure change is transmitted equally throughout the entire liquid.
    C. As the temperature of an ideal gas is elevated or reduced, the viscosity of the gas decreases or increases, respectively, in proportion to the change in temperature.
    D. The flow of a non-Newtonian fluid increases as lateral pressure exerted on the fluid decreases.
    E. The rate of gaseous effusion is directly proportional to the square root of the density and inversely proportional to the temperature.

14. Calculate the delivered flow for an oxygen delivery device operating at a flowrate of 15 liters/min and delivering 40% oxygen.

    A. 62.4 liters/min   D. 32.4 liters/min
    B. 47.4 liters/min   E. 6.0 liters/min
    C. 37.5 liters/min

15. The point at which laminar flow degenerates into turbulent flow is called the
   _____ .

   A. axial velocity   D. eddy currents
   B. boundary layer   E. critical velocity
   C. velocity profile

16. Which of the following relationships are true concerning the diagram shown in Figure
   54?

   I. $P_1 < P_2$
   II. $v_2 < v_1$
   III. $v_1 < v_2$
   IV. $P_2 < P_1$

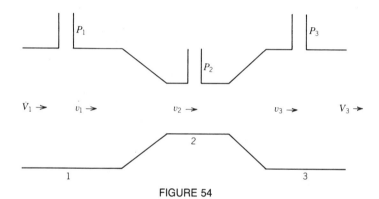

FIGURE 54

   A. I, II only   D. I, IV only
   B. III, IV only   E. II, IV only
   C. I, III only

17. Which of the following pressure measurements is *not* equivalent to 1 atm of pressure?

   A. 33 ft H_2O D. 29.9 in. H_2O
   B. 10,340 mm H_2O E. 101.3 kPa
   C. 76 cm Hg

18. The specific gravity of nitrous oxide is _____ . (N = 14 amu; 0 = 16
   amu.)

   A. 1.11   D. 1.96
   B. 1.33   E. 2.31
   C. 1.51

19. According to Poiseuille's law of laminar flow, if all the factors remain constant except
   resistance and lumen size, what is the effect on the resistance if the lumen size is reduced by one-half?

A. It increases by a factor of 4.

B. The resistance decreases 16-fold.

C. The resistance increases by a factor of 16.

D. It is halved.

E. It is doubled.

20. Calculate the total pressure in a container comprised of a P_{O_2} of 13.34 kPa, a P_{CO_2} of 54.4 cm H_2O, a P_{N_2} of 7.646 × 10^5 dynes/cm^2, and a P_{H_2O} of 47 mm Hg.

A. 760 mm Hg	D. 649 mm Hg
B. 713 mm Hg	E. 615 mm Hg
C. 662 mm Hg	

21. Which one of the following selections depicts the correct units for airway resistance?

A. cm H_2O/liter/sec	D. cm H_2O/sec
B. liter/sec/torr	E. liters/sec/cm H_2O
C. mm Hg/sec/liter	

22. What two factors can substitute for force and length when Hooke's law is applied to the lung-thorax system?

A. compliance and resistance	D. resistance and volume
B. pressure and flowrate	E. flowrate and compliance
C. pressure and volume	

23. Calculate the density of cyclopropane $(CH_2)_3$. (C = 12 amu; H = 1 amu)

A. 1.45 g/liter	D. 1.96 g/liter
B. 1.74 g/liter	E. 2.03 g/liter
C. 1.87 g/liter	

24. Determine the airway resistance for a subject breathing a 500 cc V_T at a rate of 12 breaths per minute and with an inspiratory time of 2 seconds. Mouth pressure is equal to atmospheric pressure, and intra-alveolar pressure measures −5 cm H_2O.

A. 2.5 cm H_2O/liter/sec	D. 20.0 cm H_2O/liter/sec
B. 5.0 cm H_2O/liter/sec	E. 23.6 cm H_2O/liter/sec
C. 11.6 cm H_2O/liter/sec	

25. Calculate the surface tension at the air-liquid interface of a sphere that has a 6-mm diameter and a distending pressure of 420 dynes/cm^2.

A. 31.5 dynes/cm	D. 630.0 dynes/cm
B. 63.0 dynes/cm	E. 1,260.0 dynes/cm
C. 157.5 dynes/cm	

26. Which of the following statements are true about the fraction $\Delta P/\dot{V}$?

I. It can be measured only during static conditions.

II. This ratio is increased during an asthmatic attack.

III. When this ratio is applied to a straight conducting tube, the ratio will numerically double if the length of the conducting tube doubles.

IV. Physiologically, the value of this ratio is greater in airways greater than 2 mm in diameter.

V. This ratio decreases in value if a person takes deep, slow breaths rather than rapid, shallow breaths.

A. I, II, IV only   D. I, III only

B. II, III, IV, V only   E. I, II, III, IV, V

C. II, III, IV only

27. What is the relationship between the cross-sectional area of a conducting system and the velocity of the fluid flowing through the system?

A. inverse   D. logarithmic

B. linear   E. exponential

C. sigmoid

28. Which of the following equations is the basis for helium-oxygen therapy?

A. $\dfrac{V_D}{V_T} = \dfrac{Pa_{CO_2} - P\overline{E}_{CO_2}}{Pa_{CO_2}}$

B. $A_{(trachea)}V_{(trachea)} = A_{(alveoli)}V_{(alveoli)}$

C. $D(v_2^2 - v_1^2) \propto P_1 - P_2$

D. $P_{A_{O_2}} = F_{I_{O_2}}(P_B - P_{H_2O}) - Pa_{CO_2}\left(F_{I_{O_2}} + \dfrac{1 - F_{I_{O_2}}}{R}\right)$

E. $PV = nRT$

29. Which of the following expressions are true concerning Figure 55?

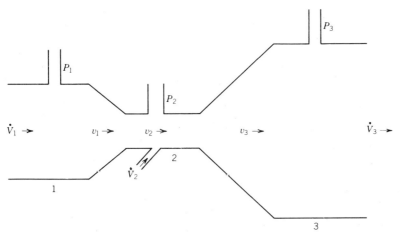

FIGURE 55

   I. $\dot{V}_2 = \dot{V}_3 - \dot{V}_1$
   II. $v_3 > v_1$
   III. $P_3 > P_2$
   IV. $v_1 = v_2$

   A. I, II, III only   D. I, III only
   B. II, III only   E. II, III, IV only
   C. I, IV only

30. Calculate the total resistance in the conducting system illustrated in Figure 56.

	ΔP FOR EACH RESISTANCE	$\dot{V}$ THROUGH EACH RESISTANCE
Resistance$_1$	15 cm H_2O	3 liters/min
Resistance$_2$	9 cm H_2O	3 liters/min
Resistance$_3$	12 cm H_2O	3 liters/min

$$\dot{V}_1 = \text{initial flowrate}$$
$$\dot{V}_f = \text{final flowrate}$$

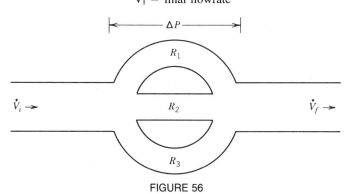

FIGURE 56

   A. 12.00 cm H_2O/liter/min   D. 1.28 cm H_2O/liter/min
   B. 4.00 cm H_2O/liter/min   E. 0.12 cm H_2O/liter/min
   C. 1.33 cm H_2O/liter/min

31. Determine the potential osmotic pressure for a 0.9% NaCl solution.

   A. 25 torr   D. 1,232 torr
   B. 52 torr   E. 5,791 torr
   C. 598 torr

32. Calculate the amount of fluid in terms of pressure (mm Hg) that is *not* reabsorbed on the venous end of the systemic capillary depicted in Figure 57.

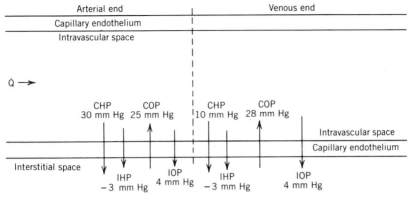

FIGURE 57

$\dot{Q}$ = perfusion (liters/min)
CHP = capillary hydrostatic pressure (mm Hg)
COP = capillary osmotic pressure (mm Hg)
IHP = interstitial hydrostatic pressure (mm Hg)
IOP = interstitial osmotic pressure (mm Hg)

A. 1 mm Hg   D. 17 mmHg
B. 12 mm Hg   E. 25 mm Hg
C. 15 mm Hg

33. Which of the following expressions represents conduction?

A. $\dfrac{1}{\Delta P/\Delta V}$ D. $\dfrac{\Delta P/\dot{V}}{1}$

B. $\dfrac{1}{\Delta P/\dot{V}}$ E. $\dfrac{\Delta V/\Delta P}{\Delta P/\dot{V}}$

C. $\dfrac{\Delta V/\Delta P}{1}$

34. A Reynold's number of 3,000 would be indicative of what form of flow pattern?

A. augmented diffusion   D. laminar
B. tracheobronchial   E. convective
C. turbulent

35. Determine the gas volume conversion factor needed to convert a gas volume from STPD to BTPS. The ambient pressure is 755 mm Hg.

A. $V_2 = 1.413\ (V_1)$ D. $V_2 = 1.073\ (V_1)$
B. $V_2 = 1.219\ (V_1)$ E. $V_2 = 1.006\ (V_1)$
C. $V_2 = 1.114\ (V_1)$

36. According to Charles' law, what would be the volume in cylinder B in Figure 58 if the temperature was decreased to $-273°C$ from that shown in cylinder A?

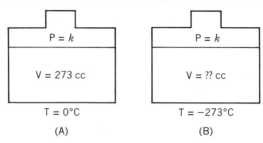

FIGURE 58

A. 0 cc   D. 431 cc
B. 137 cc   E. 546 cc
C. 273 cc

37. Which of the following statements are true concerning turbulent flow?

   I. The driving pressure required to produce turbulent flow is proportional to the square of the flowrate times a constant related to gas density.
   II. The fluid flows through the tube system essentially at uniform velocity.
   III. Movement of the fluid molecules is random, chaotic, and rapid.
   IV. Airway resistance associated with turbulent flow is greater than that with laminar flow.

   A. I, IV only   D. I, III, IV only
   B. II, III, IV only   E. I, II, III, IV
   C. II, III only

38. Calculate the barometric pressure when the height of a column of liquid is 33 in. and the density of the liquid is 0.491 lb/cu in.

   A. 8.32 psi   D. 16.20 psi
   B. 10.00 psi   E. 67.20 psi
   C. 14.70 psi

39. Calculate the density of a gas mixture having the following components 20.93% oxygen, 0.04% carbon dioxide, and 79.03% nitrogen.

   A. 4.46 g/liter   D. 2.54 g/liter
   B. 3.97 g/liter   E. 1.29 g/liter
   C. 3.14 g/liter

40. Which law is represented by the statement that at equal temperatures and pressures equal volumes of different gases contain the same number of molecules?

   A. law of continuity   D. Boyle's law
   B. Gay-Lussac's law   E. Avogadro's law
   C. Charles' law

41. Which of the following statements are true concerning viscosity?

    I. Viscosity is temperature dependent.

    II. It is a time-related property of matter

    III. Viscosity of liquids is influenced by the van der Waals forces

    IV. The unit for viscosity in the centimeter-gram-second system is the poise.

A. II, III only

B. I, III, IV only

C. II, IV only

D. I, II, IV only

E. I, II, III, IV

42. According to Gay-Lussac's law, what would be the pressure exerted by the piston in cylinder B in Figure 59 if the temperature was increased to 273°C from that in cylinder A?

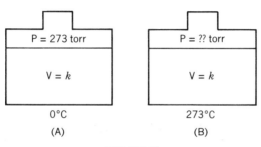

FIGURE 59

A. 673 torr

B. 546 torr

C. 499 torr

D. 452 torr

E. 273 torr

43. Calculate the relative rate of diffusion for nitrous oxide (N_2O; solubility coefficient = 0.41) and cyclopropane (C_3H_6; solubility coefficient = 0.011) in water at 38°C.

A. $r_{N_2O} = 34.47\ (r_{C_3H_6})$

B. $r_{N_2O} = 35.16\ (r_{C_3H_6})$

C. $r_{N_2O} = 36.40\ (r_{C_3H_6})$

D. $r_{N_2O} = 37.27\ (r_{C_3H_6})$

E. $r_{N_2O} = 38.30\ (r_{C_3H_6})$

44. Calculate the thoracic compliance when the total compliance measures 0.072 liter/cm H_2O and the lung compliance is 0.12 liter/cm H_2O.

A. 0.048 liter/cm H_2O

B. 0.179 liter/cm H_2O

C. 0.192 liter/cm H_2O

D. 5.56 liters/cm H_2O

E. 22.22 liters/cm H_2O

Questions 45 and 46 refer to the same information.

SPHERE X

Surface tension = 12 dynes/cm

Radius = 0.005 cm

SPHERE Y

Surface tension = 12 dynes/cm

Radius = 0.0025 cm

45. Calculate the inflation pressure for these two spheres.

    A. X = 0.12 dynes/cm²; Y = 0.06 dynes/cm²
    B. X = 0.24 dynes/cm²; Y = 0.12 dynes/cm²
    C. X = 2,400 dynes/cm²; Y = 4,800 dynes/cm²
    D. X = 4,800 dynes/cm²; Y = 9,600 dynes/cm²
    E. X = 9,600 dynes/cm²; Y = 19,200 dynes/cm²

46. If sphere X and sphere Y were in communication with each other, what would be the consequence?

    A. Sphere Y would empty into sphere X.
    B. Sphere X would empty into sphere Y.
    C. The two spheres would equilibrate.
    D. There would be *no* change in pressure.
    E. The consequence would be impossible to predetermine.

47. How many moles are contained in 98 g of H_3PO_4? (See Appendix IV.)

    A. 0.76 mole   D. 49.00 moles
    B. 1.00 mole   E. 98.00 moles
    C. 33.00 moles

48. A gas mixture contains 20% carbon dioxide, 30% oxygen, and 50% nitrogen. Calculate the partial pressure of each gas in this mixture of STPD.

    A. P_{O_2} 152 mm Hg; P_{CO_2} 228 mm Hg; P_{N_2} 380 mm Hg
    B. P_{CO_2} 152 mm Hg; P_{O_2} 228 mm Hg; P_{N_2} 380 mm Hg
    C. P_{O_2} 143 mm Hg; P_{CO_2} 214 mm Hg; P_{N_2} 356 mm Hg
    D. P_{CO_2} 143 mm Hg; P_{O_2} 214 mm Hg; P_{N_2} 356 mm Hg
    E. P_{CO_2} 152 mm Hg; P_{O_2} 182 mm Hg; P_{N_2} 213 mm Hg

49. Calculate the total alveolar volume for 300×10^6 alveoli, each of which has a radius of 0.15 mm.

    A. 2.93 liters   D. 4.24 liters
    B. 3.14 liters   E. 4.81 liters
    C. 3.80 liters

50. Calculate the alveolar surface area of the lungs, which have 300×10^6 alveoli each with a radius of 0.137 mm?

    A. 41 m²   D. 80 m²
    B. 63 m²   E. 84 m²
    C. 71 m²

ASSESSMENT ANSWER SHEET

DIRECTIONS: Darken the space under the selected answer.

	A	B	C	D	E		A	B	C	D	E
1.	[ ]	[ ]	[ ]	[ ]	[ ]	26.	[ ]	[ ]	[ ]	[ ]	[ ]
2.	[ ]	[ ]	[ ]	[ ]	[ ]	27.	[ ]	[ ]	[ ]	[ ]	[ ]
3.	[ ]	[ ]	[ ]	[ ]	[ ]	28.	[ ]	[ ]	[ ]	[ ]	[ ]
4.	[ ]	[ ]	[ ]	[ ]	[ ]	29.	[ ]	[ ]	[ ]	[ ]	[ ]
5.	[ ]	[ ]	[ ]	[ ]	[ ]	30.	[ ]	[ ]	[ ]	[ ]	[ ]
6.	[ ]	[ ]	[ ]	[ ]	[ ]	31.	[ ]	[ ]	[ ]	[ ]	[ ]
7.	[ ]	[ ]	[ ]	[ ]	[ ]	32.	[ ]	[ ]	[ ]	[ ]	[ ]
8.	[ ]	[ ]	[ ]	[ ]	[ ]	33.	[ ]	[ ]	[ ]	[ ]	[ ]
9.	[ ]	[ ]	[ ]	[ ]	[ ]	34.	[ ]	[ ]	[ ]	[ ]	[ ]
10.	[ ]	[ ]	[ ]	[ ]	[ ]	35.	[ ]	[ ]	[ ]	[ ]	[ ]
11.	[ ]	[ ]	[ ]	[ ]	[ ]	36.	[ ]	[ ]	[ ]	[ ]	[ ]
12.	[ ]	[ ]	[ ]	[ ]	[ ]	37.	[ ]	[ ]	[ ]	[ ]	[ ]
13.	[ ]	[ ]	[ ]	[ ]	[ ]	38.	[ ]	[ ]	[ ]	[ ]	[ ]
14.	[ ]	[ ]	[ ]	[ ]	[ ]	39.	[ ]	[ ]	[ ]	[ ]	[ ]
15.	[ ]	[ ]	[ ]	[ ]	[ ]	40.	[ ]	[ ]	[ ]	[ ]	[ ]
16.	[ ]	[ ]	[ ]	[ ]	[ ]	41.	[ ]	[ ]	[ ]	[ ]	[ ]
17.	[ ]	[ ]	[ ]	[ ]	[ ]	42.	[ ]	[ ]	[ ]	[ ]	[ ]
18.	[ ]	[ ]	[ ]	[ ]	[ ]	43.	[ ]	[ ]	[ ]	[ ]	[ ]
19.	[ ]	[ ]	[ ]	[ ]	[ ]	44.	[ ]	[ ]	[ ]	[ ]	[ ]
20.	[ ]	[ ]	[ ]	[ ]	[ ]	45.	[ ]	[ ]	[ ]	[ ]	[ ]
21.	[ ]	[ ]	[ ]	[ ]	[ ]	46.	[ ]	[ ]	[ ]	[ ]	[ ]
22.	[ ]	[ ]	[ ]	[ ]	[ ]	47.	[ ]	[ ]	[ ]	[ ]	[ ]
23.	[ ]	[ ]	[ ]	[ ]	[ ]	48.	[ ]	[ ]	[ ]	[ ]	[ ]
24.	[ ]	[ ]	[ ]	[ ]	[ ]	49.	[ ]	[ ]	[ ]	[ ]	[ ]
25.	[ ]	[ ]	[ ]	[ ]	[ ]	50.	[ ]	[ ]	[ ]	[ ]	[ ]

PHYSICS ANALYSES

Note: The references listed after each analysis are numbered and keyed to the reference list located at the end of this section. The first number indicates the text. The second number indicates the page where information about the question can be found. For example, (1:219,384) means that reference number 1 is to be used and that on pages 219 and 384 information about the question will be found. Frequently, it will be necessary to read beyond the page number indicated to obtain complete information. Therefore, reference to the question will be found either on the page indicated or on subsequent pages.

1. B. A Wheatstone bridge shown in Figure 60 consists of four resistors (R_1, R_2, R_3, and R_4). A galvanometer bridges the two parallel electrical circuits (ABC and ADC). The galvanometer is used to sense the voltage difference between these two circuits.

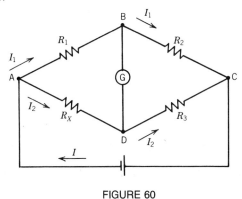

FIGURE 60

Current I is initiated by the battery and travels to point A, where it encounters R_1 and R_x. Assuming that $R_1 + R_2 = R_3 + R_x$, currents I_1 and I_2 will be equal. Furthermore, if $I_1 = I_2$, no potential difference (voltage) will exist between circuits ABC and ADC, and the galvanometer will indicate zero current between B and D. If three of the four resistances are known, the fourth can be calculated from Ohm's law, which states that

$$V = IR$$

where

$$V = \text{potential difference (volts)}$$
$$I = \text{current (amps)}$$
$$R = \text{resistance (ohms)}$$

Therefore,

$$I_1 R_1 = I_2 R_x$$

and

$$I_1 R_2 = I_2 R_3$$

Further,

$$\frac{I_1R_1}{I_1R_2} = \frac{I_2R_x}{I_2R_3}$$

or, after simplifying

$$\frac{R_1}{R_2} = \frac{R_x}{R_3}$$

$$R_xR_2 = R_1R_3 \quad \text{or} \quad R_x = R_3\left(\frac{R_1}{R_2}\right)$$

(2:197–199), (30:37–38)

2. C. Resistance can be calculated by the following expression

$$R = \frac{\Delta P}{\dot{V}}$$

where

$$R = \text{resistance (torr/liter/sec)}$$
$$\Delta P = \text{driving pressure (torr)}$$
$$\dot{V} = \text{flowrate (liters/sec)}$$

$$R_1 = \frac{\Delta P}{\dot{V}} = \frac{4 \text{ torr}}{2 \text{ liters/sec}} = 2 \text{ torr/liter/sec}$$

$$R_2 = \frac{\Delta P}{\dot{V}} = \frac{5 \text{ torr}}{2 \text{ liters/sec}} = 2.5 \text{ torr/liter/sec}$$

$$R_3 = \frac{\Delta P}{\dot{V}} = \frac{6 \text{ torr}}{2 \text{ liters/sec}} = 3 \text{ torr/liter/sec}$$

(1:144,181), (2:156), (4:30–32), (6:249–250), (8:30–39), (12:121), (29:30,270), (32:33)

3. C. In a series circuit the resistances are additive. For example, $R_1 + R_2 + R_3 = R_T$

$$\begin{array}{r}
2.0 \text{ torr/liter/sec } (R_1) \\
2.5 \text{ torr/liter/sec } (R_2) \\
+3.0 \text{ torr/liter/sec } (R_3) \\
\hline
7.5 \text{ torr/liter/sec } (R_T)
\end{array}$$

(2:155–156), (12:121), (32:33)

4. C. When a fluid flows through a conducting system in laminar fashion, it exhibits a number of characteristics. Included are

1. the fluid molecules move in horizontally (parallel), concentric layers
2. the velocity of the molecules is not uniform
3. fluid viscosity influences this particular flow pattern
4. it is thought to exist in the smaller airways of the tracheobronchial tree
5. it requires less of a driving pressure (ΔP), hence, it offers less resistance to flow than turbulent flow

(1:148), (2:145–149), (4:32–33,80), (12:122), (14:99), (29:28), (32:34)

5. E. The formula used to convert °C to °F is shown below.

$$°F = °C(1.8) + 32$$
$$= 30°C(1.8) + 32$$
$$= 54.0° + 32$$
$$= 86°$$

(1:702), (2:87–88), (4:9–10), (6:379–380)

6. D. According to Dalton's law of partial pressures, the total pressure exerted by a mixture of gases is equal to the sum of the partial pressures of the constituent gases. For example, the atmosphere is comprised of various gases.

$$P_B = P_{O_2} + P_{CO_2} + P_{N_2} + P_{H_2O}$$

When calculating the fractional concentration of one of the constituents in a gas mixture containing water vapor (P_{H_2O}), the partial pressure of the water vapor must first be subtracted from the total pressure. Therefore,

$$P_B - P_{H_2O} = P_{corrected}$$
$$760 \text{ mm Hg} - 47 \text{ mm Hg} = 713 \text{ mm Hg}$$

The fractional concentration of any of the constituent gases can be determined as follows.

$$\text{fractional concentration of gas} = \frac{\text{partial pressure of the gas}}{\text{corrected } P_B}$$

For example,

$$F_{IO_2} = \frac{P_{O_2}}{P_{corrected}}$$
$$= \frac{100 \text{ mm Hg}}{713 \text{ mm Hg}}$$
$$= 0.14$$

(2:127–130)

7. B. The expression $\dfrac{V_1}{V_2} = \dfrac{P_2}{P_1}$ represents Boyle's law, which states that when the temperature and mass of a gas are constant, the volume and pressure are inversely related. Spontaneous ventilatory efforts made against a closed glottis manifest this law. Body temperature is constant, for example, 37°C, and the mass of gas is constant because the glottis is closed.

Therefore, the diaphragm descends, decreasing intrathoracic pressure and increasing its volume. When inspiration terminates, the diaphragm ascends, increasing intrathoracic pressure and decreasing its volume.

(1:19–20,171–172), (2:13–14,120–122), (4:24,75,276–278), (8:2), (29:22,31, 56), (32:61,69,212)

8. A. STEP 1: Set up a relationship between the equivalents of 1 atm for both units of pressure.

$$\frac{1 \text{ atm in mm Hg}}{1 \text{ atm in kPa}} = \frac{760 \text{ mm Hg}}{101.33 \text{ kPa}} = 7.5 \text{ mm Hg/kPa}$$

STEP 2:   Convert 40 mm Hg to kPa.

$$\frac{40 \cancel{\text{ mm Hg}}}{7.5 \cancel{\text{ mm Hg}}\text{/kPa}} = 5.3 \text{ kPa}$$

(2:116–118)

9. D. The combined gas law, expressed below, is the basis for obtaining the volume conversion factor used for the following gas volume conversions associated with pulmonary function tests: (1) ATPS to STPD, (2) ATPS to BTPS, and (3) STPD to BTPS

$$\frac{PV}{T} = k$$

where

P = pressure (atm)
V = volume (liters)
T = absolute temperature (°K)
k = nR (number of moles times Boltzmann's constant)

STEP 1:   Refer to Appendix III to obtain the P_{H_2O} values for 26°C and 37°C, and correct the pressure readings 755 mm Hg and 760 mm Hg.

1. at 26°C, the maximum P_{H_2O} is 25.2 mm Hg

$$\begin{array}{r} 755.0 \text{ mm Hg } P_B \\ - 25.2 P_{H_2O} \\ \hline 729.8 \text{ mm Hg corrected } P_B \end{array}$$

2. at 37°C, the maximum P_{H_2O} is 47 mm Hg

$$\begin{array}{r} 760 \text{ mm Hg } P_B \\ - 47 P_{H_2O} \\ \hline 713 \text{ mm Hg corrected } P_B \end{array}$$

STEP 2:   Convert the temperature in °C to °K according to the formula

$$°K = °C + 273$$

1. °K = 26°C + 273
   = 299°K
2. °K = 37°C + 273

   = 310°K

STEP 3:   Use the combined gas law to find the gas volume correction factor from ATPS to BTPS.

$$\frac{P_1 V_1}{T_1} = \frac{P_2 V_2}{T_2}$$

$$\frac{(729.8 \text{ mm Hg})(V_1)}{299°K} = \frac{(713 \text{ mm Hg})(V_2)}{310°K}$$

$$\frac{(729.8 \text{ mm Hg})(V_1)(310°K)}{(299°K)(713 \text{ mm Hg})} = V_2$$

$$V_1 \left(\frac{226,238}{213,187}\right) = V_2$$

$$1.061(V_1) = V_2$$

The original volume, i.e., the gas collected at ATPS, needs to be mutiplied by the factor 1.061 to convert the volume to BTPS.

(1:19,26–27), (2:126–127), (4:23–25), (17:177), (29:244)

10. B. Quantitatively, Reynold's number is written as

$$R_N = \frac{v \times D \times d}{\eta}$$

where

R_N = Reynold's number

v = velocity of the fluid flowing through the tube

D = fluid density

d = tube diameter

η = fluid viscosity

The relationship among these factors is influential in determining the nature of fluid flow through a tube. A Reynold's number greater than 2,000 indicates that the flow through the tube is turbulent. Therefore, any variable in the numerator that increases in value will contribute to the presence of turbulent flow. Any increase in the denominator will tend to decrease R_N and promote laminar flow.

The following factors will tend to influence the existence of laminar flow

1. increased gas viscosity
2. decreased gas velocity
3. decreased gas density
4. decreased lumen diameter

(2:164–165), (4:33), (14:101,166), (29:29,81,246), (32:35)

11. C. Compliance is a measurement representing the degree of elasticity of an expanding or contracting body. It is expressed as a unit of volume change per unit of pressure change, i.e., liter/cm H_2O

$$C = \frac{\Delta V}{\Delta P} = \frac{\text{liter}}{\text{cm } H_2O}$$

STEP 1: Determine the volume change (ΔV). The person inspired from FRC (normal end-exhalation) and achieved a tidal volume of 500 cc. Therefore, the change in volume is 500 cc or 0.5 liter.

STEP 2: Determine the pressure change (ΔP).

$$-4 \text{ cm H}_2\text{O} - (-6.5 \text{ cm H}_2\text{O}) = \Delta P$$
$$2.5 \text{ cm H}_2\text{O} = \Delta P$$

STEP 3: Calculate the compliance (C).

$$C = \frac{\Delta V}{\Delta P} = \frac{0.5 \text{ liter}}{2.5 \text{ cm H}_2\text{O}}$$
$$C = 0.2 \text{ liter/cm H}_2\text{O}$$

(1:140–143), (2:153,169–171), (3:36), (4:28), (6:247), (12:99–105), (29:70–74), (32:21–24)

12. C. Elastance (E) is the reciprocal of compliance

$$E = \frac{\Delta P}{\Delta V} = \frac{\text{cm H}_2\text{O}}{\text{liter}}$$

or

$$E = \frac{1}{C}$$

Therefore,

$$E = \frac{1}{0.2 \text{ liter/cm H}_2\text{O}}$$
$$= 5 \text{ cm H}_2\text{O/liter}$$

(2:153,172), (4:27–28), (6:248), (29:76)

13. B. Pascal's principle states that the pressure change in a confined liquid is equally transmitted throughout the liquid when the pressure at a point in the container either increases or decreases.
(21:13)

14. A. The following relationship can be used to calculate the delivered flowrate.

$$(C_S \times \dot{V}_S) + (C_{ENT} \times \dot{V}_{ENT}) = (C_{DEL} \times \dot{V}_{DEL})$$

where

$$C_S = \text{concentration of the source gas}$$
$$\dot{V}_S = \text{flowrate of the source gas}$$
$$C_{ENT} = \text{concentration of the entrained gas}$$
$$\dot{V}_{ENT} = \text{flowrate of the entrained gas}$$
$$C_{DEL} = \text{concentration of the delivered gas}$$
$$\dot{V}_{DEL} = \text{flowrate of the delivered gas}$$

STEP 1: Use the expression $\dot{V}_S + \dot{V}_{ENT} = \dot{V}_{DEL}$ to determine the designation for $\dot{V}_{DEL}$ (lpm = liters/min).

$$\dot{V}_S = 15 \text{ lpm}$$
$$\dot{V}_{ENT} = X \text{ lpm}$$
$$\dot{V}_{DEL} = X \text{ lpm} + 15 \text{ lpm}$$

Therefore,

$$\dot{V}_S + \dot{V}_{ENT} = \dot{V}_{DEL}$$
$$15 \text{ lpm} + X \text{ lpm} = (X \text{ lpm} + 15 \text{ lpm})$$

STEP 2: Calculate the delivered flowrate using the gas entrainment formula

$$(C_S \times \dot{V}_S) + (C_{ENT} \times \dot{V}_{ENT}) = (C_{DEL} \times \dot{V}_{DEL})$$

where

$$C_S = 100\% \ O_2$$
$$\dot{V}_S = 15 \text{ lpm}$$
$$C_{ENT} = 21\% \ O_2$$
$$\dot{V}_{ENT} = X \text{ lpm}$$
$$C_{DEL} = 40\% \ O_2$$
$$\dot{V}_{DEL} = X \text{ lpm} + 15 \text{ lpm}$$
$$(100\% \times 15 \text{ lpm}) + (21\% \times X \text{ lpm}) = 40\%(X \text{ lpm} + 15 \text{ lpm})$$
$$15 \text{ lpm} + 0.21(X \text{ lpm}) = 0.40(X \text{ lpm}) + 6 \text{ lpm}$$
$$9 \text{ lpm} = 0.19(X \text{ lpm})$$
$$\frac{9 \text{ lpm}}{0.19} = X \text{ lpm}$$
$$47.4 \text{ lpm} = X = \dot{V}_{ENT}$$

STEP 3: Calculate the delivered flowrate using the following expression.

$$\dot{V}_S + \dot{V}_{ENT} = \dot{V}_{DEL}$$
$$15 \text{ lpm} + 47.4 \text{ lpm} = \dot{V}_{DEL}$$
$$62.4 \text{ lpm} = \dot{V}_{DEL}$$

(2:143–145), (4:377)

15. E. The development of laminar flow depends on both the architecture of the conducting system and certain properties of the flowing fluid. When the velocity of flow exceeds a certain value, i.e., *critical velocity*, laminar flow will convert to turbulent flow. The critical velocity is a function of the viscosity and density of the fluid. See Figure 61.
(1:148–150), (2:145–148), (4:32–33), (29:28), (32:33–35)

16. B. According to the Bernoulli effect, when a constant flow of fluid moves through a conducting system, the fluid velocity (v) varies inversely with lateral wall pressure (P). When a restriction to flow is encountered in such a system, the velocity beyond the obstruction is greater than that preceding it, and the preobstruction lateral wall pressure is greater than that beyond the obstruction.

$$P_1 - P_2 \simeq v_2^2 - v_1^2$$

(1:149–151), (2:138–141), (4:33–35), (29:246)

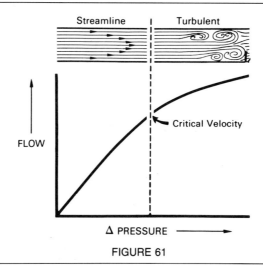

FIGURE 61

17. D. Each of the following pressure measurements is equivalent to one atmosphere (atm).

   760 mm Hg

   760 torr

   1,034 cm H_2O (10,340 mm H_2O)

   1,034 g/cm^2

   76 cm Hg

   14.7 psi

   33 ft H_2O

   29.9 in. Hg

   101.33 kPa

   1.014 $\times$ 10^6 dynes/cm^2

The International System of Units (SI) unit of pressure is the pascal (Pa). The official abbreviation SI is from the French *Le Système Internationale d'Unité*.

$$1 \text{ Pa} = 7.50 \times 10^{-3} \text{ mm Hg (torr)}$$
$$1 \text{ kilopascal (kPa)} = 1/1,000th \text{ of a pascal}$$

Therefore,

$$1 \text{ kPa} = 7.50 \text{ mm Hg (torr)}$$

Converting mm Hg or torr to kPa

$$\frac{760 \text{ mm Hg}}{7.50 \text{ mm Hg/k Pa}} = 101.33 \text{ kPa}$$

(1:11–14), (2:116–118), (4:20–21)

18. C. The density of a gas is obtained by dividing 1 gram-molecular weight of a gas by the volume (22.4 liters) 1 mole of that gas will occupy at STP.

$$\text{Density} = \frac{\text{gram-molecular weight}}{22.4 \text{ liters}}$$

STEP 1: Calculate the density of N_2O (N = 14 amu; O = 16 amu).

$$\text{Density} = \frac{44 \text{ g}}{22.4 \text{ liters}} = 1.96 \text{ g/liter}$$

STEP 2: Calculate the specific gravity for N_2O.

$$\text{specific gravity} = \frac{\text{Density of the gas}}{\text{Density of the standard*}}$$

$$\frac{1.96 \text{ g/liter}}{1.29 \text{ g/liter}} = 1.51$$

(1.7–8), (2:87), (4:19)

19. C. Poiseuille's law of laminar flow is shown below

$$\eta = \frac{\Delta P \pi r^4}{8L\dot{V}}$$

where

$$\eta = \text{viscosity index}$$
$$\Delta P = \text{driving pressure}$$
$$\pi/8 = \text{mathematical constant}$$
$$r = \text{radius to the 4th power}$$
$$L = \text{length of conducting system}$$
$$\dot{V} = \text{flowrate (volume/time)}$$

Poiseuille's law can be simplified by "lumping" a few factors together and holding them constant (k). For example, if the viscosity index (η), the mathematical constant ($\pi/8$), and length (L) will be considered constant and the equation will become

$$k = \frac{\pi}{\eta 8L}$$

$$k = \frac{\Delta P r^4}{\dot{V}}$$

In the next simplification step $\Delta P/\dot{V}$ can be depicted as resistance (R). The equation will now read.

$$k = R \, r^4 \quad \text{or} \quad R = \frac{k}{r^4}$$

*The standard for specific gravity of gases is the density of air 1.29 g/liter.

Arbitrarily affixing the following values to the factors,

$$k = 16$$
$$r = 1$$
$$R = 16$$
$$R = \frac{k}{r^4}$$
$$16 = \frac{16}{1}$$

If the radius (r) is doubled (i.e., radius = 2), then

$$R = \frac{16}{2^4}$$
$$R = \frac{16}{16} = 1$$

If the radius is halved, that is, radius = 0.5 (r^4 = 0.0625), then

$$R = \frac{16}{0.0625} = 256$$

When the radius is doubled, and all the other factors remain constant except resistance, resistance experiences a 16-fold decrease. Conversely, if the radius is halved with the same stipulations present, resistance will increase by a factor of 16.

(1:146–148), (2:160–164), (4:36–37), (29:29,81,246), (32:33–35,83–84)

20. A. The total pressure of a mixture of gases can be calculated by obtaining the sum of the individual partial pressures. Dalton's law of partial pressure can be used

$$P_T = P_1 + P_2 + P_3 + \cdots P_n$$

Before the partial pressure of the constituent gases can be added the pressure units must all be the same.

STEP 1: Convert 13.34 kPa P_{O_2} to mm Hg.

$$1 \text{ atm} = 101.33 \text{ kPa}$$
$$1 \text{ atm} = 760 \text{ mm Hg}$$

1. $\dfrac{760 \text{ mm Hg}}{101.33 \text{ kPa}} = 7.50 \text{ mm Hg/kPa}$

2. $13.34 \text{ kPa} \times 7.50 \text{ mm Hg/kPa} = 100.05 \text{ mm Hg}$

STEP 2: Convert 54.4 cm H_2O P_{CO_2} to mm Hg.

$$1 \text{ atm} = 1{,}034 \text{ cm } H_2O$$
$$1 \text{ atm} = 760 \text{ mm Hg}$$

1. $\dfrac{1{,}034 \text{ cm } H_2O}{760 \text{ mm Hg}} = 1.36 \text{ cm } H_2O/\text{mm Hg}$

2. $\dfrac{54.4 \text{ cm } H_2O}{1.36 \text{ cm } H_2O/\text{mm Hg}} = 40 \text{ mm Hg}$

STEP 3: Convert 7.646×10^5 dynes/cm^2 P_{N_2} to mm Hg.

$$1 \text{ atm} = 1.014 \times 10^6 \text{ dynes/cm}^2$$
$$1 \text{ atm} = 760 \text{ mm Hg}$$

1. $\dfrac{1.014 \times 10^6 \text{ dynes/cm}^2}{760 \text{ mm Hg}} = 1{,}334.21 \text{ dynes/cm}^2/\text{mm Hg}$

2. $\dfrac{7.646 \times 10^5 \text{ dynes/cm}^2}{1{,}334.21 \text{ dynes/cm}^2/\text{mm Hg}} = 573 \text{ mm Hg}$

STEP 4: Calculate the total pressure.

$$P_{O_2} + P_{CO_2} + P_{N_2} + P_{H_2O} = P_T$$

$$
\begin{array}{r}
100 \text{ mm Hg } P_{O_2} \\
40 \text{ mm Hg } P_{CO_2} \\
573 \text{ mm Hg } P_{N_2} \\
+\ \ 47 \text{ mm Hg } P_{H_2O} \\
\hline
760 \text{ mm Hg } P_T
\end{array}
$$

(1:11–14,700), (2:116–119,127–132), (4:22–23), (29:23), (32:69,212)

21. A. Quantitatively, airway resistance (R_{aw}) is defined as a change in pressure (ΔP) divided by the flowrate ($\dot{V}$).

$$R_{aw} = \frac{\Delta P}{\dot{V}} = \frac{\text{cm H}_2\text{O}}{\text{liter/sec}}$$

Therefore, the appropriate units for airway resistance is some unit of pressure (e.g., cm H$_2$O) per some unit of flow (e.g., liters/second), or cm H$_2$O/liter/second.

(1:145,181), (2:148,156,159), (3:36), (4:80–81), (8:30–32), (29:30,82), (32: 32–34)

22. C. Hooke's law can be applied to solid materials that are elastic. A solid is said to be elastic if it can regain its original length or shape after the removal of the force responsible for stretching or deforming it. A direct relationship exists between force and length in reference to an elastic body as shown in Figure 62. This linear relationship will be maintained until the elastic body is stretched beyond its elastic limit.

Physiologically, Hooke's law can be applied to the lung-thorax system. In this application length is replaced by volume, and force is replaced by pressure. A compliance curve, reflecting the elasticity of the lung-thorax system, can be generated by plotting changes in volume against changes in pressure. Figure 63 graphically demonstrates this relationship as lung volume increases from FRC to TLC (inspiration), and as it decreases from TLC to FRC (exhalation).

(2:165–173), (4:27–28,77–79), (29:72), (32:21–22)

23. C. The density of a gas can be calculated by dividing the gram-molecular weight by the volume occupied by the gas at standard conditions, i.e., 760 mm Hg and 0°C. The volume occupied by a gram-molecular weight of an ideal gas is 22.4 liters.

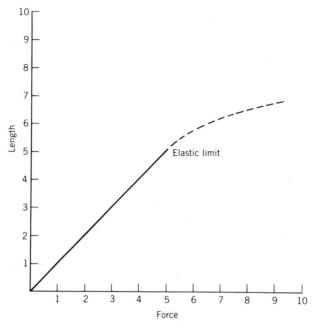

FIGURE 62

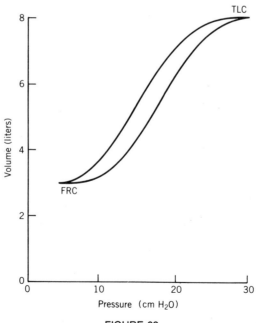

FIGURE 63

$$\text{Density} = \frac{\text{gram-molecular weight}}{22.4 \text{ liters}}$$

The molecular weight of cyclopropane $(CH_2)_3$ is 42 amu

$$\frac{42 \text{ g}}{22.4 \text{ liters}} = 1.87 \text{ g/liter}$$

(1:7–8), (2:87), (4:18–19)

24. D. STEP 1: Determine the pressure gradient.

$$\Delta P = P_m - P_{alv}$$

where

$$\Delta P = \text{pressure gradient}$$
$$P_m = \text{mouth pressure}$$
$$P_{alv} = \text{intra-alveolar pressure}$$

Mouth pressure in this case is equal to atmospheric pressure (i.e., 1,034 cm H_2O). An intra-alveolar pressure of -5 cm H_2O is equivalent to 1,029 cm H_2O. Therefore,

$$\Delta P = 1,034 \text{ cm } H_2O - 1,029 \text{ cm } H_2O$$
$$= 5 \text{ cm } H_2O$$

STEP 2: Calculate the flowrate ($\dot{V}$).

1. Convert 500 cc V_T to liter.

$$500 \text{ cc} = 0.5 \text{ liter}$$

2. The flowrate can be obtained by dividing the tidal volume by the inspiratory time (I_T).

$$\dot{V} = \frac{V_T}{I_T} = \frac{0.5 \text{ liter}}{2 \text{ seconds}}$$
$$= 0.25 \text{ liter/sec}$$

STEP 3: Apply the formula for determining airway resistance.

$$R = \frac{\Delta P}{\dot{V}} = \frac{5 \text{ cm } H_2O}{0.25 \text{ liter/sec}}$$
$$= 20 \text{ cm } H_2O/\text{liter/sec}$$

(1:144,181), (2:157–159), (4:80–82), (14:99–101), (29:30,82), (32:32–33)

25. B. Surface tension results from the imbalance of intermolecular forces existing at any gas-liquid interface. Surface tension forces can also be regarded as cohesive forces among the liquid molecules, as is shown in Figure 64. The law of LaPlace refers to spherical structures that demonstrate the interaction between the distending pressure and surface tension forces as the sphere's radius of curvature varies. The mathematical expression is shown as follows

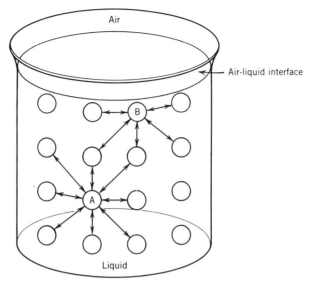

FIGURE 64

$$P = \frac{2\,ST}{r}$$

where

P = the pressure (dynes/cm^2) within the sphere acting against the surface tension forces

ST = the surface tension forces (dynes/cm)

r = the radius (cm) of the sphere

STEP 1: Express the 6 mm diameter as the radius in cm.

1. radius $= \dfrac{\text{diameter}}{2}$

$= \dfrac{6\text{ mm}}{2}$

$= 3$ mm

2. 1 mm = 0.1 cm

0.1 cm/m̶m̶ × 3 m̶m̶ = 0.3 cm

radius = 0.3 cm

STEP 2: Use the LaPlace relationship to solve for surface tension.

$$ST = \frac{Pr}{2}$$

$$= \frac{(420\text{ dynes/cm}^2)(0.3\text{ cm})}{2}$$

$$= \frac{126\text{ dynes/cm}}{2}$$

$$= 63\text{ dynes/cm}$$

(1:134–140), (2:174–176), (3:34–35), (4:28–29), (6:226,706), (8:20), (14:90, 166), (29:72,78,245), (32:26)

26. B. $\Delta P/\dot{V}$ is the quantitative expression for resistance. Resistance can be measured only during dynamic conditions.

As diaphragmatic excursions become rapid, the pressure gradient between the alveoli and the atmosphere (mouth) widens, resulting in an increased flowrate ($\dot{V}$). Consequently, airway resistance becomes greater. Slow, deep breathing reduces the airway resistance.

In the tracheobronchial tree, the airway resistance is greater in the large airways (>2 mm in diameter) than in the small airways (<2 mm in diameter). Despite their small diameter, airways <2 mm in diameter have a lower resistance than large airways because of the influence of the law of continuity on airflow.

Poiseuille's law is expressed as

$$\eta = \frac{\Delta P \pi r^4}{8L\dot{V}}$$

where,

$$\eta = \text{viscosity index}$$
$$\Delta P = \text{driving pressure}$$
$$\pi/8 = \text{mathematical constant}$$
$$r = \text{radius}$$
$$L = \text{length}$$
$$\dot{V} = \text{flowrate}$$

The relationship between airway resistance ($\Delta P/\dot{V}$) and airway length (L) can be seen by retaining these two factors in the equation and holding all the other factors constant (k).

STEP 1: Rearrange and express Poiseuille's relationship in terms of airway resistance ($\Delta P/\dot{V}$).

1. $\dfrac{\Delta P}{\dot{V}} = R$

2. $R = \dfrac{8L\eta}{\pi r^4}$

STEP 2: Identify those factors that will be held constant (k).

$$k = \pi/8, \eta, \quad \text{and} \quad r^4$$

STEP 3: Express Poiseuille's equation based on the previous considerations.

$$R = L \times k \quad \text{or} \quad \frac{R}{L} = k$$

By assigning arbitrary values to the variables (R and L) in STEP 3, one can quantitatively confirm the relationship. For example,

$$R = 4$$
$$L = 4$$
$$k = ?$$
$$R = L \times k$$
$$4 = 4 \times k$$
$$k = \frac{4}{4} = 1$$

If the length (L) of the conducting tube doubles, the resistance (R or $\Delta P/\dot{V}$) will double when all the other factors ($\pi/8$, η, and r) are held constant (k).

$$R = ?$$
$$L = 8$$
$$k = 1$$
$$\frac{R}{8} = 1$$
$$R = (8)(1) = 8$$

The converse is also true.

(1:146–148), (2:160–164), (3:37,165), (4:36–37), (6:512,1018), (14:99,166), (29:29,81,246), (32:33–35,83–84)

27. A. The law of continuity, based on the law of conservation of matter, explains the relationship between the cross-sectional area of a tube through which a fluid flows and the velocity of the flowing fluid. In quantitative terms, the product of the cross-sectional area times the velocity for a given flowrate is constant. Therefore, the two factors, cross-sectional area and velocity, are inversely related; that is, as the cross-sectional area decreases for a given flowrate the velocity of the flowing fluid increases and vice versa.

The continuity equation can be shown as

$$A \times v = k$$

where

$$A = \text{cross-sectional area (cm}^2\text{)}$$
$$v = \text{velocity (cm/sec)}$$
$$k = \text{constant}$$

(2:133–138), (4:29)

28. C. According to Bernoulli, in a constant fluid flow system the sum of the pressure energy (P), the potential energy per unit volume of fluid (Dgh), and the kinetic energy per unit of volume of fluid ($\frac{1}{2} Dv^2$) at one point in the system equals the sum of these energies at any other point. This can be shown quantitatively as

$$(\tfrac{1}{2} Dv^2)_1 + (Dgh)_1 + P_1 = (\tfrac{1}{2} Dv^2)_2 + (Dgh)_2 + P_2$$

where

$$\tfrac{1}{2} Dv^2 = \text{kinetic energy/volume}$$
$$(D = \text{density; } v = \text{velocity})$$
$$Dgh = \text{potential energy/volume (D = density;}$$
$$g = \text{acceleration due to gravity; h = height)}$$
$$P = \text{pressure energy (lateral wall pressure)}$$

By re-arranging the factors, eliminating potential energy, and simplifying the equation, the following relationship is obtained

$$\tfrac{1}{2} D(v_2^2 - v_1^2) = P_1 - P_2$$

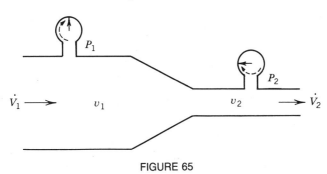

FIGURE 65

As the equation is now written, one can appreciate how the density of a gas can influence the velocity gradient and the lateral wall pressure gradient across a narrowed or partially obstructed airway. The greater the density factor, the greater the velocity gradient and the greater the lateral wall pressure (pressure energy) gradient. Any gas, regardless of its density, flowing across a stricture will develop an increased velocity gradient and an increased lateral wall pressure gradient. Note Figure 65 where $\dot{V}_1 = \dot{V}_2$. The purpose of administering a helium-oxygen mixture (e.g., 20% O_2 and 80% He) is to lessen the degree of both the velocity and lateral wall pressure gradient changes. Whether the flowing fluid is a helium-oxygen mixture or an air-oxygen mixture, lateral wall pressure drops as the fluid flows through a narrowing or a partial airway obstruction. Therefore, the lateral wall pressure gradient increases (widens) at that point. However, with a helium-oxygen mixture the lateral wall pressure drops to a lesser degree (less pressure energy converts to kinetic energy) because a helium-oxygen mixture is less dense than an air-oxygen mixture. Because lateral wall pressure drops to a lesser extent when a less dense gas is flowing, more pressure is available for airway inflation beyond the partial obstruction.
(1:149–152), (2:138–141), (4:33–35), (29:28)

29. D. Figure 66 below depicts a Venturi System. In a true Venturi system the angle of divergence must *not* exceed 15°, and the widening of the conduit distal to the narrowing must be large enough to accommodate the volume of the entrained gas, as well as that of the source gas. Consequently, the lateral wall pressure distal to the narrowing (P_3) will approximate that proximal to the narrowing (P_1).

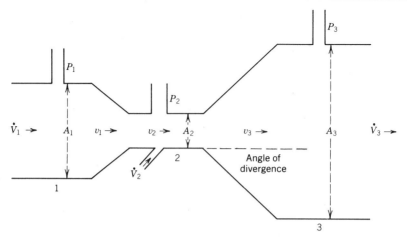

FIGURE 66

As the gas flows ($\dot{V}_1$) from its source through cross-sectional area A_1, it exerts a lateral wall pressure P_1 and has a velocity v_1. When the fluid enters the narrowing, indicated by cross-sectional area A_2, the lateral wall pressure drops as shown by P_2, and the velocity v_2 increases. This drop in lateral wall pressure (below atmospheric pressure) is used to entrain another fluid into the system. Therefore, $\dot{V}_2$ joins the flow of the source gas $\dot{V}_1$. As the entrained flow and the source gas flow traverse the tube together through the divergence, represented by the cross-sectional area A_3, the lateral wall pressure P_3 increases, and the velocity v_3 decreases. The resulting delivered flow $\dot{V}_3$, is the sum of $\dot{V}_1$ plus $\dot{V}_2$. It is, therefore, greater than each of those flowrates individually. In a Venturi system the following relationships are true.

1. $\dot{V}_1 + \dot{V}_2 = \dot{V}_3$
2. $v_1 < v_2$
3. $P_1 > P_2$
4. $P_2 < P_3$
5. $P_1 \simeq P_3$
6. $v_1 \simeq v_3$

(1:149–150), (2:142–144), (4:35)

30. D. The illustration represents three parallel resistances. The total resistance through the system can be calculated as follows

$$\frac{1}{R_T} = \frac{1}{R_1} + \frac{1}{R_2} + \frac{1}{R_3}$$

The total resistance is the sum of the reciprocal of the individual resistances.

STEP 1: Determine each of the individual resistances by using the following expression

$$R = \frac{\Delta P}{\dot{V}}$$

1. $\text{resistance}_1 = \dfrac{15 \text{ cm H}_2\text{O}}{3 \text{ liters/min}} = 5 \text{ cm H}_2\text{O/liter/min}$

2. $\text{resistance}_2 = \dfrac{9 \text{ cm H}_2\text{O}}{3 \text{ liters/min}} = 3 \text{ cm H}_2\text{O/liter/min}$

3. $\text{resistance}_3 = \dfrac{12 \text{ cm H}_2\text{O}}{3 \text{ liters/min}} = 4 \text{ cm H}_2\text{O/liter/min}$

STEP 2: Calculate the total resistance.

$$\frac{1}{5 \text{ cm H}_2\text{O/liter/min}} + \frac{1}{3 \text{ cm H}_2\text{O/liter/min}} + \frac{1}{4 \text{ cm H}_2\text{O/liter/min}} = \frac{1}{R_T}$$

0.20 liter/min/cm H$_2$O + 0.33 liter/min/cm H$_2$O

+ 0.25 liter/min/cm H$_2$O = 0.78 liter/min/cm H$_2$O

$$\frac{1}{R_T} = 0.78 \text{ liter/min/cm H}_2\text{O}$$

$$\frac{1}{0.78 \text{ liter/min/cm H}_2\text{O}} = R_T$$

$$R_T = 1.28 \text{ cm H}_2\text{O/liter/min}$$

(2:156–157), (32:33)

31. E. The potential osmotic pressure of an electrolyte solution can be obtained by using the following formula.

$$(\text{moles/liter}) \times \left(\begin{array}{c}\text{number of ionic}\\\text{species per}\\\text{molecule}\end{array}\right) \times \left(\frac{19{,}304 \text{ torr}}{\text{moles/liter}}\right) = \begin{array}{c}\text{electrolyte osmotic}\\\text{pressure (torr)}\end{array}$$

STEP 1: Determine the molecular weight of NaCl.

$$\begin{array}{l}23 \text{ amu} = \text{atomic weight of Na}\\+35 \text{ amu} = \text{atomic weight of Cl}\\\hline 58 \text{ amu} = \text{molecular weight of NaCl}\end{array}$$

STEP 2: Determine how the molecule either dissociates or ionizes into its component species.

Electrovalent (ionic) compounds are held together by an electrovalent (ionic) bond wherein electrons are transferred. Such compounds ionize. Covalent compounds are formed by sharing electrons and dissociate.

NaCl is an electrovalent (ionic) compound that ionizes into one Na$^+$ ion and one Cl$^-$ ion. One NaCl molecule, therefore, ionizes into two ions.

$$NaCl \rightleftharpoons Na^+ + Cl^-$$

STEP 3: Determine the molarity of a 0.9% NaCl solution.

1. molecular weight of NaCl = 58 amu
2. a 0.9% NaCl (W/V) solution contains 9.0 g of NaCl per liter

3. 9.0 g of NaCl = 0.15 mole of NaCl

$$\frac{9.0 \text{ g of NaCl}}{58 \text{ g/mole}} = 0.15 \text{ mole of NaCl}$$

4. molarity = moles/liter

$$= \frac{0.15 \text{ mole}}{1 \text{ liter}}$$

$$= 0.15 \ M$$

STEP 4: Calculate the potential osmotic pressure for a 0.9% NaCl solution using the equation

$$M \times \left(\begin{array}{c} \text{number of ionic} \\ \text{species per molecule} \end{array} \right) \times \left(\frac{19,304 \text{ torr}}{\text{moles/liter}} \right) = \begin{array}{c} \text{electrolyte osmotic} \\ \text{pressure (torr)} \end{array}$$

$$0.15 \ M \times 2 \times \left(\frac{19,304 \text{ torr}}{\text{moles/liter}} \right) = 5,791 \text{ torr}$$

An osmotic pressure of 5,791 torr develops when a 0.9% or 0.15 M solution of NaCl is separated from a pure H_2O solution by a membrane.

Physiologically, this quantity of osmotic pressure does not develop because all the membranes in the body are passively permeable to NaCl, Na^+ ions, and Cl^- ions. The osmotic pressure gradient that exists between the interstitial space and the vasculature results from the fact that plasma proteins are relatively impermeable across the capillary endothelium. This osmotic pressure is called the oncotic pressure, or the colloid osmotic pressure.

(1:60–63), (2:177–182), (4:10)

32. A. The four pressures (1) capillary hydrostatic pressure (CHP), (2) capillary osmotic pressure (COP), (3) interstitial hydrostatic pressure (IHP), and (4) interstitial osmotic pressure (IOP) interact and determine the direction and magnitude of fluid out of (filtration) and into (reabsorption) the vasculature at the systemic capillary level.

STEP 1: Determine the net filtration pressure at the arterial end of the systemic capillary.

1. calculate the hydrostatic pressure gradient

CHP − IHP = hydrostatic pressure gradient
30 mm Hg − (−3 mm Hg) = 30 mm Hg + 3 mm Hg
= 33 mm Hg

2. calculate the colloid osmotic pressure gradient

COP − IOP = colloid osmotic pressure gradient
25 mm Hg − 4 mm Hg = 21 mm Hg

3. subtract the colloid osmotic pressure gradient from the hydrostatic pressure gradient

33 mm Hg hydrostatic pressure gradient
−21 mm Hg colloid osmotic pressure gradient
----
12 mm Hg net filtration pressure

The net filtration pressure of 12 mm Hg indicates that there is a net movement of fluid out of the vasculature into the interstitium at the arterial end of this systemic capillary.

STEP 2: Determine the net reabsorption pressure at the venous end of the systemic capillary.

1. calculate the hydrostatic pressure gradient

$$CHP - IHP = \text{hydrostatic pressure gradient}$$
$$10 \text{ mm Hg} - (-3 \text{ mm Hg}) = 10 \text{ mm Hg} + 3 \text{ mm Hg}$$
$$= 13 \text{ mm Hg}$$

2. calculate the colloid osmotic pressure gradient

$$COP - IOP = \text{colloid osmotic pressure gradient}$$
$$28 \text{ mm Hg} - 4 \text{ mm Hg} = 24 \text{ mm Hg}$$

3. subtract the hydrostatic pressure gradient from the colloid osmotic pressure gradient

$$\begin{array}{r} 24 \text{ mm Hg colloid osmotic pressure gradient} \\ -13 \text{ mm Hg hydrostatic pressure gradient} \\ \hline 11 \text{ mm Hg net reabsorption pressure} \end{array}$$

The net reabsorption pressure of 11 mm Hg signifies that there is a net movement of fluid into the vasculature from the interstitium at the venous end of this systemic capillary.

STEP 3: Calculate the net filtration–net reabsorption pressure gradient to determine the amount of fluid expressed in pressure that does not reabsorb at the venous end of this systemic capillary.

$$\begin{array}{r} 12 \text{ mm Hg net filtration pressure} \\ -11 \text{ mm Hg net reabsorption pressure} \\ \hline 1 \text{ mm Hg filtration-reabsorption pressure} \end{array}$$

(2:186–189), (3:157), (32:100–102)

33. B. Airway conductance (G_{aw}) is the reciprocal of airway resistance (R_{aw})

$$R_{aw} = \frac{\Delta P}{\dot{V}} \quad \text{and}$$

$$G_{aw} = \frac{\dot{V}}{\Delta P}$$

Therefore,

$$R_{aw} = \frac{1}{G_{aw}} \quad \text{and}$$

$$G_{aw} = \frac{1}{R_{aw}}$$

(2:191–192), (4:32,253), (6:251), (8:32,128), (29:90,259)

34. C. A Reynold's number less than 2,000 indicates that laminar flow will prevail, whereas a Reynold's number greater than 2,000 signifies the presence of turbulent flow.

    Reynold's number, a dimensionless value, is obtained as follows

    $$R_N = \frac{\text{diameter} \times \text{density} \times \text{velocity}}{\text{viscosity}}$$

    (2:164–165), (4:33), (6:390,1018), (29:29,81,246), (32:35)

35. B. The combined gas law is used to derive gas volume correction factors from STPD to BTPS.

    $$\frac{PV}{T} = k$$

    where

    > P = pressure (mm Hg)
    > V = volume (liters)
    > T = absolute temperature (°K)
    > k = n R (number of moles times Boltzmann's constant)

    STEP 1: List the variables involved in the calculation.

STPD	BTPS
P_1 = 760 mm Hg	P_2 = 755 mm Hg
T_1 = 273°K	T_2 = 310°K
P_{H_2O} = 0 mm Hg	P_{H_2O} = 47 mm Hg
V_1	V_2

    STEP 2: Correct the final pressure (P_2) for the presence of H_2O vapor pressure.

    $$P_B - P_{H_2O} = \text{corrected } P_B$$

    or

    $$P_2 - P_{H_2O} = \text{corrected } P_B$$
    $$755 \text{ mm Hg} - 47 \text{ mm Hg} = 708 \text{ mm Hg}$$

    STEP 3: Apply the combined gas law and solve for V_2.

    $$\frac{P_1 V_1}{T_1} = \frac{P_2 V_2}{T_2}$$
    $$\frac{(760 \text{ mm Hg})(V_1)}{273°K} = \frac{(708 \text{ mm Hg})(V_2)}{310°K}$$
    $$V_2 = \frac{(760 \text{ mm Hg})(V_1)(310°K)}{(708 \text{ mm Hg})(273°K)}$$
    $$V_2 = 1.219(V_1)$$

    The factor needed to convert the gas volume from STPD to BTPS is 1.219.

Therefore, the volume (V_2) at BTPS will be 1.219 times greater than the volume (V_1) at STPD.

(1:27), (2:126–127)

36. A. Charles' law states that for a given mass of gas the volume varies directly with the absolute temperature (°K) when the pressure is constant (k). Mathematically, this relationship can be shown as

$$\frac{V}{T} = k$$

Based on this relationship, the original volume at 0°C will change 1/273 of that volume for each degree Celsius (°C) change from 0°C. For example, if the original volume at 0°C was 273 cc and the temperature decreased to −273°C, the new volume can be calculated as follows.

$$\frac{V_1}{T_1} = \frac{V_2}{T_2}$$

where

$$V_1 = 273 \text{ cc}$$
$$T_1 = 273°K \quad \text{or} \quad (0°C + 273 = 273°K)$$
$$V_2 = \text{?? cc}$$
$$T_2 = 0°K \quad \text{or} \quad [273°C + (−273) = 0°K]$$
$$\frac{273 \text{ cc}}{273°K} = \frac{V_2}{0°K}$$
$$V_2 = \frac{(273 \text{ cc})0°K}{273°K}$$
$$V_2 = 0 \text{ cc}$$

Therefore, when the temperature of the original volume at 0°C is decreased −273°C, the new volume is 0 cc. In reality this situation is not possible because of the influence of the van der Waals forces. This is just one reason why Charles' law is classified as an *ideal* gas law.

(1:20,21), (2:13,14,122–124), (4:24,273), (6:1017), (29:22)

37. E. The characteristic concentric, parallel layers of flowing gas molecules is lost when turbulent flow is present. Gas molecules travel in vortices or eddy currents and the gas velocity is essentially uniform across the velocity profile. The driving pressure needed to produce and maintain turbulent flow is proportional to the square of the flowrate times a constant related to gas density.

$$\Delta P = k \times \dot{V}^2$$

The airway resistance encountered by the flowing gas is greater in turbulent flow than in laminar flow.

(1:149), (2:147–148), (4:32,33,81), (13:12), (29:82), (32:33–35,203,209,215)

38. D. Barometric pressure (P_B) in pounds per square inch (psi) can be obtained from the following formula.

$$P_B = \left(\begin{array}{c}\text{height of the}\\\text{liquid column}\end{array}\right)(\text{density})$$

$$= (33 \text{ inches})(0.491 \text{ lb/in}^2)$$

$$= 16.20 \text{ psi}$$

(1:10–12), (2:116–117), (4:20)

39. E. The density of a mixture of gases can be determined using the following equation

$$D = \frac{[(\%)(\text{gmw})]_A + [(\%)(\text{gmw})]_B + \cdots [(\%)(\text{gmw})]_n}{22.4 \text{ liters}}$$

where

D = density of the gas mixture (g/liter)

% = concentration of each constituent in the gas mixture

gmw = gram-molecular weight of each constituent in the gas mixture (g)

STEP 1: Determine the gram-molecular weight of each constituent in the gas mixture.

CONSTITUENT	GRAM-MOLECULAR WEIGHT
Oxygen	32 g
Carbon dioxide	44 g
Nitrogen	28 g

STEP 2: Solve for the density of the mixture.

$$D = \frac{(0.2093)(32 \text{ g}) + (0.0004)(44 \text{ g}) + (0.7903)(28 \text{ g})}{22.4 \text{ liters}}$$

$$D = 1.29 \text{ g/liter}$$

(1:7–8), (4:19)

40. E. Avogadro's law states that at equal temperatures and pressures equal volumes of different gases contain the same number of molecules. Based on Avogadro's law is the fact that at STP one gram-molecular weight of a substance contains 6.023×10^{23} molecules (Avogadro's number) and occupies a volume of 22.4 liters.

(1:6), (2:132–133), (4:18), (6:1017), (29:21,22,32,125)

41. E. Viscosity is a time-related property of matter that is temperature dependent. In liquids viscosity decreases with increasing temperature. Conversely, gas viscosity increases with increasing temperature. The different units for viscosity in the various systems of units are as follows

SYSTEM OF UNITS	UNITS FOR VISCOSITY
Centimeter-gram-second (CGS)	Dyne-second/cm^2 or poise
Meter-kilogram-second (MKS)	Newton-second/m^2
International System (SI)	Pascal-second or Pas

(2:159–160), (4:33,36), (6:390), (29:27,29,81,90)

42. B. Gay-Lussac's law states that for a given mass of gas the pressure varies directly with the absolute temperature (°K) when the volume is constant (k). Mathematically,

$$\frac{P}{T} = k$$

Based on this relationship, the original pressure will change $1/273$ for each degree Celsius (°C) change from 0°C. For example, if the original pressure at 0°C was 273 torr and the temperature increased to 273°C, the new pressure can be obtained as follows

$$\frac{P_1}{T_1} = \frac{P_2}{T_2}$$

where

$$P_1 = 273 \text{ torr}$$
$$T_1 = 273°K \quad \text{or} \quad (0°C + 273 = 273°K)$$
$$P_2 = ?? \text{ torr}$$
$$T_2 = 546°K \quad \text{or} \quad (273°C + 273 = 546°K)$$

$$\frac{273 \text{ torr}}{273°K} = \frac{P_2}{546°K}$$

$$P_2 = \frac{(273 \text{ torr})(546°K)}{273°K}$$

$$P_2 = 546 \text{ torr}$$

Therefore, when the temperature of the original pressure at 0°C is increased to 273°C, the new pressure will be 546 torr.

(1:20), (2:124–125), (4:24–25), (6:1017), (29:22)

43. C. Mathematically, Graham's law of diffusion for gases in a liquid medium is shown below.

$$\frac{r_1}{r_2} = \frac{(\sqrt{MW_2})(Cs_1)}{(\sqrt{MW_1})(Cs_2)}$$

where

$$r = \text{rate of diffusion of the gas in the liquid}$$
$$MW = \text{molecular weight of the gas (gas density may substitute)}$$
$$Cs = \text{solubility coefficient of the gas}$$

STEP 1: Determine the molecular weight of N_2O and C_3H_6.

1. molecular weight of N_2O

$$N = 14$$
$$O = 16$$
$$2(14) + 16 = 44 \text{ amu}$$

2. molecular weight of C_3H_6

$$C = 12$$
$$H = 1$$
$$3(12) + 6(1) = 42 \text{ amu}$$

STEP 2: Use Graham's law of diffusion of gases in a liquid medium and solve for the relative rate of diffusion

$$\frac{r_{N_2O}}{r_{C_3H_6}} = \frac{(\sqrt{MW_{C_3H_6}})(Cs_{N_2O})}{(\sqrt{MW_{N_2O}})(Cs_{C_3H_6})}$$

$$= \frac{(\sqrt{42})(0.41)}{(\sqrt{44})(0.011)}$$

$$= \frac{(6.481)(0.41)}{(6.633)(0.011)} = \frac{2.657}{0.073}$$

$$= 36.40$$

$$r_{N_2O} = 36.40 \ (r_{C_3H_6})$$

(1:196), (2:67–69), (4:26), (27:9), (29:21,88,95), (32:122)

44. B. The formula for obtaining total compliance

$$\frac{1}{C_L} + \frac{1}{C_{CW}} = \frac{1}{C_{L\text{-}CW}}$$

where

$$C_L = \text{lung (pulmonary) compliance (liter/cm } H_2O)$$
$$C_{CW} = \text{chest wall (thorax) compliance (liter/cm } H_2O)$$
$$C_{L\text{-}CW} = \text{lung-chest wall (total) compliance (liter/cm } H_2O)$$

STEP 1: Rearrange the formula to solve for chest wall compliance (C_{CW}).

$$\frac{1}{C_{CW}} = \frac{1}{C_{L\text{-}CW}} - \frac{1}{C_L}$$

STEP 2: Insert the known values and solve for C_{CW}.

$$\frac{1}{C_{CW}} = \frac{1}{0.072 \text{ liter/cm } H_2O} - \frac{1}{0.12 \text{ liter/cm } H_2O}$$

$$= 13.89 \text{ cm } H_2O/\text{liter} - 8.33 \text{ cm } H_2O/\text{liter}$$

$$= 5.56 \text{ cm } H_2O/\text{liter}$$

$$C_{CW} = \frac{1}{5.56 \text{ cm } H_2O/\text{liter}}$$

$$= 0.179 \text{ liter/cm } H_2O$$

(1:140–143,182–184), (2:169–172), (3:36), (4:27–28,77–80), (6:247–249,1025), (8:22–26), (29:70–74,259), (32:21–23)

45. D. The law of LaPlace will allow for the computation of the inflation pressure.

$$P = \frac{2 \ ST}{r}$$

where

$$P = \text{inflation (distending) pressure (dynes/cm}^2)$$
$$ST = \text{surface tension (dynes/cm)}$$
$$r = \text{radius of the sphere (cm)}$$

STEP 1: Determine the inflation pressure of sphere X.

$$P = \frac{2(12 \text{ dynes/cm})}{0.005 \text{ cm}}$$
$$= 4{,}800 \text{ dynes/cm}^2$$

STEP 2: Determine the inflation pressure of sphere Y.

$$P = \frac{2(12 \text{ dynes/cm})}{0.0025 \text{ cm}}$$
$$= 9{,}600 \text{ dynes/cm}^2$$

The inflation pressure for sphere X is 4,800 dynes/cm^2, and the inflation pressure for sphere Y is 9,600 dynes/cm^2.

(1:134–138), (2:174–176), (3:34–35), (4:28–29,134), (6:226–706), (29:72,78, 188,245), (32:26)

46. A. Because sphere Y has the greater pressure of the two spheres, sphere Y would empty into sphere X.

(1:134–138), (2:174–176), (3:34–35), (4:28–29,134), (6:226,706), (29:72,78, 188,245), (32:26)

47. B. The number of moles of any substance can be obtained by using the expression

$$\text{moles} = \frac{\text{grams}}{\text{grams-molecular weight}}$$

STEP 1: Find the atomic weights of the constituent atoms in the H$_3$PO$_4$ molecule.

$$H = 1 \text{ amu}$$
$$P = 31 \text{ amu}$$
$$0 = 16 \text{ amu}$$

STEP 2: Determine the gram-molecular weight of H$_3$PO$_4$.

$$3(1 \text{ amu}) + 1(31 \text{ amu}) + 4(16 \text{ amu}) = 98 \text{ amu}$$

STEP 3: Use the formula for determining the number of moles.

$$\text{moles} = \frac{\text{grams}}{\text{gram-molecular weight}}$$
$$= \frac{98 \text{ g}}{98 \text{ amu}}$$
$$= 1 \text{ mole}$$

(1:6), (2:69–70), (4:18)

48. B. Because the gas mixture is at STPD, no correction for the presence of water vapor (P_{H_2O}) is necessary. Therefore,

STEP 1: Express each gas percentage as a fractional concentration.

CO_2	O_2	N_2
20% = 0.20	30% = 0.30	50% = 0.50

STEP 2: Use the formula below to obtain the partial pressure of each gas.

$$P_{gas} = F_{gas}(P_B - P_{H_2O})$$

where

P_{gas} = partial pressure of the gas
F_{gas} = fractional concentration of the gas
P_B = barometric pressure
P_{H_2O} = water vapor pressure

1. carbon dioxide

$$P_{CO_2} = 0.20 \ (760 \ mm \ Hg - 0 \ mm \ Hg)$$
$$P_{CO_2} = 152 \ mm \ Hg$$

2. oxygen

$$P_{O_2} = 0.30 \ (760 \ mm \ Hg - 0 \ mm \ Hg)$$
$$P_{O_2} = 228 \ mm \ Hg$$

3. nitrogen

$$P_{N_2} = 0.50 \ (760 \ mm \ Hg - 0 \ mm \ Hg)$$
$$P_{N_2} = 380 \ mm \ Hg$$

(1:14), (2:127–132), (4:22–23), (6:361–1017), (27:6), (29:23), (32:69,212)

49. D. The volume of a sphere can be obtained from the formula

$$V = \tfrac{4}{3} \pi r^3$$

where

V = volume of the sphere (liters)
π = pi or 3.14
r = radius (meters)

STEP 1: Convert the radius expressed in millimeters (mm) to meters (m).

$$1 \ mm = 10^{-3} \ m$$
$$(0.15 \ \cancel{mm})(10^{-3} \ m/\cancel{mm}) = 0.15 \times 10^{-3} \ m$$
$$= 1.50 \quad or \quad 10^{-4} \ m$$

STEP 2: Determine the volume of one sphere or alveolus.

$$V = \tfrac{4}{3} \pi r^3 = \tfrac{4}{3}(3.14)(1.50 \times 10^{-4} \ m)^3$$
$$= 1.413 \times 10^{-11} \ m^3$$

STEP 3: Convert 1.413×10^{-11} m³ to liters.

$$1 \text{ m}^3 = 1,000 \text{ liters} = 10^3 \text{ liters}$$

$$(1.413 \times 10^{-11} \text{ m}^3)(10^3 \text{ liters/m}^3) = 1.413 \times 10^{-8} \text{ liter}$$

The volume of one alveolus is 1.413×10^{-8} liter

STEP 4: Calculate the volume of 300×10^6 alveoli.

$$(1.413 \times 10^{-8} \text{ liter})(300 \times 10^6) = 423.9 \times 10^{-2} \text{ liters}$$

or

$$= 4.239 \text{ liters}$$

(2:135–137), (12:161–162)

50. C. The area of a sphere is provided by the formula

$$A = 4\pi r^2$$

where

$$A = \text{area of the sphere (m}^2)$$
$$\pi = pi \text{ or } 3.14$$
$$r = \text{radius (meters)}$$

STEP 1: Convert the radius expressed in millimeters (mm) to meters (m).

$$1 \text{ mm} = 10^{-3} \text{ m}$$

$$(0.137 \text{ mm})(10^{-3} \text{ m/mm}) = 0.137 \times 10^{-3} \text{ m}$$

or

$$= 1.37 \times 10^{-4} \text{ m}$$

STEP 2: Determine the surface area of one sphere or alveolus.

$$A = 4\pi r^2$$
$$A = (4)(3.14)(1.37 \times 10^{-4} \text{ m})^2$$
$$= 2.36 \times 10^{-7} \text{ m}^2$$

STEP 3: Calculate the surface area of 300×10^6 alveoli.

$$(2.36 \times 10^{-7} \text{ m}^2)(300 \times 10^6) = 70.8 \text{ m}^2$$

(2:136), (12:161–162)

REFERENCES

1. Spearman, C., and Sheldon, R., *Egan's Fundamentals of Respiratory Therapy*, 4th ed., C.V. Mosby, St. Louis, 1982.
2. Wojciechowski, W., *Respiratory Care Sciences: An Integrated Approach*, John Wiley & Sons, New York, 1985.
3. Shapiro, B., Harrison, R., Kacmarek, R., and Cane, R., *Clinical Application of Respiratory Care*, 3rd ed., Year Book Medical Publishers, Chicago, 1985.
4. Kacmarek, R., Mack, C., and Dimas, S., *The Essentials of Respiratory Therapy*, 2nd, ed., Year Book Medical Publishers, Chicago, 1985.

5. McPherson, S., *Respiratory Therapy Equipment,* 3rd ed., C.V. Mosby, St. Louis, 1985.

6. Burton, G., and Hodgkin, J., *Respiratory Care: A Guide to Clinical Practice,* 2nd ed., J.B. Lippincott, Philadelphia, 1985.

7. Frownfelter, D., *Chest Physical Therapy and Cardiopulmonary Rehabilitation, An Interdisciplinary Approach,* Year Book Medical Publishers, Chicago, 1978.

8. Cherniack, R., and Cherniack, L., *Respiration in Health and Disease,* 3rd ed., W.B. Saunders, Philadelphia, 1983.

9. Daily, E., and Schroeder, G., *Techniques in Bedside Hemodynamic Monitoring,* 3rd ed., C.V. Mosby, St. Louis, 1985.

10. Des Jardins, R., *Clinical Manifestations of Respiratory Disease,* Year Book Medical Publishers, Chicago, 1984.

11. Mitchell, R., *Synopsis of Clinical Pulmonary Disease,* 3rd ed., C.V. Mosby, St., Louis, 1982.

12. Comroe, J., *Physiology of Respiration,* 3rd ed., Year Book Medical Publishers, Chicago, 1974.

13. West, J., *Pulmonary Pathophysiology—The Essentials,* 2nd ed., Williams & Wilkins, Baltimore, 1982.

14. West, J., *Respiratory Physiology—The Essentials,* 3rd ed., Williams & Wilkins, Baltimore, 1985.

15. Martz, K., et al., *Management of the Patient-Ventilator System: A Team Approach,* 2nd ed., C.V. Mosby, St. Louis, 1984.

16. Shoup, C., and McHenry, R., *Laboratory Exercises in Respiratory Therapy,* 2nd ed., C.V. Mosby, St. Louis, 1983.

17. Ruppel, G., *Manual of Pulmonary Function Testing,* 3rd ed., C.V. Mosby, St. Louis, 1982.

18. Appelbaum, E., and Bruce, D., *Tracheal Intubation,* W.B. Saunders, Philadelphia, 1976.

19. Rau, J., *Respiratory Therapy Pharmacology,* 2nd ed., Year Book Medical Publishers, Chicago, 1984.

20. United States Department of Health, Education, and Welfare, Public Health Service, *Isolation Techniques for Use in Hospitals,* 2nd ed., Washington, D.C., 1975.

21. Brooks, S., *Integrated Basic Science,* 4th ed., C.V. Mosby, St. Louis, 1979.

22. Comroe, J., *The Lung,* Year Book Medical Publishers, Inc., Chicago, 1962.

23. Shibel, E., and Moser, K., *Respiratory Emergencies,* 2nd ed., C.V. Mosby, St. Louis, 1982.

24. Tisi, G., *Pulmonary Physiology in Clinical Medicine,* 2nd ed., Williams & Wilkins, Baltimore, 1985.

25. Cherniack, R., *Pulmonary Function Testing,* W.B. Saunders, Philadelphia, 1977.

26. Altose, M., *The Physiological Basis of Pulmonary Function Testing,* Clinical Symposia-CIBA, Vol. 31, No. 2, Summit, New Jersey, 1979.

27. Shapiro, B., Harrison, R., and Walton, J., *Clinical Application of Arterial Blood Gases,* 3rd ed., Year Book Medical Publishers, Chicago, 1982.

28. West, J., *Ventilation/Blood Flow and Gas Exchange,* 3rd ed., Blackwell Scientific Publications, 1979.

29. Slonim, N., and Hamilton, K., *Respiratory Physiology,* 4th ed., C.V. Mosby, St. Louis, 1981.

30. Rarey, K., and Youtsey, J., *Respiratory Patient Care,* Prentice-Hall, Englewood Cliffs, 1981.

31. Berne, R., and Levy, M., *Physiology,* C.V. Mosby, St. Louis, 1983.

32. Levitzky, M., *Pulmonary Physiology,* 2nd ed., McGraw-Hill, New York, 1986.

33. Wilson, P., Bell, C., and Norton, A., *Rehabilitation of the Heart and Lungs,* SensorMedics, 1980.

34. Clausen, J., and Zarins, L., *Pulmonary Function Testing Guildlines and Controversies,* Academic Press, New York, 1982.

35. Klaus, M., and Fanaroff, A., *Care of the High-Risk Neonate,* 2nd ed., W.B. Saunders, Philadelphia, 1979.

36. Lough, M., et al., *Pediatric Respiratory Therapy*, 3rd ed., Year Book Medical Publishers, Chicago, 1985.

37. Levin, D., et al., *A Practical Guide to Pediatric Intensive Care*, 2nd ed., C.V. Mosby, St. Louis, 1984.

38. O'Ryan, J., and Burns, D., *Pulmonary Rehabilitation from Hospital to Home*, Year Book Medical Publishers, Chicago, 1984.

39. Bell, C., et al., *Home Care and Rehabilitation in Respiratory Medicine*, J.B. Lippincott, Philadelphia, 1984.

40. Wilkins, R., et al., *Clinical Assessment in Respiratory Care*, C.V. Mosby, St. Louis, 1985.

41. Jones, N., and Campbell, E., *Clinical Exercise Testing*, 2nd ed., W.B. Saunders, Philadelphia, 1982.

42. Goldsmith, J., and Karotkin, E., *Assisted Ventilation of the Neonate*, W.B. Saunders, Philadelphia, 1981.

43. Blowers, M., and Sims, R., *How to Read an ECG*, 3rd ed., Medical Economics, New Jersey, 1983.

44. Eubanks, D., and Bone, R., *Comprehensive Respiratory Care*, C.V. Mosby, St. Louis, 1985.

45. Rattenborg, C., *Clinical Use of Mechanical Ventilation*, Year Book Medical Publishers, Chicago, 1981.

46. Witkowski, A. S., *Pulmonary Assessment: A Clinical Guide*, J.B. Lippincott, Philadelphia, 1985.

47. Op't Holt, Timothy B., *Assessment Based Respiratory Care*, John Wiley & Sons, New York, 1986.

CLINICAL SCIENCES

This section encompasses cardiopulmonary diseases, general medical conditions, and pediatrics and perinatology. The questions presented in these areas are intended to evaluate your understanding and knowledge of various aspects of adult, pediatric, and neonatal cardiopulmonary and general medical clinical conditions. Principles of pathophysiology, symptomology, and radiology also are included.

CARDIOPULMONARY DISEASES ASSESSMENT

PURPOSE: The purpose of this 50-item section is to evaluate your knowledge and understanding of cardiopulmonary diseases. The pathophysiology and clinical management of a variety of cardiopulmonary diseases are included.

DIRECTIONS: Each of the questions or incomplete statements below is followed by five suggested answers. Select the one which is the best in each case and then blacken the corresponding space on the answer sheet.

1. Which of the following lung diseases are classified as pneumoconioses?

    I. berylliosis
    II. baritosis
    III. histoplasmosis
    IV. silicosis

    A. I, II only
    B. II, IV only
    C. I, II, IV only
    D. I, III, IV only
    E. I, II, III, IV

2. Which of the following pulmonary pathologies are generally associated with an increase in intrapulmonary shunting?

    I. Klebsiella pneumonia
    II. pulmonary edema
    III. adult respiratory distress syndrome (ARDS)
    IV. pleural effusion

    A. I, II, III, IV
    B. II, III only
    C. III, IV only
    D. I, II only
    E. I, II, IV only

3. Which of the following pathophysiologic changes or clinical features associated with ARDS is often the first clinical manifestation of the development of this syndrome?

    A. increased lung compliance
    B. refractory hypoxemia
    C. increased pulmonary capillary permeability
    D. hypercapnia
    E. adventitious breath sounds

4. Which of the following pathophysiologic conditions contribute to the development of cor pulmonale?

    I. increased erythropoeisis

    II. hypercapnia

    III. aldosteronism

    IV. acidemia

    A. II, IV only   D. I, II, IV only

    B. I, III only   E. I, III only

    C. II, III, IV only

5. Which of the following cardiopulmonary diseases may be inherited?

    I. chronic bronchitis

    II. cystic fibrosis

    III. pulmonary emphysema

    IV. bronchiectasis

    A. I, II, III only   D. II, III, IV only

    B. II, III only   E. I, II, IV only

    C. I, III, IV only

6. A 38-year-old white female enters the emergency room displaying the following signs and symptoms: (1) chills and fever, (2) cough, (3) increased white blood cell count, and (4) pleuritic pain. The patient also complains of coughing up copious amounts of purulent, foul-smelling, foul-tasting, blood-tinged sputum. Sputum cultures indicate anaerobes and mixed flora. The patient also claims that she has not experienced any weight loss, anorexia, or dyspnea. Amphoric breath sounds can be heard upon auscultation of right anterior upper chest. Which of the following clinical conditions is the probable diagnosis?

    A. pulmonary neoplasm   D. lung abscess

    B. bronchiectasis   E. pneumomediastinum

    C. pleural effusion

7. A 33-year-old black male from South Carolina enters his physician's office complaining of general malaise, dyspnea, and a nonproductive cough. Breath sounds were found to be normal. Chest x-rays reveal bilateral hilar adenopathy and diffuse alveolar infiltrates. Pulmonary function data are shown below.

PARAMETER	PREDICTED	ACTUAL	% PREDICTED
FVC	4.65 liters	2.18 liters	47
FEV_1	3.63 liters	1.95 liters	54
FEV_1/FVC		89%	
$FEF_{25-75\%}$	4.05 liters/sec	3.00 liters/sec	74
MVV	126.0 liters/min	88.5 liters/min	70
FRC	2.65 liters	1.29 liters	49
RV	1.61 liters	0.81 liters	50
TLC	5.02 liters	2.67 liters	53
DL_{co}(ml/min/mm Hg)	22.0	15.2	69

What is the probable diagnosis for this patient?

A. sarcoidosis

B. pulmonary edema

C. asthma

D. hypersensitivity pneumonitis

E. pneumoconiosis

8. A 45-year-old white male, 5 ft. 4 in. tall and weighing 312 lb, entered the emergency room cyanotic and drowsy. Arterial blood gases on room air were immediately drawn and revealed

Pa_{O_2}: 40 mm Hg
Pa_{CO_2}: 68 mm Hg
pH: 7.32
HCO_3^-: 34 mEq/liter

His ventilatory rate was 40 breaths/min. He was then placed on a Venturi mask at 24%. Vital signs were

heart rate: 135 beats/min
blood pressure: 175/100

His measured tidal volume was 310 cc. What is the probable diagnosis for this patient?

A. adult respiratory distress syndrome

B. pulmonary infarction

C. bronchial asthma

D. Pickwickian syndrome

E. interstitial lung disease

9. Which of the following clinical interventions are appropriate for the treatment of carbon monoxide poisoning?

I. The administration of oxygen under normobaric conditions.

II. The administration of oxygen under hyperbaric conditions.

III. The administration of carbogen (5% CO_2 and 95% O_2) to increase the minute ventilation.

IV. Endotracheal intubation of an apneic victim along with hyperventilation via a manual resuscitator and oxygen administration.

A. II, IV only

B. I, III, IV only

C. I, II, IV only

D. I, II, III only

E. I, II, III, IV

10. A 38-year-old white female was hospitalized and was convalescing comfortably from fractures of bones in both legs resulting from a skiing accident. Before this mishap, the victim had no cardiopulmonary disease and a nonsmoking history.

Two days later, the patient suddenly became dyspneic, tachypneic, and cyanotic. Adventitious breath sounds—rales and rhonchi—were heard upon auscultation of the chest. The patient exhibited a diminished sensorium and petechiae on her chest and neck. What is the probable diagnosis?

A. fat embolization

B. acute myocardial infarction

C. tension pneumothorax

D. aspiration pneumonitis

E. pulmonary edema

11. Which of the following statements accurately compare/contrast the clinical manifestations of a viral pneumonia and a bacterial pneumonia?

   I. A viral pneumonia is of gradual onset, whereas bacterial pneumonia occurs suddenly.

   II. A bacterial pneumonia is generally associated with a leukocyte count of greater than $10,000/mm^3$, whereas a viral pneumonia usually has a white blood cell count of less than $10,000/mm^3$.

   III. Both forms of pneumonia cause thick, purulent sputum to be produced.

   IV. A viral pneumonia rarely causes pleuritic pain, whereas a bacterial pneumonia is occasionally associated with pleuritic pain.

   A. I, II, III, IV
   B. I, II only
   C. I, II, IV only
   D. III, IV only
   E. II, III only

12. A 27-year-old Vietnamese male was fishing in a boat in the Gulf of Mexico off the Alabama coast. He was proceeding to shore in response to weather forecasts warning of the impending arrival of Hurricane Elena when his boat capsized. He was soon retrieved from the water by a passing Coast Guard Vessel. Resuscitation was begun.

   He was immediately air-evacuated to the University of South Alabama Medical Center where he immediately received O_2 and $NaHCO_3$, and was placed on intermittent mandatory ventilation with the following settings

$$V_T: \quad 800 \text{ cc}$$
$$F_{I_{O_2}}: \quad 0.40$$
$$\text{ventilatory rate:} \quad 5 \text{ breaths/min}$$

   He had a spontaneous ventilatory rate of 12 breaths/min and a spontaneous V_T of 400 cc. When the ventilator cycled on to deliver the 800 cc tidal volume, the peak inspiratory pressure consistently registered 30 cm H_2O.

   Arterial blood gases while on the ventilator were as follows:

$$Pa_{O_2}: \quad 95 \text{ mm Hg}$$
$$Pa_{CO_2}: \quad 44 \text{ mm Hg}$$
$$pH: \quad 7.38$$
$$HCO_3^-: \quad 26 \text{ mEq/liter}$$

   Twenty-four hours after admission, the patient's ventilatory rate increased to 26 breaths/min, his heart rate increased to 130 beats/min, and he became cyanotic. The peak inspiratory pressure (PIP) during the mandatory breaths increased to 50 cm H_2O. Arterial blood gases at this time were

$$Pa_{O_2}: \quad 41 \text{ mm Hg}$$
$$Pa_{CO_2}: \quad 29 \text{ mm Hg}$$
$$pH: \quad 7.50$$
$$HCO_3^-: \quad 22 \text{ mEq/liter}$$

   The $F_{I_{O_2}}$ was increased to 0.80. The patient was sedated. The ventilator was changed to the control mode with a rate of 12 breaths/min. Arterial blood gases 20 minutes after these changes were instituted were

$$Pa_{O_2}: \quad 55 \text{ mm Hg}$$
$$Pa_{CO_2}: \quad 45 \text{ mm Hg}$$
$$pH: \quad 7.38$$
$$HCO_3^-: \quad 24 \text{ mEq/liter}$$

What clinical condition is the probable cause of the patients's problems?

A. pulmonary embolism

B. adult respiratory distress syndrome

C. spontaneous pneumothorax

D. ventilator malfunction

E. aspiration pneumonitis

Questions 13, 14, and 15 refer to the scenario described below.

A 62-year-old female had completed a 6-hour airplane flight. She immediately experienced pain in the calf of her left leg and noted that the area was slightly swollen and tender to the touch. That night she was awakened by a sudden pain in the left midlateral chest. The pain was sharp and became more intense during deep breathing and coughing. She also experienced an acute shortness of breath. A few hours later she coughed up a small amount of clear, blood-tinged sputum.

Examination by her physician revealed decreased movement and decreased breath sounds on the left side of the chest where friction rubs also were perceived. The ankle and calf were slightly swollen with the calf warm and tender. A positive Homan's sign was observed. (This sign consists of pain in the calf when the foot is dorsiflexed).

The chest roentgenogram showed a triangular shadow in the left middle chest with its base along the pleural lining. A slight pleural effusion was also observed.

13. What may be this patient's clinical problem?

A. myocardial infarction

B. pulmonary embolism

C. coronary thrombosis

D. spontaneous pneumothorax

E. bronchopulmonary fistula

14. What does the triangular shadow in the left midchest with its base on the pleural lining signify?

A. acute pleuritis

B. adult respiratory distress syndrome

C. pulmonary edema

D. pulmonary infarction

E. hemoptysis

15. What was the significance of the painful legs?

A. atherosclerosis

B. arteriosclerosis

C. acute vasculitis

D. leg cramps

E. thromboembolism

16. A 42-year-old black female in ventilatory failure entered the emergency room at approximately 5:00 PM. She was ultimately admitted to the respiratory intensive care unit and placed on a mechanical ventilator. Her arterial blood gas values in the Emergency Room were

Pa_{O_2}:   55 mm Hg
Pa_{CO_2}:   60 mm Hg
pH: 7.22
HCO_3^-:   29 mEq/liter

The patient's husband informed the medical personnel that his wife complained of general fatigue and muscle weakness, especially in her legs. The husband also described his wife as experiencing diplopia, ptosis, dysphonia, and dysphagia. He expressed that these signs and symptoms were rarely present in early morning hours or after his wife took a nap. They seemed to appear more regularly late in the day.

Medical personnel also were informed that the patient had not had any bacterial or viral infections for a few years. What is the probable diagnosis of this patient?

A. Guillain-Barré syndrome   D. amyotrophic lateral sclerosis
B. infectious polyneuritis   E. acute poliomyelitis
C. myasthenia gravis

17. Four persons attending the Senior Bowl at Ladd Stadium in Mobile, Alabama were stricken with food poisoning and were subsequently treated at the University of South Alabama Medical Center for various degrees of ventilatory failure associated with ventilatory muscle paralysis. What microorganism is most likely the cause of this situation?

A. *Clostridium perfringens*   D. *Proteus vulgaris*
B. *Clostridium botulinum*   E. *Bacillus anthracis*
C. *Proteus mirabilis*

18. Which of the following drugs is the best medication to use to distinguish between a myasthenic crisis and a cholinergic crisis?

A. edrophonium chloride   D. *d*-Tubocurarine
B. neostigmine methylsulfate   E. succinylcholine
C. pyridostigmine

19. Which of the following factors are commonly used for assessing a patient's perfusion state?

I. sensorium
II. capillary refill
III. $\dot{Q}s/\dot{Q}_T$
IV. V_D/V_T

A. I, II, III, IV   D. I, IV only
B. I, II, III only   E. I, II only
C. II, III only

20. Which disease entity is a common complication of silicosis?

A. Streptococcus pneumonia   D. tuberculosis
B. sarcoidosis   E. bronchogenic carcinoma
C. Klebsiella pneumonia

21. Which of the following pulmonary diseases can cause lung cavitations?

    I. coccidioidomycosis
    II. aspergillosis
    III. histoplasmosis
    IV. blastomycosis

    A. I, IV only
    B. II, III, IV only
    C. I, III only

    D. I, III, IV only
    E. I, II, III, IV

22. Which of the following diseases can be classified as environmental lung diseases endemic to a certain geographic area?

    I. blastomycosis
    II. nocardiosis
    III. cryptococcosis
    IV. histoplasmosis
    V. aspergillosis

    A. I, II, III only
    B. I, IV only
    C. II, IV, V only

    D. I, III only
    E. I, II, III, IV, V

23. Which disease entities can be classified as restrictive lung diseases?

    I. Guillain-Barré syndrome
    II. Freidländer's pneumonia
    III. kyphoscoliosis
    IV. asbestosis

    A. I, II, III, IV
    B. I, III only
    C. I, III, IV only

    D. I, II, III only
    E. II, IV only

24. Which of the following statements accurately describe farmer's lung?

    I. acute presentation may be characterized with chills, fever, diaphoresis, malaise, nausea, headache, and anorexia occuring 4 to 6 hours after exposure
    II. only about 5% of farm personnel develop clinical pulmonary symptoms
    III. caused by the inhalation of microbial spores generally produced by *Histoplasma capsulatum* which flourish in moldy hay or silage
    IV. treatment amounts to avoidance of the offending antigen

    A. I, IV only
    B. I, II, IV only
    C. I, III, IV only

    D. II, III only
    E. I, II, III, IV

25. Which of the following entities are usually associated with the development of an empyema?

    I. staphylococcal pneumonia
    II. asbestosis
    III. actinomycosis
    IV. coccidioidomycosis

A. I, III, IV only   D. I, IV only
B. II, IV only   E. II, III only
C. I, III only

26. Which of the following clinical manifestations refer to pectus excavatum?

    I. It is a posterior chest wall deformity.
    II. Exercise intolerance sometimes exists along with chest pain.
    III. On lateral x-ray the xiphoid aspect of the sternum is shown pointing toward the spine.
    IV. No blood gas or acid-base disorders generally exist.

A. I, II, III, IV   D. I, II, III only
B. I, III only   E. II, III, IV only
C. II, IV only

27. Which of the following clinical signs and symptoms are associated with sleep apnea?

    I. excessive daytime sleepiness
    II. hypertension
    III. nocturnal enuresis
    IV. abnormal motor activity during sleep

A. I, II, III, IV
B. III, IV only   D. I, II only
C. I, III only   E. I, III, IV only

28. Which variety of pneumonia is associated with the highest incidence of mortality?

A. Klebsiella pneumonia   D. Pseudomonas pneumonia
B. staphylococcal pneumonia   E. Hemophilus pneumonia
C. streptococcal pneumonia

29. About 85% of the occurrence of _____ is said to be viral origin.

A. epiglottitis   D. laryngotracheobronchitis
B. bronchiolitis   E. pneumonitis
C. tracheitis

30. How does the cerebrospiral fluid (CSF) of a normal person compare with that of a chronic bronchitic?

A. A chronic bronchitic has less than normal amounts of HCO_3^- in his CSF.
B. A normal person has CSF [HCO_3^-] less than that of a chronic bronchitic.
C. Both persons have identical CSF [HCO_3^-].

D. A chronic bronchitic has CSF P_{CO_2} less than that of a normal person.

E. Both persons have an identical CSF P_{CO_2}.

31. Patients suffering from extrinsic asthma will have _____ .

   A. bronchospasm from allergens that either cannot be identified or are difficult to isolate

   B. elevated IgE serum levels

   C. normal IgE serum levels

   D. prolonged inspiration during an asthmatic episode

   E. little mucosal inflammation during an attack

32. Which microorganism is responsible for the development of Friedländer's pneumonia?

   A. *Pseudomonas aeruginosa*   D. *Streptococcus pneumoniae*

   B. *Klebsiella pneumoniae*   E. *Hemophilus influenzae*

   C. *Staphylococcus pneumoniae*

33. Assuming that a patient is infected with *Blastomyces dermatitidis,* what are the possible courses of the disease?

   I. The person may develop acute pulmonary symptoms.

   II. If the patient develops acute pulmonary symptoms, the disease may resolve shortly thereafter.

   III. If the patient develops acute pulmonary symptoms, the disease may become progressive.

   IV. Pharmacologic treatment often includes the administration of amphotericin B.

   A. I, III, IV only   D. II, III, IV only

   B. I, II only   E. I, II, III, IV

   C. I, III only

34. Which of the following pathologic changes are generally associated with an acute asthmatic attack?

   I. squamous cell metaplasia

   II. respiratory mucosal edema

   III. hyperactivity of the mucus-secreting glands

   IV. bronchospasm

   A. I, II, III, IV   D. II, III, IV only

   B. I, III, IV only   E. III, IV only

   C. II, III only

35. Which clinical features could be classfied as (a) sign(s) of pulmonary disease?

   I. chest pain

   II. abnormal chest wall movement

III. digital clubbing
IV. dyspnea
 V. chest wall deformity

A. I, II, III, IV, V
B. II, III, V only
C. I, IV only

D. I only
E. II, III, IV, V only

36. The presence of sputum production for, at least, 3 months for, at least, 2 successive years lends evidence to the existence of which disease entity?

A. pulmonary emphysema
B. chronic bronchitis
C. bronchial asthma
D. bronchiectasis
E. chronic obstructive pulmonary disease (COPD)

37. A chronic necrotizing infection of the bronchi and bronchioles leading to, or associated with, abnormal dilatation of these airways describes which disease entity?

A. chronic bronchitis
B. bronchiectasis
C. pneumoconiosis

D. cystic fibrosis
E. laryngotracheobronchitis

38. Which statements are true about kyphoscoliosis?

 I. It is a combination of both lateral and posterior curvature of the lumbar spine.
 II. Ninety percent of kyphoscoliosis patients exhibit severe symptoms of this affliction.
III. Pneumonia is a frequent complication because of the inability of the patient to generate an effective cough.
IV. One portion of lung may be compressed while another portion is overdistended.

A. I, III, IV only
B. I, II only
C. I, III only

D. III, IV only
E. I, II, III, IV

39. Which clinical situations are characterized by lung parenchymal destruction and/or alteration?

 I. asthma
 II. chronic bronchitis
III. pulmonary emphysema
IV. asbestosis
 V. Pickwickian syndrome

A. I, II, III, IV, V
B. II, III, IV only
C. III, IV only

D. I, III, V only
E. II, III, V only

40. The *distinctive* clinical feature in making the diagnosis of Pickwickian syndrome is
_____ .

    A. gross obesity
    B. daytime somnolence
    C. CO_2 retention
    D. hypoxemia
    E. small lung volumes

41. Infant respiratory distress syndrome (IRDS) is characterized by which of the following clinical presentations and/or pathophysiologic manifestations?

    I. hyaline membrane formation
    II. expiratory grunting
    III. glottic closure during exhalation
    IV. inactive or absent pulmonary surfactant

    A. I, II, IV only
    B. II, III only
    C. II, IV only
    D. I, III, IV only
    E. I, II, III, IV

42. Which of the following lung diseases result from the inhalation of thermophilic actinomycetes?

    I. farmer's lung
    II. coccidioidomycosis
    III. cryptococcosis
    IV. actinomycosis
    V. bagassosis

    A. I, V only
    B. I, IV only
    C. I, II, III only
    D. II, III only
    E. I, II, V only

43. Which of the following infectious lung diseases can be called opportunistic, i.e., the
responsible microorganism invades a susceptible host such as someone on immuno-
suppressive therapy?

    I. blastomycosis
    II. histoplasmosis
    III. candidiasis
    IV. cryptococcosis

    A. I, II, III, IV
    B. I, III only
    C. III, IV only
    D. II, IV only
    E. II, III only

44. Which of the following clinical conditions can cause high-pressure pulmonary edema?

    I. mitral valve stenosis
    II. left ventricular failure
    III. right ventricular failure
    IV. adult respiratory distress syndrome

A. II, III only

B. I, IV only

C. I, II, IV only

D. I, II only

E. I, II, III only

45. Which of the following situations is the *primary* cause of hypoxemia in a chronic bronchitic patient?

A. diffusion impairment

B. pulmonary infiltrates

C. alveolar septal destruction

D. $\dot{V}_A/\dot{Q}_C$ abnormalities

E. anatomic shunting

46. Which of the following radiographic findings are characteristic of pulmonary emphysema?

I. reduced vascular markings

II. increased anteroposterior chest diameter

III. fluid in the intrapleural space

IV. decreased radiolucency

A. II, IV only

B. I, III only

C. I, II only

D. I, II, IV only

E. I, II, III only

47. Which statement(s) accurately describe(s) a transudate?

I. A transudate is the fluid that normally filters from the vasculature into the interstitium at the capillary level.

II. A transudate is the fluid that enters the interstitium as a result of an imbalance of pressures that interact at the capillary level.

III. A transudate has a large protein content and a high specific gravity.

IV. A transudate is fluid that accumulates in the interstitial spaces during cardiogenic pulmonary edema.

A. II, IV only

B. I only

C. III, IV only

D. II only

E. II, III only

48. Which of the following diseases commonly exhibit digital clubbing?

I. chronic bronchitis

II. cystic fibrosis

III. bronchogenic carcinoma

IV. bronchiectasis

A. I, II, IV only

B. II, III, IV only

C. II, III only

D. I, IV only

E. I, II, III, IV

49. The presence of lymph fluid in the intrapleural space is called a(n) _____ .

A. empyema

B. fibrothorax

C. hemothorax

D. pneumothorax

E. chylothorax

50. Which of the following statements accurately describe tuberculosis?

   I. The primary infection is called the *Ghon complex*.

   II. In most persons the primary tuberculosis infection heals, forming scar tissue.

   III. In the later stage of the disease tubercle bacilli spread to other organ systems.

   IV. The lower lobes of the lungs are generally the initial site of infection by *Mycobacterium tuberculosis*.

   A. II, IV only

   B. I, II, IV only

   C. I, II only

   D. III, IV only

   E. I, III, IV only

ASSESSMENT ANSWER SHEET

DIRECTIONS: Darken the space under the selected answer.

	A	B	C	D	E		A	B	C	D	E
1.	[ ]	[ ]	[ ]	[ ]	[ ]	26.	[ ]	[ ]	[ ]	[ ]	[ ]
2.	[ ]	[ ]	[ ]	[ ]	[ ]	27.	[ ]	[ ]	[ ]	[ ]	[ ]
3.	[ ]	[ ]	[ ]	[ ]	[ ]	28.	[ ]	[ ]	[ ]	[ ]	[ ]
4.	[ ]	[ ]	[ ]	[ ]	[ ]	29.	[ ]	[ ]	[ ]	[ ]	[ ]
5.	[ ]	[ ]	[ ]	[ ]	[ ]	30.	[ ]	[ ]	[ ]	[ ]	[ ]
6.	[ ]	[ ]	[ ]	[ ]	[ ]	31.	[ ]	[ ]	[ ]	[ ]	[ ]
7.	[ ]	[ ]	[ ]	[ ]	[ ]	32.	[ ]	[ ]	[ ]	[ ]	[ ]
8.	[ ]	[ ]	[ ]	[ ]	[ ]	33.	[ ]	[ ]	[ ]	[ ]	[ ]
9.	[ ]	[ ]	[ ]	[ ]	[ ]	34.	[ ]	[ ]	[ ]	[ ]	[ ]
10.	[ ]	[ ]	[ ]	[ ]	[ ]	35.	[ ]	[ ]	[ ]	[ ]	[ ]
11.	[ ]	[ ]	[ ]	[ ]	[ ]	36.	[ ]	[ ]	[ ]	[ ]	[ ]
12.	[ ]	[ ]	[ ]	[ ]	[ ]	37.	[ ]	[ ]	[ ]	[ ]	[ ]
13.	[ ]	[ ]	[ ]	[ ]	[ ]	38.	[ ]	[ ]	[ ]	[ ]	[ ]
14.	[ ]	[ ]	[ ]	[ ]	[ ]	39.	[ ]	[ ]	[ ]	[ ]	[ ]
15.	[ ]	[ ]	[ ]	[ ]	[ ]	40.	[ ]	[ ]	[ ]	[ ]	[ ]
16.	[ ]	[ ]	[ ]	[ ]	[ ]	41.	[ ]	[ ]	[ ]	[ ]	[ ]
17.	[ ]	[ ]	[ ]	[ ]	[ ]	42.	[ ]	[ ]	[ ]	[ ]	[ ]
18.	[ ]	[ ]	[ ]	[ ]	[ ]	43.	[ ]	[ ]	[ ]	[ ]	[ ]
19.	[ ]	[ ]	[ ]	[ ]	[ ]	44.	[ ]	[ ]	[ ]	[ ]	[ ]
20.	[ ]	[ ]	[ ]	[ ]	[ ]	45.	[ ]	[ ]	[ ]	[ ]	[ ]
21.	[ ]	[ ]	[ ]	[ ]	[ ]	46.	[ ]	[ ]	[ ]	[ ]	[ ]
22.	[ ]	[ ]	[ ]	[ ]	[ ]	47.	[ ]	[ ]	[ ]	[ ]	[ ]
23.	[ ]	[ ]	[ ]	[ ]	[ ]	48.	[ ]	[ ]	[ ]	[ ]	[ ]
24.	[ ]	[ ]	[ ]	[ ]	[ ]	49.	[ ]	[ ]	[ ]	[ ]	[ ]
25.	[ ]	[ ]	[ ]	[ ]	[ ]	50.	[ ]	[ ]	[ ]	[ ]	[ ]

CARDIOPULMONARY DISEASES ANALYSES

Note: The references listed after each analysis are numbered and keyed to the reference list located at the end of this section. The first number indicates the text. The second number indicates the page where information about the question can be found. For example, (1:219, 384) means that reference number 1 is to be used and that on pages 219 and 384 information about the question will be found. Frequently, it will be necessary to read beyond the page number indicated to obtain complete information. Therefore, reference to the question will be found either on the page indicated or on subsequent pages.

1. C. A pneumoconiosis is a lung disease that is caused by the inhalation of inorganic matter. Most pneumoconioses are occupationally acquired. A number of factors determines if a person will contract a lung disease of this variety. These factors include (1) duration of exposure, (2) intensity of exposure, (3) particle size, and (4) individual susceptibility to lung disease. The following list indicates the type of pneumoconiosis and the related causative agent.

PNEUMOCONIOSIS	CAUSATIVE AGENT
berylliosis	beryllium
baritosis	barium
silicosis	silica
asbestosis	asbestos
stannosis	tin
siderosis	iron
talcosis	talc
bysinnosis	cotton
coal worker's pneumoconiosis (CWP)	coal

   (8:311–312), (11:242), (13:143)

2. A. Ordinarily, the presence of hypoxemia is associated with varying degrees of shunting. There are a number of different types of shunt. For example, an *anatomic shunt* includes blood that does not enter the pulmonary capillary network. *Intrapulmonary shunting* is comprised of two components: *capillary shunting* and *venous admixture* (perfusion in excess of ventilation).

   A number of pulmonary diseases are associated with increased intrapulmonary shunting. Any pneumonia increases intrapulmonary shunting because of the presence of secretions impeding airflow, causing either partial or complete airway obstruction. The increased intrapulmonary shunting caused by pulmonary edema results from vascular fluid occupying alveoli. Adult respiratory distress syndrome (ARDS) produces an exudation of vascular fluid into the alveolar spaces. A pleural effusion can compress alveoli and prevent air from entering alveoli, thereby depriving venous blood from becoming oxygenated.

   (13:22,29,175), (27:209–210)

3. B. Adult respiratory distress syndrome often follows a variety of indirect and direct lung insults. For example, acute pancreatitis, massive trauma, oxygen toxicity,

near drowning, and inhalation of noxious gases are some clinical conditions known to precede the development of ARDS. The patient usually experiences a latent period (24 to 48 hours) after the initial insult. During that time he is generally stable and appears to be recovering.

The clinical picture then deteriorates. The patient appears to be in respiratory distress (tachypnea, sternal retractions, and dyspnea). Arterial blood gases at this point characteristically reveal a decreased Pa_{O_2}, a normal or decreased Pa_{CO_2}, a normal or decreased pH, and a normal or increased HCO_3^-. The Pa_{O_2} is unresponsive to oxygen therapy (refractory hypoxemia). The refractory hypoxemia is caused by the increased intrapulmonary shunting and $\dot{V}A/\dot{Q}C$ mismatching (perfusion in excess of ventilation).

As the syndrome advances, other clinical features include decreased lung compliance caused by inactivation of surfactant and increased pulmonary capillary permeability. Adventitious breath sounds (rales and rhonchi) become prominant as more vascular fluid enters the alveoli. When consolidation and atelectasis ensue, vesicular breath sounds fail to develop in the affected area and are replaced by bronchial sounds. Percussion over such an area reveals a dull sound.
(3:482–483), (4:321–322), (6:854), (11:66), (13:158,164–165), (24:211–212, 215–218)

4. D. Cor pulmonale is the term used to describe right ventricular failure that results from a pulmonary disease. Right ventricular failure caused by left ventricular failure does not apply to that term.

Cor pulmonale usually results from a combination of events. When lung disease develops, the person generally exhibits hypoxemia with normocapnia. The hypoxemia arises basically from $\dot{V}A/\dot{Q}C$ mismatching. The hypoxemia causes an increase in the red blood cell (RBC) production as the hormone *erythropoietin* stimulates the bone marrow to manufacture more RBCs. Consequently, blood viscosity increases. The hypoxemia creates two situations that contribute to the development of cor pulmonale—pulmonary vasoconstriction and increased blood viscosity.

As the person's pulmonary status deteriorates, hypercapnia develops accompanied by acidemia. The blood gas (hypoxemia and hypercapnia) and acid-base (acidemia) alterations cause a more pronounced pulmonary vasconstriction than any one of these alterations alone.

What the right ventricle is ultimately faced with is pumping a more viscous liquid through more narrowed conduits. The increased work causes the right ventricle to experience hypertrophy and hyperplasia.
(1:261–262,266–268), (4:304), (10:118–119), (11:83,98–99), (13:133)

5. B. Cystic fibrosis is an inherited autosomal recessive disorder characterized by dysfunction of the exocrine glands. Heterozygotes (carriers) do not exhibit the clinical features of this disease. Two heterozygotes are required to produce a child with cystic fibrosis. When both parents are carriers, there is a 25% chance that the offspring will have cystic fibrosis, a 25% chance that the child will be normal, and a 50% chance that the child will be a carrier.

Similarly, pulmonary emphysema can be caused by an alpha₁ antitrypsin deficiency. This deficiency is inherited when carrier parents produce a homozygote having this abnormal gene. Heterozygotes, generally, do not develop emphysema from alpha$_1$ antitrypsin deficiency, although they do have less alpha$_1$ antitrypsin than normal.

The theory is that trypsin or a protease destroys lung tissue and that alpha$_1$ antitrypsin negates the deleterious influences of the proteases or trypsin.

(3:300,305), (6:765–766,799), (8:153–154,288,295–298), (10:134–135, 330–355), (13:152–153), (24:153–154)

6. D. The early clinical presentation of lung abscess resembles that of pneumonia: cough, pleuritic pain, leukocytosis (increased white blood cell count), fever, chills, and general malaise. The abscess often produces large amounts of foul-smelling, foul-tasting, blood-tinged sputum. The sputum produced in brochiectasis generally is foul-smelling and separates into distinct layers upon settling. Weight loss and anoxeria are usually associated with pulmonary neoplasms. Amphoric breath sounds are characteristic of cavitations associated with lung abscesses. Amphoric breath sounds resemble the sound produced as air is blown over the mouth of an empty pop bottle.

(6:286,319), (11:14,181–186)

7. A. Sarcoidosis is a systemic granulomatous disease of unkown etiology. The disease is prevalent among blacks in the Southeast. Although clinical manifestations of sarcoidosis are varied because this disease is a multisystem disorder, pulmonary signs and symptoms are frequent.

Ordinarily, the patient will have an unremarkable physical examination. Breath and voice sounds are usually normal. However, if advanced fibrosis is present, bronchial breath sounds will predominate. Coughing is a common complaint, but sputum production is uncommon. The patient also expresses being fatigued and having general malaise. Dyspnea at rest and on exertion may occur. Radiologically, bilateral hilar adenopathy with or without alveolar or pulmonary interstitial infiltrates are observed.

Pulmonary function studies in sarcoidosis patients ordinarily reflect a restrictive disease.

(6:328,331,798), (8:261,313), (11:261–266), (13:26,104–106), (24:181–182, 184–185)

8. D. Persons who are grossly obese often present with the restrictive abnormality described as Pickwickian syndrome (idiopathic central hypoventilation). It is important to point out that not all grossly obese people are Pickwickians. The hallmark of this disorder is hypercapnia. Grossly obese non-Pickwickian person's are generally hypoxemic with a normocapnia. Pickwickians are concurrently hypoxemic and hypercapnic. Their blood gas and acid-base status are essentially the same as those of a COPD patient.

The increased mass on the chest wall from the large amount of adipose tissue and the infringement of the abdominal viscera into the thoracic cavity account for the restrictive nature of this disorder. The hypoxemia is attributed to $\dot{V}A/\dot{Q}c$ inequalities, whereas the hypercapnia results from a decreased minute alveolar ventilation ($\dot{V}A$). Pickwickians who have no complicating lung disease essentially have a normal lung parenchyma and a normal tracheobronchial tree.

Treatment of this condition amounts to having the patient lose a number of pounds. In many cases a small weight loss is all that is needed to alleviate the CO_2 retention and to improve the $\dot{V}A$. Once the patient returns to a normocapnic state, he is no longer classified as Pickwickian.

(6:278,287), (11:230–231), (24:108–109)

9. C. Carbon monoxide (CO) is a tasteless, odorless gas. It can be breathed unknowingly and cause dangerous consequences. Carbon monoxide in the blood shifts the oxyhemoglobin dissociation curve to the left, thereby interferring with the release of oxygen at the tissue level. It also interferes with oxygen transport because hemoglobin has an affinity for CO 210 times greater than it has for O_2.

Treatment of CO poisoning centers around oxygen administration and hyperventilation. Therefore, it would be appropriate to administer either hyperbaric or normobaric O_2 to a carbon monoxide poisoning victim depending on the carboxyhemoglobin (COHb) level in the blood. Similarly, if a CO inhalation victim was apneic, it would be appropriate to intubate, oxygenate, and hyperventilate to help remove the CO from the blood as rapidly as possible. Oxygen administration greatly reduces the half-life of CO in the blood.

It would be inappropriate to administer carbon dioxide to increase ventilation because it might aggravate an existing metabolic acidosis (lactic acidosis).

(3:535–538), (4:91,332–333), (6:262–263,889–890), (8:81,184), (12:40,53,187, 192), (4:71–72), (27:24,256)

10. A. Persons who experience long bone fractures are prone to the development of fat embolization. The clinical features of this condition include acute onset, refractory hypoxemia, diaphoresis, dyspenea, tachypnea, tachycardia, cyanosis, diminished sensorium and petechiae, and pulmonary infiltrates.

A couple of theories are thought to be responsible for the development of fat embolization. One is that fat from the site of the fracture enters circulation. The other theory advocates that fat is mobilized from the fracture site and coalesces into large globules after it enters circulation.

(3:475), (6:327,928–929), (8:246,368)

11. C. There are a number of distinct differences between a viral pneumonia and a bacterial pneumonia. Characteristics of a viral pneumonia include (1) rare pleuritic pain, (2) gradual onset, (3) low-grade fever, (4) rarely causes chills, (4) thin, mucoid sputum, and (5) a leukocyte count of less than 10,000/mm³. Characteristics of a bacterial pneumonia include (1) occasional pleuritic pain, (2) rapid, sudden onset, (3) high-grade fever, (4) thick, purulent sputum, and (5) a leukocyte count greater than 10,000/mm³ of blood.

(3:204–208), (4:324), (6:286,296,327–328,872), (8:300–307), (11:37,47)

12. B. Adult respiratory distress syndrome is a common sequelae of near drowning. It is not uncommon for such a patient to be stablized for 24 to 48 hours, then deteriorate suddenly. The abrupt deterioration is actually the early stage of ARDS. The patient experiences refractory hypoxemia, decreased lung compliance, tachypnea, and chest x-rays showing bilateral alveolar infiltrates (honeycomb effect).

Near drowning victims must be watched very closely during this 24 to 48 hour latent period because the onset of ARDS is rapid. The usual primary concern when initially treating near drowing victims is the correction of hypoxemia and acidemia. Oxygen, obviously, should be administered. The mixed acidemia—respiratory and metabolic—is ordinarily treated with ventilation and sodium bicarbonate ($NaHCO_3$) administration.

(3:482–483), (4:321), (6:854), (11:271)

13. B. One of the three factors that facilitates the formation of a clot in a blood vessel is stagnation of blood or venous stasis. This elderly woman was confined to an airplane seat for 6 hours. This amount of immobility can place an elderly person, such as this woman, at risk for developing a thromboembolism. The clinical manifestations of pulmonary embolism are nonspecific. Generally, dyspnea and the angina-like chest pain are the most common symptoms. The sudden onset of this clinical disorder is also noteworthy.

The other clues to suspecting this diagnosis is the presence of pain, tenderness, and swelling of the extremities. Decreased breath sounds, reduced chest movement, and friction rubs on the affected side are important signs. Chest roentgenographs commonly reveal a pleural effusion. Hemoptysis, although uncommon, is important to the diagnosis when present.

It should be mentioned here that pulmonary thromboembolism (PTE) can only be definitively diagnosed via a positive pulmonary angiogram. It can be suspected by a positive perfusion scan. Clinical signs and symptoms alone are *not* definitively diagnostic.

(4:325–326), (6:821–822), (8:328–331), (10:227), (11:114), (13:124), (24:193–207)

14. D. The presence of a pulmonary infarction on a chest roentgenogram sometimes reveals an opacity that takes on a triangular, conical, wedge shape. The apex of the triangle is directed toward the hilum and the base lies along the pleural lining. A pleural effusion is a common radiographic finding associated with a pulmonary embolism.

(6:822), (8:331), (13:126), (24:203–204)

15. E. The vast majority of pulmonary emboli originate from the deep veins of the lower extremities. Three factors are involved in the formation of a thrombus: (1) vessel wall damage or abnormality, (2) stasis or stagnation of blood, and (3) a state of hypercoagulability.

The positive Homan's sign, along with the tender, warm, swollen calf and ankle all indicated that the pathogenesis of the pulmonary embolism was the dislodgement of a deep leg vein thrombus or thromboembolism.

(4:325), (6:816–817), (8:328), (11:114–121), (13:124), (24:201–202)

16. C. Myasthenia gravis is a neuromuscular disease that is thought to be autoimmune in nature. However, the specific etiology and pathogenesis have not been completely identified.

The disease is characterized by general fatigability and striated muscle weakness, especially of the extremities. The patient frequently complains of double vision (diplopia), drooping eyelids (ptosis), difficult and slurred speech (dysphonia), and difficulty chewing and swallowing (dysphagia). Generally, these clinical manifestations are not present in the morning hours after a night's sleep or any time after the patient rests. They usually occur late in the day or when the patient undergoes physical or emotional stress.

The disease process results from the fact that the striated muscles ineffectively ·contract because of inadequate stimulation at the neuromuscular junction. Under normal circumstances acetylcholine is released from motor nerve endings and reacts with special receptors on the muscle end plate or the muscle cell membrane. After other physiologic events, the striated muscle ultimately contracts. The enzyme acetylcholinesterase then inactivates the remaining acetylcholine at the neuromuscular junction to allow the muscle fibers to repolarize.

In the case of myasthenia gravis, it appears that there may be autoantibodies against acetylcholine receptors on the muscle end plate or muscle cell membrane. In an effort to increase the stimulation of striated muscles, patients with this disease are treated with anticholinesterase medication, e.g., neostigmine or Mestinon. Anticholinesterases inactivate acetylcholinesterase at the neuromuscular junction, thereby allowing the acetylcholine to remain longer causing increased muscle stimulation. Muscle stimulation is not restored to normal. Muscle strength is somewhere around 80% of normal.

(3:340–341), (4:328–329), (6:236,837,844), (8:367,370), (13:111), (24:183,188)

17. B. *Clostridium botulinum* is the microorganism responsible for causing botulism, which generally results from eating improperly canned or preserved foods. The toxins produced by these bacteria cause muscle paralysis by preventing the release of acetylcholine at neuromuscular junctions. The ventilatory failure occurs acutely and often requires treatment by mechanical ventilation.

(2:276), (4:368), (6:836,844)

18. A. Myasthenia gravis is treated with anticholinesterase medication. Long-term anticholinesterase medications include neostigmine methylsulfate and pyridostigmine (Mestinon). During the course of treatment these patients can experience myasthenic and/or cholinergic crises. A myasthenic crisis takes place if the patient either is delinquent in taking his medication, or is receiving an inadequate dosage. A cholinergic crisis occurs when the muscle cell membrane essentially becomes desensitized to acetylcholine. In either crisis the signs and symptoms are the same, i.e., muscle weakness and ventilatory failure.

The Tensilon test distinguishes between these two crises. Tensilon (edrophonium chloride) is a fast- and short-acting anticholinesterase medication. When Tensilon is administered and the patient improves, the patient is having a myasthenic crisis. If the patient does not improve after the Tensilon administration, the crisis is a cholinergic one.

Once the type of crisis has been identified, appropriate treatment can be instituted. A myasthenic crisis usually can be terminated by increasing the patient's dosage of anticholinesterase medication, or by urging the patient to be more diligent in taking his medication. A cholinergic crisis often requires mechanically ventilating the patient and withholding his anticholinesterase medication to allow the muscle cell membranes at the neuromuscular junctions to again become responsive to acetylcholine.

(3:340–341), (4:328–329), (6:236,837,844), (8:367,370), (13:111), (24:183,188)

19. E. When one evaluates the cardiovascular system, the blood pressure is measured, the heart rate (pulse) is taken, and the perfusion status is determined. The perfusion status is assessed by (1) observing the patient's skin color, (2) noting skin texture, (3) checking capillary refill, (4) noting the patient's sensorium (level of consciousness), and (5) measuring or observing the extent of urine output. (3:188–189), (4:298), (6:942)

20. D. Tuberculosis is a common complication of silicosis. Silicosis is a pneumoconiosis caused by the chronic inhalation of silicon dioxide or free crystalline silica particles. Therapeutic measures are usually taken to prevent the incidence of complicating tuberculosis. For example, silicosis patients having a positive tuberculin test despite not having active tuberculosis are placed on prophylactic isoniazid (INH) therapy. (11:247,248), (13:146)

21. E. Cavitations or cavities are holes in the lung parenchyma. They are radiolucent lesions encircled by denser tissue. Fungal diseases frequently cause lung cavities to develop. Each of the fungal diseases listed often produce cavities in the lungs. (6:314,319), (8:305–306)

22. B. Both blastomycosis and histoplasmosis are fungus diseases of the lung. Each is endemic to specific geographic areas. Blastomycosis is prevalant in the central and southeastern United States and is caused by inhaling the microorganism *Blastomyces dermatitidis,* which resides in the soil. It is also called North American blastomycosis. A South American blastomycosis is caused by the microorganism *Paracoccidioides brasiliensis.*

    Histoplasmosis, caused by the fungus *Histoplasma capsulatum,* predominates in river valleys. Areas endemic to the United States include the river valleys in Ohio, Mississippi, Potomac, Delaware, Hudson, and St. Lawrence. Infection generally occurs after inhaling airborne spores. These spores become airborne when the soil, in which they reside, is disturbed. Bird droppings are responsible for the presence of this microorganism. (6:314), (8:305), (11:167–169,171)

23. A. Neuromuscular disorders, such as Guillain-Barré syndrome and myasthenia gravis, are restrictive diseases. Infectious diseases, such as bacterial and viral pneumonias and fungal infections, produce a restrictive pattern. Skeletal wall deformities, e.g., kyphoscoliosis and ankylosing spondylitis, are also restrictive conditions. The pneumoconioses (asbestosis, silicosis, byssinosis) generally produce a restrictive abnormality, as well. (4:314–333), (6:236), (24:184)

24. B. According to Coombs and Gell, immune reactions are classified into four categories: (1) type I (immediate hypersensitivity)—rapid onset after exposure to the antigen; (2) type II hypersensitivity—circulating antibodies attacking tissue antigens (autoimmune diseases); (3) type III hypersensitivity—reactions developing after 6 to 8 hours often caused by antigen-antibody interaction; and (4) type IV hypersensitivity (delayed)—reactivity to antigens mediated by T-lymphocytes,

achieving peak intensity about 24 hours after intradermal injection of the antigen to a sensitized person.

IMMUNE REACTION	CLINICAL EXAMPLE
Type I	Asthma
Type II	Goodpasture's syndrome
Type III	Farmer's lung
Type IV	Tuberculin testing

Farmer's lung, also classified as a hypersensitivity pneumonitis, is caused by the inhalation of an organic dust. The causative agent is *Micropolyspora faeni,* which is found in moldy hay. The acute form of farmer's lung is manifested by the onset of chills, fever, diaphoresis, general malaise, nausea, headache, and anorexia 4 to 6 hours after exposure. The acute form generally requires no treatment as the signs and symptoms spontaneously subside. Steroids sometimes are used in the management of this disorder. Essentially, treatment amounts to avoidance of the offending antigen. A very small percentage of farm personnel (about 5%) are affected by this microorganism.
(8:159,314), (13:106)

25. C. Empyema is the term used to describe pleural fluid that is grossly purulent or contains pyogenic microorganisms. Staphylococcal pneumonia, caused by the bacterium *Staphylococcus aureus,* and the fungus-like infection, actinomycosis, caused by the bacterium *Actinomyces israelii,* cause an infectious lung disease that can progress to pleural involvement producing an empyema. The empyema is usually treated by thoracentesis and appropriate antibiotic therapy.
(4:317,569–570), (6:311,322,437,761,765–766), (8:301,343), (11:35,43,44,175)

26. E. *Pectus excavatum,* also known as funnel chest, is an anterior chest wall deformity. Because the xiphoid is directed posteriorly while the ribs continue to ossify and grow, a depression of the anterior chest wall occurs. Ordinarily, no ventilatory complications occur. Arterial blood gases and the acid-base status are usually normal. In severe deformities, exercise may not be well tolerated.
Pectus carinatum, known as pigeon breast, is characterized by an anterior protrusion of both the sternum and its associated costal cartilages.
Both of these chest wall deformities have a familial occurrence.
(4:290), (8:355), (11:312), (24:183,187–188)

27. A. Sleep apnea is classified into three categories (1) central apnea, (2) obstructive apnea, and (3) mixed apnea. In central apnea the termination of airflow through the lungs results from a lack of ventilatory effort. In obstructive apnea the termination of airflow into and out of the lungs results from an upper airway obstruction (relaxation of the genioglossus muscle during sleep). Both abdominal and thoracic movements are present. The mixed variety is a combination of the other two.
Signs and symptoms of sleep apnea include:

1. excessive daytime sleepiness
2. personality changes

   3. sexual problems
   4. nocturnal enuresis
   5. snoring
   6. abnormal motor activity during sleep
   7. hypertension
   8. deteriorating intellectual capacity
   9. morning headaches
  10. sudden death during sleep

(6:992–997), (8:372), (11:225–233)

28. A. Klebsiella pneumonia, caused by Friedländer's bacillus (*Klebsiella pneumoniae*) is associated with a mortality rate of approximately 50%. Cephalosporins, chloramphenicol, gentamicin, or tobramycin are commonly used in treating Klebsiella pneumonia.

29. D. Laryngotracheobronchitis (LTB), or subglottic croup, is viral in origin in about 85% of the cases. The most common causative agent is the parainfluenza virus. Supraglottic croup, or epiglottitis, is primarily caused by bacterial infection by *Hemophilus influenzae* type B.
(4:354–355), (6:776–777), (8:274)

30. B. A CO_2 retainer will have more HCO_3^- in his CSF than someone who has a Pa_{CO_2} of 40 mm Hg. CO_2 passes freely across the blood-brain barrier (BBB). The Pa_{CO_2} and CSF CO_2 are, for all practical purposes, in equilibrium. As the Pa_{CO_2} changes, so does the CSF CO_2.
A CO_2 retainer (COPD patient) experiences active transport of HCO_3^- into the CSF to buffer the effect of the increased CO_2. HCO_3^- will be actively transported into the CSF until the pH there returns to 7.32. Therefore, a CO_2 retainer has a greater CSF HCO_3^- concentration than a normal person has.
(1:225–227), (4:92–94), (8:97–98), (12:59–61), (14:116–118)

31. B. Patients having extrinsic (allergic) asthma have an elevated serum immunoglobulin E (IgE) level, whereas those suffering from intrinsic (idiopathic) asthma have normal serum IgE levels.
Sensitized mast cells have antigen-specific IgE molecules fixed to and circumscribing the cell surface. When exposure to the appropriate antigen occurs, in the form of bridging two IgE molecules of the same specificity, the antigen-antibody reaction triggers the biochemical sequence that ultimately leads to mast cell degranulation. Figure 67 illustrates a sensitized mast cell (A), and an antigen-antibody reaction (B) occurring on the mast cell surface.
The antigen-antibody reaction increases cell membrane permeability, allowing for the release of stored vasoactive mediators into the pulmonary interstitium. The mediators (histamine, prostaglandins, serotonin, bradykinin, slow-reacting substance of anaphylaxis [SRS-A], eosinophil chemotactic factor of anaphylaxis [ECF-A], etc.) stimulate their respective receptor sites located on the bronchial smooth muscle cells, and trigger a chain of biochemical events responsible for de-

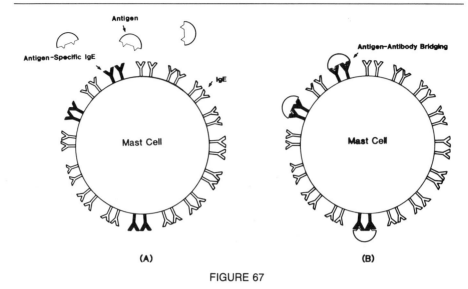

FIGURE 67

creasing their intracellular levels of cyclic AMP. The net physiologic response is bronchospasm.

(2:257–259), (4:310), (6:794,797), (8:278), (13:83)

32. B. *Klebsiella pneumoniae* is a gram-negative rod (bacillus) that is responsible for the development of Friedländer's pneumonia.

(4:573), (6:311), (8:249,301), (11:45)

33. E. *Blastomyces dermatitidis* is the microorganism responsible for the pulmonary fungal infection blastomycosis. *Blastomyces dermatitidis* is a dimorphic fungus. It becomes a budding yeast in the host, but exists as a mold in the soil.

The disease runs an unpredictable course. Once infected, a person can present with acute pulmonary symptoms (e.g., productive cough, chest pain, hemoptysis). The symptoms can resolve spontaneously or after medical treatment, usually with amphotericin B. The disease can progress to involve the skin and central nervous system.

(8:306), (11:171)

34. D. An acute asthmatic episode is associated with (1) diffuse bronchospasm, (2) respiratory mucosal edema, and (3) increased activity of the mucus-secreting glands.

(4:311), (6:792), (8:281), (10:159), (11:52–53), (13:80), (24:171)

35. B. There is a distinct difference between a sign and a symptom. A sign can be observed or otherwise objectively determined by the practitioner. A symptom is a subjective complaint conveyed by the patient to the clinician. For example, signs of pulmonary disease include (1) digital clubbing, (2) chest wall movement, (3) chest wall deformity, (4) tachypnea, (5) bradypnea, (6) hemoptysis, etc. Dyspnea is a symptom. The clinician cannot on her own perception ascertain the presence or absence of dyspnea. The clinician can only *assume* its presence or absence by

observing the patient. The presence or absence of dyspnea can only be communicated by the patient to the clinician.

(8:163,166,196)

36. B. Chronic bronchitis is diagnosed clinically as the presence of excessive mucus production for, at least, 3 months a year for, at least, 2 successive years. The hallmarks of the disease are hypertrophy and hyperplasia of mucus-secreting glands—goblet cells and submucosal glands. Inflammatory changes also occur throughout the tracheobronchial tree.

(3:505), (4:306), (6:790), (11:97), (13:64), (24:135)

37. B. Bronchiectasis is a chronic necrotizing disease of the bronchi and bronchioles. Abnormal dilation, inflammation, and destruction of the walls of the bronchi and bronchioles are associated with this chronic lung disease. Mucociliary clearance is impaired. Consequently, secretions stagnate and lead to increased infections.

Three types of bronchiectasis are pathologically described, i.e., saccular, tubular (cylindrical), and cystic. Saccular bronchiectasis is characterized by irregular dilatations, narrowings, and bronchial wall destruction. Tubular or cylindrical bronchiestasis lacks the normal airway tapering and is characterized by more regular dilatations. Cystic bronchiectasis generally presents with irregular airway dilatations having bulbous terminations.

A number of etiologic factors are associated with the development of bronchiectasis. Some of the causes are repeated airway infections, atelectasis, and airway obstruction (foreign body or disease process). The affected airways become abnormally dilated. Hemoptysis is a common complication resulting from the local hyperemia from the bronchial circulation.

(4:308), (6:802), (8:292), (11:177)

38. D. Kyphoscoliosis is a deformity of the thoracic spine. The spine is deformed both laterally and posteriorly. The distorted thoracic cage prevents normal lung expansion. Therefore, this condition is classified as a restrictive abnormality. The reduced lung volumes prevent kyphoscoliosis patients from generating an effective cough. Bronchial hygiene is compromised, resulting in frequent pulmonary infections. The hypoxemia associated with this condition arises from the $\dot{V}_A/\dot{Q}_C$ abnormalities caused by a combination of lung compression and lung overdistension. Likewise, the pulmonary vasculature is often reduced because of the compression effect of the thorax.

(4:328), (6:1009), (8:353–355), (13:110–111)

39. C. Pulmonary emphysema and asbestosis manifest themselves clinically by altering lung parenchymal tissue. Pulmonary emphysema can be either centrilobular or panlobular, depending upon what portion of the acinus is involved. Centrilobular emphysema involves the respiratory bronchioles. Panlobular emphysema affects the entire acinus. The disease is characterized by alveolar wall and capillary bed destruction leading to decreased lung elastance, increased lung compliance, air trapping, and $\dot{V}_A/\dot{Q}_C$ abnormalities.

In asbestosis, asbestos fibers have invaded the tracheobronchial tree. The fibers cannot be cleared by alveolar macrophages. The nature of the fiber is such that macrophage ingestion is prohibited. Consequently, the fibers become enveloped by proteinaceous material, which can eventually lead to diffuse interstitial fibrosis. Bronchogenic carcinoma is a common complication of asbestosis.

(4:305–306,314–315), (6:798), (8:153,197,246,286–292), (11:97–99,248–249), (13:26,61–64,146), (24:149–164,184)

40. C. Carbon dioxide retention is the distinguishing clinical manifestation when diagnosing Pickwickian syndrome (alveolar hypoventilation syndrome). The other features are not as confirming. For example, not all grossly obese people are Pickwickian. Furthermore, daytime somnolence does not confirm the presence of this syndrome. Extremely obese people may have difficulty sleeping at night; consequently, they may slumber off during the day at uncommon times. As a rule, grossly obese people have some degree of hypoxemia because of reduced lung volumes caused by the compression of lung tissue by the adipose tissue.

Ventilatory failure and impending ventilatory failure are confirmed on the basis of the Pa_{CO_2}.

(4:330–331), (6:287), (8:360–362), (11:230–231), (13:26), (24:108–109)

41. E. Infants presenting with infant respiratory distress syndrome (IRDS) or hyaline membrane disease (HMD) are usually infants of less than 35 weeks' gestation and of low birth weight (1.0 to 1.5 kg). Depending on the degree of prematurity, pulmonary surfactant may be completely absent, or it may be present in inadequate amounts.

Numerous clinical signs appear. These manifestations include tachypnea, nasal flaring, and sternal retractions. Expiratory grunting, which is also present, manifests an attempt to keep the airways open to facilitate the ensuing inspiration.

(3:483), (4:335–336), (8:227,316–319), (13:167), (35:185–187)

42. A. The inhalation of organic material or dust can produce an infectious lung disease called *extrinsic allergic alveolitis* or *hypersensitivity pneumonitis*. The inhalation of these organic dusts produces infiltrative lesions and is not associated with bronchospasm. The type of microorganisms implicated in this disorder is known as thermophilic actinomycetes.

Farmer's lung, caused by the thermophilic actinomycete *Micropolyspora faeni,* usually results from the inhalation of spores that become airborne when moldy hay or grain is disturbed. Bagassosis is caused by the inhalation of the microorganism *Thermoactinomyces vulgaris.* This microorganism is often found in moldy bagasse. Bagasse is the fibrous residue of sugar cane from which the juice has been removed. When bagasse is exposed to hot, humid weather, mold forms. The offending antigen can then be inhaled when moldy bagasse is disturbed.

The clinical manifestations of these diseases vary as exposure conditions vary. Generally, the acute form is characterized by dyspnea, general malaise, anorexia, chills, fever, and nonproductive cough 4 to 6 hours after exposure. The episode runs its course for about 12 to 48 hours, then subsides. A chronic form can develop if exposure to the precipitin continues.

(8:159,198,257,314), (11:129–131), (13:106), (24:184–185)

43. C. A microorganism that causes disease only in a debilitated host, or does so with increased severity or frequency, is called an *opportunist. Cryptococcus neoformans,*

the yeast that produces cryptococcosis, and *Candida albicans,* the fungus responsible for causing candidiasis, are considered opportunists.

(2:291), (4:578), (8:253,305,306), (11:173–175)

44. D. High-pressure (cardiogenic) pulmonary edema is described as fluid in the pulmonary interstitium and alveoli as a result of an increased pulmonary capillary hydrostatic pressure. In this condition the integrity of the alveolar-capillary membrane is unaltered. The cause of the transudation of fluid out of the vasculature is an elevated capillary hydrostatic pressure. Both mitral valve stenosis and left ventricular failure cause the pulmonary capillary hydrostatic pressure to exceed the pulmonary capillary osmotic pressure. A transudation of fluid results.

Adult respiratory distress syndrome is often described as permeability (non-cardiogenic) pulmonary edema because it is associated with an exudative process leading to vascular fluid entering the pulmonary interstitium. The pulmonary capillary hydrostatic pressure in these instances is generally normal. The integrity of the alveolar-capillary membrane becomes compromised, thereby allowing vascular fluid to leak into the pulmonary insterstitium.

(2:177–193),   (3:315,477–478,484,491),   (4:318–320),   (6:327,854–874), (8:335–340), (10:211), (11:268–272), (13:116)

45. D. Varying degrees of partial airways obstruction contribute to the development of low ventilation/perfusion units. Low $\dot{V}A/\dot{Q}C$ units are responsible for the hypoxemia that occurs in chronic bronchitis.

Low $\dot{V}A/\dot{Q}C$ units (perfusion in excess of ventilation) are also termed *shunt effect.* When a patient breathes room air, shunt effects act as capillary shunts. Shunt effect regions are amenable to oxygen therapy, whereas capillary shunts are not. Increased sputum production and airway inflammatory changes are responsible for the reduced ventilation to the gas exchange units, thereby resulting in low $\dot{V}A/\dot{Q}C$ abnormalities.

(3:195), (4:302,376), (8:282–286), (11:98), (13:74,159), (24:138–139)

46. C. Roentgenographic manifestations of pulmonary emphysema vary with the type (panlobular or centrilobular) and severity of emphysema. However, classically, this form of COPD usually presents with hyperlucency, flattened diaphragm, increased anteroposterior (A-P) diameter, decreased vascular markings, and air between the sternum and the heart (increased retrosternal space).

When cor pulmonale and pulmonary hypertension co-exist, vascular markings increase.

(4:302), (8:290–291)

47. A. A transudate is fluid that accumulates in the interstitium whenever an imbalance of pressures occurs at the capillary level. The four factors responsible for determining the magnitude and direction of fluid movement into (reabsorption) and out of (filtration) the vasculature are (1) the capillary hydrostatic pressure, (2) the capillary osmotic pressure, (3) the interstitial hydrostatic pressure, and (4) the interstitial osmotic pressure.

An exudate has a higher protein content than a transudate, consequently it also has a higher specific gravity (>1.018). An exudate occurs when the permeability of the capillary endothelium increases. This situation develops with ARDS.

High pressure (cardiogenic) pulmonary edema produces a transuadate as the pulmonary capillary hydrostatic pressure exceeds the pulmonary capillary osmotic pressure.

(2:177–193), (8:247), (11:193)

48. B. Digital clubbing refers to the painless, nontender, bulbous enlargment of the terminal phalanges of the fingers and toes. Certain lung diseases are associated with digital clubbing. These include cystic fibrosis, bronchiectasis, bronchogenic carcinoma, and lung abscess.

Clubbing is present when the angle between the nail and the proximal skin increases to or beyond 180°. The normal angle for fingers is about 160°. Figure 68 depicts a normal configuration, and Figure 69 illustrates digital clubbing.

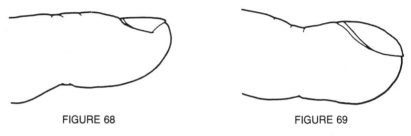

FIGURE 68   FIGURE 69

(1:284–286), (4:309,352–353), (8:189–192)

49. E. The presence of pure lymph fluid in the intrapleural space is called a *chylothorax*. Pure lymph fluid is termed *chyle*. A chylothorax often results from the obstruction of the thoracic duct. The thoracic duct, the largest lymph vessel in the body, rejoins venous circulation at the junction of the left internal jugular vein and the left subclavian vein.

(4:317), (6:322), (8:344–345), (11:192)

50. A. The Ghon complex is described as the combination of the primary tuberculous infection site and lymph node involvement. Normal persons who become infected by *Mycobacterium tuberculosis* usually heal completely from the primary tuberculosis via scarring and calcifying. The lower lobes are the usual initial infection site. Soon after the primary infection occurs, some tubercle bacilli hematogenously spread to other organ systems that have high tissue oxygen tensions. These organ systems ordinarily include the kidneys, brain, ends of long bones, and the lung apices. Like the primary infection, metastatic foci (secondary infection sites) usually completely heal by scarring and calcifying.

(11:136–155), (13:151–152)

REFERENCES

1. Spearman, C., and Sheldon, R., *Egan's Fundamentals of Respiratory Therapy,* 4th ed., C.V. Mosby, St. Louis, 1982.
2. Wojciechowski, W., *Respiratory Care Sciences: An Integrated Approach,* John Wiley & Sons, New York, 1985.

3. Shapiro, B., Harrison, R., Kacmarek, R., and Cane, R., *Clinical Application of Respiratory Care,* 3rd ed., Year Book Medical Publishers, Chicago, 1985.

4. Kacmarek, R., Mack, C., and Dimas, S., *The Essentials of Respiratory Therapy,* 2nd ed., Year Book Medical Publishers, Chicago, 1985.

5. McPherson, S., *Respiratory Therapy Equipment,* 3rd ed., C.V. Mosby, St. Louis, 1985.

6. Burton, G., and Hodgkin, J., *Respiratory Care: A Guide to Clinical Practice,* 2nd ed., J.B. Lippincott, Philadelphia, 1985.

7. Frownfelter, D., *Chest Physical Therapy and Cardiopulmonary Rehabilitation, An Interdisciplinary Approach,* Year Book Medical Publishers, Chicago, 1978.

8. Cherniack, R., and Cherniack, L., *Respiration in Health and Disease,* 3rd ed., W.B. Saunders, Philadelphia, 1983.

9. Daily, E., and Schroeder, G., *Techniques in Bedside Hemodynamic Monitoring,* 3rd ed., C.V. Mosby, St. Louis, 1985.

10. Des Jardins, R., *Clinical Manifestations of Respiratory Disease,* Year Book Medical Publishers, Chicago, 1984.

11. Mitchell, R., *Synopsis of Clinical Pulmonary Disease,* 3rd ed., C.V. Mosby, St., Louis, 1982.

12. Comroe, J., *Physiology of Respiration,* 3rd ed., Year Book Medical Publishers, Chicago, 1974.

13. West, J., *Pulmonary Pathophysiology—The Essentials,* 2nd ed., Williams & Wilkins, Baltimore, 1982.

14. West, J., *Respiratory Physiology—The Essentials,* 3rd ed., Williams & Wilkins, Baltimore, 1985.

15. Martz, K., et al., *Management of the Patient-Ventilator System: A Team Approach,* 2nd ed., C.V. Mosby, St. Louis, 1984.

16. Shoup, C., and McHenry, R., *Laboratory Exercises in Respiratory Therapy,* 2nd ed., C.V. Mosby, St. Louis, 1983.

17. Ruppel, G., *Manual of Pulmonary Function Testing,* 3rd ed., C.V. Mosby, St. Louis, 1982.

18. Appelbaum, E., and Bruce, D., *Tracheal Intubation,* W.B. Saunders, Philadelphia, 1976.

19. Rau, J., *Respiratory Therapy Pharmacology,* 2nd ed., Year Book Medical Publishers, Chicago, 1984.

20. United States Department of Health, Education, and Welfare, Public Health Service, *Isolation Techniques for Use in Hospitals,* 2nd ed., Washington, D. C., 1975.

21. Brooks, S., *Integrated Basic Science,* 4th ed., C.V. Mosby, St. Louis, 1979.

22. Comroe, J., *The Lung,* Year Book Medical Publishers, Chicago, 1962.

23. Shibel, E., and Moser, K., *Respiratory Emergencies,* 2nd ed., C.V. Mosby, St. Louis, 1982.

24. Tisi, G., *Pulmonary Physiology in Clinical Medicine,* 2nd ed., Williams & Wilkins, Baltimore, 1985.

25. Cherniack, R., *Pulmonary Function Testing,* W.B. Saunders, Philadelphia, 1977.

26. Altose, M., *The Physiological Basis of Pulmonary Function Testing,* Clinical Symposia-CIBA, Vol. 31, No. 2, Summit, New Jersey, 1979.

27. Shapiro, B., Harrison, R., and Walton, J., *Clinical Application of Arterial Blood Gases,* 3rd ed., Year Book Medical Publishers, Chicago, 1982.

28. West, J., *Ventilation/Blood Flow and Gas Exchange,* 3rd ed., Blackwell Scientific Publications, 1979.

29. Slonim, N., and Hamilton, K., *Respiratory Physiology,* 4th ed., C.V. Mosby, St. Louis, 1981.

30. Rarey, K., and Youtsey, J., *Respiratory Patient Care,* Prentice-Hall, Englewood Cliffs, 1981.

31. Berne, R., and Levy, M., *Physiology,* C.V. Mosby, St. Louis, 1983.

32. Levitzky, M., *Pulmonary Physiology,* 2nd ed., McGraw-Hill, New York, 1986.

33. Wilson, P., Bell, C., and Norton, A., *Rehabilitation of the Heart and Lungs,* SensorMedics, 1980.

34. Clausen, J., and Zarins, L., *Pulmonary Function Testing Guildlines and Controversies,* Academic Press, New York, 1982.

35. Klaus, M., and Fanaroff, A., *Care of the High-Risk Neonate,* 2nd ed., W.B. Saunders, Philadelphia, 1979.

36. Lough, M., et al., *Pediatric Respiratory Therapy,* 3rd ed., Year Book Medical Publishers, Chicago, 1985.

37. Levin, D., et al., *A Practical Guide to Pediatric Intensive Care,* 2nd ed., C.V. Mosby, St. Louis, 1984.

38. O'Ryan, J., and Burns, D., *Pulmonary Rehabilitation from Hospital to Home,* Year Book Medical Publishers, Chicago, 1984.

39. Bell, C., et al., *Home Care and Rehabilitation in Respiratory Medicine,* J.B. Lippincott, Philadelphia, 1984.

40. Wilkins, R., et al., *Clinical Assessment in Respiratory Care,* C.V. Mosby, St. Louis, 1985.

41. Jones, N., and Campbell, E., *Clinical Exercise Testing,* 2nd ed., W.B., Saunders, Philadelphia, 1982.

42. Goldsmith, J., and Karotkin, E., *Assisted Ventilation of the Neonate,* W.B. Saunders, Philadelphia, 1981.

43. Blowers, M., and Sims, R., *How to Read an ECG,* 3rd ed., Medical Economics, New Jersey, 1983.

44. Eubanks, D., and Bone, R., *Comprehensive Respiratory Care,* C.V. Mosby, St. Louis, 1985.

45. Rattenborg, C., *Clinical Use of Mechanical Ventilation,* Year Book Medical Publishers, Chicago, 1981.

46. Witkowski, S., *Pulmonary Assessment: A Clinical Guide,* J.B. Lippincott, Philadelphia, 1985.

47. Op't Holt, Timothy B., *Assessment Based Respiratory Care,* John Wiley & Sons, New York, 1986.

PEDIATRICS AND PERINATOLOGY ASSESSMENT

PURPOSE: The purpose of this 50-item assessment is to evaluate the degree of your understanding and knowledge of pediatric and neonatal diagnostic procedures and interpretation and cardiopulmonary diseases. The pathophysiology, symptomatology, diagnosis, and management of various diseases will be included.

DIRECTIONS: Each of the questions or incomplete statements is followed by five suggested answers. Select the one which is the best in each case and then blacken the corresponding space on the answer sheet.

1. Persistent fetal circulation may involve which of the following anatomic shunts?

    I. patent umbilical arteries

    II. patent foramen ovale

    III. patent umbilical vein

    IV. patent ductus venosus

    V. patent ductus arteriosus

A. II, V only
B. I, III only
C. II, IV only

D. I, III, V only
E. II, IV, V only

2. At what point in intrauterine life does the production of pulmonary surfactant usually begin?

A. between 22 to 24 weeks' gestation
B. between 24 to 26 weeks' gestation
C. between 26 to 28 weeks' gestation

D. between 28 to 30 weeks' gestation
E. between 30 to 32 weeks' gestation

3. A 26-year-old diabetic primagravida has just given birth to a 1,200-g male infant of 33 weeks' gestation. Observation of the infant indicates that he is grunting on exhalation, has nasal flaring, sternal and intercostal retractions, and is cyanotic. His ventilatory rate is 20 breaths/min. Auscultation of the chest reveals diminished breath sounds. The chest roentgenogram shows an asymmetric reticulogranular pattern and a general loss of lung volume. What is the probable diagnosis of this neonate?

A. primary apnea
B. hyaline membrane disease
C. Wilson-Mikity syndrome

D. epiglottitis
E. laryngotracheobronchitis

4. Bronchiolitis in children between the ages 6 to 18 months is generally caused by which microorganism?

A. adenovirus
B. parainfluenza virus
C. *Staphylococcus aureus*

D. respiratory syncytial virus
E. *Hemophilus influenzae*

5. Which of the following statements are true concerning whooping cough?

I. The condition usually occurs in three stages—
catarrhal, paroxysmal, and convalescent.
II. *Bordetella pertussis* is the most common causative agent.
III. Hyperimmune globulin is used in the treatment of this disease.
IV. Between coughing spells the infant is generally symptom free.

A. II, III, IV only
B. I, IV only
C. III, IV only

D. II, III only
E. I, II, III, IV

6. Which of the following factors affect the heat transfer from the surface of an infant's body to the external environment?

I. radiation
II. condensation
III. convection
IV. diffusion

A. I, II, III only

D. I, III, IV only

B. II, IV only

E. II, III, IV only

C. I, III only

7. A 3-year-old child is admitted to the Emergency Room presenting the following clinical signs: a brassy, barking cough; inspiratory and expiratory stridor; and a fiery red,
swollen, edematous epiglottis. Which microorganism is most likely the cause of this
condition?

A. *Hemophilus influenzae,* type B

D. *Diplococcus pneumoniae*

B. *Staphylococcus aureus*

E. Respiratory syncytial virus

C. *Pseudomonas aeruginosa*

8. Which of the following cardiac anomalies are included in the congenital heart abnormality described as tetralogy of Fallot?

  I. ventricular septal defect

 II. atrial septal defect

III. aortic valve stenosis

IV. pulmonic valve stenosis

A. I, III only

D. I, IV only

B. II, III only

E. I, II, III, IV

C. I, II, IV only

9. Which of the following measurements is *most* responsible for the development of
retrolental fibroplasia?

A. $P_{A_{O_2}}$

D. $F_{I_{O_2}}$

B. $S_{a_{O_2}}$

E. $P_{a_{O_2}}$

C. $P_{I_{O_2}}$

10. The lecithin/sphingomyelin (L/S) ratio is most closely related to which of the following disease condition?

A. bronchiolitis

D. Wilson-Mikity syndrome

B. retrolental fibroplasia

E. bronchopulmonary dysplasia

C. infant respiratory distress syndrome

11. The presence of meconium in the amniotic fluid is usually indicative of
_____ .

A. necrotizing enterocolitis

B. an intrauterine asphyxial episode

C. persistent fetal circulation

D. an infant's predisposition toward the development of bronchopulmonary dysplasia

E. a congenital heart defect

12. Which of the following circulatory channels are extracardiac shunts in fetal circulation?

   I. fossa ovalis

  II. foramen ovale

 III. ductus venosus

 IV. ductus arteriosus

A. I, II, III, IV   D. I, II only

B. II, IV only   E. II, III, IV only

C. III, IV only

13. A reliable sweat chloride test shows a sodium concentration _____ , or a chloride concentration of _____ .

A. >30 mEq/liter; >70 mEq/liter   D. >60 mEq/liter; >70 mEq/liter

B. >40 mEq/liter; >40 mEq/liter   E. >70 mEq/liter; >60 mEq/liter

C. >40 mEq/liter; >50 mEq/liter

14. Which of the following clinical signs are included in the Apgar score for clinically evaluating a neonate?

   I. heart rate

  II. ventilatory rate

 III. color

 IV. reflex irritability

  V. muscle tone

A. I, II, III, IV, V   D. I, III, IV, V only

B. I, II, III only   E. I, IV, V only

C. II, IV, V only

Questions 15 and 16 refer to Figure 70.

15. Which child or children will inherit cystic fibrosis from its(their) parents?

A. children 2 and 3   D. children 1 and 4

B. child 2   E. child 1

C. child 3

16. What is the percent chance that a child will *not* inherit cystic fibrosis based on the diagram?

A. 100%   D. 25%

B. 75%   E. 20%

C. 50%

17. During intrauterine development from what structure do the lungs arise?

A. hyoid bone   D. thoracic aorta

B. stomach   E. trachea

C. esophagus

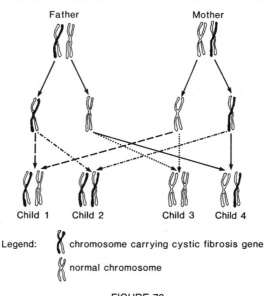

Father   Mother

Child 1   Child 2   Child 3   Child 4

Legend: chromosome carrying cystic fibrosis gene

normal chromosome

FIGURE 70

18. Which of the following clinical findings establish the diagnosis of esophageal atresia?

    I. an elevated pulmonary capillary wedge pressure
    II. an inability to pass a nasogastric tube
    III. radiographic identification of a blind esophageal pouch
    IV. an inability to create a good seal when performing bag-mask ventilation

    A. II, III only   D. III, IV only
    B. I, IV only   E. I, II only
    C. I, II, III only

19. Which of the following L/S ratios would reflect the highest probability of a neonate being born with hyaline membrane disease?

    A. 3.5:1   D. 1.5:1
    B. 3:1   E. 1:1.5
    C. 2:1

20. Which of the following statements accurately describe the congenital heart defect coarctation of the aorta?

    I. It can occur as a preductal or postductal obstruction.
    II. It is a purely cyanotic anomaly.
    III. It is characterized by a narrowed aortic lumen
    IV. It is caused by a fibrous ring that forms around the aortic valve.

A. II, III only

B. I, II, III only

C. II, III, IV only

D. I, III, IV only

E. I, III only

21. During delivery what should be done if the hypopharynx of a meconium-stained infant has not been suctioned before ventilations begin?

A. A DeLee suction catheter should be inserted into the infant's lower airway.

B. An oropharyngeal airway should be inserted to ensure a patent airway.

C. Approximately 1 to 2 cc of normal saline should be instilled into the infant's airway and deep suctioning should be performed.

D. The infant should be intubated and suctioned immediately.

E. Once the infant has been delivered, a few cubic centimeters of normal saline should be instilled and then promptly suctioned.

22. A newborn weighing 1,100 g at a gestational age of 33 weeks had Apgar scores of 5 and 5 at 1 and 5 minutes, respectively. She developed IRDS within 24 hours and required CPAP with an F_{IO_2} of 0.70. She also had an umbilical artery catheter inserted. She progressed enough warranting the discontinuation of the CPAP, oxygen, and arterial line after 2 days. On the third day she was placed on standard formula. Four days later, she had abdominal distention, blood-tinged stools, and vomiting. What is this infant's probable diagnosis?

A. septicemia

B. meconium aspiration

C. necrotizing enterocolitis

D. esophageal atresia

E. neonatal polycythemia.

23. Which of the following statements accurately describe the Wilson-Mikity syndrome?

I. It usually occurs during the first hours of extrauterine life.

II. The chest radiograph is usually normal at birth.

III. It generally occurs in premature infants weighing less than 1,500 g.

IV. Its frequency of occurrence is directly dependent upon the L/S ratio.

A. II, III only

B. III, IV only

C. I, III, IV only

D. II, III, IV only

E. I, III only

24. Which of the following therapeutic modalities, and/or pharmacologic agents are used in the treatment of persistent fetal circulation?

I. tolazoline hydrochloride

II. wide spectrum antibiotics

III. mechanical ventilation

IV. oxygenation

A. II, III, IV only

B. III, IV only

C. I, II only

D. I, III, IV only

E. I, II, III, IV

25. Which of the following congenital cardiac anomalies produce cyanosis?

    I. patent ductus arteriosus
    II. ventricular septal defects
    III. truncus arteriosus
    IV. tricuspid atresia

    A. III, IV only
    B. I, II, III only
    C. I, III, IV only

    D. II, III, IV only
    E. I, II, III, IV

26. Why does blood drawn from an umbilical artery catheter in neonates with a patent ductus arteriosus sometimes reflect a low arterial oxygen saturation?

    A. Because of anatomic differences among neonates.
    B. Because air embolization is a frequent complication when drawing blood from the catheter.
    C. Because of the location of the arterial catheter.
    D. Because fibrin frequently accumulates at the tip of the arterial catheter.
    E. Because of excessive loss of hemoglobin caused by frequent sampling.

27. Which of the following pharmacologic agents and therapeutic interventions are useful in the treatment of bronchopulmonary dysplasia?

    I. digitalis
    II. oxygen
    III. furosemide
    IV. mechanical ventilation
    V. chest physiotherapy and suctioning

    A. I, II only
    B. II, III only
    C. II, IV, V only

    D. I, II, IV, V only
    E. I, II, III, IV, V

28. Which of the following chest radiographic findings are consistent with bronchiolitis?

    I. hyperinflation
    II. hyperlucency
    III. sternal bowing
    IV. patchy hilar infiltrates

    A. I, II only
    B. II, III, IV only
    C. I, II, III only

    D. II, IV only
    E. I, II, III, IV

29. A chest roentgenogram described as demonstrating "pneumatosis intestinalis" represents which abnormality?

A. necrotizing enterocolitis
B. gastroschisis
C. esophageal atresia

D. omphalocele
E. diaphragmatic hernia

30. Which of the following statements accurately describe bronchiolitis?

    I. Bronchiolitis usually occurs only once during infancy.
    II. The disease usually has a rapid onset, high fever, and a persistent productive cough.
    III. The disease is sometimes thought to be asthma.
    IV. Bronchiolitis occurs more frequently during the winter.

    A. I, IV only
    B. I, III, IV only
    C. II, III, IV only

    D. I, II, III only
    E. I, II, III, IV

31. Which of the following disease entities is consistent with the radiographic and physical findings listed below?

    1. mild to moderate airway obstruction
    2. signs of anxiety
    3. normal pharynx
    4. normal lateral neck x-ray
    5. normal epiglottis
    6. anteroposterior chest x-ray, indicates subglottic narrowing
    7. barking cough and stridor

    A. acute epiglottitis
    B. asthma
    C. pneumonia

    D. bronchiolitis
    E. acute laryngotracheobronchitis

32. Which of the following congenital cardiac anomalies is characterized by oxygenated blood returning from the lungs to the right atrium by one or more pulmonary veins?

    A. transposition of the great vessels
    B. truncus arteriosus
    C. coarctation of the aorta

    D. tetralogy of Fallot
    E. anomalous venous return

33. Which of the following statements accurately describe epiglottitis?

    I. The child ordinarily goes to bed feeling well, but awakens later febrile and dyspneic.
    II. It is often recommended to turn on a hot shower to allow the child to breathe the steam.
    III. The child often drools in association with this condition.
    IV. Nebulized racemic epinephrine is useful in treating this disease.

A. I, III only

B. II, III, IV only

C. I, II, III only

D. II, IV only

E. I, III, IV only

34. Which of the following clinical conditions are complications of cystic fibrosis?

   I. aspiration pneumonitis

   II. bronchiectasis

   III. pneumothoraces

   IV. cor pulmonale

A. II, III only

B. II, IV only

C. II, III, IV only

D. I, III, IV only

E. I, II, III only

35. Which of the following pathologic changes are associated with pneumonia?

   I. mucosal edema

   II. luminal and intra-alveolar secretions

   III. capillary shunting

   IV. pulmonary vasoconstriction

A. I, II only

B. II, III, IV only

C. III, IV only

D. I, II, III only

E. I, II, III, IV

36. Which of the following congenital cardiac abnormalities produce an increased pulmonary capillary hydrostatic pressure?

   I. tetralogy of Fallot

   II. ventricular septal defect

   III. coarctation of the aorta

   IV. transposition of the great vessels

A. II, III, IV only

B. I, III, IV only

C. III, IV only

D. I, II only

E. I, II, III, IV

37. Which congenital heart anomaly(ies) does(do) *not* produce hypoxemia?

   I. tetralogy of Fallot

   II. patent ductus arteriosus

   III. truncus arteriosus

   IV. ventricular septal defect

A. II only

B. I, III, IV only

C. II, IV only

D. I, II, III only

E. I, IV only

BREATHING NOMOGRAM

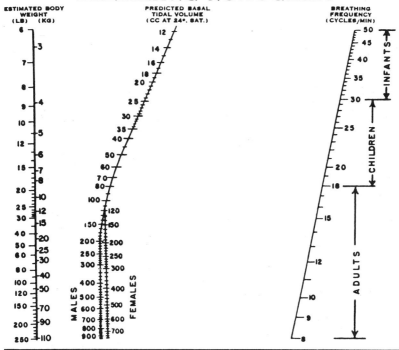

| ESTIMATED BODY WEIGHT (LB) (KG) | PREDICTED BASAL TIDAL VOLUME (CC AT 24°, SAT.) | BREATHING FREQUENCY (CYCLES/MIN) |

CORRECTIONS TO BE APPLIED TO PREDICTED BASAL TIDAL VOLUME

Using English System Measurements:
Daily activity (i.e. patients not in coma): add 10%.
Fever: add 5% for each degree above 99° F. (rectal).
Altitude: add 5% for each 2000 feet above sea level.
Tracheotomy (or endotracheal tube): subtract a volume equal to one-half body weight in lbs.
Metabolic Acidosis during Anesthesia: add 20%.
Dead Space of Anesthesia Apparatus: Add volume of apparatus and mask dead space.

Using Metric System Measurements:
Daily activity: add 10%.
Fever: add 9% for each degree above 37° C. (rectal).
Altitude: add 8% for each 1000 M above sea level.
Tracheotomy (or endotracheal tube): subtract 1 cc./kg. of body weight.
Metabolic Acidosis during Anesthesia: add 20%.
Dead Space of Anesthesia Apparatus: Add volume of apparatus and mask dead space.

REFERENCE: EDWARD P. RADFORD, JR., BENJAMIN G. FERRIS, JR., and BERTRAND C. KRIETE: Clinical Use of a Nomogram to Estimate Proper Ventilation during Artificial Respiration. NEW ENGLAND JOURNAL OF MEDICINE, 251:877-884 (November 25), 1954.

FIGURE 71

38. Using the nomogram (Figure 71), determine the predicted tidal volume for a tracheotomized, 3,000-g infant breathing at a rate of 37 breaths/min.

A. 12 cc   D. 20 cc

B. 15 cc   E. 22 cc

C. 18 cc

39. Right ventricular hypertrophy produced secondarily from a chronic pulmonary disease is called _____ .

A. right ventricular failure   D. hyperplasia

B. increased pulmonary vascular resistance   E. cor pulmonale

C. cardiomegaly

40. The Silverman scale is useful for evaluating which of the following conditions?

A. cyanosis   D. pulmonary surfactant

B. respiratory distress   E. meconium aspiration

C. congenital cardiac defects

41. Which of the following clinical aspects are used in compiling the Silverman score?

   I. heart sounds

  II. capillary refill

 III. expiratory grunting

 IV. amniocentesis

  V. xiphoid retractions

A. I, II only   D. III, V only

B. II, IV only   E. II, III, V only

C. I, III, IV only

42. Generally, the intrapleural pressure generated to initiate a neonate's first breath is

_____ .

A. -3 to -5 cm H_2O D. -40 to -100 cm H_2O

B. -10 to -20 cm H_2O E. -100 to -130 cm H_2O

C. -20 to -40 cm H_2O

43. Which of the following diagnostic evaluations can be accomplished via amniocentesis?

   I. L/S ratios

  II. meconium levels

 III. placenta location

 IV. chromosomal makeup

A. I, II, IV only   D. I, II, III only

B. II, III only   E. I, II, III, IV

C. I, IV only

44. Which of the following statements accurately describe fetal circulation?

   I. Blood flow to the pulmonary vasculature is low.

  II. Blood flow passes from the right ventricle to the left ventricle through the foramen ovale.

 III. The ductus arteriosus allows fetal blood to pass from the pulmonary veins to the aorta.

 IV. The vascular pressures on the right side of circulation are greater than those on the left.

A. I, IV only
B. II, IV only
C. II, III, IV only

D. I, II, III only
E. I, II, IV only

45. Which of the following diseases are ordinarily associated with digital clubbing?

  I. asthma
 II. cystic fibrosis
III. bronchiolitis
IV. congenital cardiac anomalies
 V. epiglottitis

A. I, III only
B. II, IV only
C. II, III, IV, V only

D. II, IV, V only
E. I, II, III only

46. Which of the following congenital cardiac anomalies produce left-to-right shunts?

  I. atrial septal defect
 II. preductal coarctation of the aorta
III. patent ductus arteriosus
IV. tetralogy of Fallot

A. I, II, III only
B. I, II only
C. I, III only

D. III, IV only
E. II, III, IV only

Questions 47 and 48 are based on the same information.

A neonate is observed at one minute after birth. Her heart is 110 beats/min. Her ventilatory rate is 40 breaths/min; she is also crying. She is exhibiting peripheral cyanosis. Some flexion of her extremities is displayed. The nurse has passed a suction catheter down the neonate's nose, causing the infant to sneeze.

47. What should the baby girl's Apgar score be?

A. 0
B. 4
C. 6

D. 8
E. 10

48. Based on this 1-minute Apgar score, what action should be taken at this time?

A Bag-mask ventilation along with supplemental oxygen is indicated to alleviate the peripheral cyanosis.
B. Suctioning should precede the bag-mask ventilation and oxygen administration.
C. No resuscitation measures appear necessary.
D. Cardiopulmonary resuscitation is indicated immediately.
E. The neonate needs only supplemental oxygen.

49. What is the name of the structure that remains after anatomic closure of the ductus arteriosus?

    A. foramen ovale   D. ligamentum arteriosus
    B. ostium primum   E. fossa arteriosus
    C. fossa ovalis

50. Which of the following statements accurately describe acute laryngotracheobronchitis?

      I. Antibiotics are usually of no value in treating this disease.
     II. This condition sometimes necessitates a tracheostomy.
    III. Aerosol therapy should be avoided because it only worsens the condition by inducing fluid overload.
     IV. Physical examination of the pharynx must be avoided because further airway obstruction can result.

    A. I, II, III, IV   D. I, II, III only
    B. III, IV only   E. I, II only
    C. I, II, IV only

ASSESSMENT ANSWER SHEET

DIRECTIONS: Darken the space under the selected answer.

	A	B	C	D	E		A	B	C	D	E
1.	[ ]	[ ]	[ ]	[ ]	[ ]	26.	[ ]	[ ]	[ ]	[ ]	[ ]
2.	[ ]	[ ]	[ ]	[ ]	[ ]	27.	[ ]	[ ]	[ ]	[ ]	[ ]
3.	[ ]	[ ]	[ ]	[ ]	[ ]	28.	[ ]	[ ]	[ ]	[ ]	[ ]
4.	[ ]	[ ]	[ ]	[ ]	[ ]	29.	[ ]	[ ]	[ ]	[ ]	[ ]
5.	[ ]	[ ]	[ ]	[ ]	[ ]	30.	[ ]	[ ]	[ ]	[ ]	[ ]
6.	[ ]	[ ]	[ ]	[ ]	[ ]	31.	[ ]	[ ]	[ ]	[ ]	[ ]
7.	[ ]	[ ]	[ ]	[ ]	[ ]	32.	[ ]	[ ]	[ ]	[ ]	[ ]
8.	[ ]	[ ]	[ ]	[ ]	[ ]	33.	[ ]	[ ]	[ ]	[ ]	[ ]
9.	[ ]	[ ]	[ ]	[ ]	[ ]	34.	[ ]	[ ]	[ ]	[ ]	[ ]
10.	[ ]	[ ]	[ ]	[ ]	[ ]	35.	[ ]	[ ]	[ ]	[ ]	[ ]
11.	[ ]	[ ]	[ ]	[ ]	[ ]	36.	[ ]	[ ]	[ ]	[ ]	[ ]
12.	[ ]	[ ]	[ ]	[ ]	[ ]	37.	[ ]	[ ]	[ ]	[ ]	[ ]
13.	[ ]	[ ]	[ ]	[ ]	[ ]	38.	[ ]	[ ]	[ ]	[ ]	[ ]
14.	[ ]	[ ]	[ ]	[ ]	[ ]	39.	[ ]	[ ]	[ ]	[ ]	[ ]
15.	[ ]	[ ]	[ ]	[ ]	[ ]	40.	[ ]	[ ]	[ ]	[ ]	[ ]
16.	[ ]	[ ]	[ ]	[ ]	[ ]	41.	[ ]	[ ]	[ ]	[ ]	[ ]
17.	[ ]	[ ]	[ ]	[ ]	[ ]	42.	[ ]	[ ]	[ ]	[ ]	[ ]
18.	[ ]	[ ]	[ ]	[ ]	[ ]	43.	[ ]	[ ]	[ ]	[ ]	[ ]
19.	[ ]	[ ]	[ ]	[ ]	[ ]	44.	[ ]	[ ]	[ ]	[ ]	[ ]
20.	[ ]	[ ]	[ ]	[ ]	[ ]	45.	[ ]	[ ]	[ ]	[ ]	[ ]
21.	[ ]	[ ]	[ ]	[ ]	[ ]	46.	[ ]	[ ]	[ ]	[ ]	[ ]
22.	[ ]	[ ]	[ ]	[ ]	[ ]	47.	[ ]	[ ]	[ ]	[ ]	[ ]
23.	[ ]	[ ]	[ ]	[ ]	[ ]	48.	[ ]	[ ]	[ ]	[ ]	[ ]
24.	[ ]	[ ]	[ ]	[ ]	[ ]	49.	[ ]	[ ]	[ ]	[ ]	[ ]
25.	[ ]	[ ]	[ ]	[ ]	[ ]	50.	[ ]	[ ]	[ ]	[ ]	[ ]

PEDIATRICS AND PERINATOLOGY ANALYSES

Note: The references listed after each analysis are numbered and keyed to the reference list located at the end of this section. The first number indicates the text. The second number indicates the page where information about the question will be found. For example, (1:219,384) means that reference number 1 is to be used and that on pages 219 and 384 information about the question will be found. Frequently, it will be necessary to read beyond the page number indicated to obtain complete information. Therefore, reference to the question will be found either on the page indicated or on subsequent pages.

1. A. Persistent fetal circulation (Figure 71A) is characterized by pulmonary hypertension with right-to-left shunting through persistent fetal channels which may include a patent ductus arteriosus, a patent foramen ovale, or both. Normally, closure of the ductus arteriosus begins immediately at birth. The process is usually completed during the first 24 hours of postnatal life. The foramen ovale functionally closes in the immediate postnatal period, but anatomic closure takes several months or longer.

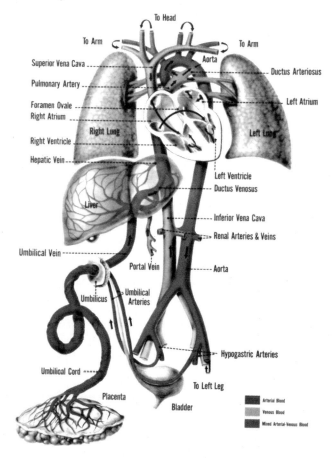

FIGURE 71A

The mechanism for closure of the ductus arteriosus is oxygenation. As the neonate begins breathing, the oxygen in the inspired air entering the blood causes vaso-constriction of this structure. Hypoxemia and/or acidemia in the first few days of life can cause the ductus arteriosus to re-open. The foramen ovale closes in re-sponse to increasing left heart pressures and decreasing right heart pressures. Pre-sistent pulmonary hypertension maintains high right heart pressures, which can in-terfere with closure of the foramen ovale after birth.

(8:119,122–113), (34:298–299)

2. A. The production of pulmonary surfactant begins during intrautarine life at approxi-mately 22 to 24 weeks' gestation. The biochemical synthesis of this phospholipid molecule relies on the presence of two metabolic pathways—the methyltrans-ferase system (22 to 24 weeks) and the phosphocholine transferase system (35 weeks).

(2:232), (6:705), (36:16)

3. B. Hyaline membrane disease (HMD) or infant respiratory distress syndrome (IRDS) occurs commonly in premature infants whose mothers either experience bleeding or are diabetic. Clinical manifestations of this disease include (1) expiratory grunt-ing, (2) nasal flaring, (3) sternal and intercostal retractions, (4) cyanosis, (5) di-minished breath sounds, and (6) rapid or slow ventilatory rate. Chest x-rays often show a ground-glass or reticulogranular appearance with decreased lung volume.

(6:712–714), (35:183–187), (36:47–53)

4. D. Bronchiolitis in children (6 to 18 months) is usually caused by the respiratory syn-cytial virus (RSV). Other viruses, for example, adenovirus and parainfluenza, are sometimes the causative factor.

(3:353), (6:779), (36:94–97)

5. E. *Bordetella pertussis* is the most common causative agent responsible for the de-velopment of whooping cough or pertussis. Other responsible microorganisms are *Bordetella parapertussis* and adenovirus.

The disease occurs in three stages. The *catarrhal* stage is characterized as an up-per airway infection, which then progresses to the *paroxysmal* stage. The paroxys-mal stage is marked by the "whoop." The whoop occurs during the vigorous in-spiratory effort that follows the brief, recurring coughs taking place during the previous exhalation. Also during the paroxysmal stage, the infants are treated with hyperimmune globulin. Between coughing episodes the infant is relatively symp-tom free. In fact, it is recommended that a sleeping infant be allowed to rest be-tween paroxysms because feeding or crying can trigger another episode.

The *convalescent* stage follows the 4- to 6-week paroxysmal stage. Paroxysms oc-cur with much less frequency during this stage.

(6:780)

6. C. Infants lose body heat via two gradients—internal and external. The internal gra-dient refers to the heat loss from within the infant's body and the infant's body surface. Physiologic mechanisms, e.g., vasoconstriction and vasodilatation, change the internal gradient by altering blood flow to the skin.

The external gradient refers to the heat transfer from the infant's body surface to the surrounding environment. Four physical factors influence this gradient: radiation, conduction, convection, and evaporation.

(35:96–97), (37:120)

7. A. Acute epiglottitis is a supraglottic airway obstruction. The presenting patient is usually febrile, exhibiting inspiratory and expiratory stridor and ventilatory distress. Visualization of the pharynx will reveal a fiery red, swollen, edematous epiglottis. The origin of acute epiglottitis is usually caused by the bacterial microorganism *Hempophilus influenzae* type B.

(4:354–355), (6:776), (8:274), (36:84–85), (37:202–207,545)

8. D. The congenital cardiac anomaly described as tetralogy of Fallot shown in Figure 71B is characterized by the combination of the following four defects (1) ventricular septal defect, (2) pulmonic valve stenosis, (3) overriding aorta, and (4) right ventricular hypertrophy. The severity of symptoms depends on the degree of the pulmonic valve stenosis, the size of the ventricular septal defect, and the extent to which the aorta overrides the ventricular septal defect.

(4:344), (37:245)

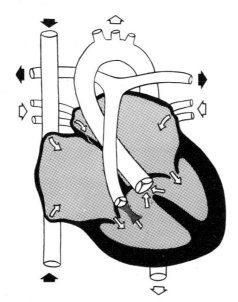

FIGURE 71B

9. E. The amount of oxygen dissolved in the arterial blood, i.e., the Pa_{O_2}, influences the development of retrolental fibroplasia (RLF). The development of this condition is also influenced by the immaturity of the neonate and the duration of exposure to the high Pa_{O_2}. The specific value of Pa_{O_2} that will cause RLF is not known; however, clinical experience has shown that the incidence of RLF is drastically reduced when the Pa_{O_2} is maintained between 60 and 100 mm Hg.

(1:457–458), (2:254), (4:372–373), (6:401,701), (35:176,179,216), (36:54,133), (37:226)

10. C. Assessing the lecithin/sphingomyelin (L/S) ratio via amniocentesis provides a measure of lung maturity. Before 35 weeks' gestation, sphingomyelin (another phospholipid) predominates, thus rendering an L/S ratio less than 2. At approximately 35 weeks' gestation lecithin production increases and its concentration in the amniotic fluid begins to exceed that of sphingomyelin. An L/S ratio 2:1 or greater reflects lung maturation sufficient to support extrauterine life. Such an L/S ratio indicates less than a 5% risk for the development of IRDS, whereas a ratio of 1:1 or less is associated with a greater than 90% risk. A transitional L/S ratio (1.5:1) indicates a 50% probability of risk.

(2:232), (4:167,335), (6:706,717,723), (35:7–8,20), (36:17)

11. B. Meconium, (fetal intestinal tract fluid), in the amniotic fluid usually indicates that the fetus has experienced an episode of asphyxia *in utero*. Postterm infants are at greatest risk of meconium aspiration.

(4:337), (6:731–732), (35:35,190), (36:65–66), (37:233)

12. C. The ductus venosus and ductus arteriosus are the two extracardiac shunts in fetal circulation. The ductus venosus allows oxygenated blood from the placenta to bypass the portal (liver) circulation. The blood then enters the inferior vena cava as it courses its way to the right atrium.

The other extracardiac shunt is the ductus arteriosus which allows poorly oxygenated blood to pass from the pulmonary artery to the aorta below the point where blood is supplied to the brain and heart. Both of these extracardiac shunts are highlighted in Figure 71C.

The foramen ovale is the opening between the right and left atria in the heart. The fossa ovalis is the slight depression between the right and left atria that remains from the closure of the foramen ovale.

(4:108,167–169), (8:118–120), (14:140–142), (36:20–22)

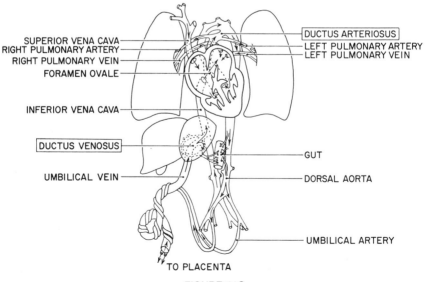

FIGURE 71C

13. D. The sodium and chloride content of sweat in children with cystic fibrosis is two to five times greater than that of normal children and occurs in 98% of affected children. For diagnostic purposes, the quantitative test is performed on sweat obtained by iontophoresis of pilocarpine in which a small electric current carries the cholinergic drug pilocarpine into a small patch of skin to stimulate the local sweat glands.

Normally, the sweat chloride content ranges between about 10 to 40 mEq/liter. A chloride concentration greater than 70 mEq/liter and a sodium concentration greater than 60 mEq/liter are diagnostic of cystic fibrosis.

(6:762)

14. D. The purpose of the Apgar score is to clinically evaluate the cardiopulmonary status of a newborn. The Apgar score is comprised of the following clinical signs (1) heart rate, (2) respiratory (ventilatory) effort, (3) muscle tone, (4) reflex irritability, and (5) color. Ventilatory rate is *not* one of the clinical signs included; ventilatory effort is. The Apgar scale is shown in Table 2. The Apgar score is based on a scale of 0 to 10. Apgar score ranges and their corresponding clinical interventions are listed in Table 3. Apgar scores should be determined at 1 and 5 minutes after birth.

(6:709–710), (35:31–34), (36:32–33), (JAMA, August 1, 1980, Vol. 244, No. 5, 495–496)

15. B. When both parents are carriers (heterozygotes) of the cystic fibrosis gene, there is a one in four (25%) chance with each conception that the offspring will inherit the disease.

(36:99)

TABLE 2

Sign	Score		
	0	1	2
Heart rate	Absent	<100 bpm	>100 bpm
Ventilatory effort	Absent	Weak, irregular	Good, crying
Muscle tone	Flaccid, limp	Some flexion of extremities	Active, well flexed
Reflex irritability	No response	Grimace	Cough, sneeze
Color	Peripheral and central cyanosis	Peripheral cyanosis	Completely pink

TABLE 3

Apgar Score	Evaluation
7–10	Resuscitative measures are not needed
4–6	Mild to moderate asphyxia, suctioning and oxygenation indicated; ventilation considered
0–3	Cardiopulmonary resuscitation indicated

16. B. At each conception one chromosome from each parent is inherited by the offspring. Therefore, the various outcomes and their chances of occurrence are as follows:

OUTCOME	PROBABILITY
Cystic fibrosis	25%
Carrier (no disease)	50%
Normal (noncarrier)	25%

Because carriers of the cystic fibrosis gene do not present the clinical manifestations of this disease, there is a 75% chance that the offspring of heterozygote (carrier) parents will not inherit cystic fibrosis.
(36:99)

17. C. At about the 20th to 24th day of intrauterine life, the lungs begin as a bud or outpouching arising from the esophagus (Figure 71D). The left and right lungs begin to differentiate at about the 26th to 28th day.
(4:166), (36:4–5)

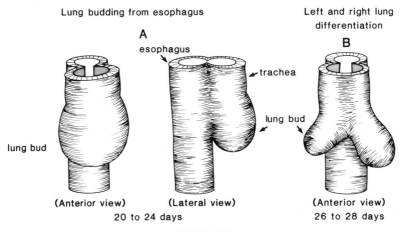

Lung budding from esophagus

Left and right lung differentiation

A

esophagus

trachea

lung bud

lung bud

B

lung bud

(Anterior view)   (Lateral view)   (Anterior view)
20 to 24 days   26 to 28 days

FIGURE 71D

18. A. Esophageal atresia can be confirmed (1) by an inability to pass a nasogastric (NG) tube, and (2) by radiographically indentifying a blind esophageal pouch. Figure 72 illustrates an esophageal atresia. Note the esophageal pouch which is commonly observed radiographically and prevents the passage of an NG tube.
(6:737–738), (37:350–351)

19. E. An L/S ratio of 2:1 or greater reflects lung maturation sufficient to support extrauterine life. Such a ratio represents less than a 5% risk for the development of hyaline membrane disease (HMD). An L/S ratio of 1:1 or less is associated with a greater than 90% risk. A transitional L/S ratio, i.e., 1.5:1, reflects a 50% probability of risk.
(2:232), (4:167,335), (6:706,717,723), (35:7–8,20), (36:17)

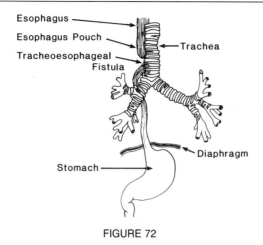

Esophagus

Esophagus Pouch

Tracheoesophageal
Fistula

Trachea

Diaphragm

Stomach

FIGURE 72

20. E. Coarctation of the aorta is a congenital cardiac anomaly characterized as a narrowed aortic lumen (Figure 72A).

The narrowing (partial obstruction) can occur before the ductus arteriosus
(preductal) or it can be located beyond the ductus arteriosus (postductal). If the
narrowing is preductal, cyanosis will occur. A postductal coarctation does not
produce cyanosis.

A fibrous ring around the aortic valve describes the condition known as subaortic
stenosis. It is not associated with coarctation of the aorta.

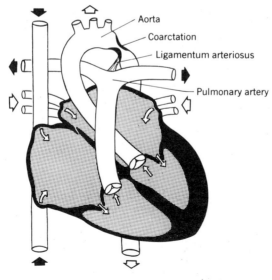

Aorta

Coarctation

Ligamentum arteriosus

Pulmonary artery

FIGURE 72A

(4:342–343), (35:313–314)

21. D. The hypopharynx of meconium-stained infants should be suctioned immediately to prevent aspiration. Ideally, the physician will suction the hypopharynx of such infants before ventilations begin. If the meconium is not suctioned from the hypopharynx before the infant begins to breathe, the infant should be intubated and suctioned immediately.
   (JAMA, August 1, 1980, Vol. 244, No. 5, 496)

22. C. Enterocolitis is usually seen in neonates that are low birth weight and premature. They also present with low Apgar scores.
   Necrotizing enterocolitis is an ischemic condition of the gut that seems to occur in neonates of low birth weight and early gestational age. Its etiology is unknown, but a number of mechanisms have been considered, e.g., a lack of maternal milk, hyperosmolar feedings, and umbilical artery catheters. Clinical features of this disorder include abdominal distention, bloody stools, lethargy, gastric retention, and vomiting.
   (35:136–137), (37:347–349)

23. A. The Wilson-Mikity syndrome or pulmonary dysmaturity usually occurs 1 to 5 weeks after birth. The chest radiograph is normal at birth but deteriorates later as the disorder becomes clinically manifest. Infants usually weigh less than 1,500 g and are premature. This condition (etiology unknown) has no association with IRDS or bronchopulmonary dysplasia.
   (4:338,339), (6:727–728)

24. D. Treatment for persistent fetal circulation, characterized by pulmonary hypertension, may include mechanical ventilation, high concentrations of oxygen, and tolazoline hydrochloride (Priscoline).
   The mechanical ventilation is intended to improve alveolar minute ventilation or in some instances to hyperventilate the infant and normalize the Pa_{CO_2}. High concentrations of oxygen are administered to vasodilate the pulmonary vasculature. Tolazoline, an alpha-adrenergic blocker, is a potent vasodilator, and is administered to reduce the pulmonary hypertension. Because tolazoline is a nonspecific vasodilator, its administration must be viewed with caution and should be withheld from a shocky infant until good blood pressure and cardiac output are assured.
   (4:337–338)

25. A. Truncus arteriosus and tricuspid atresia both produce cyanosis. Truncus arteriosus is characterized by a ventricular septal defect (VSD) communicating with a common vessel. The aorta and pulmonary artery normally undergo separation embryologically. Failure of this normal separation to occur produces a single arterial trunk that overrides the ventricles (Figure 73). Tricuspid atresia is characterized by a narrowing of the tricuspid valve which communicates the right atrium with the right ventricle. Additionally, an atrial septal defect (ASD) and a VSD co-exist. As blood flow enters the right atrium, it passes through the ASD into the left atrium. There it mixes with oxygenated blood from the pulmonary veins. Once it enters the left ventricle, the blood courses one of two routes. Some of the blood flow leaves via the aorta, and the remainder passes through the VSD to the right ventricle and into the pulmonary vasculature. Consequently, the right ventricle is

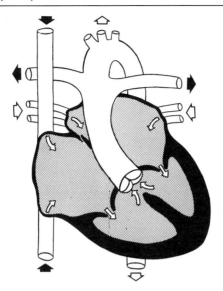

FIGURE 73. Truncus arteriosus: Note the VSD and the failure of the aorta and pulmonary artery to separate into two distinct vessels.

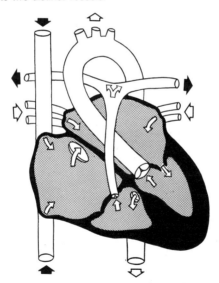

FIGURE 74. Tricuspid artesia: Note the ASD, VSD, small right ventricle, large left ventricle, and reduced pulmonary perfusion.

very small; the left ventricle becomes large and pulmonary perfusion is diminished (Figure 74). A patent ductus arteriosus and a VSD *by themselves* do not produce cyanosis because in both situations blood is shunted from left to right. (4:339–341,343–346)

26. C. Blood drawn from an umbilical artery catheter in neonates with a patent ductus arteriosus sometimes reflects a low arterial saturation because the arterial catheter is located distal to the patent ductus arteriosus. The blood at the catheter site is

sometimes less oxygenated because of the venous admixture caused by a patent ductus arteriosus that is associated with right-to-left shunting.
(4:337,339,340), (9:161)

27. E. Once bronchopulmonary dysplasia (BPD) is clinically manifest, the congestive right ventricular failure is treated with medications that will increase the myocardial contractility, e.g., digitalis. The administration of diuretics, for example, furosemide (Lasix) helps prevent fluid retention. Oxygen is usually required, often in high concentrations. Mechanical ventilation may be required as well. When the infant is intubated bronchial hygiene and airway care, i.e., chest physiotherapy and tracheobronchial suctioning, are paramount.

Mild BPD may not require as much support as the more severe forms. There is a wide spectrum of disability associated with BPD. Therefore, high levels of support are not necessary in all cases.
(6:727), (35:195)

28. C. Roentgenographically, bronchiolitis is characterized by hyperinflation, flattened diaphragm, increased anteroposterior (A-P) diameter, and general hyperlucency.
(6:779)

29. A. Necrotizing enterocolitis is an ischemic disease of the gut occurring in low birth weight, immature infants, who may have suffered asphyxia, hyaline membrane disease, patent ductus arteriosus, polycythemia, and/or sepsis. It is postulated that necrotizing enterocolitis results from a circulatory system reflex causing ischemia of the gut to maintain circulation to the brain. Among a variety of signs and symptoms pneumatosis intestinalis, or air within the intestinal wall, presents during gastric radiography.
(35:137), (37:347)

30. B. Bronchiolitis, an acute viral infection that occurs frequently in the winter, is characterized by a gradual (several days) worsening of signs and symptoms. Initially, the disease produces nasal symptoms, such as rhinorrhea. Cough and low-grade fever are also present. A few days later, the infant becomes tachypneic, dyspneic, and tachycardic. Intercostal retractions, wheezing, and hyperinflated chest are also present.

To differentiate bronchiolitis from asthma, it is suggested that an aerosolized bronchodilator or intramuscular epinephrine, or both, be administered. Once these medications prove to be of no value, they should be discontinued.
(4:353–354), (6:779), (8:277), (36:91,94–97)

31. E. Acute laryngotracheobronchitis (LTB) is an infection that produces mild to moderate upper airway obstruction in children 6 months to 3 years of age. Radiographs of the neck are ordinarily unremarkable in that the pharynx and epiglottis appear normal. An A-P chest film, however, generally indicates subglottic narrowing. The barking cough and stridor manifest themselves a few days after the initial presentation of upper respiratory signs and symptoms (rhinorrhea, cough, and fever). As the barking cough and stridor develop, the child exhibits more apprehension which, in turn, aggravates the dyspnea.
(4:354), (6:776), (8:274), (36:86–88)

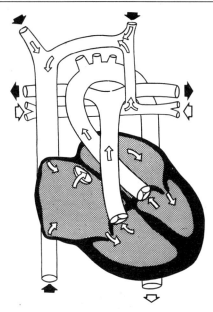

FIGURE 75

32. E. The congenital cardiac defect known as anomalous venous return is characterized by the return of oxygenated blood from the lungs to the right atrium via one or more pulmonary veins. A surgically induced communication between the right and left atria is required for survival of the infant (Figure 75).
(4:347–348), (36:111–112)

33. A. Epiglottitis manifests itself as an inflammatory process affecting the entire laryngeal inlet, i.e., the epiglottis, aryepiglottic folds, and adjacent tissue. The offending microorganism is usually *Hemophilus influenzae* type B. It can have a rapid onset. In fact, the child, usually between 3 and 6 years old, may go to bed perfectly well, but awaken later with a high-grade fever, dyspnea, drooling, dysphonia (or aphonia), dysphagia, and inspiratory stridor.

Unlike acute laryngotracheobronchitis (LTB), heated and unheated aerosols are ineffective for relieving the obstruction. Similarly, epiglottitis is not treatable with nebulized racemic epinephrine (Micronephrine, Vaponephrin).
(4:354–355), (6:469–470,776), (8:274–275), (36:84–88,217)

34. C. The bronchiectasis often results from the chronic airway obstruction. The abnormal dilatation of the bronchial walls associated with this complication results from chronic inflammatory changes involving the bronchial mucosal and submucosal layers.

The cor pulmonale develops in response to the pulmonary hypertension and the increased pulmonary vascular resistance both of which cause the right ventricle to increase work. The co-existence of hypoxemia, hypercapnia, and acidemia is the primary reason pulmonary hypertension occurs. Each of these conditions by itself causes pulmonary vasoconstriction. However, when two or more are present simultaneously, the pulmonary vasoconstriction is potentiated.

The hypoxemia has an additional contributory effect. Hypoxemia stimulates the kidneys to release the hormone erythropoietin into the blood. This hormone stimulates the bone marrow to produce more erythrocytes (red blood cells) in an attempt to increase the blood's oxygen-carrying capacity. As a result, the blood becomes more viscous.

The right ventricle, therefore, has the job of pumping a more viscous fluid through more narrowed vessels. This increased strain on the right ventricle increases the muscle mass of that heart chamber.

Pneumothoraces can occur as a result of lung parenchymal changes caused by the chronic nature of cystic fibrosis. Blebs and bullae develop as the lungs become emphysematous.

(4:352–353), (6:768), (8:295–298), (36:84–85)

35. E. Pneumonias are considered shunt-producing diseases because the associated increased secretions often produce atelectasis by obstructing the airways. The presence of the secretions and capillary shunting account for the hypoxemia which produces pulmonary vasoconstriction. The infectious process, of course, causes mucosal edema and the secretions that reside in the airways and alveoli.

(6:730–731), (8:307), (36:102–103)

36. A. A ventricular septal defect (VSD) produces a left-to-right shunt in extrauterine life because the high vascular pressures inside the left ventricle cause blood to move into the right ventricle across the defect. Consequently, the right ventricle pumps more blood into the pulmonary vasculature. The increased pulmonary blood volume produces a high pulmonary vascular hydrostatic pressure (Figure 75A). Coarctation of the aorta is characterized by either pre- or postductal (ductus arteriosus) narrowing of the aorta. The narrowing of this vessel prevents the left ventricle from completely emptying during ventricular systole. Therefore, the left

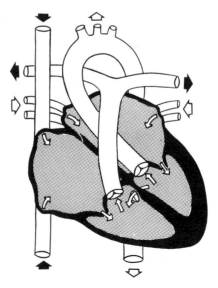

FIGURE 75A

atrium cannot deposit its entire blood volume into the left ventricle. Blood volume then increases in the pulmonary vascular bed as the right ventricle continues to place its normal output there, and as the outflow from the pulmonary vasculature is impeded. The result is an increased pulmonary capillary hydrostatic pressure (Figure 75B).

The congenital cardiac anomaly, described as transposition of the great vessels (Figure 75C), is characterized by the right ventricle pumping blood out the aorta and the left ventricle depositing its output through the pulmonary artery. In this defect the two circulation networks (systemic and pulmonary) are in parallel rather than in series, which is how they normally are. Consequently, the pulmonary blood volume increases producing an increased pulmonary capillary hydrostatic pressure.

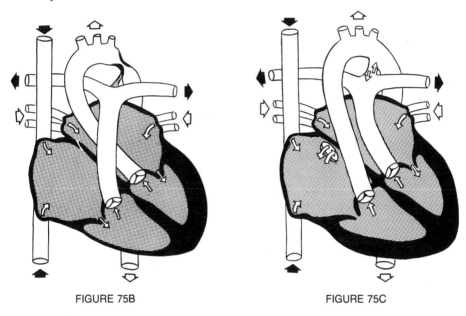

FIGURE 75B   FIGURE 75C

(4:341,342–343,346), (36:111–115)

37. C. Neither a patent ductus arteriosus (PDA) nor a ventricular septal defect (VSD) by itself produces hypoxemia. In the case of a PDA, oxygenated blood from the aorta is shunted into the pulmonary artery for passage through the lungs once again. Blood flow through the pulmonary vasculature is increased and gas exchange is normal. Pulmonary hypertension develops.

Similarly, for a VSD, oxygenated blood flows from the left ventricle to the right ventricle, then out the pulmonary artery to the lungs. Once again, oxygenation is not the problem, but pulmonary hypertension is.

Patients with truncus arteriosus are hypoxemic because only one great artery arises from both left and right ventricles. In this situation oxygenated and unoxygenated blood mix.

In tetralogy of Fallot (VSD, pulmonic valve stenosis, right ventricular hypertrophy, and overriding aorta), pulmonic valve stenosis prevents normal ejection of

BREATHING NOMOGRAM

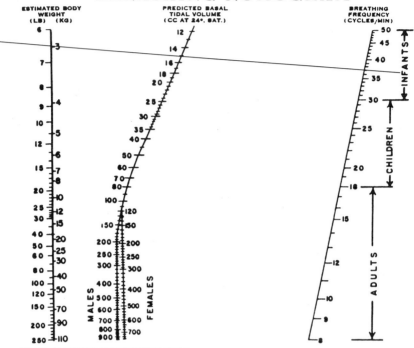

| ESTIMATED BODY WEIGHT (LB) (KG) | PREDICTED BASAL TIDAL VOLUME (CC AT 24°, SAT.) | BREATHING FREQUENCY (CYCLES/MIN) |

CORRECTIONS TO BE APPLIED TO PREDICTED BASAL TIDAL VOLUME

Using English System Measurements:
Daily activity (i.e. patients not in coma): add 10%.
Fever: add 5% for each degree above 99° F. (rectal).
Altitude: add 5% for each 2000 feet above sea level.
Tracheotomy (or endotracheal tube): subtract a volume equal to one-half body weight in lbs.
Metabolic Acidosis during Anesthesia: add 20%.
Dead Space of Anesthesia Apparatus: Add volume of apparatus and mask dead space.

Using Metric System Measurements:
Daily activity: add 10%.
Fever: add 9% for each degree above 37° C. (rectal).
Altitude: add 8% for each 1000 M above sea level.
Tracheotomy (or endotracheal tube): subtract 1 cc./kg. of body weight.
Metabolic Acidosis during Anesthesia: add 20%.
Dead Space of Anesthesia Apparatus: Add volume of apparatus and mask dead space.

REFERENCE: EDWARD P. RADFORD, JR., BENJAMIN G. FERRIS, JR., and BERTRAND C. KRIETE: Clinical Use of a Nomogram to Estimate Proper Ventilation during Artificial Respiration. NEW ENGLAND JOURNAL OF MEDICINE, 251:877-884 (November 25), 1954.

FIGURE 76

blood from the right ventricle. Therefore, pressure in the right ventricle exceeds that in the left ventricle and blood flows across the VSD from right to left, bypassing pulmonary circulation. Hypoxemia occurs.

(4:339–341,344–346), (36:111–115)

38. A. The Radford nomogram is used for estimating a person's tidal volume when the person's body weight and ventilatory rate are known. The nomogram is shown in Figure 76.

STEP 1: Convert 3,000 g to kilograms. Since 1 kg = 1,000 g or 10^3 g, then

$$3,000 \, \cancel{g} \left(\frac{1 \text{ kg}}{10^3 \, \cancel{g}} \right) =$$

$$\frac{3,000}{1,000} (1 \text{ kg}) = 3 \text{ kg}$$

STEP 2: Use a straight edge to connect the point 3 kg on the weight scale and 37 breaths/min on the ventilatory rate scale. The straight edge intersects the tidal volume scale at the point indicating 15 cc.

STEP 3: Using metric system units, employ the correction factor for tracheotomized patients, i.e., subtract 1 cc/kg of body weight. Since the patient weighs 3 kg,

$$3 \, \cancel{\text{kg}} \times 1 \text{ cc/}\cancel{\text{kg}} = 3 \text{ cc}$$

Therefore,

15 cc VT from nomogram
$-$ 3 cc tracheotomy correction factor
12 cc estimated VT

N Engl J Med, November 25, 1954, Vol. 251, No. 22.

39. E. Cor pulmonale refers to the condition of right ventricular hypertrophy secondary to a pulmonary disease. Pulmonary diseases that produce chronic pulmonary hypertension are associated with cor pulmonale. Right ventricular hypertrophy, or right ventricular failure, secondary to left ventricular failure is *not* cor pulmonale. (1:261–262), (4:304), (6:405–406), (8:188)

40. B. The Silverman score provides a means of assessing the degree of respiratory distress of a neonate. Scores range from 0 to 10. Scores of 0 to 3 indicate little or no respiratory distress. Scores ranging from 4 to 6 indicate moderate respiratory distress. Scores of 7 to 10 represent severe respiratory distress. The clinical signs evaluated and the points assigned are shown in Table 4.

TABLE 4

Sign	Score		
	0	1	2
Upper chest movement	Synchronized movement	Lag of upper chest or inspiration	Asynchronized movement
Lower chest movement	No retractions	Occasional retractions	Many retractions
Xiphoid retractions	No retractions	Occasional retractions	Many retractions
Dilation of nares	Absent	Minimal dilation	Maximal dilation
Expiratory grunting	Absent	Perceived only with aid of stethoscope	Perceived with unaided ear

(4:171–172)

41. D. The Silverman score is a method whereby a neonate's ventilatory status is assessed. The scale ranges from 0 to 10, which 0 being the best score. The clinical signs evaluated are as follows:

1.   upper chest movements
2.   lower chest movements
3.   xiphoid retractions
4.   dilation of nares
5.   expiratory grunting

(4:171–172)

42. D. *In utero,* the fetal lung contains a volume of liquid approximately equal to the functional residual capacity (FRC) of a newborn. During birth some of this liquid is normally squeezed from the lungs and out the oropharynx. The remaining liquid is reabsorbed into the vasculature, i.e., pulmonary capillaries and lymphatics.

When the neonate generates its first transairway (P_{mouth}-$P_{alveoli}$) pressure, it does so with great effort and energy expenditure. The pressure ordinarily generated by a neonate to initiate the first lung inflation ranges from -40 to -100 cm H_2O.

(4:170–171), (8:120–122), (14:142–143)

43. A. Amniocentesis is a procedure whereby a transabdominal perforation (usually with a needle) of the amniotic sac is performed for the purpose of obtaining a sample of amniotic fluid. Amniocentesis provides for prenatal diagnosis of certain genetically transmitted chromosomal disorders, the L/S ratio levels, and meconium levels.

(4:175)

44. A. Fetal circulation (Figure 77) is very different from adult circulation.

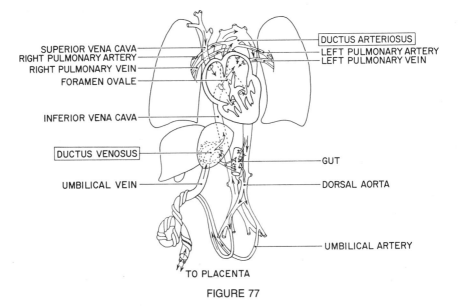

FIGURE 77

In utero, the placenta functions as the gas exchange organ. Oxygenated blood flows through the umbilical vein. This blood flow then is shunted through the portal circulation via the ductus venosus and on into the inferior vena cava. Before entering the right atrium, this oxygenated blood mixes with venous blood flowing through the superior vena cava. This mixture then passes into the right atrium. At this point, approximately, one-half of the blood flow is diverted to the left atrium via the foramen ovale (i.e., the opening between the two atria), and the remaining half passes into the right ventricle.

The blood from the left atrium passes into the left ventricle. This oxygenated blood perfuses the fetal brain. Blood from the right ventricle flows out the pulmonary artery and bypasses the lung via the ductus arteriosus, the communication between the pulmonary artery and aorta. The umbilical arteries then return fetal venous blood to the placenta for oxygenation.

(4:167–169), (8:118–120), (14:140–142), (36:20–21)

45. B. Digital clubbing refers to the painless enlargement of the terminal portions of the fingers and toes that develops from a variety of pulmonary and nonpulmonary disorders.

Cardiac anomalies that produce cyanosis cause clubbing, e.g., coarctation of the aorta (preductal), tricuspid atresia, tetralogy of Fallot, truncus arteriosus, anomalous venous return, and transposition of the great vessels.

Pulmonary disorders that usually cause digital clubbing include cystic fibrosis, bronchiectasis, interstitial fibrosis, bronchogenic carcinoma, and chronic bronchitis.

(1:284–286), (4:301,306,316,347,353), (8:189–191)

46. C. Congenital cardiac anomalies produce shunting in either direction, i.e., right to left or left to right. Left-to-right shunting, such as atrial septal defects, patent ductus arteriosus, ventricular septal defects, and coarctation of the aorta (postductal), does *not* produce cyanosis.

Right-to-left cardiac defects include tricuspid atresia, tetralogy of Fallot, truncus arteriosus, and coarctation of the aorta (preductal).

The direction of the shunt is determined by the vascular pressure gradient that exists across the communication. The flow of blood moves form an area of high vascular pressure to one of low vascular pressure.

(4:347), (36:111–115)

47. D. The Apgar score is used to evaluate the clinical status of neonates at 1 and 5 minutes after birth. The highest possible score is 10, and the lowest is 0. The score obtained helps determine the need for resuscitation measures. The Apgar score is shown in Table 5. Based on the clinical information presented in the question, the Apgar score is determined as follows:

1. heart rate of 110 beats/min: 2 points
2. a good ventilatory effort accompanied by crying: 2 points
3. color reflected peripheral cyanosis; central color assumed to be good because not mentioned: 1 point
4. muscle tone indicated by some flexion of the extremities: 1 point

TABLE 5

Sign	Rating		
	0	1	2
Heart Rate	Absent	<100/min	>100 min
Ventilatory effort	Absent	Slow, irregular	Good, crying
Muscle tone	Limp	Some flexion	Active motion
Reflex irritability	No response	Grimace	Cough or sneeze
Color	Central and peripheral cyanosis	Peripheral cyanosis	Completely pink

    5. reflex irritability represented by the sneeze caused by passage of suction catheter into nose: 2 points

        Apgar score 8

    (6:709–710), (35:31–34), (36:32–33), (JAMA, August 1, 1980, Vol. 244, No. 5, 495–496)

48. C. There appears to be no need to perform any resuscitation measures at this time because an Apgar score in the range of 7 to 10 generally indicates that the infant has a stable cardiopulmonary status. However, the Apgar score at 5 minutes after birth might indicate otherwise. The infant can deteriorate between Apgar evaluations.

    To summarize, Apgar scores ranging from 7 to 10 indicate no immediate need to resuscitate; 4 to 6 suggest that the infant to be suctioned, oxygenated, and possibly ventilated; and 0 to 3 indicate the need for cardiopulmonary resuscitation.

    (4:171), (6:709–710), (35:31–34), (36:32–33), (JAMA, August 1, 1980, Vol. 244, No. 5, 495–496)

49. D. Anatomic closure of the ductus arteriosus usually occurs about 3 weeks after birth. The remnant of the ductus arteriosus is called the *ligamentum arteriosus*.

    (4:170)

50. E. Acute laryngotracheobronchitis (LTB) is viral in origin about 85% of the time. The viruses implicated in this disease are usually the parainfluenza viruses 1, 2, and 3, along with adenoviruses and the respiratory syncytial virus (RSV). Consequently, antibiotics are usually ineffective.

    Aerosol therapy seems to be effective in lessening the symptoms of this disease. Frequently, parents are advised to sit in the bathroom with their child while a hot shower is steaming the room. Relief is often temporarily obtained. Unheated aerosols are preferred because the heat produced by the running hot water is undesirable for a febrile child. In fact, nebulized racemic epinephrine (Micronephrine, Vaponephrin) is often administered in the hospitalized patient.

    Severe froms of LTB sometimes necessitate intubation or tracheostomy. Unlike epiglottitis, laryngoscopy, or other methods of physically examining the pharynx and larynx will ordinarily not worsen the airway obstruction.

    (4:354), (6:776–777), (8:274), (36:86–88)

REFERENCES

1. Spearman, C., and Sheldon, R., *Egan's Fundamentals of Respiratory Therapy,* 4th ed., C.V. Mosby, St. Louis, 1982.
2. Wojciechowski, W., *Respiratory Care Sciences: An Integrated Approach,* John Wiley & Sons, New York, 1985.
3. Shapiro, B., Harrison, R., Kacmarek, R., and Cane, R., *Clinical Application of Respiratory Care,* 3rd ed., Year Book Medical Publishers, Chicago, 1985.
4. Kacmarek, R., Mack, C., and Dimas, S., *The Essentials of Respiratory Therapy,* 2nd ed., Year Book Medical Publishers, Chicago, 1985.
5. McPherson, S., *Respiratory Therapy Equipment,* 3rd ed., C.V. Mosby, St. Louis, 1985.
6. Burton, G., and Hodgkin, J., *Respiratory Care: A Guide to Clinical Practice,* 2nd ed., J.B. Lippincott, Philadelphia, 1985.
7. Frownfelter, D., *Chest Physical Therapy and Cardiopulmonary Rehabilitation, An Interdisciplinary Approach,* Year Book Medical Publishers, Chicago, 1978.
8. Cherniack, R., and Cherniack, L., *Respiration in Health and Disease,* 3rd ed., W.B. Saunders, Philadelphia, 1983.
9. Daily, E., and Schroeder, G., *Techniques in Bedside Hemodynamic Monitoring,* 3rd ed., C.V. Mosby, St. Louis, 1985.
10. Des Jardins, R., *Clinical Manifestations of Respiratory Disease,* Year Book Medical Publishers, Chicago, 1984.
11. Mitchell, R., *Synopsis of Clinical Pulmonary Disease,* 3rd ed., C.V. Mosby, St., Louis, 1982.
12. Comroe, J., *Physiology of Respiration,* 3rd ed., Year Book Medical Publishers, Chicago, 1974.
13. West, J., *Pulmonary Pathophysiology—The Essentials,* 2nd ed., Williams & Wilkins, Baltimore, 1982.
14. West, J., *Respiratory Physiology—The Essentials,* 3rd ed., Williams & Wilkins, Baltimore, 1985.
15. Martz, K., et al., *Management of the Patient-Ventilator System: A Team Approach,* 2nd ed., C.V. Mosby, St. Louis, 1984.
16. Shoup, C., and McHenry, R., *Laboratory Exercises in Respiratory Therapy,* 2nd ed., C.V. Mosby, St. Louis, 1983.
17. Ruppel, G., *Manual of Pulmonary Function Testing,* 3rd ed., C.V. Mosby, St. Louis, 1982.
18. Appelbaum, E., and Bruce, D., *Tracheal Intubation,* W.B. Saunders, Philadelphia, 1976.
19. Rau, J., *Respiratory Therapy Pharmacology,* 2nd ed., Year Book Medical Publishers, Chicago, 1984.
20. United States Department of Health, Education, and Welfare, Public Health Service, *Isolation Techniques for Use in Hospitals,* 2nd ed., Washington, D.C., 1975.
21. Brooks, S., *Integrated Basic Science,* 4th ed., C.V. Mosby, St. Louis, 1979.
22. Comroe, J., *The Lung,* Year Book Medical Publishers, Chicago, 1962.
23. Shibel, E., and Moser, K., *Respiratory Emergencies,* 2nd ed., C.V. Mosby, St. Louis, 1982.
24. Tisi, G., *Pulmonary Physiology in Clinical Medicine,* 2nd ed., Williams & Wilkins, Baltimore, 1985.
25. Cherniack, R., *Pulmonary Function Testing,* W.B. Saunders, Philadelphia, 1977.
26. Altose, M., *The Physiological Basis of Pulmonary Function Testing,* Clinical Symposia-CIBA, Vol. 31, No. 2, Summit, New Jersey, 1979.
27. Shipiro, B., Harrison, R., and Walton, J., *Clinical Application of Arterial Blood Gases,* 3rd ed., Year Book Medical Publishers, Chicago, 1982.
28. West, J., *Ventilation/Blood Flow and Gas Exchange,* 3rd ed., Blackwell Scientific Publications, 1979.

29. Slonim, N., and Hamilton, K., *Respiratory Physiology,* 4th ed., C.V. Mosby, St. Louis, 1981.

30. Rarey, K., and Youtsey, J., *Respiratory Patient Care,* Prentice-Hall, Englewood Cliffs, 1981.

31. Berne, R., and Levy, M., *Physiology,* C.V. Mosby, St. Louis, 1983.

32. Levitzky, M., *Pulmonary Physiology,* 2nd ed., McGraw-Hill, New York, 1986.

33. Wilson, P., Bell, C., and Norton, A., *Rehabilitation of the Heart and Lungs,* SensorMedics, 1980.

34. Clausen, J., and Zarins, L., *Pulmonary Function Testing Guildlines and Controversies,* Academic Press, New York, 1982.

35. Klaus, M., and Fanaroff, A., *Care of the High-Risk Neonate,* 2nd ed., W.B. Saunders, Philadelphia, 1979.

36. Lough, M., et al., *Pediatric Respiratory Therapy,* 3rd ed., Year Book Medical Publishers, Chicago, 1985.

37. Levin, D., et al., *A Practical Guide to Pediatric Intensive Care,* 2nd ed., C.V. Mosby, St. Louis, 1984.

38. O'Ryan, J., and Burns, D., *Pulmonary Rehabilitation from Hospital to Home,* Year Book Medical Publishers, Chicago, 1984.

39. Bell, C., et al., *Home Care and Rehabilitation in Respiratory Medicine,* J.B. Lippincott, Philadelphia, 1984.

40. Wilkins, R., et al., *Clinical Assessment in Respiratory Care,* C.V. Mosby, St. Louis, 1985.

41. Jones, N., and Campbell, E., *Clinical Exercise Testing,* 2nd ed., W.B., Saunders, Philadelphia, 1982.

42. Goldsmith, J., and Karotkin, E., *Assisted Ventilation of the Neonate,* W.B. Saunders, Philadelphia, 1981.

43. Blowers, M., and Sims, R., *How to Read an ECG,* 3rd ed., Medical Economics, New Jersey, 1983.

44. Eubanks, D., and Bone, R., *Comprehensive Respiratory Care,* C.V. Mosby, St. Louis, 1985.

45. Rattenborg, C., *Clinical Use of Mechanical Ventilation,* Year Book Medical Publishers, Chicago, 1981.

46. Witkowski, A.S., *Pulmonary Assessment: A Clinical Guide,* J.B. Lippincott, Philadelphia, 1985.

47. Op't Holt, Timothy B., *Assessment Based Respiratory Care,* John Wiley & Sons, New York, 1986.

SECTION 4

RESPIRATORY CARE CONTENT AREAS

This portion of the book has been subdivided into the following 11 clinical content areas.

1. Oxygen/gas therapy
2. Aerosol/humidity therapy
3. Hyperinflation therapy
4. Chest physiotherapy
5. Cardiopulmonary resuscitation
6. Airway management
7. Mechanical ventilation management
8. Cardiopulmonary evaluation/cardiopulmonary monitoring and interpretation
9. Cardiopulmonary diagnostics and interpretation
10. Pediatrics and perinatology
11. Cardiopulmonary rehabilitation and home care

The questions presented in these areas will pertain to concepts and knowledge of clinical practice, as well as to actual clinical situations.

OXYGEN/GAS THERAPY ASSESSMENT

PURPOSE: The purpose of this 50-item section is to give you the opportunity to evaluate your understanding and comprehension in the areas of oxygen and gas therapy. You will be required to make clinical judgments and decisions concerning various oxygen and medical gas delivery appliances, compressed gas cylinders, regulators, flowmeters, safety systems, gas mixtures, and oxygen analyzers. You will also be confronted with mathematical problems about duration of flow of compressed gas cylinders, room air entrainment, and gas transport in the blood.

DIRECTIONS: Each of the questions or incomplete statements is followed by five suggested answers. Select the one which is the best in each case and then blacken the corresponding space on the answer sheet.

1. A gas mixture of 95% O_2 and 5% CO_2 usually is contained in what color of cylinder?

A. black	D. red
B. brown	E. gray and green
C. brown and green	

Questions 2, 3, and 4 refer to the same data.

2. Calculate the factor that relates cylinder volume to cylinder pressure for a compressed gas cylinder having a 244-cu ft capacity.

A. 0.11 liter/psig	D. 2.50 liters/psig
B. 0.28 liter/psig	E. 3.14 liters/psig
C. 2.41 liters/psig	

3. What size cylinder would this be?

A. A   D. K
B. D   E. G
C. E

4. Calculate the duration of flow for this cylinder when it is three-fourths full and operating an aerosol device at 12 liters/min.

A. 7.1 hours   D. 39 minutes
B. 5.5 hours   E. 15 minutes
C. 4.3 hours

5. Which of the following statements accurately describe the Diameter Index Safety System (DISS)?

I. It is designed for indexing devices operating < 200 psig.
II. It uses internal and external threading for the attachment of appliances.
III. The point at which an oxygen appliance attaches to a pressure regulator represents DISS.
IV. This system is similar to the American Standard System.

A. I, II, III only   D. I, II only
B. II, IV only   E. I, II, III, IV
C. II, III, IV only

6. Which statements are true about the device illustrated in Figure 78?

I. The diagram depicts a high-pressure adjustable gas regulator.
II. The Thorpe tube presented is shown as an uncompensated flowmeter.
III. The Bourdon gauge shown is usually used to indicate liter flow in this situation.
IV. The diagram displays a single-stage regulator.
V. The pressure in the pressure chamber will be vented via a safety vent in the event that pressure exceeds 200 psig.

A. I, II, V only   D. II, III only
B. I, IV, V only   E. IV, V only
C. II, IV only

7. When compressed gas cylinders are hydrostatically tested, how is the elastic expansion calculated?

A. permanent expansion times total expansion
B. total expansion minus permanent expansion
C. total expansion divided by permanent expansion
D. permanent expansion divided by total expansion
E. permanent expansion minus total expansion

8. Which of the following statements are true about a single-stage compressed gas regulator?

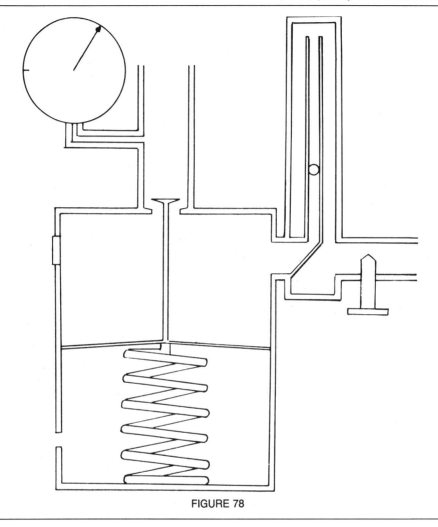

FIGURE 78

I. This type of device is manufactured as either adjustable or preset.

II. This device has either two Bourdon gauges, or one Bourdon gauge and a Thorpe tube.

III. Single-stage regulators essentially reduce high pressures to 50 psig.

IV. Generally, the device has a safety relief device incorporated into it.

A. I, II, III, IV   D. II, IV only
B. I, III only   E. I, III, IV only
C. III, IV only

9. IPPB therapy with an 80%-20% helium-oxygen mixture is theoretically best suited for which type(s) of patient?

I. a patient having an acute asthmatic attack

II. a preoperative orientation patient

III. a patient in acute pulmonary edema

IV. a chronic bronchitic experiencing a superimposed pulmonary infection

V. a recent postoperative pneumonectomy patient

A. III, V only   D. III, IV, V only

B. I, IV only   E. I, III, IV only

C. I, II, III only

10. When would you change a full K cylinder of oxygen functioning as the gas source for a nebulizer operating at 15 liters/min?

A. 10 hours   D. 7 hours

B. 9 hours   E. 1 hour

C. 8 hours

11. You have received a written order from a physician requesting IPPB therapy with He-O_2 for a patient. The mixture you are asked to use is 80%-20%. You proceed immediately to the cylinder storage area to select the appropriate tank to administer the therapy. What color of tank should you be looking for?

A. orange   D. black and green

B. light blue   E. brown and green

C. gray and green

12. To what flowrate would you need to dial an oxygen flowmeter in order to deliver 15 liters/min of an 80%-20% He-O_2 gas mixture to a patient?

A. 8 liters/min   D. 12 liters/min

B. 9 liters/min   E. 15 liters/min

C. 10 liters/min

13. Which gases and/or gas mixtures would support combustion?

I. He-O_2

II. N_2O

III. O_2-CO_2

IV. N_2

V. CO_2

A. I, II, III only   D. II, III, V only

B. II, III only   E. I, II, III, IV only

C. I, II only

14. Which of the following statements correctly refer to the illustration shown in Figure 79?

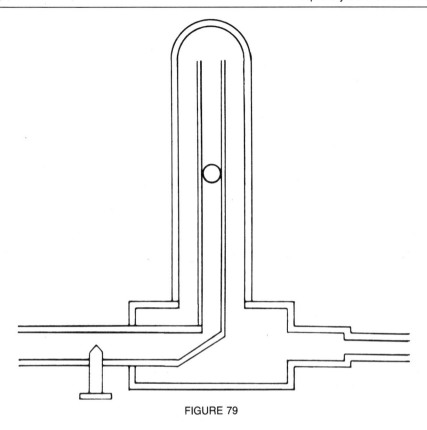

FIGURE 79

I. Gas will cease flowing into the tube if the back pressure exceeds 50 psig.

II. When experiencing back pressure resistance caused by the attachment of an oxygen delivery device, the patient will receive a flowrate higher than that shown on the flowmeter.

III. When an unrestricted gas flows through the device shown above, the pressure below the ball is greater than the pressure above the ball.

IV. From the illustration one can infer that the device is at 50 psig from the source to the ball, and at 14.7 psig from the ball to the outlet.

V. The precise gas flow through the tube will always be indicated despite any restrictions resulting from the attachment of appliances.

A. I, II only   D. III, V only

B. I, II, III only   E. III, IV only

C. I, III only

15. Which properties refer to carbon dioxide gas at normal atmospheric conditions?

    I. colorless

    II. odorless

    III. a density of 1.43 g/liter

    IV. a specific gravity of 1.52

A. I, II, III, IV
B. I, II, IV only
C. I, II, III only

D. I, III, IV only
E. II, III only

16. What does the 3AA marking on a compressed gas cylinder shoulder mean?

A. The cylinder contains a liquid.
B. The cylinder is constructed of steel alloys.
C. The cylinder can be operated only at low working pressures.
D. The cylinder can be tested every 10 years.
E. The cylinder will accommodate only PISS regulators.

17. Which of the following regulatory agencies establishes the regulations governing the storage of compressed gas cylinders?

A. NFPA
B. ANSI
C. CGA

D. DOT
E. ICC

18. Which of the following statements correctly describe the Pin Index Safety System?

I. It is designed to prevent the wrong cylinder from being attached to a given yoke connection.
II. Under normal clinical and operational situations this system is foolproof.
III. All cylinders serviced at 2,200 psig are indexed according to this system.
IV. Three holes are drilled in the face of the valve, and their exact positions vary according to the gas or gases contained in the cylinder.

A. I, II, III only
B. II, III, IV only
C. I, II only

D. I, III only
E. I, III, IV only

19. How should the reservoir bag on a partial re-breathing bag be set up when this oxygen delivery appliance is clinically used on a patient?

A. The reservoir bag should completely deflate upon exhalation.
B. The reservoir bag should remain somewhat inflated upon exhalation.
C. The reservoir bag should completely deflate during inspiration.
D. The reservoir bag should remain somewhat inflated during inspiration.
E. The partial re-breathing mask is a high-flow oxygen delivery system; therefore, any of these situations would be acceptable.

20. Which parameter is *most* responsible for the development of retrolental fibroplasia?

A. $F_{I_{O_2}}$
B. $P_{A_{O_2}}$
C. Sa_{O_2}

D. Pa_{O_2}
E. $P_{I_{O_2}}$

21. At $-297.3°F$, 16 cu ft of liquid oxygen is equivalent to _____ cu ft of gaseous oxygen at ambient temperature and pressure?

A. 53.7

D. 22,000.0

B. 4,756.8

E. 65,536.0

C. 13,769.6

22. Calculate the alveolar-arterial oxygen tension gradient in a patient receiving 100% oxygen at sea level. This patient's arterial blood gases are indicated below. (Assume a normal respiratory quotient.)

Pa_{O_2}:   250 mm Hg
Pa_{CO_2}:   49 mm Hg
  pH: 7.33

A. 664 mm Hg

D. 365 mm Hg

B. 615 mm Hg

E. 201 mm Hg

C. 414 mm Hg

23. A Coronary Care Unit patient with a V_T 500 cc and a ventilatory rate of 18 breaths/min is suspected of having had a myocardial infarction. What type of O_2 device would you recommend for this patient?

A. a Venturi mask at 30% O_2

D. a nasal catheter at 6 liters/min

B. a nasal cannula at 1 liter/min

E. an aerosol mask at 40%

C. a simple mask at 7 liters/min

24. When the $F_{I_{O_2}}$ inside a mist tent is analyzed, from which site should the sampled gas be taken?

A. where the oxygen is entering the tent, to determine how much oxygen is being deposited into the device

B. anywhere on the surface of the mattress because, at this point, the gases have been well mixed

C. near the opening at the top of the tent, to take the patient's exhaled carbon dioxide into account

D. on the mattress surface near the patient's head, to determine the amount of oxygen the patient is breathing

E. anywhere in the delivery tubing, to determine if the device is functioning properly

25. What is the minimum flowrate that could be set on the flowmeter to provide an adequate flow to a patient on a 28% Venturi mask? The patient's ventilatory status is indicated below.

Ventilatory rate: 20 breaths/min
Inspiratory time: 1 sec
Expiratory time: 2 sec
    Tidal volume: 500 cc

A. 2 liters/min   D. 5 liters/min

B. 3 liters/min   E. 6 liters/min

C. 4 liters/min

26. A 65-year-old COPD patient is admitted to the Emergency Room complaining of shortness of breath. His family informs the physician that the patient recently caught the flu and that his condition has worsened during the past few days. He appears dyspneic and has an irregular ventilatory pattern. His V_T is 400 cc, and his radial pulse is 122 beats/min. The patient is lucid and responds to questioning. Room air blood gases reveal:

Pa_{O_2}:   50 torr

Pa_{CO_2}: 68 torr

pH: 7.29

Sa_{O_2}:   75%

[Hb]:   18 g%

A nasal cannula with a flowrate of 6 liters/min is installed for this patient per physician's orders. Upon your return to this patient's room after being away for about 20 minutes, you observe the patient appears to be asleep. His ventilatory rate is now 10 breaths/min; his tidal volume has fallen to 300 cc. He responds lethargically as you call his name. He is confused, does not respond well to questioning, and slumbers off to sleep again.

Which statement(s) correctly describe(s) this situation?

   I. The fact that this patient is no longer tachypneic is a sign of improvement.

  II. His somnolence and reduced sensorium indicate CO_2 narcosis.

 III. The oxygen administered to this patient is being provided by the appropriate device for this situation.

  IV. The patient should be left alone (i.e., *not* awakened) because this is the first time in a few days that he has been able to rest.

A. I, IV only   D. I only

B. III, IV only   E. I, III, IV only

C. II only

27. Which of the following statements accurately relate to the oxygen appliance illustrated in Figure 80?

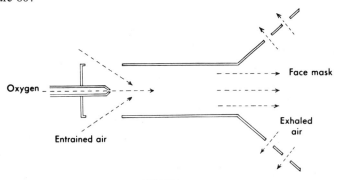

FIGURE 80

    I. It is the preferred oxygen device for patients in acute pulmonary edema.

    II. It has the capability of delivering an F_{IO_2} range from 0.21 to 0.90.

    III. Precise and consistent F_{IO_2}s can be delivered to the patient by this device regardless of the patient's inspiratory time.

    IV. Under most conditions this system provides a flowrate sufficient to meet a peak flowrate consistent with the patient's ventilatory pattern.

    V. A disadvantage of this oxygen apparatus is that it does *not* provide an oxygen reservoir capable of meeting increased patient ventilatory demands.

A. I, II, V only

B. I, II only

C. II, V only

D. III, IV only

E. I, II, V only

28. Which of the following statements are *not* true about the Beckman D2 oxygen analyzer?

    I. Under normal room air conditions the magnetic force exactly balances the torque of the quartz fiber and the dumbbell remains stationary.

    II. The degree of rotation of the dumbbell is proportional to the partial pressure of oxygen in the gas sampled.

    III. The basic principle of operation depends upon the diamagnetic property of the oxygen molecule.

    IV. The gas analyzed must be humidified.

    V. Once the analyzer is factory calibrated, it is *not* influenced by variances in pressure resulting from geographic relocation.

A. I, II, IV only

B. III, IV, V only

C. IV, V only

D. I, II, III only

E. I, II only

29. Which of the following oxygen therapy devices are considered high-flow oxygen delivery systems?

    I. Venturi mask

    II. nasal catheter

    III. Briggs adapter with reservoir tubing

    IV. partial re-breathing mask

A. I, III only

B. I, III, IV only

C. II, IV only

D. II, III, IV only

E. I, IV only

30. When should a full E cylinder of O_2 operating a therapeutic appliance at 5 liters/min and delivering an F_{IO_2} of 0.4 need to be changed before its contents are depleted?

A. 1 hour

B. 1 hour and 30 minutes

C. 2 hours

D. 2 hours and 15 minutes

E. 3 hours

Questions 31 and 32 refer to the same patient.

31. A 340-lb, 5 ft 4 in., 38-year-old female was admitted to the hospital lethargic and somnolent. The following blood gas data were obtained:

   Pa_{O_2}:   49 mm Hg
   Pa_{CO_2}: 76 mm Hg
   pH: 7.33

   Which condition is this patient most likely experiencing?

   A. alveolar hypoventilation syndrome   D. pulmonary fibrosis
   B. emotional stress or anxiety   E. status asthmaticus
   C. pulmonary embolism

32. Which therapeutic procedure would you institute immediately?

   A. a Venturi mask at 24% O_2
   B. ultrasonic nebulization with normal saline prn
   C. q4h IPPB with Isuprel
   D. q4h postural drainage
   E. tracheostomy

33. One night Mr. Al Cohol, "professional" jogger, celebrated after his record-setting time of 24 minutes in the 10-km run through the azalea-filled streets of Mobile, Alabama. The otherwise tee-totaling Mr. Cohol consumed mass quantities of piñã coladas. At the conclusion of the revelry, Mr. Cohol drove home, pulled into the garage, closed the garage with the automatic door control, and fell asleep in the car with the car engine running.

   About $1\frac{1}{2}$ hours later Mrs. Joy Cohol, Al's wife, removed him from the toxic environs. Soon thereafter, he was taken to the hospital.

   Assume that all of the hemoglobin oxygen-binding sites are unavailable for oxygen transport; therefore, tissue oxygenation can be achieved only via the dissolved route.

   Which of the following mechanisms of oxygenation would need to be used to provide this patient's tissues with 5 vol% oxygen?

   A. One hundred percent O_2 under normobaric conditions via a non-rebreathing mask
   B. Endotracheal intubation with 100% O_2 administered through a volume ventilator under ambient conditions
   C. Tracheotomy with 100% O_2 administered by means of a volume ventilator at 2 atm of pressure in a hyperbaric chamber
   D. Eighty percent O_2 under 3 atm of pressure
   E. Four atmospheres of pressure with an $F_{I_{O_2}}$ of 0.5

34. The oxygen tension of a fluid can be measured by a(n) _____.

   A. Clark electrode   D. CO-oximeter
   B. Sanz electrode   E. hygrometer
   C. Severinghaus electrode

35. Which of the following statements accurately compare certain aspects of the galvanic and polarographic oxygen analyzers?

    I. The galvanic electrode uses batteries to polarize the electrode.

    II. The polarographic analyzer has a quicker response time.

    III. Neither analyzer should be used in an operating room.

    IV. The polarographic analyzer is *not* accurate when experiencing marked increases in system pressure.

    V. Electrodes used in polarographic analyzers do *not* last as long as those in galvanic analyzers.

A. II, IV, V only   D. IV, V only

B. I, III, IV only   E. I, II, III, IV, V

C. II, V only

36. Which statements accurately describe a nasal cannula?

    I. It delivers a fixed F_{IO_2} consistently, regardless of the patient's ventilatory pattern.

    II. It can deliver a low oxygen concentration (i.e., 24%).

    III. It should *not* be used if the patient is a mouth breather because, in such instances, the patient would receive more therapeutic oxygen.

    IV. This device should *not* be operated at 10 liters/min.

    V. In some circumstances humidification with the use of this apparatus may be omitted.

A. II, IV only   D. II, III, IV only

B. I, III only   E. I, II, III, IV, V

C. II, IV, V only

37. The five parts of Figure 81 (pages 291–292) depict air entrainment devices operating with oxygen as their source gas. Assuming that they are functioning under the same ambient conditions, as well as experiencing the same O_2 source flowrate, select the device that would deliver the lowest F_{IO_2}.

38. Which of the following laws would be manifested if the oxygen liter flow operating a simple O_2 mask was increased from 5 liters/min to 7 liters/min in an attempt to raise the arterial partial pressure of oxygen in a patient's blood?

    I. law of LaPlace

    II. Henry's law of solubility

    III. Avogadro's law

    IV. Dalton's law of partial pressure

    V. Poiseuille's law of laminar flow

A. I, II, V only   D. III, V only

B. II, IV, V only   E. II, IV only

C. I, III only

39. Identify the component labeled "3" in Figure 82.

A. It is the component that prevents gas from entering the chamber when the internal pressure exceeds the adjusted pressure.

B. It is the flexible diaphragm that is forced downward against the upward force exerted by the spring.

C. It is a safety relief device that provides a means for gas escape.

D. It is an impactor.

E. It is the area where the lateral wall pressure drops and the gas velocity increases.

40. Which mathematical relationship(s) represent(s) the therapeutic advantage of using an 80%-20% (He-O_2) mixture on a patient experiencing diffuse airway obstruction?

   I. $P_a - P_b = D(v_b^2 - v_a^2)$

  II. $P = \dfrac{2ST}{r}$

  III. $\eta = \dfrac{(P_1 - P_2)\pi r^4}{\dot{V}L8}$

  IV. $\dfrac{P_1}{V_2} = \dfrac{P_2}{V_1}$

A.

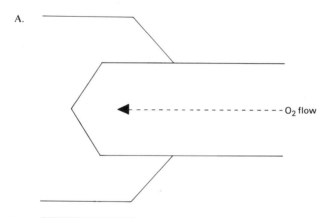

B.

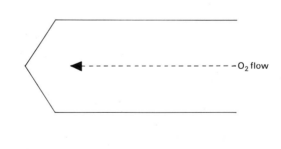

FIGURE 81

C.

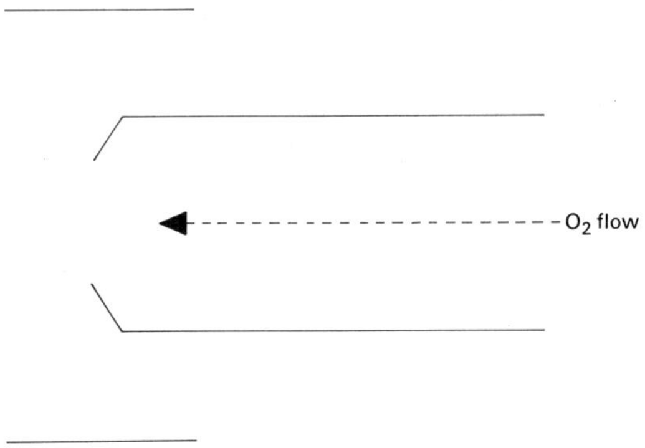

O_2 flow

D.

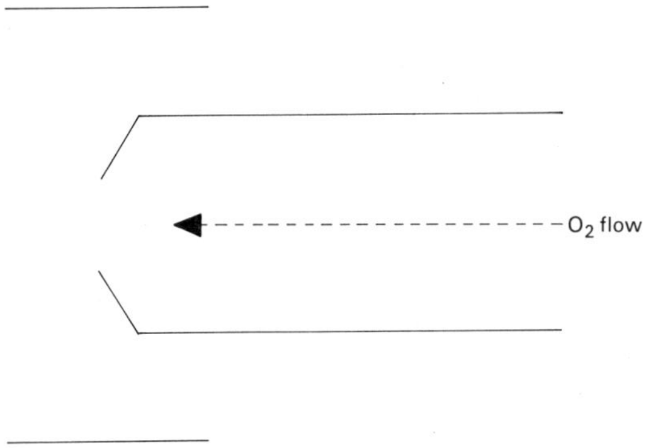

O_2 flow

E.

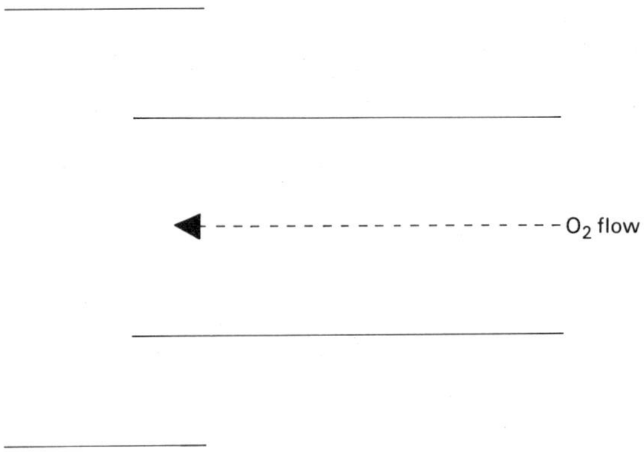

O_2 flow

FIGURE 81 (*continued*)

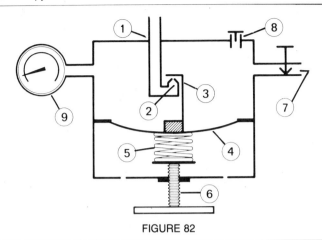

FIGURE 82

A. II only   D. III, IV only
B. I only   E. I, III only
C. I, IV only

Questions 41 and 42 refer to the same information.

41. A Puritan-Bennett all-purpose nebulizer operating at 10 liters/min, delivering an F_{IO_2} of 0.70, produces what total liter flow?

A. 3 liters/min   D. 16 liters/min
B. 4 liters/min   E. 20 liters/min
C. 6 liters/min

42. Determine the air/O_2 ratio in Problem 41.

A. 0.3:1.0   D. 1.6:1.0
B. 0.4:1.0   E. 2:1.0
C. 0.6:1.0

43. Calculate the theoretical maximum P_{AO_2} that can be achieved by a normal person breathing an F_{IO_2} of 1.0 at 1 atm under normal resting conditions. Assume a $\dot{V}_A/\dot{Q}_C$ of 1.0.

A. 730 mm Hg   D. 673 mm Hg
B. 720 mm Hg   E. 616 mm Hg
C. 713 mm Hg

44. Calculate the partial pressure exerted by oxygen in the alveoli under the following conditions:

Body temperature: 93.2°F
Pressure: 1 atm
Water vapor: 40 torr
Alveolar oxygen %: 14%

A. 101 cm H_2O
B. 106 cm H_2O
C. 137 cm H_2O

D. 137 mm Hg
E. 106 mm Hg

45. Calculate the $F_{I_{O_2}}$ being delivered to a 150-lb man (ideal body weight) via a nasal cannula operating at 3 liters/min under the following conditions:

Ventilatory rate:	20 breaths/min
V_T:	500 cc
Inspiratory time:	1 second
Expiratory time:	2 seconds
Anatomic reservoir volume:	50 cc

A. 0.28
B. 0.32
C. 0.36

D. 0.40
E. 0.44

46. Which of the following factors will cause the $F_{I_{O_2}}$ of a low-flow system oxygen delivery device to increase?

I. a large tidal volume
II. a slow ventilatory rate
III. a decreased $\dot{V}_E$
IV. a fast ventilatory rate
V. a small tidal volume

A. II, III, V only
B. I, IV only
C. I, II, III only

D. IV, V only
E. II, V only

47. Calculate the arterial-venous oxygen content difference at pH 7.20 using Figure 83. This patient has 13 g% Hb, Pa_{O_2} 100 torr, and $P\bar{v}_{O_2}$ 40 torr.

A. 5.00 vol%
B. 5.75 vol%
C. 6.60 vol%

D. 7.01 vol%
E. 7.34 vol%

48. Calculate the partial pressure of oxygen in a sample of normal atmospheric air at STPD.

A. 673 mm Hg
B. 250 mm Hg
C. 159 mm Hg

D. 149 mm Hg
E. 100 mm Hg

49. Which of the following pathophysiologic occurrences are amenable to oxygen therapy?

I. capillary shunting
II. low $\dot{V}_A/\dot{Q}_C$ units
III. diffusion impairments
IV. perfusion in excess of ventilation

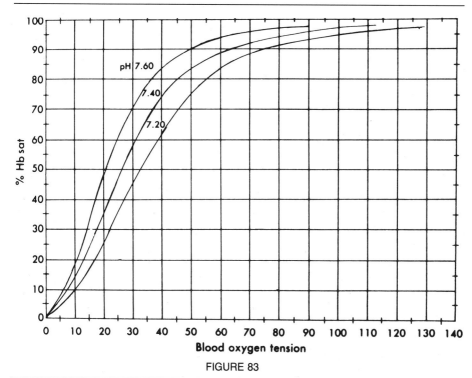

FIGURE 83

A. II, III, IV only   D. III, IV only
B. I, II only   E. I, III only
C. II, IV only

50. Based on the patient information given below, what type of tissue hypoxia is this patient most likely experiencing?

Pa_{O_2}:   91 mm Hg
Pa_{CO_2}:   33 mm Hg
pH: 7.44
Sa_{O_2}:   96%
Hb: 7 g%
$P\bar{v}_{O_2}$:   32 mm Hg
FI_{O_2}:   0.2093
V_T: 500 cc
f: 14 breaths/minute

A. hypoxic hypoxia   D. anemic hypoxia
B. stagnant hypoxia   E. circulatory hypoxia
C. histotoxic hypoxia

ASSESSMENT ANSWER SHEET

DIRECTIONS: Darken the space under the selected answer.

	A	B	C	D	E						
1.	[ ]	[ ]	[ ]	[ ]	[ ]	26.	[ ]	[ ]	[ ]	[ ]	[ ]
2.	[ ]	[ ]	[ ]	[ ]	[ ]	27.	[ ]	[ ]	[ ]	[ ]	[ ]
3.	[ ]	[ ]	[ ]	[ ]	[ ]	28.	[ ]	[ ]	[ ]	[ ]	[ ]
4.	[ ]	[ ]	[ ]	[ ]	[ ]	29.	[ ]	[ ]	[ ]	[ ]	[ ]
5.	[ ]	[ ]	[ ]	[ ]	[ ]	30.	[ ]	[ ]	[ ]	[ ]	[ ]
6.	[ ]	[ ]	[ ]	[ ]	[ ]	31.	[ ]	[ ]	[ ]	[ ]	[ ]
7.	[ ]	[ ]	[ ]	[ ]	[ ]	32.	[ ]	[ ]	[ ]	[ ]	[ ]
8.	[ ]	[ ]	[ ]	[ ]	[ ]	33.	[ ]	[ ]	[ ]	[ ]	[ ]
9.	[ ]	[ ]	[ ]	[ ]	[ ]	34.	[ ]	[ ]	[ ]	[ ]	[ ]
10.	[ ]	[ ]	[ ]	[ ]	[ ]	35.	[ ]	[ ]	[ ]	[ ]	[ ]
11.	[ ]	[ ]	[ ]	[ ]	[ ]	36.	[ ]	[ ]	[ ]	[ ]	[ ]
12.	[ ]	[ ]	[ ]	[ ]	[ ]	37.	[ ]	[ ]	[ ]	[ ]	[ ]
13.	[ ]	[ ]	[ ]	[ ]	[ ]	38.	[ ]	[ ]	[ ]	[ ]	[ ]
14.	[ ]	[ ]	[ ]	[ ]	[ ]	39.	[ ]	[ ]	[ ]	[ ]	[ ]
15.	[ ]	[ ]	[ ]	[ ]	[ ]	40.	[ ]	[ ]	[ ]	[ ]	[ ]
16.	[ ]	[ ]	[ ]	[ ]	[ ]	41.	[ ]	[ ]	[ ]	[ ]	[ ]
17.	[ ]	[ ]	[ ]	[ ]	[ ]	42.	[ ]	[ ]	[ ]	[ ]	[ ]
18.	[ ]	[ ]	[ ]	[ ]	[ ]	43.	[ ]	[ ]	[ ]	[ ]	[ ]
19.	[ ]	[ ]	[ ]	[ ]	[ ]	44.	[ ]	[ ]	[ ]	[ ]	[ ]
20.	[ ]	[ ]	[ ]	[ ]	[ ]	45.	[ ]	[ ]	[ ]	[ ]	[ ]
21.	[ ]	[ ]	[ ]	[ ]	[ ]	46.	[ ]	[ ]	[ ]	[ ]	[ ]
22.	[ ]	[ ]	[ ]	[ ]	[ ]	47.	[ ]	[ ]	[ ]	[ ]	[ ]
23.	[ ]	[ ]	[ ]	[ ]	[ ]	48.	[ ]	[ ]	[ ]	[ ]	[ ]
24.	[ ]	[ ]	[ ]	[ ]	[ ]	49.	[ ]	[ ]	[ ]	[ ]	[ ]
25.	[ ]	[ ]	[ ]	[ ]	[ ]	50.	[ ]	[ ]	[ ]	[ ]	[ ]

OXYGEN/GAS THERAPY ANALYSES

Note: The references listed after each analysis are numbered and keyed to the reference list located at the end of this section. The first number indicates the text. The second number indicates the page where information about the question can be found. For example, (1:219,384) means that reference number 1 is to be used and that on pages 219 and 384 information about the question will be found. Frequently, it will be necessary to read beyond the page number indicated to obtain complete information. Therefore, reference to the question will be found either on the page indicated or on subsequent pages.

1. E. The Bureau of Standards of the United States Department of Commerce has adopted a color code for medical gases for anesthesia. Because these color codes listed below serve only as guides, the practitioner is reminded and urged to read the identification label on the cylinder. Table 6 lists the color code for compressed gas cylinders.

   TABLE 6

Color	Gas
Green	Oxygen
Gray	Carbon dioxide
Light blue	Nitrous oxide
Orange	Cyclopropane
Brown	Helium
Red	Ethylene
Gray and green	Carbon dioxide and oxygen
Brown and green	Helium and oxygen
Yellow	air

   (1:428), (4:361), (5:42), (6:349,397)

2. E. The factor that relates pressure drop to gas volume (liters/psig) can be determined as follows

   $$\frac{\left(\begin{array}{l}\text{cu ft of gas}\\\text{in full cylinder}\end{array}\right)\left(\begin{array}{l}\text{conversion factor from}\\\text{cu ft to liters}\end{array}\right)}{\text{pressure in a full cylinder}} = \text{liters/psig}$$

   Insert the known values into the formula.

   $$\frac{244 \text{ cu ft} \times 28.3 \text{ liters/cu ft}}{2,200 \text{ psig}} = 3.14 \text{ liters/psig}$$

   (1:431), (4:360)

3. D. Table 7 lists cylinder sizes commonly used in clinical medicine and their corresponding factor.
   (1:432), (4:360)

TABLE 7

Cylinder size	Factor
D	0.16 lites/psig
E	0.28 liters/psig
G	2.41 liters/psig
H or K	3.14 liters/psig

4. A. The duration of flow for the compressed gas cylinder given in the problem can be obtained as follows.

STEP 1: Use the formula below for calculating flow duration from a compressed gas cylinder.

$$\frac{(\text{gauge pressure})\left(\begin{array}{l}\text{factor relating pressure}\\ \text{drop to gas volume}\end{array}\right)}{\text{liter flow}} = \text{duration of flow}$$

STEP 2: Determine the pressure (psig) of a compressed gas cylinder that is 3/4, or 75%, full.

$$\begin{array}{r} 2{,}200 \text{ psig (pressure in full cylinder)} \\ \times \quad 75\% \\ \hline 1{,}650 \text{ psig (pressure in 3/4-full cylinder)} \end{array}$$

STEP 3: Insert the known values into the flow duration formula.

$$\frac{1{,}650 \text{ psig} \times 3.14 \text{ liters/psig}}{12 \text{ liters/min}} = 431 \text{ min}$$

STEP 4: Convert 431 min to hours.
Since 60 min = 1 hr,

$$\frac{431 \text{ min}}{60 \text{ min/hr}} = 7.1 \text{ hr}$$

(1:432), (4:360–361)

5. E. The Diameter Index Safety System (DISS) is quite similar to the American Standard Safety System (Figure 84). DISS is used for indexing low pressure sources, that is, < 200 psig. It is designed to prevent the accidental interchanging of threaded connectors (regulators) and medical gases. DISS is *not* a cylinder safety system because it governs the attachment of therapeutic appliances to pressure regulators.

It accomplishes its indexing by a variety of internally and externally threaded outlets and connectors.

(1:438–439), (4:367–368), (5:45,47,65), (6:355,356)

6. E. Figure 78 illustrates a preset regulator. This device has only one stage; however, it contains two chambers. The pressure chamber is designed to vent at pressures

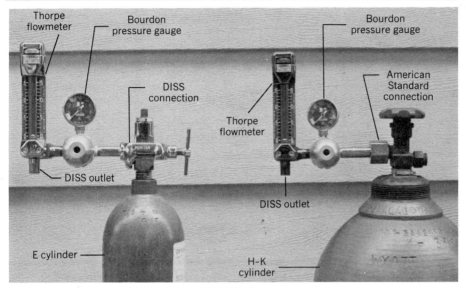

FIGURE 84

exceeding 200 psig via a safety relief device. The ambient chamber houses the spring having a preset tension. The Bourdon gauge shown is used to indicate the remaining pressure in the cylinder, whereas the compensated Thorpe tube displays the source gas flow.

(1:441–442), (4:362–363), (5:87–90)

7. B. When a compressed gas cylinder is hydrostatically tested, it is immersed in a water jacket. The cylinder causes water to be displaced and establishes a reference point (Figure 84A).

Once a reference point has been established, the empty cylinder is exposed to 5/3 of its working pressure (2,010 psig × 5/3) while still immersed in the water

HYDROSTATIC TESTING

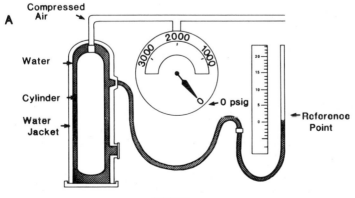

FIGURE 84A

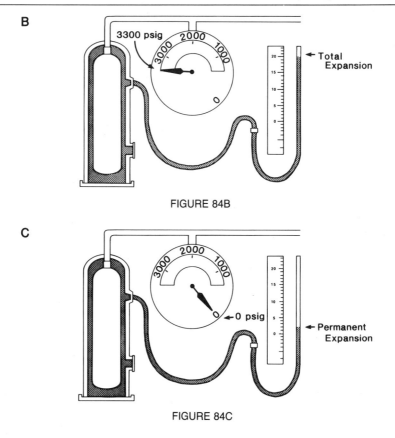

FIGURE 84B

FIGURE 84C

jacket. As this amount of pressure is applied to the cylinder, the cylinder expands and displaces more water (Figure 84B).

The volume of water displaced above the reference point at this time is called the *total expansion*. When the 5/3 of the working pressure is removed, the cylinder "contracts" and some of the displaced water volume recedes. However, the water level usually recedes to a point above the level before the application of pressure (reference point). This new level is termed the *permanent expansion* (Figure 84C).

The elastic expansion is calculated by subtracting the permanent expansion from the total expansion.

(4:361), (6:347–348)

8. A. Basically, a compressed gas regulator incorporates a reducing valve and a flowmeter. The purpose of a compressed gas regulator is to reduce high-pressure gas to a clinical working pressure and to provide a means of controlling and measuring gas flow.

Single-stage compressed gas regulators may be preset at 50 psig or adjusted to any pressure up to 50 psig.

Two Bourdon gauges may be incorporated on a regulator. One gauge functions to measure tank pressure, while the other is calibrated to reflect gas flow. Some preset regulators use a Thorpe tube to measure gas flow.

A safety relief device is generally located in the pressure chamber in the regulator. (1:440–443), (4:361–362), (5:74–78)

9. B. In the face of significant airway obstruction, gas flow may be improved by using a lower density gas mixture, such as an 80%-20% He-O_2 mixture. This expectation is based on the following considerations. The factors in Reynold's equation are shown below.

$$\text{Reynold's number} = \frac{\text{density} \times \text{velocity} \times \text{diameter}}{\text{viscosity}}$$

Reducing the density of the gas flowing through a tube (airway) system tends to promote laminar flow. A gas flowing in a laminar fashion encounters less airway resistance.

Also, Bernoulli stated that the summation of energies involved in the entire conduction system at any two points within that system would be equal. For example, with gas flowing as a result of a pressure gradient throughout the tracheobronchial tree, the summation of the kinetic energy and the pressure energy at one point in the system will equal the summation of the same two factors at another point in the system.

$$\text{Kinetic energy} = \tfrac{1}{2}Dv^2$$

where

$$D = \text{density (mass/volume)}$$
$$v = \text{velocity}$$
$$\text{Pressure energy} = P$$

where

$$P = \text{lateral wall pressure}$$

According to Bernoulli

$$\tfrac{1}{2}Dv_a^2 + P_a = \tfrac{1}{2}Dv_b^2 + P_b$$

Transposing the equation,

$$P_a - P_b = \tfrac{1}{2}Dv_b^2 - \tfrac{1}{2}Dv_a^2$$
$$P_a - P_b = \tfrac{1}{2}D(v_b^2 - v_a^2)$$

As a gas flow encounters a partial obstruction, a velocity increase will occur. However, if a less dense (D) gas is used, the velocity increase across the obstruction will not be as great as that of a gas of larger density. Therefore, theoretically a greater volume of a He-O_2 mixture would move beyond a partial obstruction than would that of an air-O_2 mixture. Therefore, persons experiencing an obstructive episode, for example, asthma or chronic bronchitis, may benefit from He-O_2 therapy. (1:149–152), (2:138–141,164–165), (4:33–35), (5:24–28,33)

10. D. STEP 1: Obtain the factor relating pressure drop to gas volume for a K cylinder of oxygen.

$$\text{K cylinder of oxygen factor} = 3.14 \text{ liters/psig}$$

STEP 2: Use the following formula.

$$\frac{\text{(pressure gauge reading)(cylinder factor)}}{\text{flowrate}} = \text{duration of flow}$$

$$\frac{(2,200 \text{ psig})(3.14 \text{ liters/psig})}{15 \text{ liters/min}} = 460.5 \text{ min}$$

STEP 3: Convert 460.5 minutes to hours.
Because 60 minutes equal 1 hour,

$$\frac{460.5 \text{ min}}{60 \text{ min/hr}} = 7.68 \text{ hours}$$

The tendency here is for one to round off the figure to the next whole number, that is, 8. However, clinically this is incorrect and dangerous because the calculated duration of flow from the cylinder would then be overestimated. One should attend to changing the cylinder at a time less than that arrived at by calculation, to ensure that the cylinder gas is not depleted before the cylinder is changed. In this instance, the best selection was to change the cylinder after 7 hours in use.
(1:432), (4:360–361)

11. E. A cylinder containing a mixture of helium and oxygen bears the colors brown and green.
(1:428), (4:361), (5:42), (6:349)

12. A. When an 80%-20% He-O_2 mixture is being administered, a flowmeter specifically calibrated for this mixture should be used. If, however, one is not available and an oxygen flowmeter is used, the flowrate needed must be divided by 1.8. The value obtained is the flowrate to which the oxygen flowmeter must be dialed. The 1.8 factor arises from the fact that the He-O_2 mixture (80%-20%) flows through restrictions 1.8 times easier than 100% oxygen. This relationship can be shown mathematically by comparing the densities of these two gases.

$$\frac{\text{He-}O_2 \text{ (80\%-20\%) density}}{O_2 \text{ (100\%) density}} = \frac{\sqrt{0.429}}{\sqrt{1.439}} = \frac{1.182 \text{ g/liter}}{0.655 \text{ g/liter}} = 1.8$$

Therefore,

$$\frac{15 \text{ liters/min (desired flowrate)}}{1.8} = 8.3 \text{ liters/min } O_2 \text{ flowrate setting}$$

(1:483,484), (6:342)

13. A. The following gases support combustion; oxygen, nitrous oxide, air, oxygen/nitrogen mixture, oxygen/carbon dioxide mixture, helium/oxygen mixture.
(1:425), (4:358)

14. B. Figure 79 depicts an uncompensated Thorpe tube. The portions of the tube distal to (downstream from) the needle valve are calibrated against atmospheric pressure without any restrictions provided by attached appliances. Therefore, when used clinically, these flowmeters will indicate a flow less than what the patient may actually be receiving. The pressure above the ball (float) is less than that below it,

based on the inverse relationship between lateral wall pressure and velocity, as described by Bernoulli.

(1:445,446), (4:364–366), (5:78–81)

15. B. Carbon dioxide gas is colorless and odorless at normal atmospheric conditions. It has a molecular weight of 44 amu.

$$\frac{44 \text{ g}}{22.4 \text{ liters}} = 1.96 \text{ g/liter density}$$

Using air as the standard, CO_2 has a specific gravity of

$$\frac{1.96 \text{ g/liter}}{1.29 \text{ g/liter}} = 1.52$$

(6:342)

16. B. The 3AA designation, located next to the Department of Transportation's acronym, DOT, indicates that the cylinder is seamless, and constructed of high-quality, heat-treated steel alloy chrome molybdenum.

(1:425–426), (4:358), (5:36), (6:346)

17. A. The National Fire Protection Association (NFPA) recommends standards for the storage of compressed gas cylinders. The American National Standards Institute (ANSI) coordinates voluntary developments of United States standards. The Compressed Gas Association (CGA) recommends standards and safety systems for compressed gas cylinders. The Department of Transportation (DOT) regulates the transport of compressed gas cylinders. The DOT took over this responsibility from the Interstate Commerce Commission (ICC) in 1967.

(1:423–424), (4:359), (5:36,40,45), (6:342,351–354)

18. C. The Pin Index Safety System, shown in Figure 85, is designed to prevent the wrong medical gas from being administered to a patient. The flat face of the valve

PIN INDEX SAFETY SYSTEM

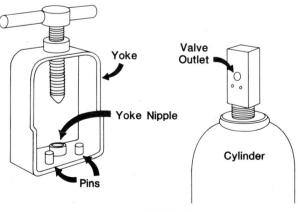

FIGURE 85

TABLE 8

Gas Mixture	Pin Combination
Oxygen	2 and 5
Carbon dioxide-oxygen ($\leq$ 7% CO_2)	2 and 6
Helium-oxygen ($\leq$ 80% He)	2 and 4
Ethylene	1 and 3
Nitrous oxide	3 and 5
Cyclopropane	3 and 6
Helium-oxygen (> 80% He)	4 and 6
Carbon dioxide-oxygen (> 7% CO_2)	1 and 6
Air	1 and 5

has two holes bored into itself. Metal projections on the yoke adapter must fit into the recesses on the valve face in order for the cylinder to become functional.

The Pin Index Safety System has nine pin-hole combinations for nine specific gases (Table 8).

Figure 86 shows the location of the holes on the valve face.

This safety system is foolproof under normal operating conditions. However, some people engage in the practice of breaking off the two metal projections on the yoke connection so that that connection can be conveniently secured to any Pin Indexed cylinder. This practice should be discouraged. This safety system is designed for small cylinders up to and including size E.

(1:436–438), (4:366), (5:45,46), (6:355,356)

19. D. The reservoir bag on a partial re-breathing mask must not be allowed to become deflated completely during a patient's inspiration. During inspiration the patient breathes oxygen-enriched gas from the reservoir bag and from the oxygen source. When the patient exhales, the first $\frac{1}{3}$ of his exhaled volume enters the reservoir

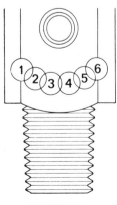

FIGURE 86

bag. The carbon dioxide-laden gas is directed out of the mask through the mask's ports because the reservoir bag is full by the time CO_2-rich gas from the patient's lungs reaches the mask area. The amount of re-breathed CO_2 is negligible because the initial third of a person's exhalation is essentially anatomic dead space gas.

This oxygen appliance should be operated at a flowrate between 7 and 10 liters/min. The F_{IO_2} attainable under ideal conditions is between 0.70 and 0.80+.

(1:466–468), (3:184,186–187), (4:379), (5:92,93), (6:410)

20. D. The amount of oxygen dissolved in the arterial blood (Pa_{O_2}) is the major factor contributing to the development of retrolental fibroplasia (RLF) in newborns receiving oxygen therapy. Although no particular Pa_{O_2} has been established for the development of RLF, RLF is thought to occur in neonates when their Pa_{O_2} is in the 60 to 80 torr range.

(1:457–458), (2:254), (4:372–373), (6:401,702)

21. C. One cubic foot of liquid oxygen at its boiling point ($-297.3°F$) is equal to 860.6 cu ft of oxygen gas at ambient pressure and temperature. Therefore, 16.6 cu ft of liquid oxygen would convert to 13,769.6 cu ft of gaseous oxygen at the conditions specified.

$$\frac{\begin{array}{r} 860.6 \text{ cu ft of gaseous } O_2/\text{cu ft of liquid } O_2 \\ \times \quad 16.6 \text{ cu ft of liquid } O_2 \end{array}}{13{,}769.6 \text{ cu ft of gaseous } O_2}$$

(1:433–434), (5:50)

22. C. STEP 1: Calculate the $P_{A_{O_2}}$ using the alveolar air equation.

$$P_{A_{O_2}} = (P_B - P_{H_2O})F_{IO_2} - P_{A_{CO_2}}{}^*\left(F_{IO_2} + \frac{1 - F_{IO_2}}{R}\right)^\dagger$$
$$= (760 \text{ mm Hg} - 47 \text{ mm Hg})1.0 - 49 \text{ mm Hg}(1.0)$$
$$= (713 \text{ mm Hg})1.0 - 49 \text{ mm Hg}$$
$$= 664 \text{ mm Hg}$$

STEP 2: Subtract the Pa_{O_2} from the $P_{A_{O_2}}$ to obtain the $P(A-a)O_2$.

$$\frac{\begin{array}{r} 664 \text{ mm Hg } P_{A_{O_2}} \\ - \quad 250 \text{ mm Hg } Pa_{O_2} \end{array}}{414 \text{ mm Hg } P(A-a)O_2}$$

(1:303–306,717), (2:19,22), (4:220), (6:260,999)

23. B. The patient is not in ventilatory distress or failure. However, the purpose of administering the oxygen is to reduce the work of the heart and to help prevent lethal

---

*The Pa_{CO_2} can substitute for the $P_{A_{CO_2}}$ because complete equilibration across the alveolar-capillary membrane is assumed.

†Whenever the F_{IO_2} is 1.00, the expression $\left(F_{IO_2} + \dfrac{1 - F_{IO_2}}{R}\right)$ will always equal 1.00, regardless of the value of the respiratory quotient R.

dysrhythmias from developing. Based on the ventilatory conditions specified, this patient can use a low-flow oxygen device. The criteria for using such a device are (1) a consistent ventilatory pattern, (2) a VT of 300 cc to 700 cc, and (3) a ventilatory rate of less than 25 breaths/min. The nasal cannula at 1 liter/min would provide an F_{IO_2} of 0.24.

(1:460–463), (3:182–185), (4:377–379), (6:407)

24. D. Because oxygen is more dense (1.43 g/liter) than air (1.29 g/liter), and because oxygen has a greater specific gravity (1.11) than air (1.00), it tends to "settle" toward the lower aspects of the enclosure. Hence, any oxygen concentration measurements should be performed as close to the patient's face as possible, as well as on the surface of the mattress.

(5:97–101)

25. B. STEP 1: Calculate the patient's inspiratory flowrate.

1. $\dfrac{500 \text{ cc}}{1 \text{ sec}} = 500 \text{ cc/sec} = 0.5 \text{ liter/sec}$

2. Because 60 sec = 1 min,
   then,

$$(0.5 \text{ liter/sec})(60 \text{ sec/min}) = 30 \text{ liters/min}$$

STEP 2: Divide the inspiratory flowrate by the air/O_2 ratio at 28% (air/O_2 ratio at 28% = 10/1).

$$\frac{30 \text{ liters/min}}{10} = 3 \text{ liters/min}$$

At 3 liters/min the patient would receive a total flow of 33 liters/min. Therefore, 3 liters/min represents the minimum oxygen flowmeter setting for the Venturi mask set at 28% O_2 for this patient.

(3:181–182), (4:377), (6:407)

26. C. This patient was administered an inappropriate oxygen device. He did not adhere to the low-flow oxygen delivery system criteria—(1) a regular ventilatory pattern, (2) a ventilatory rate not greater than 25 breaths/min, and (3) a tidal volume of 300 cc to 700 cc. In fact, his ventilatory pattern was not regular; his ventilatory rate was 40 breaths/min. Therefore, he should have been given a Venturi mask at a low F_{IO_2}, perhaps 0.24.

Under the conditions stipulated for a low-flow oxygen device, a cannula at 6 liters/min can be expected to deliver 44% oxygen. With the clinical conditions presented here, the F_{IO_2} would even be greater because low-flow systems will provide a higher F_{IO_2} as the tidal volume (VT) or minute ventilation ($\dot{V}E$) decreases.

The high oxygen concentration received by this COPD patient obliterated his hypoxic stimulus, causing hypercarbia and CO_2 narcosis.

(1:450–451), (3:129,182,185–187,512–516), (4:303,377–379), (6:402,403), (27:177)

27. D. Figure 80 outlines the features of a Venturi mask. Despite the fact that this oxygen delivery device generally is used for the administration of low oxygen percentages, it is classified as a high-flow system. The patient's ventilatory pattern does not alter the F_{IO_2} being delivered. The range of F_{IO_2} available via the Venturi mask differs among manufacturers. Ordinarily, it can deliver an F_{IO_2} between 0.24 and 0.50.

(1:470–473), (3:180–182), (4:375,377), (5:104–109), (6:409)

28. B. The Beckman D2 oxygen analyzer functions according to the principle of paramagnetic susceptibility displayed by the oxygen molecule. This principle, described by Dr. Linus Pauling, states that oxygen molecules are attracted by a magnetic field. This behavior is the opposite of the diamagnetic activity, that is, repelled by a magnetic field, displayed by most molecules.

The gas sampled by this analyzer must be anhydrous. Otherwise, the moisture that would enter the area where the analysis takes place inside the device would adhere to the quartz fiber and to the glass dumbbell and interfere with their movement.

This analyzer is factory calibrated for the general atmospheric pressure that exists in the geographic area to which the analyzer is to be sent. Therefore, transporting the device to an area that will vary in atmospheric pressure will result in inaccurate readings.

(1:476), (2:194–197), (4:414), (5:205–207)

29. A. A high-flow oxygen delivery system is one that can provide the patient with all his inspiratory needs. Both the Venturi mask and the Briggs adapter (T-piece) can supply a complete inspiratory atmosphere to the patient. Gas provided by each of these two devices can supply an adequate flowrate, an adequate F_{IO_2}, and adequate humidity.

(3:180–182), (4:375,377)

30. B. STEP 1:

$$\frac{2,200 \ \text{psig} \times 0.28 \ \text{liter/psig}}{5 \ \text{liters/min}} = 123 \ \text{min}$$

STEP 2:

$$\frac{123 \ \text{min}}{60 \ \text{min/hr}} = 2.0 \ \text{hr}$$

This E cylinder should be changed after approximately 1 hour and 30 minutes of service under these conditions.

(1:432), (4:360–361)

31. A. Grossly obese persons often present with a variety of clinical manifestations known as alveolar hypoventilation syndrome (Pickwickian syndrome). These clinical manifestations include lethargy, somnolence, pulmonary hypertension, and congestive heart failure. The excessive weight carried by these persons creates a restrictive breathing condition. Diaphragmatic and thoracic excursions are limited. Arterial blood gases reveal alveolar hypoventilation, either partially compensated or noncompensated respiratory acidosis, depending on the severity of the restric-

tive condition and the resultant effects of the increased work of breathing. It is a condition producing a low $\dot{V}_A/\dot{Q}c$ ratio due almost entirely to poor alveolar ventilation.

(4:330–331), (6:287), (13:25)

32. A. The ordinarily high CO_2 of the Pickwickian patient has, in essence, produced the same effects as a chronic CO_2 retainer breathing in response to a hypoxic drive. The starting baseline for O_2 administration is a low F_{IO_2}. Of course, O_2 administration should be correlated to arterial blood gas analyses and O_2 percentage adjusted accordingly to the patient's expected normals. The first therapeutic intervention should be directed toward relieving the hypoxia and the work of breathing. In the absence of further complications (i.e., pulmonary infection), the implementation of IPPB, aerosol therapy, or CPT is not indicated at the onset. Assessment should be performed to determine if the immediate O_2 therapy has relieved the patient's distress and improved alveolar ventilation. If it has not, consideration should be given to mechanical ventilatory support (intermittent or continuous).

(4:330–331), (6:287), (8:361), (13:26)

33. D. The normal arterial-venous difference is 5 vol%. This value represents the amount of oxygen removed from the arterial blood by the tissues. Normally, this oxygen need is easily fulfilled by both oxygen transport mechanisms, that is, $KHbO_2$ (combined O_2) and Pa_{O_2} (dissolved O_2). In this situation the ability of the Hb to transport oxygen to the tissues is impaired. Hence, the only way in which oxygen can be carried for tissue utilization is in the dissolved state.

Administering 100% O_2 at 1 atm (normobaric conditions) can (theoretically) elevate the Pa_{O_2} only to 673 torr.

$$[P_B - (Pa_{CO_2} + P_{H_2O})] \, F_{IO_2} \times 0.003 \text{ ml } O_2/\text{ ml plasma/torr } P_{O_2}$$
$$= \text{vol\% (dissolved } O_2)*$$

For example,

$$[760 \text{ torr} - (40 \text{ torr} + 47 \text{ torr})] \, 1.0 \times 0.003 = 2.01 \text{ vol\% (dissolved } O_2)$$

This amount of O_2 administration falls short of the tissue's needs. However, an F_{IO_2} of 0.80 at 3 atm is sufficient to provide the tissue O_2 needs of 5 vol%.

$$[(3 \text{ atm} \times 760 \text{ torr}) - (40 \text{ torr} + 47 \text{ torr})]0.8 \times 0.003$$
$$= 5.2 \text{ vol\% dissolved } O_2$$

(1:305–306), (2:535–538), (4:91,332–331), (13:179), (29:123–124,208), (32:215)

34. A. Although the readout is sometimes given as a percent, the P_{O_2} of a liquid or a gas is measured by a Clark electrode via the polarographic principle.

(2:94), (4:415–416), (5:208–210), (6:978–980)

---

*For the derivation of the conversion factor 0.003 vol%/torr, consult Wojciechowski, W., *Respiratory Care Sciences: An Integrated Approach,* John Wiley & Sons, New York, 1985, pages 63–64.

35. A. Galvanic cell oxygen analyzers depend on electrochemical reactions caused by oxygen combining with water to form hydroxyl ions, which break down into lead oxide, water, and electrons at the lead electrode. No external polarizing voltage is associated with the galvanic cell analyzer as opposed to the polarographic type. Because polarographic analyzers are battery operated, their response time is quicker and their electrodes wear out sooner. Both devices are adversely affected by marked increases in system pressure.

    (2:89–97), (4:415–418), (5:208–210), (6:978–980)

36. A. The nasal cannula is classified as a low-flow oxygen device. The F_{IO_2} it delivers will vary according to the patient's ventilatory pattern. Under ideal conditions (V_T 300 cc to 700 cc; f ≤ 25 breaths/min; normal ventilatory pattern), it delivers a constant F_{IO_2}. For example, at 1 liter/min an F_{IO_2} of 0.24 may be expected. The maximum flow is 6 liters/min because at that point the anatomic and appliance reservoirs are already filled with oxygen. Patient discomfort and nasal mucosal drying are other considerations. One study has indicated that a patient would receive less oxygen if she is a mouth breather.

    (1:460–463), (3:182–187), (4:377–379), (5:94–97)

37. B. According to the Bernoulli principle, lateral wall pressure and gas velocity are inversely related. In the figures illustrated the oxygen delivery device rendering the lowest F_{IO_2} is the one that restricts the oxygen source flow the most. Restricting the source gas flow has the effect of reducing the lateral wall pressure around the area of the restriction, thereby increasing the entrained (room air) gas flow and diluting the source gas (lower F_{IO_2}).

    (1:149–153), (2:138–141), (4:33–35), (5:24–28)

38. E. Henry's law of solubility states that the amount of gas that will dissolve in a liquid is directly proportional to the partial pressure of that gas above the surface of the liquid and inversely proportional to the temperature. Therefore, assuming adequate alveolar ventilation and unimpeded gas diffusion across the alveolar-capillary membrane, the more oxygen (P_{O_2}), for example, that enters the alveoli, the more oxygen that will dissolve in the plasma.

    Dalton's law of partial pressures states that the total pressure exerted by a gas is the sum of the partial pressures of the constituent gases. Generally, representative alveolar air is composed of P_{O_2} 100 torr, P_{CO_2} 40 torr, P_{H_2O} 47 torr, and P_{N_2} 573 torr (P_B 760 torr). Elevating the F_{IO_2} will alter the partial pressures of two of the constituent gases (oxygen and nitrogen). However, the rise in P_{O_2} and the drop in P_{N_2} will not affect the P_B (760 torr).

    (1:196), (2:16,20,63–67,127–132), (4:22,26)

39. A. Figure 82 indicates an adjustable pressure regulator. Number 3 in the diagram represents the valve (seat) that covers the opening in the pressure chamber when the source gas pressure exceeds that which is set by the adjustable control, that is, the spring in the ambient chamber.

    (1:441–442), (4:362–363), (5:74–75)

40. B. According to Bernoulli, the sum of all the energy at one point in a conduction system will equal the sum of all the energy at another point in that system. P_a and P_b

represent the pressure energy at those two respective points. Similarly, $\frac{1}{2}Dv_a^2$ and $\frac{1}{2}Dv_b^2$ represent the kinetic energy of the flowing gas at those two points. Bernoulli states that

$$P_a + \tfrac{1}{2}Dv_a^2 = P_b + \tfrac{1}{2}Dv_b^2$$

After the equation is factored and the factor $\frac{1}{2}$ is eliminated because it is a constant, the resulting relationship is

$$P_a - P_b = D(v_b^2 - v_a^2)$$

The relationship indicates that the lateral wall pressure gradient across a partial obstruction between points a and b can be lessened if a gas of lower density is flowing.
(1:149–153), (2:138–141), (4:33–35), (5:24–28)

41. D. STEP 1: Use the following formula

$$(C_S \times \dot{V}_S) + (C_{ENT} \times \dot{V}_{ENT}) = (C_{DEL} \times \dot{V}_{DEL})$$

where

$$C_S = \text{concentration of the source gas}$$
$$\dot{V}_S = \text{flowrate of the source gas}$$
$$C_{ENT} = \text{concentration of the entrained gas}$$
$$\dot{V}_{ENT} = \text{flowrate of the entrained gas}$$
$$C_{DEL} = \text{concentration of the delivered gas}$$
$$\dot{V}_{DEL} = \text{flowrate of the delivered gas}$$

STEP 2: Establish symbols for unknown values.
Since $\dot{V}_{DEL} = \dot{V}_S + \dot{V}_{ENT}$,
therefore,

$$\dot{V}_S = 10 \text{ lpm}$$
$$\dot{V}_{ENT} = X \text{ lpm}$$
$$\dot{V}_{DEL} = 10 \text{ lpm} + X \text{ lpm}$$

STEP 3: Insert values into the air entrainment formula.

$$(100\% \text{ O}_2 \times 10 \text{ lpm}) + (21\% \text{ O}_2 \times X \text{ lpm})$$
$$= 70\% \text{ O}_2(10 \text{ lpm} + X \text{ lpm})$$
$$1{,}000 + 21X = 700 + 70X$$
$$1{,}000 - 700 = 70X - 21X$$
$$300 = 49X$$
$$X = 6.1 \text{ lpm}$$

Approximately, 6 liters/min of room air are entrained.

STEP 4: The question asked for the calculation of the total delivered flowrate $(\dot{V}_{DEL})$.

Therefore, from STEP 2

$$\dot{V}_{DEL} = \dot{V}_S + \dot{V}_{VENT}$$
$$= 10 \text{ lpm} + 6 \text{ lpm}$$
$$= 16 \text{ lpm}$$

(2:142–145), (4:377), (5:11)

42. C. The air-oxygen ratio can be computed as follows

$$\frac{\text{air flowrate}}{\text{oxygen flowrate}} = \frac{6 \text{ liters/min}}{10 \text{ liters/min}} = \frac{0.6}{1.0} = 0.6:1.0$$

(2:7–8), (4:377), (5:107)

43. D. Theoretically, all the perfusion would come into contact with all the ventilation. Gas exchange would be perfect in this perfect lung. An F_{IO_2} of 1.0 would result in the washout of all the nitrogen. The only gases that would remain in the lungs along with the oxygen would be CO_2 and H_2O.

$$\begin{array}{r} 760 \text{ torr } P_B \\ - \quad 47 \text{ torr } P_{H_2O} \\ \hline 713 \text{ torr corrected } P_B \\ - \quad 40 \text{ torr } P_{CO_2} \\ \hline 673 \text{ torr } P_{O_2} \text{ (theoretical maximum)} \end{array}$$

This relationship can be verified by the alveolar air equation.

$$P_{AO_2} = (P_B - P_{H_2O})F_{IO_2} - Pa_{CO_2}\left(F_{IO_2} + \frac{1 - F_{IO_2}}{R}\right)$$
$$= (760 \text{ torr} - 47 \text{ torr})1.0 - 40 \text{ torr } (1)*$$
$$= 713 \text{ torr} - 40 \text{ torr}$$
$$= 673 \text{ torr}$$

(1:305–306), (2:19,22,131–132)

44. C. STEP 1: Determine the corrected barametric pressure.

$$P_B - P_{H_2O} = \text{corrected } P_B$$
$$760 \text{ torr} - 40 \text{ torr} = 720 \text{ torr corrected } P_B$$

STEP 2: Calculate the alveolar oxygen tension (P_{AO_2}) expressed in torr.

$$\begin{array}{r} 720 \text{ torr corrected } P_B \\ \times \ 0.14 \ O_2 \text{ in the alveoli } (F_{AO_2}) \\ \hline 101 \text{ torr } P_{AO_2} \end{array}$$

*Note that whenever the F_{IO_2} is 1.0, the expression $\left(F_{IO_2} + \frac{1 - F_{IO_2}}{R}\right)$ will always equal 1.0, regardless of the value of the respiratory quotient R. Normally, R = 0.8.

STEP 3: Obtain the conversion factor from torr to cm H_2O.

$$\frac{1 \text{ atm in cm } H_2O}{1 \text{ atm in torr}} = \frac{1{,}034 \text{ cm } H_2O}{760 \text{ torr}} = 1.36 \text{ cm } H_2O/\text{torr}$$

STEP 4: Convert the P_{AO_2} expressed in torr to cm H_2O.

$$P_{AO_2} = (101 \text{ ~~torr~~ } P_{AO_2})(1.36 \text{ cm } H_2O/\text{~~torr~~}) = 137 \text{ cm } H_2O$$

(1:12–14,25), (2:116–118,126–132), (4:20–23)

45. B. The nasal cavity, oral cavity, oropharynx, and nasopharynx comprise the anatomic reservoir.

STEP 1: Determine the volume of oxygen inspired each breath.

1. A flowrate of 3 liters/min equals 3,000 ml/min, or

$$\frac{3{,}000 \text{ ml/~~min~~}}{60 \text{ sec/~~min~~}} = 50 \text{ ml/sec}$$

Therefore, 50 ml of oxygen will be delivered by the cannula to the patient in 1 second.

2. Most of the patient's exhaled flow occurs during the first 75%, or 1.5 seconds, of exhalation. During the remaining 0.5 second of expiratory time, the anatomic reservoir (50 cc) becomes half filled because in a 0.5-second time, a flowrate of 50 ml/sec provides 25 cc of O_2.

STEP 2: Determine the portion of the 500 cc V_T that is comprised of 100% oxygen.

During the 1-second inspiratory time, 25 ml of 100% oxygen occupy the anatomic reservoir, and 50 ml of 100% oxygen are provided by the cannula (flowrate 50 ml/sec). Therefore, 75 ml of 100% oxygen (25 ml + 50 ml) are included within the 500 cc tidal volume.

$$\begin{array}{r} 25 \text{ ml of 100\% oxygen anatomic reservoir} \\ + \ 50 \text{ ml of 100\% oxygen provided by cannula} \\ \hline 75 \text{ ml of 100\% oxygen comprise 500 cc } V_T \end{array}$$

The remaining 425 cc of V_T will contain 20% oxygen (approximate room air concentration).

STEP 3: Compute the volume of oxygen within the remaining 425 cc of tidal volume.

1.
$$\begin{array}{r} 500 \text{ cc } V_T \\ - \ 75 \text{ cc 100\% oxygen} \\ \hline 425 \text{ cc of } V_T \text{ containing 20.93\% } O_2 \text{ (rounded off to 20\%)} \end{array}$$

2.
$$\begin{array}{r} 425 \text{ cc} \\ \times \ 20\% \ O_2 \\ \hline 85 \text{ cc of } O_2 \end{array}$$

STEP 4: Calculate the F_{IO_2}.

1. Because the 500 cc V_T contains 160 cc of 100% oxygen:

$$
\begin{array}{r}
50 \text{ cc } O_2 \\
25 \text{ cc } O_2 \\
+\quad 85 \text{ cc } O_2 \\
\hline
160 \text{ cc } O_2
\end{array}
$$

2. Therefore,

$$\frac{160 \text{ cc}}{500 \text{ cc}} = 0.32$$

(3:183–185), (4:378), (27:175–177)

46. A. A low-flow oxygen delivery system requires the following three criteria in order to provide a precise and constant F_{IO_2}:

1. a regular ventilatory pattern
2. a V_T between 300 cc and 700 cc
3. a ventilatory rate not greater than 25 breaths/min

However, a change in any or all these criteria outside the stated ranges will alter the F_{IO_2}.

The F_{IO_2} of a low-flow system will increase if

1. the V_T gets smaller
2. the ventilatory rate slows
3. the minute ventilation ($\dot{V}_E$) diminishes

The F_{IO_2} of a low-flow system will decrease if

1. the V_T gets larger
2. the ventilatory rate increases
3. the minute ventilation ($\dot{V}_E$) increases

(3:182–186), (4:378), (27:177)

47. B. STEP 1: Find the Sa_{O_2} at pH 7.20 that corresponds to a Pa_{O_2} of 100 torr. From the oxyhemoglobin dissociation curve an Sa_{O_2} of 94% corresponds to a Pa_{O_2} of 100 torr at pH 7.20.

STEP 2: Calculate the dissolved arterial oxygen expressed in vol%.

$$Pa_{O_2} \times 0.003 \text{ vol\%/torr} = \text{dissolved arterial } O_2 \text{ in vol\%}$$
$$(100 \text{ torr})(0.003 \text{ vol\%/torr}) = 0.3 \text{ vol\%}$$

STEP 3: Determine combined arterial oxygen.

$$Sa_{O_2} \times [Hb] \times 1.34 \text{ ml } O_2/g \text{ Hb} = \text{combined arterial } O_2$$
$$94\% \times 13 \text{ g\%} \times 1.34 \text{ ml } O_2/g \text{ Hb} = 16.37 \text{ vol\%}$$

STEP 4: Compute the total arterial oxygen content.

$$\text{combined arterial } O_2 + \text{dissolved arterial } O_2 = \text{total arterial } O_2 \text{ content}$$
$$16.37 \text{ vol\%} + 0.3 \text{ vol\%} = 16.67 \text{ vol\%}$$

STEP 5: Find the $S\bar{v}_{O_2}$ at pH 7.20 that corresponds to a $P\bar{v}_{O_2}$ of 40 torr. From the oxyhemoglobin dissociation curve an $S\bar{v}_{O_2}$ of 62% corresponds to a $P\bar{v}_{O_2}$ of 40 torr at pH 7.20.

STEP 6: Calculate the dissolved venous oxygen expressed in vol%.

$$P\bar{v}_{O_2} \times 0.003 \text{ vol\%/torr} = \text{dissolved venous } O_2 \text{ in vol\%}$$
$$(40 \text{ torr})(0.003 \text{ vol\%/torr}) = 0.12 \text{ vol\%}$$

STEP 7: Determine the combined venous oxygen.

$$S\bar{v}_{O_2} \times [Hb] \times 1.34 \text{ ml } O_2/g \text{ Hb} = \text{combined venous } O_2$$
$$62\% \times 13 \text{ g\%} \times 1.34 \text{ ml } O_2/g \text{ Hb} = 10.80 \text{ vol\%}$$

STEP 8: Compute the total venous oxygen content.

$$\text{combined venous } O_2 + \text{dissolved venous } O_2 = \text{total venous } O_2 \text{ content}$$
$$10.80 \text{ vol\%} + 0.12 \text{ vol\%} = 10.92 \text{ vol\%}$$

STEP 9: Calculate the arterial-venous difference.

$$\text{total arterial } O_2 \text{ content} - \text{total venous } O_2 \text{ content} = \text{a-v difference}$$
$$16.67 \text{ vol\%} - 10.92 \text{ vol\%} = 5.75 \text{ vol\%}$$

(1:205–208), (29:125), (32:93,135–137,207)

48. C. The initials STPD represent the conditions of standard temperature and standard pressure of a dry gas sample. Standard temperature is 0°C; standard pressure is 760 mm Hg. Atmospheric air contains 20.93% oxygen. Therefore, atmospheric P_{O_2} (P_{IO_2}) can be calculated by multiplying the standard pressure by the F_{IO_2}.

$$\frac{760 \text{ mm Hg} \times 0.2093 \, F_{IO_2}}{159 \text{ mm Hg } P_{O_2} \text{ or } P_{IO_2}}$$

When water vapor is present, it must be subtracted from the total pressure before the corrected barometric pressure is multiplied by the F_{IO_2}.

(1:13–14,18), (2:126–127), (4:21,22–23)

49. A. Low $\dot{V}A/\dot{Q}c$ units, or areas where perfusion exceeds ventilation and diffusion impairments are all amenable to oxygen therapy. Capillary shunting, lung units receiving perfusion but not ventilation, cannot be corrected by oxygen therapy. A collapsed or completely obstructed alveolus will not gas exchange regardless of the F_{IO_2} breathed.

Figures 87 and 88 illustrate how low $\dot{V}A/\dot{Q}c$ lung units (perfusion in excess of ventilation, shunt effect) can increase blood oxygenation when subjected to higher F_{IO_2}s.

In Figure 87, when room air is breathed, the low $\dot{V}A/\dot{Q}c$ alveolus mimics a capillary shunt, and a venous admixture ultimately combines with blood that has normally exchanged. The result can produce hypoxemia. Oxygenation can be improved, as in Figure 88, when the F_{IO_2} is increased (e.g., 1.0). Oxygen molecules displace nitrogen molecules, and more oxygen molecules move past the partial obstruction, thereby improving oxygenation to the distal alveolus. Arterial oxygenation, consequently, improves.

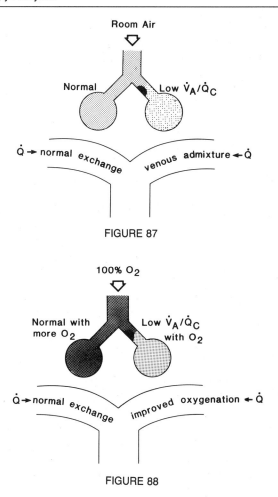

Room Air

Normal

Low $\dot{V}_A/\dot{Q}_C$

$\dot{Q} \rightarrow$ normal exchange   venous admixture $\leftarrow \dot{Q}$

FIGURE 87

100% O_2

Normal with
more O_2

Low $\dot{V}_A/\dot{Q}_C$
with O_2

$\dot{Q} \rightarrow$ normal exchange   improved oxygenation $\leftarrow \dot{Q}$

FIGURE 88

Depending on the nature of the diffusion impairment, an increased $F_{I_{O_2}}$ ordinarily corrects the hypoxemia, as reflected by a lower $P(A-a)O_2$.
(1:298–308), (3:193–208), (4:375–377)

50. D. The patient's Pa_{O_2} is within the normal range; therefore, hypoxic hypoxia can be ruled out. The fact that the Pa_{O_2} and Sa_{O_2} are normal eliminates the possibility of stagnant or circulatory hypoxia. The normal ventilatory status (V_T 500 cc; f 14 breaths/min) helps eliminate histotoxic hypoxia as a possible cause. Also, in histotoxic hypoxia the Pa_{O_2} would essentially equal the $P\bar{v}_{O_2}$. The low hemoglobin concentration (7 g%) indicates the presence of anemic hypoxia. The normal hemoglobin concentration range is 12 g% to 16 g%.

Hypoxic hypoxia is defined as inadequate tissue oxygenation caused by fewer than normal oxygen molecules diffusing across the alveolar-capillary membrane (e.g., COPD). Stagnant or circulatory hypoxia is described as inadequate tissue oxygenation caused by insufficient blood supply (e.g., congestive heart failure). Histotoxic hypoxia results from an inability of the tissues to use the oxygen carried in the blood (e.g., cyanide poisoning). Anemic hypoxia results from a low oxygen-carrying capacity in the blood (e.g., carbon monoxide poisoning and anemia). (1:277–287), (4:370–371), (6:404), (8:80–81,365)

REFERENCES

1. Spearman, C., and Sheldon, R., *Egan's Fundamentals of Respiratory Therapy*, 4th ed., C.V. Mosby, St. Louis, 1982.

2. Wojciechowski, W., *Respiratory Care Sciences: An Integrated Approach*, John Wiley & Sons, New York, 1985.

3. Shapiro, B., Harrison, R., Kacmarek, R., and Cane, R., *Clinical Application of Respiratory Care*, 3rd ed., Year Book Medical Publishers, Chicago, 1985.

4. Kacmarek, R., Mack, C., and Dimas, S., *The Essentials of Respiratory Therapy*, 2nd ed., Year Book Medical Publishers, Chicago, 1985.

5. McPherson, S., *Respiratory Therapy Equipment*, 3rd ed., C.V. Mosby, St. Louis, 1985.

6. Burton, G., and Hodgkin, J., *Respiratory Care: A Guide to Clinical Practice*, 2nd ed., J.B. Lippincott, Philadelphia, 1985.

7. Frownfelter, D., *Chest Physical Therapy and Cardiopulmonary Rehabilitation, An Interdisciplinary Approach*, Year Book Medical Publishers, Chicago, 1978.

8. Cherniack, R., and Cherniack, L., *Respiration in Health and Disease*, 3rd ed., W.B. Saunders, Philadelphia, 1983.

9. Daily, E., and Schroeder, G., *Techniques in Bedside Hemodynamic Monitoring*, 3rd ed., C.V. Mosby, St. Louis, 1985.

10. Des Jardins, *Clinical Manifestations of Respiratory Disease*, Year Book Medical Publishers, Chicago, 1984.

11. Mitchell, R., *Synopsis of Clinical Pulmonary Disease*, 3rd ed., C.V. Mosby, St. Louis, 1982.

12. Comroe, J., *Physiology of Respiration*, 3rd ed., Year Book Medical Publishers, Chicago, 1974.

13. West, J., *Pulmonary Pathophysiology—The Essentials*, 2nd ed., Williams & Wilkins, Baltimore, 1982.

14. West, J., *Respiratory Physiology—The Essentials*, 3rd ed., Williams & Wilkins, Baltimore, 1985.

15. Martz, K., et al., *Management of the Patient-Ventilator System: A Team Approach*, 2nd ed., C.V. Mosby, St. Louis, 1984.

16. Shoup, C., and McHenry, R., *Laboratory Exercises in Respiratory Therapy*, 2nd ed., C.V. Mosby, St. Louis, 1983.

17. Ruppel, G., *Manual of Pulmonary Function Testing*, 3rd ed., C.V. Mosby, St. Louis, 1982.

18. Appelbaum, E., and Bruce, D., *Tracheal Intubation*, W.B. Saunders, Philadelphia, 1976.

19. Rau, J., *Respiratory Therapy Pharmacology*, 2nd ed., Year Book Medical Publishers, Chicago, 1984.

20. United States Department of Health, Education, and Welfare, Public Health Service, *Isolation Techniques for Use in Hospitals*, 2nd ed., Washington, D.C., 1975.

21. Brooks, S., *Integrated Basic Science*, 4th ed., C.V. Mosby, St. Louis, 1979.

22. Comroe, J., *The Lung*, Year Book Medical Publishers, Chicago, 1962.

23. Shibel, E., and Moser, K., *Respiratory Emergencies*, 2nd ed., C.V. Mosby, St. Louis, 1982.

24. Tisi, G., *Pulmonary Physiology in Clinical Medicine*, 2nd ed., Williams & Wilkins, Baltimore, 1985.

25. Cherniack, R., *Pulmonary Function Testing*, W.B. Saunders, Philadelphia, 1977.

26. Altose, M., *The Physiological Basis of Pulmonary Function Testing*, Clinical Symposia-CIBA, Vol. 31, No. 2, Summit, New Jersey, 1979.

27. Shapiro, B., Harrison, R., and Walton, J., *Clinical Application of Arterial Blood Gases,* 3rd ed., Year Book Medical Publishers, Chicago, 1982.

28. West, J., *Ventilation/Blood Flow and Gas Exchange,* 3rd ed., Blackwell Scientific Publications, 1979.

29. Slonim, N., and Hamilton, K., *Respiratory Physiology,* 4th ed., C.V. Mosby, St. Louis, 1981.

30. Rarey, K., and Youtsey, J., *Respiratory Patient Care,* Prentice-Hall, Englewood Cliffs, 1981.

31. Berne, R., and Levy, M., *Physiology,* C.V. Mosby, St. Louis, 1983.

32. Levitzky, M., *Pulmonary Physiology,* 2nd ed., McGraw-Hill, New York, 1986.

33. Wilson, P., Bell, C., and Norton, A., *Rehabilitation of the Heart and Lungs,* SensorMedics, 1980.

34. Clausen, J., and Zarins, L., *Pulmonary Function Testing Guildlines and Controversies,* Academic Press, New York, 1982.

35. Klaus, M., and Fanaroff, A., *Care of the High-Risk Neonate,* 2nd ed., W.B. Saunders, Philadelphia, 1979.

36. Lough, M., et al., *Pediatric Respiratory Therapy,* 3rd ed., Year Book Medical Publishers, Chicago, 1985.

37. Levin, D., et al., *A Practical Guide to Pediatric Intensive Care,* 2nd ed., C.V. Mosby, St. Louis, 1984.

38. O'Ryan, J., and Burns, D., *Pulmonary Rehabilitation from Hospital to Home,* Year Book Medical Publishers, Chicago, 1984.

39. Bell, C., et al., *Home Care and Rehabilitation in Respiratory Medicine,* J.B. Lippincott, Philadelphia, 1984.

40. Wilkins, R., et al., *Clinical Assessment in Respiratory Care,* C.V. Mosby, St. Louis, 1985.

41. Jones, N., and Campbell, E., *Clinical Exercise Testing,* 2nd ed., W.B. Saunders, Philadelphia, 1982.

42. Goldsmith, J., and Karotkin, E., *Assisted Ventilation of the Neonate,* W.B. Saunders, Philadelphia, 1981.

43. Blowers, M., and Sims, R., *How to Read an ECG,* 3rd ed., Medical Economics, New Jersey, 1983.

44. Eubanks, D., and Bone, R., *Comprehensive Respiratory Care,* C.V. Mosby, St. Louis, 1985.

45. Rattenborg, C., *Clinical Use of Mechanical Ventilation,* Year Book Medical Publishers, Chicago, 1981.

46. Witkowski, A.S., *Pulmonary Assessment: A Clinical Guide,* J.B. Lippincott, Philadelphia, 1985.

47. Op't Holt, Timothy B., *Assessment Based Respiratory Care,* John Wiley & Sons, New York, 1986.

AEROSOL/HUMIDITY THERAPY ASSESSMENT

PURPOSE: The purpose of this 65-item section is to give you an opportunity to review and assess your knowledge and understanding in the clinical area of aerosol therapy. The questions pertain to (1) indications and contraindications of aerosol/humidity therapy, (2) ensuring effective aerosol delivery to the lungs, (3) concepts of aerosol particle behavior, (4) aerosol/humidity delivery equipment, (5) physical laws describing equipment operation, (6) medications used in conjunction with aerosol therapy, and (7) calculations concerning relative humidity, body humidity, and humidity deficit. Calculation problems concerning gas flowrates, fractional concentration of inspired oxygen, and partial pressure of inspired oxygen are also included.

DIRECTIONS: Each of the questions or incomplete statements is followed by five suggested answers. Select the one which is the best in each case and then blacken the corresponding space on the answer sheet.

1. Which of the following statements represent disadvantages of aerosol therapy?

   I. Small amounts of the nebulized medication are delivered to the lungs.

   II. Bronchospasm may be induced.

   III. The exact amount of medication received by the patient cannot be determined.

   IV. It cannot be administered to a comatose patient.

   A. I, II, III, IV

   B. II, IV only

   C. III, IV only

   D. I, II, III only

   E. I, II only

2. In what ways can temperature affect the aerosol content delivered to the patient?

   I. Heating the nebulizer increases the absolute humidity.

   II. Nebulizers operated without heating will produce aerosols at less than room temperature.

   III. As "cold" aerosol travels through the tubing some warming occurs, resulting in an increased absolute humidity.

   IV. A heated aerosol will cool as it travels toward the patient.

   A. I, II, III, IV

   B. II, III only

   C. I, IV only

   D. III, IV only

   E. II, IV only

3. The term *hydrophilic* refers to particles that _____ .

   A. are therapeutically administered

   B. penetrate down to the alveoli

   C. impact out in the nose

   D. absorb moisture

   E. are $<1.0\mu$ in diameter

4. At about what diameter do aerosol particles begin to enter the small airways?

   A. 10μ

   B. 5μ

   C. 3μ

   D. 2μ

   E. 1μ

5. For what clinical purposes are bland aerosols best suited?

   I. to mobilize secretions

   II. to induce sputum production

   III. to stimulate mucokinesis

   IV. to bronchodilate

   A. II, III only

   B. I, IV only

   C. II, III, IV only

   D. I, III only

   E. I, II, III only

6. What is the affect of gravity on aerosol deposition?

   A. As particle size decreases, gravitational effect increases.
   B. Gravity renders larger particles less stable and causes them to deposit sooner than smaller particles.
   C. The relationship between gravitational effect and particle size is inverse.
   D. Deposition of aerosol particles distal to the lobar bronchi is *not* affected by gravity.
   E. Gravity renders smaller particles less stable and causes them to deposit in the large airways.

7. Which ventilatory patterns or breathing maneuvers provide for more effective delivery to the lungs of a nebulized medication?

   I. inspiratory hold
   II. mouth breathing
   III. deep inspirations
   IV. pursed-lip breathing

   A. I, II, III only   D. I, IV only
   B. II, III only   E. I, II, III, IV
   C. II, III, IV only

8. Which conditions could result as a consequence of a humidity deficit existing in a patient's tracheobronchial tree?

   I. tenacious secretions
   II. decreased bronchial clearance
   III. increased conductance
   IV. increased work of breathing
   V. atelectasis

   A. I, II, III, IV, V   D. IV, V only
   B. II, IV only   E. I, II, III, IV only
   C. I, II, IV, V only

Questions 9 and 10 refer to the same patient.

9. Calculate the P_{IO_2} to which a patient is exposed when receiving aerosol therapy via a nebulizer operating at 10 liters/min and entraining 15 liters/min of room air. (Assume that the inspired gas is 100% saturated at body temperature under normal ambient conditions.)

   A. 485 torr   D. 330 torr
   B. 395 torr   E. 295 torr
   C. 375 torr

10. Compute the air-oxygen ratio in Question 9.

A. 0.6:1.0
B. 1.0:0.6
C. 1.0:1.5

D. 1.5:1.0
E. 1.85:1.0

11. The concept of *directional divergence* is most closely associated with the term _____ .

A. inertial impaction
B. ventilatory pattern
C. kinetic activity

D. clearance
E. aerosol stability

12. A sol dispersed in a gas is called a(n) _____ .

A. gel
B. colloid
C. dispersion

D. aerosol
E. evaporative suspension

13. What are some of the mechanisms for clearing aerosol particles from the respiratory tract?

I. exhalation
II. mucociliary blanket function
III. alveolar macrophage activity
IV. alveolar type II cells

A. I, II, III, IV
B. II, III only
C. I, II, III only

D. I, III only
E. I, II, IV only

14. Which of the following statements accurately describe an ultrasonic nebulizer?

I. Electric energy is converted to mechanical energy.
II. The energy transformation produces a temperature change from 3°C to 10°C above that of room temperature.
III. The accompanying temperature increase eliminates the need for heating the reservoir to increase the humidity.
IV. The water in the couplant is the water that is nebulized for patient inhalation.

A. I, II, IV only
B. II, III only
C. III, IV only

D. I, II only
E. I, II, III, IV

15. What is the hallmark difference between atomizers and nebulizers.

A. Atomizers are small volume dispensers of aerosols, whereas nebulizers are large volume dispensers.
B. Nebulizers incorporate a Bernoulli effect, but atomizers do *not*.
C. Atomizers generate aerosols of uniform particle size; nebulizers do *not*.

D. All atomizers are hand-held; nebulizers are *not*.

E. Nebulizers incorporate baffles; atomizers do *not*.

16. Which type of aerosol generator has the greatest risk of producing bronchospasm?

A. hand-held nebulizer   D. centrifugal nebulizer

B. ultrasonic nebulizer   E. jet nebulizer

C. all-purpose nebulizer

17. For what therapeutic purposes are hand-held nebulizers best indicated?

I. For short-term administration of bronchodilators

II. For use with patients who can coordinate breathing phases to ensure optimum inhalation of the aerosol

III. For patients who have a diminished tidal volume and vital capacity

IV. For the humidification of the tracheobronchial tree of an intubated patient

A. II, III only   D. I, II only

B. III, IV only   E. I, II, III, IV

C. I, III, IV only

18. Which statements correctly relate to the nebulizer operating according to the Babington principle?

I. Particles are produced by physically vibrating the solution to be nebulized.

II. It can operate efficiently at low source pressures.

III. It incorporates the principle of centrifugal force.

IV. It is reported that about half the particles produced are $< 5\mu$ in diameter.

A. II, III, IV only   D. II, III only

B. I, II only   E. I, III, IV only

C. II, IV only

19. A jet nebulizer incorporates which physical concept(s)?

I. Dalton's law of partial pressure

II. Henry's law of solubility

III. Bernoulli principle

IV. Venturi effect

V. Graham's law of diffusion

A. III only   D. I, II, V only

B. II, III, IV only   E. III, V only

C. III, IV only

20. Why is heating an ultrasonic nebulizer *not* necessary?

A. because the temperature in the nebulizing chamber rises from 3°C to 10°C above ambient during its operation

B. because the particles are of a smaller and more uniform size

C. because of the high aerosol output

D. because it would interfere with the vibrating transducer

E. because the frictional heat produced by the blower motor is transferred to the couplant

21. Which statements accurately describe the relationship between the temperature of delivered aerosols and the factors that may affect their temperature?

   I. Aerosol temperature varies directly with the water level in the reservoir in an im-
mersion heater nebulizer system.

   II. Higher flowrates of gas powering the nebulizer produce temperature drops in the
reservoir.

   III. As the aerosol travels from an unheated nebulizer through the delivery tube to the
patient, the temperature of the aerosol increases.

   IV. The delivered water content of unheated nebulizers is nearly the same as that
with heated nebulizers.

   A. II, IV only   D. I, II, III only

   B. I, III only   E. I, II, III, IV

   C. II, III only

22. Which inhalational medications would be useful in the treatment of an asthmatic
episode?

   I. cromolyn sodium

   II. isoproterenol

   III. isoetharine

   IV. Mucomyst

   V. atropine

   A. II, III, V only   D. II, III only

   B. I, II, III only   E. I, IV, V only

   C. II, IV only

23. Which clinical conditions are indications for aerosol therapy administration?

   I. post-extubation

   II. sputum induction

   III. relief of bronchospasm

   IV. retained secretions

   A. I, II, IV only   D. I, II only

   B. II, III, IV only   E. I, II, III, IV

   C. I, III only

24. The delivered aerosol density will _____ if the total flow from an aerosol
device does *not* equal or exceed the patient's inspiratory flowrate.

A. be unaffected

B. decrease

C. increase

D. decrease for ultrasonic nebulizers

E. be unaffected for devices operating according to the Babington principle

25. Which nebulizer operates primarily as a sidestream nebulizer?

A. Puritan All-Purpose nebulizer

B. Bennett Slip/Stream nebulizer

C. Bennett Twin nebulizer

D. Bird Micronebulizer

E. Hydro-Sphere

26. A tube attached to the distal end of a Briggs adapter, while on a patient receiving continuous O_2 aerosol therapy via a jet nebulizer, serves what purpose?

A. It increases the F_{IO_2}.

B. It increases the delivered flowrate.

C. The tube decreases the delivered flowrate.

D. The tube maintains a uniform F_{IO_2}.

E. It increases the mechanical dead space.

27. What is the advantage of aerosolized medication?

A. The onset of drug action is *not* rapid, thus allowing the patient to tolerate the medication.

B. Minute doses can be administered providing maximal respiratory effect with minimal side effects on the other body systems.

C. Repeated doses can be given without the threat of patient intolerance.

D. Personnel *not* trained in IM or IV drug administration can easily give medications via the inhalational route.

E. All patients can tolerate aerosolized drugs, whereas *not* all can accept orally or parenterally administered agents.

28. The application of Stoke's law is most closely associated with the effect of _____ on aerosol stability.

A. inertial impaction

B. ventilatory pattern

C. temperature

D. time

E. gravity

29. Which variable most influences aerosol penetration and deposition within the tracheobronchial tree?

A. the temperature of the aerosol particles

B. the patient's ventilatory pattern

C. the ambient temperature

D. the density of the aerosol produced by the device.

E. the amount of room air entrained.

30. Which statements apply to ultrasonic nebulizers?

    I. They incorporate a piezoelectric transducer.

    II. Baffles are used to create uniform particle size.

    III. They can be used in-line with an IPPB unit for concurrent administration.

    IV. They can be operated only at an $F_{I_{O_2}}$ equal to that of room air.

    V. They have a total output greater than that of most conventional jet nebulizers.

    A. I, II, III, IV, V   D. II, III, V only

    B. I, II, V only   E. I, III, V only

    C. I, III, IV only

31. How can one determine the adequacy of the flowrate from an aerosol delivery device?

    A. Measure the patient's $\dot{V}E$ and multiply it by 3.

    B. Note the aerosol mist exiting the delivery device as the patient inhales.

    C. Determine the V_T and multiply it by 5.

    D. Multiply the patient's ventilatory rate by the V_T.

    E. Measure the temperature of the patient's expirate.

32. Which of the following equipment is commonly used with a nebulizer?

    I. oxyhoods

    II. incubators

    III. mist tents

    IV. Briggs adaptors

    V. tracheostomy masks

    A. III, IV, V only   D. II, III, IV, V only

    B. IV, V only   E. I, II, III, IV, V

    C. I, III, IV, V only

33. A hand-held nebulizer is best suited for a patient requiring _____ .

    A. aerosol therapy for secretion mobilization

    B. sputum induction

    C. administration of medication

    D. aerosol therapy to reduce sputum viscosity

    E. dense mist therapy

34. Which medications would be useful for reducing respiratory mucosal edema?

    I. isoproterenol

    II. isoetharine

    III. racemic epinephrine

    IV. ephedrine

    V. phenylephrine

A. I, II only

B. I, II, III, IV only

C. III, V only

D. III, IV, V only

E. II, III, V only

35. What are some disadvantages of administering medication via aerosolization?

    I. Latent onset of therapeutic effect.

    II. Increased expense compared with the oral route of administration.

    III. Administration of imprecise dosage.

    IV. Increased risk of systemic side effects.

A. I, II, III, IV

B. II, III, IV only

C. II, III only

D. I, IV only

E. I, II, IV only

36. Which jet nebulizer setting would have the greatest aerosol output?

A. 10 liters/min on 100% O_2

B. 10 liters/min on 70% O_2

C. 10 liters/min on 60% O_2

D. 10 liters/min on 40% O_2

E. 10 liters/min on 30% O_2

37. The Bird micronebulizer exemplifies what type(s) of nebulizers?

    I. impeller

    II. sidestream

    III. ultrasonic

    IV. mainstream

A. II only

B. I only

C. II, IV only

D. III only

E. I, IV only

38. Reservoir nebulizers are used for which of the following purposes?

    I. continuous use

    II. prolonged intermittent use

    III. medication delivery

    IV. bland aerosol administration

A. I, II, III, IV

B. I, II, IV only

C. I, III, IV only

D. I, II only

E. II, IV only

39. Another name for a centrifugal nebulizer is a(n) _____ .

A. Pitot tube

B. Babington nebulizer

C. ultrasonic nebulizer

D. room humidifier

E. inert gas-powered nebulizer

40. How is the principle of kinetic activity applied to a gaseous suspension of aerosol particles?

  A. The phenomenon has a significant effect on aerosol deposition in the tracheobronchial tree.
  B. Diffusion deposition in the alveoli decreases as the velocity of the aerosol particles increases.
  C. Aerosol particles of 0.1μ in diameter exhibit activity similar to Brownian movement.
  D. The forces of gravity and kinetic activity are cumulative for particles of 0.1μ in diameter.
  E. Kinetic activity tends to make a gas a better vehicle for the delivery of medication.

41. Which conditions or situations are associated with decreased aerosol stability?

   I. coalescence
   II. exposure to air saturated with water vapor and warmer than the aerosol
   III. baffling
   IV. traversing through a tortuous tube
   V. exposure to air less than 100% relative humidity

  A. I, II, IV, V only   D. II, III, IV only
  B. I, III only   E. I, II, III, IV, V
  C. I, III, V only

42. Which of the following statements best describes the device illustrated in Figure 89?

  A. The illustration shows a Babington nebulizer.
  B. The illustration shows a conventional jet nebulizer.
  C. The diagram depicts a single-stage pressure regulating device.
  D. The illustration shows a portion of a chest drainage system.
  E. The diagram shows an ultrasonic nebulizer.

43. What means of humidification would best be indicated for a patient with an artificial airway in place?

   I. cool humidification
   II. heated aerosol
   III. cool water vapor
   IV. heated humidification

  A. I, II only   D. II only
  B. II, IV only   E. III only
  C. I only

44. Aside from aerosol therapy, what other therapeutic measures can the therapist use to aid in removing secretions from the respiratory tract?

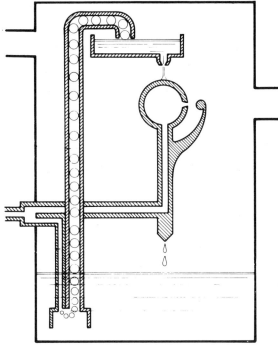

FIGURE 89

I. Chest physiotherapy can be used to aid in the drainage and removal of secretions.
II. Instruction in appropriate cough techniques aid in clearance.
III. Proper breathing patterns help to ensure maximum penetration of aerosols.
IV. Tracheobronchial suctioning can be used to evacuate liquified secretions.

A. I, II, III, IV   D. II, III, IV only
B. I, II only   E. I, II, IV only
C. II, III only

45. What factor accounts for or controls the particle size produced by an ultrasonic nebulizer?

A. the amplitude
B. the current
C. the water level in the coupling chamber
D. the frequency of the electrical energy
E. the quality of the piezoelectric disc

46. Which statement is true of devices used to deliver medication via volatile propellants?

A. Administration of bronchodilators by this method is *not* very effective.
B. High dosages are difficult to achieve in a single application.

C. Overdosage is *not* a major source of concern.
D. Patient misuse seldom causes side effects.
E. The propellant itself can cause side effects.

47. What is the effect on the reservoir water temperature as oxygen flows through an un-heated jet nebulizer?

A. The water temperature remains constant.
B. The temperature of the water increases.
C. The water temperature decreases.
D. The reservoir water temperature initially decreases; then it gradually rises.
E. The water temperature in the reservoir equilibrates with ambient temperature.

48. Calculate the humidity deficit if a humidifier is delivering 25 mg of water per liter of inspired gas.

A. 18.8 mg/liter
B. 25.0 mg/liter
C. 42.9 mg/liter
D. 57.0 mg/liter
E. 68.8 mg/liter

49. Which of the following methods of delivering oxygen with high humidity would be the best for an intubated patient?

A. An unheated Puritan-Bennett nebulizer attached to a Briggs adaptor.
B. An unheated cascade humidifier with the tower removed attached to a tracheostomy collar.
C. A heated Ohio nebulizer attached to a T-piece.
D. A Puritan-Bennett bubble jet humidifier attached to a tracheostomy collar.
E. A sterile, disposable Aquapak bubble humidifier attached to a T-piece.

50. Under which of the following operating conditions would aerosol density be the greatest for a jet nebulizer?

A. 10 liters/min on 100% O_2
B. 10 liters/min on 70% O_2
C. 10 liters/min on 40% O_2
D. 10 liters/min on 30% O_2
E. Altering the FI_{O_2} setting will *not* significantly affect the aerosol density.

51. A liter of air at 37°C has a relative humidity of 65%. What increase in absolute humidity would be necessary to attain saturation?

A. 12.4 mg/liter
B. 15.3 mg/liter
C. 24.9 mg/liter
D. 37.0 mg/liter
E. 43.8 mg/liter

52. Assuming a fixed water content in a closed system, a temperature increase will result in a(n) _____ in the percent relative humidity.

A. increase
B. decrease
C. alteration

D. fluctuation
E. equilibration

53. Which type of humidifier provides the least amount of humidity?

A. unheated jet humidifier
B. cascade humidifier
C. bubble-through humidifier

D. unheated pass-over humidifier
E. heated pass-over humidifier

54. What factors affect the efficiency of a humidifier?

    I. the surface area of the gas-liquid interface
   II. the duration of contact between the liquid and the gas
  III. the temperature of the liquid
  IV. the size of the bubbles moving through the liquid

A. II, III only
B. I, III only
C. I, II, III only

D. II, IV only
E. I, II, III, IV

55. In reference to Figure 90, what function is served by the pinhole located in the middle portion of the cascade tower?

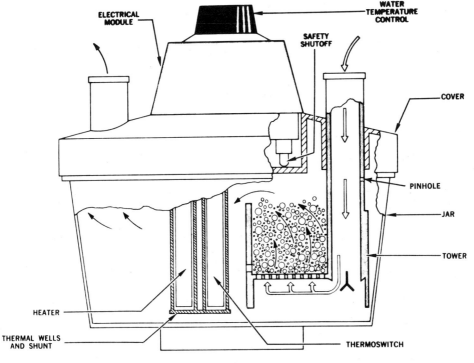

FIGURE 90

A. It allows the patient to generate less effort to initiate inspiration when assisting the mechanical ventilator.

B. It provides a means for more airflow through the cascade, facilitating source gas humidification.

C. It functions to help regulate the dialed-in oxygen percentage on the machine.

D. It indicates the level to which water should be added to the humidifier.

E. It allows the cascade tower to expand without cracking when warm gases pass through the cascade.

56. The amount of water vapor in a volume of inspired air at 37°C compared with the amount of water vapor in air saturated at 37°C is (can be) referred to as the _____ .

    I. humidity deficit
   II. relative humidity
  III. absolute humidity
  IV. body humidity
   V. comparative humidity

A. I only
B. II, IV only
C. III only

D. IV only
E. III, V only

57. Which mathematical expression represents the calculation of humidity deficit?

A. $\dfrac{\text{Content of inspired room air}}{\text{Capacity of alveolar air}}$

B. $\dfrac{\text{Content (inspired ambient air)}}{-\ \text{Capacity (alveolar air)}}$

C. $\dfrac{\text{Content (inspired ambient air)}}{+\ \text{Capacity (alveolar air)}}$

D. $\dfrac{\text{Capacity (alveolar air)}}{-\ \text{Content (inspired ambient air)}}$

E. $\dfrac{\text{Content (inspired room air)}}{\times\ \text{Capacity (alveolar air)}}$

58. Calculate the amount of water in a sample of air that has a relative humidity of 54% at 30°C under standard pressure conditions. The capacity of air at 30°C is 32 torr.

A. 728 torr
B. 59 torr
C. 20 torr

D. 17 torr
E. 10 torr

59. Which of the following statement(s) is(are) true about unheated bubble-diffusion humidifiers?

    I. They produce unstable particles.
   II. The humidity produced from these devices is acceptable for use on a patient with a tracheostomy.
  III. The lower the flowrate, the higher the water content of the bubbles.
  IV. The size of the bubbles produced has *no* influence on the relative humidity.
   V. The water level in the reservoir influences the humidity output.

A. III only   D. III, V only
B. IV only   E. I, II, V only
C. II, III, V only

60. At room temperature, 20°C, air has the potential for holding 18 g of H_2O/m^3. If the air contains 14 mg of H_2O/liter at a particular time, what is the percent relative humidity at that instant?

A. 4%   D. 66%
B. 17%   E. 78%
C. 53%

61. Which of the following statements accurately describe the mucociliary blanket?

   I. The cilia are bathed in the sol layer, while their whipping action moves the uppermost gel layer.
   II. The cilia are rigid during their cephalad stroke and become flaccid during their recovery stroke.
   III. Smoke, alcohol, and hypoxemia impair ciliary activity.
   IV. The mucociliary blanket is useful for removing impurities in the inspired air from the lungs.

A. II, III, IV only   D. II, IV only
B. I, II only   E. I, II, III, IV
C. III, IV only

62. Which statements are true about humidification devices?

   I. As the oxygen flowrate is increased on an unheated humidifier, the relative humidity produced by the device increases.
   II. The Hydro-Sphere has a greater particle output when powered by compressed air, as compared with being driven by 100% oxygen.
   III. The percent relative humidity increases when the source gas flowrate is increased on an unheated jet nebulizer.
   IV. Heating elements improve the output performance of both humidifiers and nebulizers.

A. III, IV only   D. II, IV only
B. I, III only   E. I, II only
C. II, III, IV only

63. Calculate the P_{IO_2} for someone in a hyperbaric chamber breathing an FI_{O_2} of 0.55 at 3 atmospheres of pressure. This normothermic patient has a normal Pa_{CO_2} and respiratory quotient.

A. 418 mm Hg   D. 2,233 mm Hg
B. 1,228 mm Hg   E. 2,280 mm Hg
C. 1,254 mm Hg

64. Calculate the humidity deficit of a patient with a normal temperature breathing gas that is 57% humidified at body temperature.

    A. 26.7 mg/liter   D. 18.8 g/m³
    B. 24.9 g/m³   E. 6.0 mg/liter
    C. 20.2 mg/liter

65. Which of the following circumstances would result in the presence of a humidity deficit?

      I. inspired air at 41°F with 50% relative humidity

     II. inspired gas having an absolute humidity of 43.8 mg of H_2O/liter

    III. inspiration of fully saturated air at a temperature of 20°C

    IV. inspired gas at a temperature of 37°C and a relative humidity of 90%

     V. inspired air at 100% body humidity

    A. I, II, III, IV, V   D. I, III, IV only
    B. I, II, III, IV only   E. III, V only
    C. I, II, IV only

ASSESSMENT ANSWER SHEET

DIRECTIONS: Darken the space under the selected answer.

	A	B	C	D	E		A	B	C	D	E
1.	[ ]	[ ]	[ ]	[ ]	[ ]	28.	[ ]	[ ]	[ ]	[ ]	[ ]
2.	[ ]	[ ]	[ ]	[ ]	[ ]	29.	[ ]	[ ]	[ ]	[ ]	[ ]
3.	[ ]	[ ]	[ ]	[ ]	[ ]	30.	[ ]	[ ]	[ ]	[ ]	[ ]
4.	[ ]	[ ]	[ ]	[ ]	[ ]	31.	[ ]	[ ]	[ ]	[ ]	[ ]
5.	[ ]	[ ]	[ ]	[ ]	[ ]	32.	[ ]	[ ]	[ ]	[ ]	[ ]
6.	[ ]	[ ]	[ ]	[ ]	[ ]	33.	[ ]	[ ]	[ ]	[ ]	[ ]
7.	[ ]	[ ]	[ ]	[ ]	[ ]	34.	[ ]	[ ]	[ ]	[ ]	[ ]
8.	[ ]	[ ]	[ ]	[ ]	[ ]	35.	[ ]	[ ]	[ ]	[ ]	[ ]
9.	[ ]	[ ]	[ ]	[ ]	[ ]	36.	[ ]	[ ]	[ ]	[ ]	[ ]
10.	[ ]	[ ]	[ ]	[ ]	[ ]	37.	[ ]	[ ]	[ ]	[ ]	[ ]
11.	[ ]	[ ]	[ ]	[ ]	[ ]	38.	[ ]	[ ]	[ ]	[ ]	[ ]
12.	[ ]	[ ]	[ ]	[ ]	[ ]	39.	[ ]	[ ]	[ ]	[ ]	[ ]
13.	[ ]	[ ]	[ ]	[ ]	[ ]	40.	[ ]	[ ]	[ ]	[ ]	[ ]
14.	[ ]	[ ]	[ ]	[ ]	[ ]	41.	[ ]	[ ]	[ ]	[ ]	[ ]
15.	[ ]	[ ]	[ ]	[ ]	[ ]	42.	[ ]	[ ]	[ ]	[ ]	[ ]
16.	[ ]	[ ]	[ ]	[ ]	[ ]	43.	[ ]	[ ]	[ ]	[ ]	[ ]
17.	[ ]	[ ]	[ ]	[ ]	[ ]	44.	[ ]	[ ]	[ ]	[ ]	[ ]
18.	[ ]	[ ]	[ ]	[ ]	[ ]	45.	[ ]	[ ]	[ ]	[ ]	[ ]
19.	[ ]	[ ]	[ ]	[ ]	[ ]	46.	[ ]	[ ]	[ ]	[ ]	[ ]
20.	[ ]	[ ]	[ ]	[ ]	[ ]	47.	[ ]	[ ]	[ ]	[ ]	[ ]
21.	[ ]	[ ]	[ ]	[ ]	[ ]	48.	[ ]	[ ]	[ ]	[ ]	[ ]
22.	[ ]	[ ]	[ ]	[ ]	[ ]	49.	[ ]	[ ]	[ ]	[ ]	[ ]
23.	[ ]	[ ]	[ ]	[ ]	[ ]	50.	[ ]	[ ]	[ ]	[ ]	[ ]
24.	[ ]	[ ]	[ ]	[ ]	[ ]	51.	[ ]	[ ]	[ ]	[ ]	[ ]
25.	[ ]	[ ]	[ ]	[ ]	[ ]	52.	[ ]	[ ]	[ ]	[ ]	[ ]
26.	[ ]	[ ]	[ ]	[ ]	[ ]	53.	[ ]	[ ]	[ ]	[ ]	[ ]
27.	[ ]	[ ]	[ ]	[ ]	[ ]	54.	[ ]	[ ]	[ ]	[ ]	[ ]

55. [ ]   [ ]   [ ]   [ ]   [ ]   61. [ ]   [ ]   [ ]   [ ]   [ ]

56. [ ]   [ ]   [ ]   [ ]   [ ]   62. [ ]   [ ]   [ ]   [ ]   [ ]

57. [ ]   [ ]   [ ]   [ ]   [ ]   63. [ ]   [ ]   [ ]   [ ]   [ ]

58. [ ]   [ ]   [ ]   [ ]   [ ]   64. [ ]   [ ]   [ ]   [ ]   [ ]

59. [ ]   [ ]   [ ]   [ ]   [ ]   65. [ ]   [ ]   [ ]   [ ]   [ ]

60. [ ]   [ ]   [ ]   [ ]   [ ]

AEROSOL/HUMIDITY THERAPY ANALYSES

Note: The references listed after each analysis are numbered and keyed to the reference list located at the end of this section. The first number indicates the text. The second number indicates the page where information about the question can be found. For example, (1:219,384) means that reference number 1 is to be used and that on pages 219 and 384 information about the question will be found. Frequently, it will be necessary to read beyond the page number indicated to obtain complete information. Therefore, reference to the question will be found either on the page indicated or on subsequent pages.

1. D. Eighty percent of the medication is lost in the device, 10% does not penetrate beyond the trachea, and only 10% is delivered to the lungs. The drug is randomly nebulized—reconcentration can occur. The small particles can irritate the nasal mucosa. Expense increases when compared with other modes of medication administration. A cooperative patient is also required.
   (1:374), (5:142,159), (6:456), (24:25)

2. A. Cool aerosols will pick up some heat from the ambient air. The higher temperature accelerates the evaporation process, thereby increasing the absolute humidity of the aerosol. Heated aerosols will lose heat to the cooler ambient temperature.
   (1:341,366), (3:91), (5:128,142), (6:379)

3. D. The term *hydrophilic* refers to substances that have the ability to absorb water. The term can be applied to aerosol particles, as well as to dried secretions in the respiratory tract. The term *hygroscopic* also refers to the same property.
   (1:346), (3:160), (5:140)

4. C. Particles around 3μ in diameter begin to enter the small airways with increased frequency. Particles are said to begin entering the alveoli around 2μ.
   (1:353), (5:137)

5. E. Aerosols that are believed to be soothing or lacking in physically or chemically active ingredients are termed "bland." The saline and water solutions, as well as other "wetting agents," are commonly administered bland aerosols. Sputum induction is most often accomplished via bland aerosol therapy.
   (1:355–358), (5:142), (6:379)

6. B. Deposition is the result of an aerosol's eventual instability, causing the particles to fall out on nearby surfaces. Gravity will increase deposition of suspended particles in direct relationship to particle mass; as particle size increases, so does deposition. Particle sizes of 2μ or less may enter the alveoli because gravitational effects are less than on larger particles. Particles of this size continue to be subject to the effects of gravity.
   (1:348), (13:96), (5:137), (6:390)

7. E. Performing an inspiratory hold provides for a more even distribution of the medication, as well as increasing the time available for penetration and deposition. Nasal breathing is accompanied by turbulent air movement and increased contact

between the nasal mucosa and the medication, in addition to the nasal filtering apparatus; therefore, mouth breathing is preferred. Deep inspirations favor increased aerosol penetration. Pursed-lip breathing extends the time of exhalation, providing the opportunity for more particle deposition.

(1:351), (3:107), (5:142), (6:457), (24:24)

8. C. Secretions will thicken, consequently, overburdening the mucociliary blanket. Air distribution throughout the lungs will be impaired by the presence of retained secretions and airway resistance will increase. Certain lung units will receive less ventilation, resulting in atelectasis. Conductance is the reciprocal of resistance. As airway resistance increases, conductance decreases.

(1:354), (3:106), (6:374,457)

9. C. The following steps show how the P_{IO_2} can be calculated.
STEP 1: Determine the delivered flow from the formula

$$\dot{V}_{DEL} = \dot{V}_S + \dot{V}_{ENT}$$

where

$\dot{V}_{DEL}$ = flowrate of the delivered gas
$\dot{V}_S$ = flowrate of the source gas
$\dot{V}_{ENT}$ = flowrate of the entrained gas

$\dot{V}_{DEL}$ = 10 liters/min + 15 liters/min
= 25 liters/min

STEP 2: Determine the concentration of the delivered gas from the formula

$$(C_S \times \dot{V}_S) + (C_{ENT} \times \dot{V}_{ENT}) = (C_{DEL} \times \dot{V}_{DEL})$$

where

C_S = concentration of the source gas
$\dot{V}_S$ = flowrate of the source gas
C_{ENT} = concentration of the entrained gas
$\dot{V}_{ENT}$ = flowrate of the entrained gas
C_{DEL} = concentration of the delivered gas
$\dot{V}_{DEL}$ = flowrate of the delivered gas

$(100\% \times 10$ liters/min$) + (21\% \times 15$ liters/min$)$
$= (C_{DEL})(25$ liters/min$)$
$1{,}000 + 315 = 25\ (C_{DEL})$
$\dfrac{1{,}315}{25} = C_{DEL}$
$52.6\% = C_{DEL}$

The F_{IO_2} is 0.526.
STEP 3: Calculate the P_{IO_2}.

1.   760 torr P_B
− 47 torr P_{H_2O}
_____
713 torr corrected P_B

2.   713 torr corrected P_B

$$\frac{\times \; 0.526 \; F_{IO_2}}{375 \text{ torr } P_{IO_2}}$$

(2:142–145), (4:377), (5:151), (6:259,998)

10. D. The air-oxygen ratio can be obtained by dividing the flowrate of the entrained gas ($\dot{V}_{ENT}$) by the flowrate of the source gas ($\dot{V}_S$). For example,

$$\frac{\text{air}}{\text{oxygen}} = \frac{\dot{V}_{ENT}}{\dot{V}_S} = \frac{15 \text{ liters/min}}{10 \text{ liters/min}} = \frac{1.5}{1.0} = 1.5{:}1.0$$

(2:142–145), (4:377), (5:107,151)

11. A. Particles suspended in an airstream tend to continue a straight course when the stream encounters a sudden change in direction. The divergence of the particles' path from that of the airstream is referred to as *directional divergence* or "sideways slip." The inertia of liquid particles moving in a straight line is greater than the inertia on gas molecules.
(1:350), (3:97), (5:140)

12. D. A *sol* is a colloidal dispersion of a solid (dispersed or discontinuous phase) in a liquid (dispersion or continuous phase). A colloidal system of either a liquid or solid dispersed in any gas is an *aerosol.*
(1:346), (3:95), (5:137), (6:358,390)

13. C. Clearance of aerosol particles from the respiratory tract can be accomplished in a variety of ways. Ciliary mucus transport is responsible for cleansing the upper tract. In the lobular lung units, pulmonary tissue clearance can be accomplished via encapsulation, macrophage activity, and lymphatic drainage. Exhalation is responsible for a significant amount of aerosol clearance. Alveolar type II cells, responsible for surfactant production, do not contribute to clearance of aerosol particles.
(1:352), (3:18,20,100), (6:371)

14. D. An ultrasonic nebulizer contains a piezoelectric transducer that has the ability to convert electric energy to mechanical energy. The couplant (water bath) is the medium that provides the focusing of the vibrational waves against a pliable diaphragm that supports the nebulized liquid. As the electric energy is transformed into mechanical energy, a temperature increase varying from 3°C to 10°C in the nebulizing liquid occurs. Again, the couplant is the medium through which the vibrational energy is conducted. It is not the nebulized liquid. Heating the reservoir to increase the humidity is unnecessary because the output (6 cc/min) from the ultrasonic nebulizer is high. Unheated jet nebulizers range in output somewhere between 0.5 to 5.0 cc/min.
(1:369), (3:104), (5:156), (6:387)

15. E. Both nebulizers and atomizers dispense aerosols. Nebulizers, however, incorporate some baffling structure or mechanism which causes large particles to re-de-

posit into the solution or to break up into smaller particles. The result of baffling in nebulizers is to produce an aerosol of more uniform particle size.
(3:100), (5:143), (6:385)

16. B. The occurrence of bronchospasm increases as the density of the mist increases and with particle size concentrating in the therapeutic range of 0.5μ to 3μ. The ultrasonic nebulizer produces a water content greater than 100 mg/liter with 90% of its particles in the therapeutically effective range. The ultrasonic nebulizer is unique in this regard compared with the other nebulizers, i.e., hand-held, jet, and all-purpose.
(3:104,108), (5:156), (6:387)

17. D. Aerosol delivery is the method by which medication is delivered to the tracheobronchial tree. Effective administration requires a cooperative patient who can operate the device, e.g., be able to use the thumb to block the T-tube before inhaling. The patient must be capable of inspiring slightly greater than his normal V_T to ensure effective penetration of the aerosol.
(1:363), (3:107), (6:391)

18. C. The hydrosphere nebulizer, which operates according to the Babington principle, functions at source pressures between 10 psi and 50 psi, produces aerosol particles in the range of 1μ to 10μ in diameter (97% of its output), and produces 50% of its particles below 5μ in diameter.
(1:368), (3:103), (5:155), (6:387)

19. A. A jet nebulizer takes advantage of the inverse relationship between the lateral wall pressure and the velocity of the flowing gas. As a consequence, the lateral wall pressure decreases as gas moves through a constriction with increased velocity. Because lateral wall pressure drops, another gas can enter the main gas flow. This entrainment phenomenon does not constitute a true Venturi, however. A true Venturi requires precise architectural specifications; the angle of dilatation should not exceed 15°, and the cross-sectional area distal to the restriction site must be large enough to accommodate the entrained volume. In a true Venturi the prerestriction lateral wall pressure is closely achieved in the postrestriction area. Because the Venturi architectural requirements are *not* present in respiratory therapy equipment, it is erroneous to include the Venturi principle as one of the operational principles of a jet nebulizer. The word *Venturi* is used in the loosest sense of the term when applied to respiratory therapy equipment.
(1:359), (2:138–143), (3:101), (5:143), (6:387)

20. C. Because an ultrasonic nebulizer produces such a large aerosol output, heating the unit to yield a greater amount of humidity is not necessary. Therefore, the unit can be operated effectively at room temperature.
(1:369), (3:104), (5:156), (6:387)

21. D. As flowrates increase, the temperature of the water in the reservoir decreases, thus reducing the temperature of delivered aerosols. Heated nebulizers with low water levels may allow for excessive temperatures. As the water level decreases, there is less water present to absorb the heat being produced. A larger volume of water will absorb more heat. Servo-controlled heat nebulizers maintain a constant tem-

perature. Some warming of the aerosol may occur as it travels through the delivery tube from heated nebulizers.
(1:366), (5:153)

22. A. Isoproterenol and isoetharine are administered in aerosolized form as bronchodilators. Atropine, an anticholinergic bronchodilator, can be administered via the inhalational route. Cromolyn sodium is useful in the prophylactic treatment of certain forms of asthma, but it is ineffective in the treatment of an asthmatic episode. Mucomyst can induce bronchospasm; therefore, it would be contraindicated.
(1:398–400,407,412), (3:119–122), (6:462,470,472,481,483), (24:124,158,171)

23. E. Aerosols are particulate water in a carrier gas. The absorption of particulate water by retained secretions reduces the viscosity and enhances the mobilization of secretions via the mucus blanket. Sputum induction is best achieved with bland aerosol administration. Patients who have recently been extubated may benefit from the "soothing" effect of the aerosol to reduce mucosal edema. Bronchospasm may be precipitated by the foreign aerosol particles unless a bronchodilator is being administered.
(1:354,357), (3:106)

24. B. As the patient's need for an increased flowrate occurs, more room air is drawn into the system, thus decreasing the F_{IO_2} and the relative humidity of the inspired gas. The amount of aerosol per liter of gas decreases with air entrainment.
(1:366), (5:152)

25. C. The Puritan-Bennett Twin nebulizer is a sidestream nebulizer with the aerosol injected into the main gas stream. The Puritan-Bennett Slip/Stream nebulizer is primarily a mainstream nebulizer; the main flow of gas is directed through the nebulizer vial. The Puritan-Bennett All-Purpose Nebulizer is a mainstream nebulizer. The Bird Micronebulizer can function as either a mainstream or a sidestream nebulizer.
(3:102), (5:145)

26. D. This type of tubing is termed *reservoir tubing*. It reduces the amount of room air drawn through its distal end by the patient's inspirations. Depending on its length, the room air dilution may be eliminated.
(16:69)

27. B. Small amounts of inhalational agents can be administered, resulting in rapid onset. Despite the lack of total specificity of topical medications, fewer side effects on other body systems are associated with them.
(6:457), (24:25)

28. E. Stoke's law can be represented by the equation: settling rate $\cong$ (density) (diameter)^2. As particle size increases, gravity has a greater influence and the particles settle out of suspension more quickly.
(1:348), (3:96), (5:137), (6:369)

29. B. The following factors influence the penetration and deposition of aerosol particles within the tracheobronchial tree.

1. gravity
2. kinetic activity of the aerosol
3. inertial impaction
4. physical nature of the aerosol
5. ventilatory pattern

(1:348–352), (4:391–392), (30:56)

30. E. An ultrasonic nebulizer converts electrical energy to mechanical energy. The piezoelectric transducer is responsible for causing this phenomenon. An ultrasonic nebulizer is often used in-line with positive pressure ventilation. The output of many ultrasonic nebulizers is as high as 6 ml of H_2O/min.
(1:369), (3:104), (5:156), (6:387)

31. B. If aerosol particles can be seen exiting the device during the patient's inspiratory phase, the flowrate of the device is sufficient to meet the patient's inspiratory needs at that time.
(16:69), (5:152)

32. C. Nebulizers are commonly used with infant oxyhoods, Briggs adapters, mist tents, and tracheostomy masks.
(16:68)

33. C. Secretion mobilization, reduction of mucus viscosity, and sputum induction generally require longer term therapy with relatively dense mist production. The hand-held nebulizer is a small volume nebulizer intended primarily to administer medications.
(1:363), (5:145), (6:391–393)

34. D. Racemic epinephrine, ephedrine, and phenylephrine all elicit an alpha-adrenergic response.
(1:398), (3:120), (6:469–478), (24:326)

35. C. Topical administration of medication results in a rapid therapeutic effect. Actually, systemic side effects are said to be minimized via the aerosolized route of administration. Aerosolized drug administration generally is more expensive when compared with other methods. The time involved of skilled personnel and equipment for administration are the cost-contributing factors. It is difficult to deliver precise dosages of aerosolized drugs.
(1:374), (3:111), (6:456)

36. E. With the air entrainment port opened to 30% oxygen, more air is entrained into the device and the output of aerosol is increased. Aerosol output increases as air entrainment increases.
(1:366), (5:152), (16:64)

37. C. The Bird micronebulizer can be classified as either a mainstream or a sidestream nebulizer because this device functions in either capacity.
(5:145–149)

38. A. Reservoir nebulizers have large fluid capacities. Therefore, they can be used for extended periods without frequent refilling. Reservoir nebulizers are often used with tents for prolonged intermittent use. While reservoir type nebulizers are occasionally used to administer medications, they are most often used to aerosolize water or saline.

    (1:365), (3:102), (5:149)

39. D. Most room humidifiers operate on the principle of centrifugal force. A spinning disk throws the water outward and aerosol particles are produced.

    (1:369), (5:155)

40. C. The continual motion of a molecule and its subsequent rapid, random movement is called *kinetic activity* ($\frac{1}{2} Dv^2$). The smaller the aerosol particle, the more likely it is to display behavior similar to that of a molecule. Particles of 0.1μ in diameter, the size that can enter the alveoli, are likely to be influenced by kinetic activity. The random collisions cause diffusion deposition of these small particles on the alveolar surface.

    (1:349), (3:96), (5:140)

41. A. Coalescence results in a more gravity-influenced situation, thus an increased tendency to settle. Saturated air is a poor vehicle for the transport of additional particles. Turbulence, resulting from movement through a tortuous tube, causes increased particle settling. Exposure to air less than 100% relative humidity results in evaporation. Baffling increases particle stability by reducing the particle size.

    (1:347–351), (3:95–100), (5:137–142), (24:21)

42. A. Figure 89 illustrates a hydrosphere that operates according to the Babington principle.

    (1:368), (3:103), (5:155), (6:387)

43. B. For patients with artificial airways, the primary goal is to provide gases near 100% body humidity. Heated aerosol (heated humidification) would best accomplish this goal. The particulate water tends to keep secretions liquified reducing the risk of airway obstruction. Some clinicians, however, would argue that heated aerosols increase risk of infection and bronchospasm when compared with heated humidity from a cascade humidifier or other heated humidifier supplying high output molecular water.

    (1:355), (3:106)

44. A. Liquifying secretions to reduce mucus viscosity is only one method of secretion removal. Other modalities, such as chest physiotherapy, coughing, breathing techniques, and tracheobronchial suctioning, should also be considered.

    (1:356), (3:106,150)

45. D. The frequency determines the particle size, the amplitude, or strength of the sound waves and also determines aerosol output by increasing or decreasing the number of particles produced.

    (1:370), (3:104), (5:156), (6:387)

46. E. Patients must be carefully instructed in the use of inert gas-powered nebulizers. They must keep the dose only to the prescribed level. These nebulizers have remained popular and are an effective means of administering high dosages of bronchodilators in a single use or application. There is some concern regarding the propellants for the device, especially the hazard of cardiac disturbance.
(1:362), (6:393)

47. C. Because of evaporation (cooling), the gas passing through the nebulizer cools the temperature of the water reservoir below ambient or room temperature.
(1:366)

48. A. Alveolar gas at 37°C contains 43.8 mg of water per liter (capacity). The humidity deficit represents the amount of water rendered by the respiratory mucosa to the inspired gas to produce 100% body humidity. If the inspired gas contained 25.0 mg of water per liter (content), the humidity deficit would be 18.8 mg/liter. The calculation is

$$\text{capacity} - \text{content} = \text{humidity deficit}$$
$$43.8 \text{ mg/liter} - 25.0 \text{ mg/liter} = 18.8 \text{ mg/liter}$$

(1:17,336–338), (2:14–15), (4:21–22), (29:24–25,47), (30:44–46)

49. C. Because an intubated patient cannot adequately humidify and heat inspired gas, gas delivered to the airways of such a patient should essentially be 100% humidified at body temperature (100% body humidity). The best device to use to accomplish this condition is a heated nebulizer or a heated cascade humidifier. Unheated nebulizers, bubble humidifiers, and unheated cascade humidifiers provide insufficient humidity.
(1:339–340,344), (30:47,67–68)

50. A. Increasing room air entrainment, i.e., lowering the oxygen percentage delivered, with a jet nebulizer will increase the aerosol output and increase the total flow of gas. However, the aerosol density or amount of aerosol per liter of gas actually decreases with increased air entrainment.
(1:366), (5:152), (16:64)

51. B. Air saturated at 37°C contains 43.8 mg of H_2O/liter, or 43.8 g of H_2O/m^3. Because

$$\frac{\text{content}}{\text{capacity}} \times 100 = \text{percent relative humidity}$$

the content for gas at 37°C having a relative humidity of 65% can be calculated as follows

$$(\text{capacity})(\text{percent relative humidity}) = \text{content}$$
$$43.8 \text{ mg/liter} \times \frac{65}{100} = 28.47 \text{ mg/liter}$$

To calculate the amount of water needed to saturate this volume of gas, subtract the content from the capacity.

$$\begin{array}{r} 43.8 \text{ mg/liter} \\ - \ 28.5 \text{ mg/liter} \\ \hline 15.3 \text{ mg/liter} \end{array}$$

(1:17,337–338), (2:14–15), (4:21–22), (5:119–123), (6:381–383)

52. B. Assuming a closed system, as the temperature rises, the capacity of the gas to hold moisture increases; however, the content does *not* change. Therefore, if the capacity increases with the content remaining constant, the percent relative humidity will decrease.

$$\frac{\text{content}}{\text{capacity}} \times 100 = \text{percent relative humidity}$$

(1:17,337–338), (2:14–15), (4:21–22), (5:119–123), (6:381–383)

53. D. Unheated pass-over humidifiers represent the least effective type of humidifier. The general range of relative humidity produced by this humidifier is 10% to 20%. Bubble-diffusion (unheated) humidifiers can produce about a 40% relative humidity under ambient conditions.
(1:341–346), (5:124–135), (6:384–389)

54. E. The larger the gas-liquid interface (increased surface area), the greater the amount of humidity picked up by the gas. The more time the gas remains in contact with the liquid, the more humidity it will contain. Elevating the liquid temperature increases the vapor content of the gas. Many minute bubbles are more efficient for humidification than a few large ones.
(1:340–341), (5:123–124), (6:384)

55. A. A Puritan-Bennett cascade humidifier is shown in Figure 90. The pinhole in the upper portion of the cascade tower allows the patient to bypass drawing against the water to begin an assisted inspiration.
(5:129–131)

56. B. The information in the stem satisfies the definition of both relative humidity and body humidity. Actually, body humidity is relative humidity expressed at body temperature. Both are calculated as the content divided by the capacity, multiplied by 100. However, the only difference between the two types of humidity is that the capacity used for the calculation of body humidity is always 43.8 mg/liter (capacity at 37°C).
(1:17,337–338), (4:21–22), (5:119–123), (6:381)

57. D. The water vapor capacity of air at 37°C (43.8 mg/liter, 43.8 g/m^3, or 47 mm Hg) minus the amount of moisture present in the inspired gas represents the amount of water given up by the respiratory mucosa (humidity deficit) to achieve 100% body humidity.
(1:337–338), (6:383)

58. D. Because the percent relative humidity can be obtained from the expression

$$\frac{content}{capacity} \times 100 = \text{percent relative humidity}$$

the content can be calculated by rearranging the equation as follows

$$content = (capacity)(\text{percent relative humidity})$$
$$= (32 \text{ torr})\left(\frac{54}{100}\right)$$
$$= 17.3 \text{ torr}$$

(1:337–338), (2:14–15), (4:21–22), (5:119–123), (6:381–383)

59. D. Lowering the flowrate of the gas through the reservoir increases the contact time between the therapeutic gas and reservoir, providing for more evaporation. If the water level in the reservoir jar is low, the gas bubbling through will not spend adequate time in contact with the water; hence, less evaporation will occur.
(1:340–341), (5:123–124)

60. E. The equation to be used to calculate the percent relative humidity is

$$\frac{content}{capacity} \times 100 = \text{percent relative humidity}$$
$$\frac{14 \text{ mg/liter}}{18 \text{ mg/liter}} \times 100 = 78\%$$

(1:337–338), (2:14–15), (4:21–22), (5:119–123), (6:381–383)

61. E. Portions of the respiratory mucosa are lined by pseudostratified ciliated columnar epithelium and ciliated cuboidal epithelium (generations 0 through 15, inclusively). The cellular structures house goblet cells that secrete mucus. In addition, the submucosal glands contribute to this fluid layer, which bathes the cilia. The mucus blanket has a watery component (sol) in which the cilia are totally immersed. The gel layer, atop the watery component, functions as a trap for foreign particles and prevents the desiccation of the respiratory mucosa. Note the mucociliary blanket in Figure 91.

The cilia move in a cephalad (toward the head) direction. They are so efficient that no retrograde motion occurs during their recovery stroke. They are rigid when they whip forward (effective stroke) and become flaccid during the recovery stroke. Certain noxious chemicals and environmental factors impair ciliary activity, for example, tobacco smoke, alcohol, and hypoxemia. Figure 92 depicts ciliary motion and mucus flow.
(1:352), (4:40–42), (6:372–374)

62. A. Increasing the O_2 flowrate through an unheated humidifier decreases the contact time between the H_2O in the reservoir and the flowing gas. Increasing the O_2 flowrate through an unheated jet nebulizer increases the activity at the baffle, resulting in an increased amount of evaporation in the device. Heating the reservoir raises the P_{H_2O} of the source gas because increasing the temperature increases the capacity of the gas to hold moisture.
(1:340–341), (5:123–124)

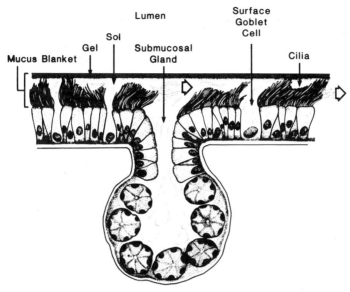

FIGURE 91

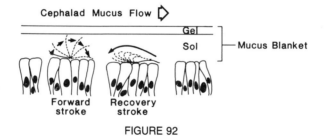

FIGURE 92

63. B. STEP 1: Use the formula shown below.

$$(P_B - P_{H_2O})FI_{O_2} = PI_{O_2}$$

STEP 2: Determine the barometric pressure (P_B) inside the chamber.

$$(760 \text{ mm Hg/atm})(3 \text{ atm}) = 2{,}280 \text{ mm Hg}$$

The pressure inside the hyperbaric chamber is 2,280 mm Hg.

STEP 3: Obtain the corrected barometric pressure ($P_B - P_{H_2O}$).

$$(2{,}280 \text{ mm Hg} - 47 \text{ mm Hg}) = 2{,}233 \text{ mm Hg}$$

STEP 4: Calculate the partial pressure of the inspired oxygen (PI_{O_2}).

$$(\text{corrected } P_B)(FI_{O_2}) = PI_{O_2}$$
$$(2{,}233 \text{ mm Hg})(0.55) = 1{,}228.2 \text{ mm Hg}$$

(12:278–280), (13:179), (14:138), (29:123–124,208)

64. D. At normal body temperature (37°C) each liter of air has the capacity of holding 43.8 mg of water. Because the gas is 57% humidified,

$$
\begin{array}{r}
43.8 \text{ mg/liter (capacity)} \\
\times \quad 57\% \text{ relative humidity} \\
\hline
25.0 \text{ mg/liter (content)}
\end{array}
$$

$$
\begin{array}{r}
43.8 \text{ mg/liter (capacity)} \\
- \quad 25.0 \text{ mg/liter (content)} \\
\hline
- \quad 18.8 \text{ mg/liter (humidity deficit)}
\end{array}
$$

The unit mg/liter is equivalent to g/m^3. Therefore,

$$18.8 \text{ mg/liter} = 18.8 \text{ g/m}^3$$

(1:337–338), (6:383)

65. D. Humidity deficit is defined as the amount of water that the respiratory mucosa must supply to the inspired air to achieve 100% saturation in the alveoli. Therefore, air at 41°F at 100% relative humidity still would not hold 43.8 mg of H_2O/liter. Fully saturated air at 20°C would, likewise, contain less than 43.8 mg of H_2O/liter. Inspired gas at 37°C and 90% relative humidity would have under 43.8 mg of H_2O/liter.

(1:337–338), (6:383)

REFERENCES

1. Spearman, C., and Sheldon, R., *Egan's Fundamentals of Respiratory Therapy*, 4th ed., C.V. Mosby, St. Louis, 1982.
2. Wojciechowski, W., *Respiratory Care Sciences: An Integrated Approach*, John Wiley & Sons, New York, 1985.
3. Shapiro, B., Harrison, R., Kacmarek, R., and Cane, R., *Clinical Application of Respiratory Care*, 3rd ed., Year Book Medical Publishers, Chicago, 1985.
4. Kacmarek, R., Mack, C., and Dimas, S., *The Essentials of Respiratory Therapy*, 2nd ed., Year Book Medical Publishers, Chicago, 1985.
5. McPherson, S., *Respiratory Therapy Equipment*, 3rd ed., C.V. Mosby, St. Louis, 1985.
6. Burton, G., and Hodgkin, J., *Respiratory Care: A Guide to Clinical Practice*, 2nd ed., J.B. Lippincott, Philadelphia, 1985.
7. Frownfelter, D., *Chest Physical Therapy and Cardiopulmonary Rehabilitation, An Interdisciplinary Approach*, Year Book Medical Publishers, Chicago, 1978.
8. Cherniack, R., and Cherniack, L., *Respiration in Health and Disease*, 3rd ed., W.B. Saunders, Philadelphia, 1983.
9. Daily, E., and Schroeder, G., *Techniques in Bedside Hemodynamic Monitoring*, 3rd ed., C.V. Mosby, St. Louis, 1985.
10. Des Jardins, R., *Clinical Manifestations of Respiratory Disease*, Year Book Medical Publishers, Chicago, 1984.
11. Mitchell, R., *Synopsis of Clinical Pulmonary Disease*, 3rd ed., C.V. Mosby, St. Louis, 1982.
12. Comroe, J., *Physiology of Respiration*, 3rd ed., Year Book Medical Publishers, Chicago, 1974.
13. West, J., *Pulmonary Pathophysiology—The Essentials*, 2nd ed., Williams & Wilkins, Baltimore, 1982.

14. West, J., *Respiratory Physiology—The Essentials,* 3rd ed., Williams & Wilkins, Baltimore, 1985.

15. Martz, K., et al., *Management of the Patient-Ventilator System: A Team Approach,* 2nd ed., C.V. Mosby, St. Louis, 1984.

16. Shoup, C., and McHenry, R., *Laboratory Exercises in Respiratory Therapy,* 2nd ed., C.V. Mosby, St. Louis, 1983.

17. Ruppel, G., *Manual of Pulmonary Function Testing,* 3rd ed., C.V. Mosby, St. Louis, 1982.

18. Appelbaum, E., and Bruce, D., *Tracheal Intubation,* W.B. Saunders, Philadelphia, 1976.

19. Rau, J., *Respiratory Therapy Pharmacology,* 2nd ed., Year Book Medical Publishers, Chicago, 1984.

20. United States Department of Health, Education, and Welfare, Public Health Service, *Isolation Techniques for Use in Hospitals,* 2nd ed., Washington, D.C., 1975.

21. Brooks, S., *Integrated Basic Science,* 4th ed., C.V. Mosby, St. Louis, 1979.

22. Comroe, J., *The Lung,* Year Book Medical Publishers, Chicago, 1962.

23. Shibel, E., and Moser, K., *Respiratory Emergencies,* 2nd ed., C.V. Mosby, St. Louis, 1982.

24. Tisi, G., *Pulmonary Physiology in Clinical Medicine,* 2nd ed., Williams & Wilkins, Baltimore, 1985.

25. Cherniack, R., *Pulmonary Function Testing,* W.B. Saunders, Philadelphia, 1977.

26. Altose, M., *The Physiological Basis of Pulmonary Function Testing,* Clinical Symposia-CIBA, Vol. 31, No. 2, Summit, New Jersey, 1979.

27. Shapiro, B., Harrison, R., and Walton, J., *Clinical Application of Arterial Blood Gases,* 3rd ed., Year Book Medical Publishers, Chicago, 1982.

28. West, J., *Ventilation/Blood Flow and Gas Exchange,* 3rd ed., Blackwell Scientific Publications, 1979.

29. Slonim, N., and Hamilton, K., *Respiratory Physiology,* 4th ed., C.V. Mosby, St. Louis, 1981.

30. Rarey, K., and Youtsey, J., *Respiratory Patient Care,* Prentice-Hall, Englewood Cliffs, 1981.

31. Berne, R., and Levy, M., *Physiology,* C.V. Mosby, St. Louis, 1983.

32. Levitzky, M., *Pulmonary Physiology,* 2nd ed., McGraw-Hill, New York, 1986.

33. Wilson, P., Bell, C., and Norton, A., *Rehabilitation of the Heart and Lungs,* SensorMedics, 1980.

34. Clausen, J., and Zarins, L., *Pulmonary Function Testing Guidelines and Controversies,* Academic Press, New York, 1982.

35. Klaus, M., and Fanaroff, A., *Care of the High-Risk Neonate,* 2nd ed., W.B. Saunders, Philadelphia, 1979.

36. Lough, M., et al., *Pediatric Respiratory Therapy,* 3rd ed., Year Book Medical Publishers, Chicago, 1985.

37. Levin, D., et al., *A Practical Guide to Pediatric Intensive Care,* 2nd ed., C.V. Mosby, St. Louis, 1984.

38. O'Ryan, J., and Burns, D., *Pulmonary Rehabilitation from Hospital to Home,* Year Book Medical Publishers, Chicago, 1984.

39. Bell, C., et al., *Home Care and Rehabilitation in Respiratory Medicine,* J.B. Lippincott, Philadelphia, 1984.

40. Wilkins, R., et al., *Clinical Assessment in Respiratory Care,* C.V. Mosby, St. Louis, 1985.

41. Jones, N., and Campbell, E., *Clinical Exercise Testing,* 2nd ed., W.B. Saunders, Philadelphia, 1982.

42. Goldsmith, J., and Karotkin, E., *Assisted Ventilation of the Neonate,* W.B. Saunders, Philadelphia, 1981.

43. Blowers, M., and Sims, R., *How to Read an ECG,* 3rd ed., Medical Economics, New Jersey, 1983.

44. Eubanks, D., and Bone, R., *Comprehensive Respiratory Care,* C.V. Mosby, St. Louis, 1985.

45. Rattenborg, C., *Clinical Use of Mechanical Ventilation,* Year Book Medical Publishers, Chicago, 1981.

46. Witkowski, A.S., *Pulmonary Assessment: A Clinical Guide,* J.B. Lippincott, Philadelphia, 1985.

47. Op't Holt, Timothy B., *Assessment Based Respiratory Care,* John Wiley & Sons, New York, 1986.

HYPERINFLATION THERAPY ASSESSMENT

PURPOSE: The purpose of this 45-item section is to provide you with the opportunity to assess your knowledge and understanding of the forms of hyperinflation therapy which include intermittent positive pressure breathing (IPPB) and incentive spirometry.

DIRECTIONS: Each of the questions or incomplete statements is followed by five suggested answers. Select the one which is the best in each case and then blacken the corresponding space on the answer sheet.

1. An emphysema patient to whom you are administering an IPPB treatment experiences air trapping from generating a forceful cough that terminates at mid-expiration. This patient cannot create an adequate intrathoracic pressure to overcome this air trapping and produce an inspiration, nor can he complete his previous exhalation. What action should you take?

   A. Get a mask and deliver positive pressure to the patient's airways.
   B. Attempt to coach the patient into relaxing and spontaneously breathing slowly and deeply.
   C. Have the patient breathe a bronchodilator administered via a hand-held nebulizer.
   D. Perform the Heimlich maneuver on this patient.
   E. Get a manual resuscitator and a mask, and administer hand-compressed ventilations at a rate of 12 per minute until the patient is relieved.

2. Which of the following patient responses during an IPPB treatment warrant the termination of the treatment?

   I. tachycardia
   II. hypotension
   III. hemoptysis
   IV. substernal pain
   V. paresthesia

   A. I, II, III, IV only   D. II, III only
   B. I, II, III only   E. I, II, III, IV, V
   C. I, II, III, V only

3. What is the rationale for administering an IPPB treatment in-line with an ultrasonic nebulizer?

A. This is an attempt to create greater irritation to the patient's airways, thus inducing him to cough.

B. The mean particle size produced with this setup is smaller than that produced by the ultrasonic nebulizer functioning alone.

C. The patient is less prone to hyperventilate when these two modalities are concomitantly administered because of the soothing effect of the aerosol particles on the tracheobronchial tree.

D. The aerosol particles can generally penetrate and deposit deeper in the tracheobronchial tree with the assistance of the positive pressure.

E. The risk of insensible H_2O loss is reduced by this method.

4. Which therapeutic modality(ies) *may* be considered (a) method(s) of intermittent lung hyperinflation?

   I. incentive spirometry
   II. periodic CPAP
   III. IPPB
   IV. periodic PEEP

A. I, II, III, IV
B. I, III only
C. II, IV only
D. I, II, III only
E. III only

5. Why is incentive spirometry a less expensive therapeutic modality than IPPB therapy?

   I. The equipment used for incentive spirometry is less expensive.
   II. Incentive spirometry does *not* require a respiratory care practitioner in attendance after the initial treatment.
   III. Incentive spirometry takes less time to administer than IPPB.

A. I only
B. I, II only
C. II, III only
D. III only
E. I, II, III

6. Which statements are true about the five alveolar units depicted in Figure 93? (Assume that positive pressure ventilation is being applied via a constant flow generator.)

$$\dot{V} = \text{gas flowrate}$$
$$R = \text{airway resistance}$$
$$C = \text{pulmonary compliance}$$

   I. Alveolus A would fill faster than alveolus C.
   II. Alveolus D would take longer to fill than alveolus E.
   III. Alveolus E would take longer to fill than alveolus C.
   IV. Alveolus A would fill faster than all the other alveoli shown.
   V. Alveolus B would require the shortest time to fill compared with all the other alveoli shown.

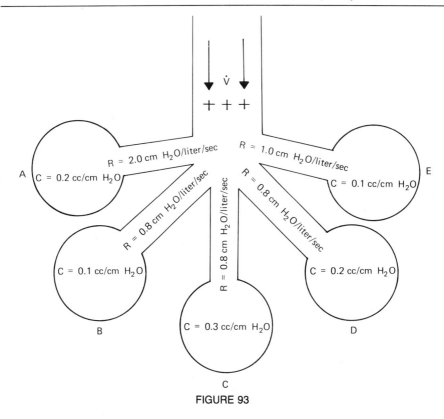

FIGURE 93

A. I, III, V only   D. I, IV only
B. II, V only   E. II, III, V only
C. II, IV, V only

7. What aspect(s) of the patient should be monitored during the administration of an IPPB treatment?

    I. the patient's ventilatory rate before, during, and after the treatment
   II. the patient's sensorium
  III. the patient's pupil status
  IV. the patient's apical pulse
   V. the patient's chest should be auscultated

A. I, II, V only   D. I, II, IV, V only
B. I, IV, V only   E. I, II, III, IV, V
C. IV only

8. For maximum effectiveness, how often should incentive spirometry be performed?

A. 20 minutes, four times a day   D. 5 minutes hourly
B. 10 breaths, four times a day   E. 10 breaths hourly
C. 10 minutes every hour

9. What are the major concerns when using CO_2 rebreathing devices as a means of hyperinflation therapy?

  I. controlling the concentration of CO_2 in the re-breathing system
  II. preventing hypercapnia
  III. avoiding hypoxemia
  IV. forestalling the development of tachypnea

  A. I, II, III, IV   D. I, IV only
  B. I, II, III only   E. I, II, IV only
  C. II, III only

10. What are some of the therapeutic goals of incentive spirometry?

  I. to prevent postoperative atelectasis
  II. to prevent tracheal malacia
  III. to prevent hypostatic pneumonia
  IV. to promote deep breathing

  A. I, III, IV only   D. I, IV only
  B. II, III, IV only   E. I, II, III, IV
  C. II, IV only

11. In which clinical situations or conditions would the use of PEEP be *generally* contraindicated?

  I. cerebrovascular hypertension
  II. flail chest
  III. treated tension pneumothorax
  IV. cor pulmonale
  V. cardiovascular collapse

  A. I, II, III, IV, V   D. I, IV, V only
  B. I, III, IV, V only   E. I, V only
  C. II, IV, V only

12. Which of the following statements correctly refer to IPPB therapy?

  I. A patient's Pa_{O_2} may be elevated by IPPB therapy despite the use of room air.
  II. A decrease in Pa_{CO_2} may be observed as a result of IPPB therapy.
  III. IPPB therapy may reinflate atelectatic areas.
  IV. IPPB therapy may increase the functional residual capacity.

  A. I, II, III, IV   D. II, III, IV only
  B. III, IV only   E. I, II only
  C. I, II, III only

13. What is the rationale for having negative pressure exhalation available on certain IPPB devices?

  A. to help alleviate the exudative process associated with pulmonary edema

B. to prevent patient ventilatory fatigue during therapy, that is, to switch from passive exhalation to negative pressure exhalation

C. to improve venous return

D. to bronchodilate the airways throughout the tracheobronchial tree

E. to prevent air trapping when administering IPPB to an emphysematous patient

14. Which statement(s) represent(s) the rationale for incentive spirometry?

    I. to replace IPPB therapy that has been scientifically disproved

    II. to prevent alveolar collapse

    III. to increase the patient's Pa_{O_2}

    IV. to simulate the patient's sigh mechanism

A. I, II, III, IV   D. II, IV only

B. II only   E. II, III, IV only

C. I, IV only

15. If the preset pressure is being prematurely achieved when an IPPB treatment is being administered to a patient, what action(s) should be taken?

    I. Increase the machine sensitivity.

    II. Reduce the flowrate.

    III. Increase the pressure limit.

    IV. Institute negative pressure on exhalation.

A. I, II, III only   D. III only

B. II, IV only   E. II, III only

C. II only

16. What is the prescribed CO_2-O_2 mixture used for CO_2-induced hyperventilation therapy?

A. 20%-80%   D. 5%-95%

B. 15%-85%   E. 2%-98%

C. 10%-90%

17. Approximately, what percentage of pharmacologic agents aerosolized via IPPB will be retained in the body?

A. 5% to 10%   D. 50% to 60%

B. 10% to 20%   E. 75% to 90%

C. 20% to 40%

18. Which of the following conditions can be considered contraindications for IPPB therapy?

    I. hemoptysis

    II. increased intracranial pressure

    III. decreased cardiac output

    IV. untreated tension pneumothorax

A. I, IV only   D. II, III only
B. I, III only   E. I, II, III, IV
C. II, III, IV only

19. Which hemodynamic changes may be associated with the use of IPPB therapy?

    I. Initially, left ventricular output will increase, that is, for only a few beats after its application.
    II. Right ventricular cardiac output decreases.
    III. During exhalation after a positive pressure inhalation, total thoracic blood volume decreases.
    IV. After prolonged application of IPPB (e.g., 10 minutes), left ventricular output will be decreased during exhalation.

    A. I, II, III, IV   D. II, III only
    B. II, IV only   E. I, II, IV only
    C. I, II, III only

20. The expiratory retard cap available on the Bird Mark VIII may be useful for the treatment of which clinical conditions?

    I. pulmonary edema
    II. preoperative pulmonary hygiene
    III. cystic fibrosis
    IV. pulmonary emphysema
    V. pulmonary fibrosis

    A. I, II, III, IV, V   D. I, IV only
    B. II, IV, V only   E. II, III, IV only
    C. I, III, V only

21. Of the amount of aerosolized normal saline retained in the body after an IPPB treatment, what is the anatomically distributed percentage?

    I. At least, 20% of the aerosol is retained in the lungs.
    II. At least, 10% of the aerosol is deposited in the mouth and pharynx.
    III. Approximately, 5% of the aerosol is swallowed, entering the gastrointestinal tract resulting in systemic absorption.
    IV. Nearly 5% of the aerosol deposits in the mouth and pharynx.
    V. Approximately, 8% of the aerosol is retained in the lungs.

    A. I, II only   D. I, IV only
    B. III, IV, V only   E. I, II, III, IV, V
    C. III, IV only

22. What are considered preferred written physician orders for IPPB therapy?

    A. Standing orders to facilitate the appropriate utilization of IPPB by physicians of various specialties.

B. Orders that specify the therapeutic outcomes, but leave the frequency and other machine settings to the therapist's discretion.

C. An order, such as IPPB four times a day, is sufficient in most circumstances.

D. An order specifying frequency, F_{IO_2}, maximum inspiratory pressure, duration of therapy, medication dosage, and treatment objectives.

E. An order for IPPB therapy listing medication dosage and other parameters properly left to the therapist's discretion.

23. Generally, what are the postoperative indications for IPPB for patients unable to perform deep breathing exercises?

   I. to reduce venous return

  II. to facilitate secretion removal

 III. to prevent atelectasis

 IV. to reduce arterial carbon dioxide tension

A. I, II, III, IV   D. II, III only

B. I, III, IV only   E. I, III, IV only

C. II, III, IV only

24. Which patient(s) would be likely to experience gastric insufflation from an IPPB treatment?

   I. a patient having a treated pneumothorax, that is, with chest tubes in place, while receiving an IPPB treatment via a mask

  II. a comatose patient with a nasogastric tube in place receiving a mask IPPB treatment

 III. a pulmonary emphysema patient prone to air trapping

 IV. a patient being treated postoperatively after open-heart surgery

A. I, III only   D. I, II only

B. II only   E. III, IV only

C. I only

25. What is(are) (some of) the intended role(s) of IPPB therapy in the treatment of acute cardiogenic (high pressure) pulmonary edema?

   I. to elevate the mean intrathoracic pressure, to reduce the flow of blood to the right side of the heart

  II. to increase the cardiac output from the left side of the heart

 III. to elevate the intra-alveolar pressure, in turn, elevating systemic arterial pressure, to increase renal output

 IV. to elevate the Pa_{O_2} to dilate the pulmonary artery

  V. to alleviate the general hypoxemic condition of the patient

A. I, V only   D. II, III, IV only

B. I, II, IV, V only   E. I, III, IV, V only

C. I only

26. How can the use of IPPB produce a decreased Pa_{CO_2}?

    I. by increasing the ventilation of low compliance lung units
    II. by reducing the work of breathing
    III. by delivering increased tidal volumes
    IV. by administering a high F_{IO_2}

    A. I, II, III, IV   D. I, IV only
    B. II, III only   E. III, IV only
    C. I, II, III only

27. For home IPPB therapy where the primary objective is the delivery of positive pressure to improve minute ventilation, what might be a preferred ventilator to use?

    A. Bird Mark VII   D. Bennett PV-3P
    B. Bennett PR-2   E. Bennett AP-5
    C. Bennett TV-2P

28. When one is administering IPPB therapy to a patient, why should the patient be instructed to perform an inspiratory hold?

    I. to allow for a better distribution of the inspired gas
    II. to provide more time for medication to settle out of suspension in the inspired gas
    III. to facilitate venous return
    IV. to allow gas flow to move beyond partial airway obstructions

    A. I, II only   D. I, II, IV only
    B. II, III, IV only   E. I, II, III, IV
    C. I, III, IV only

29. Which of the following situations may result in premature attainment of the preset pressure?

    I. sudden development of a pneumothorax in the patient
    II. hyperventilation by the patient
    III. a decreased lung elastance in the patient
    IV. having the inspiratory nebulizer turned to its maximum output

    A. I, II, III, IV   D. II, IV only
    B. I, III, IV only   E. I, II, III only
    C. I, II only

30. Which of the following clinical presentations may be contraindications for IPPB therapy?

    I. loss of sensorium
    II. hypotension
    III. evidence of hyperinflation
    IV. hypoxemia

A. I, II, III, IV
B. II, IV only
C. I, II, III only

D. II, III, only
E. I, III only

31. What is the proper protocol for administering IPPB therapy to a hospitalized patient?

    A. The therapist should be in attendance during the administration of IPPB for all patients.
    B. Once the patient has demonstrated a clear understanding and capability to take a proper treatment, the therapist's presence is *not* required.
    C. Patients who are experienced with IPPB therapy, e.g., COPD patient with home units, do *not* require the presence of a therapist during treatment administration.
    D. The therapist can determine if the patient requires supervision during IPPB therapy.
    E. The therapist should be present only when the physician's order specifies the therapist's presence.

32. Which of the following incentive spirometry device(s) is(are) electronically powered?

    I. Spirocare
    II. TRIFLO II
    III. Bartlett-Edwards

    A. I only
    B. II, III only
    C. I, II only

    D. III only
    E. I, II, III

33. While administering an IPPB treatment with a Puritan-Bennett PR-2 to a patient, the therapist notices that the machine pressure gauge deflects to -2 cm H_2O before the machine is cycled on by the patient. What should the therapist do in this situation?

    A. Stop the treatment to allow the patient to relax and slow down her ventilations.
    B. Do nothing.
    C. Adjust the sensitivity control to allow the machine to cycle on easier.
    D. Reduce the preset pressure because it is probably too high for the patient to tolerate.
    E. Terminate the treatment because the patient's inspiratory effort is adequate; therefore, IPPB probably is *not* indicated.

34. Which statement(s) is(are) true about the relationship between IPPB therapy and body fluid balance?

    I. IPPB administration causes a decrease in circulating antidiuretic hormone (ADH) levels.
    II. IPPB may contribute to the development of both peripheral edema and pulmonary congestion.
    III. IPPB may be associated with a vascular increase in Na^+ concentration when 0.9 NaCl is nebulized.

IV. IPPB may facilitate the drainage of pulmonary congestion via the lymphatic system in the lungs.

A. I only

B. II, III only

C. II, IV only

D. II, III, IV only

E. I, II, III, IV

35. A physician has ordered IPPB therapy for a tuberculosis patient who is in strict isolation. What precautions should be taken before and after the treatment?

    I. A gown should be put on.

  II. Equipment should be properly bagged and left in the room.

 III. All items that were worn should be discarded outside the patient's room.

 IV. A cap should be worn to cover the hair.

A. I, II, III, IV

B. I, IV only

C. I, II, III only

D. I, II, IV only

E. II, III only

36. What is(are) (an) appropriate patient instruction(s) for incentive spirometry therapy?

    I. Perform a sustained inspiratory maneuver.

  II. Sustain a deep inspiration for 5 to 15 seconds.

 III. Repeatedly perform deep, sustained inspirations 8 to 10 times per hour.

 IV. Attempt successively larger inspiratory efforts.

A. I, II, III, IV

B. I, IV only

C. II, III, IV only

D. I only

E. II, IV only

37. What type of ventilatory pattern should a patient with COPD assume during an IPPB treatment?

A. high flow inspiratory phase with expiratory retard

B. slow inspiration with end-inspiratory breathholding and a maximum expiratory effort to residual volume

C. low inspiratory flowrate and a slow exhalation

D. high inspiratory flow and nonforced exhalation

E. high inspiratory flow with expiratory retard

38. Which of the following statements are true about the Bird Mark VII?

    I. When the air-mix plunger is in the *in* position, 100% source gas flows through the machine.

  II. Pressure exerted by the patient back toward the machine increases the F_{IO_2} of the device if the air-mix control is pulled out.

 III. This device is classified as a pressure generator when the air-mix control is pushed in.

 IV. When functioning on air-mix, the nebulizer, if operating, will elevate the F_{IO_2}.

A. I, IV only

B. II, III only

C. I, III, IV only

D. II, IV only

E. I, II, IV only

39. Which of the following statements are true concerning the TRIFLO II incentive spirometer pictured in Figure 94.

    I. When the patient exhales through the mouthpiece, the balls in the three chambers will sequentially rise from left to right, depending on the expiratory flowrate generated.

    II. The magnitude of the patient's inspiratory effort generated through the mouthpiece will determine the number of balls that rise to the tops of their respective chambers.

    III. It is advantageous for the patient to sustain the elevation of the three balls for 3 to 5 seconds.

    IV. The chamber on the far left requires less of a flowrate to cause elevation of the ball than the chamber on the far right.

A. I, III, IV only

B. II, III, IV only

C. II, III only

D. I, III only

E. II, IV only

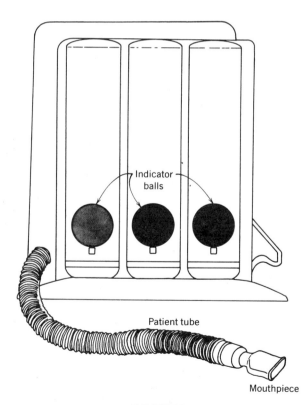

Indicator balls

Patient tube

Mouthpiece

FIGURE 94

40. Which of the following incentive spirometers are volume displacement devices?

    I. Spirocare (model 108B)

    II. Volurex

    III. VOLDYNE®

    IV. Argyle Tru-Vol

    A. II, III, IV only   D. I, II, IV only

    B. I, III only   E. I, II, III, IV

    C. III, IV only

41. Estimate the inspired volume achieved by a 120-lb female patient who is performing incentive spirometry with the Airlife Air™ incentive spirometer. The patient sustained an inspiratory flowrate of 400 cc/sec for 3 seconds.

    A. 350 cc   D. 1,145 cc

    B. 400 cc   E. 1,200 cc

    C. 1,050 cc

42. While administering an IPPB treatment with a Puritan-Bennett PR-2 via O_2 to a patient in the Emergency Room, you notice that the patient is displaying decreased sensorium. What might be the cause of this response?

    A. Relief from hypoxemia usually relaxes the patients; therefore, this is quite common and *not* an event of great concern.

    B. The patient may be experiencing CO_2 narcosis.

    C. The decreased peripheral chemoreceptor stimulation to the medulla often initiates drowsiness.

    D. The patient probably has developed a spontaneous pneumothorax.

    E. The patient is probably being overwhelmed by secretions and requires suctioning.

43. When using a pressure-cycled ventilator, what initial pressure limit is often suggested for a patient receiving an IPPB treatment for the first time?

    A. 5 to 10 cm H_2O

    B. 10 to 15 cm H_2O

    C. 15 to 20 cm H_2O

    D. It is *not* necessary to begin the therapy with any specific pressure limit.

    E. The physician should state in the treatment order the pressures to be used.

44. Which of the following physiologic changes may be associated with IPPB therapy?

    I. The intrathoracic pressure decreases during inspiration.

    II. The blood volume in the thorax decreases during inspiration.

    III. The right ventricular output decreases during inspiration.

    IV. Reduced pulmonary vascular blood volume occurs during inspiration.

    A. I, II, III, IV   D. I, III only

    B. II, III, IV only   E. II, IV only

    C. I, IV only

45. What is the preferred patient position for IPPB therapy?

    A. seated upright   D. supine

    B. prone   E. lateral decubitus

    C. Trendelenburg

ASSESSMENT ANSWER SHEET

DIRECTIONS: Darken the space under the selected answer.

	A	B	C	D	E		A	B	C	D	E
1.	[ ]	[ ]	[ ]	[ ]	[ ]	24.	[ ]	[ ]	[ ]	[ ]	[ ]
2.	[ ]	[ ]	[ ]	[ ]	[ ]	25.	[ ]	[ ]	[ ]	[ ]	[ ]
3.	[ ]	[ ]	[ ]	[ ]	[ ]	26.	[ ]	[ ]	[ ]	[ ]	[ ]
4.	[ ]	[ ]	[ ]	[ ]	[ ]	27.	[ ]	[ ]	[ ]	[ ]	[ ]
5.	[ ]	[ ]	[ ]	[ ]	[ ]	28.	[ ]	[ ]	[ ]	[ ]	[ ]
6.	[ ]	[ ]	[ ]	[ ]	[ ]	29.	[ ]	[ ]	[ ]	[ ]	[ ]
7.	[ ]	[ ]	[ ]	[ ]	[ ]	30.	[ ]	[ ]	[ ]	[ ]	[ ]
8.	[ ]	[ ]	[ ]	[ ]	[ ]	31.	[ ]	[ ]	[ ]	[ ]	[ ]
9.	[ ]	[ ]	[ ]	[ ]	[ ]	32.	[ ]	[ ]	[ ]	[ ]	[ ]
10.	[ ]	[ ]	[ ]	[ ]	[ ]	33.	[ ]	[ ]	[ ]	[ ]	[ ]
11.	[ ]	[ ]	[ ]	[ ]	[ ]	34.	[ ]	[ ]	[ ]	[ ]	[ ]
12.	[ ]	[ ]	[ ]	[ ]	[ ]	35.	[ ]	[ ]	[ ]	[ ]	[ ]
13.	[ ]	[ ]	[ ]	[ ]	[ ]	36.	[ ]	[ ]	[ ]	[ ]	[ ]
14.	[ ]	[ ]	[ ]	[ ]	[ ]	37.	[ ]	[ ]	[ ]	[ ]	[ ]
15.	[ ]	[ ]	[ ]	[ ]	[ ]	38.	[ ]	[ ]	[ ]	[ ]	[ ]
16.	[ ]	[ ]	[ ]	[ ]	[ ]	39.	[ ]	[ ]	[ ]	[ ]	[ ]
17.	[ ]	[ ]	[ ]	[ ]	[ ]	40.	[ ]	[ ]	[ ]	[ ]	[ ]
18.	[ ]	[ ]	[ ]	[ ]	[ ]	41.	[ ]	[ ]	[ ]	[ ]	[ ]
19.	[ ]	[ ]	[ ]	[ ]	[ ]	42.	[ ]	[ ]	[ ]	[ ]	[ ]
20.	[ ]	[ ]	[ ]	[ ]	[ ]	43.	[ ]	[ ]	[ ]	[ ]	[ ]
21.	[ ]	[ ]	[ ]	[ ]	[ ]	44.	[ ]	[ ]	[ ]	[ ]	[ ]
22.	[ ]	[ ]	[ ]	[ ]	[ ]	45.	[ ]	[ ]	[ ]	[ ]	[ ]
23.	[ ]	[ ]	[ ]	[ ]	[ ]						

HYPERINFLATION THERAPY ANALYSES

Note: The references listed after each analysis are numbered and keyed to the reference list located at the end of this section. The first number indicates the text. The second number indicates the page where information about the question can be found. For example, (1:219,384) means that reference number 1 is to be used and that on pages 219 and 384 information about the question will be found. Frequently, it will be necessary to read beyond the page number indicated to obtain complete information. Therefore, reference to the question will be found either on the page indicated or on subsequent pages.

1. D. The respiratory care practitioner should approach the patient from the back side, place her fist on the patient's epigastrium, place her other hand on top of the hand held in a fist, and apply successive compressions to the epigastrium until the patient is relieved. Essentially, the practitioner should perform the Heimlich maneuver in this situation.

   It is also imperative to instruct this type of patient not to generate a cough from the maximum end-inspiratory (total lung capacity) position. Rather, coughing from the mid-inspiratory position may prevent the build up of too great an intrathoracic pressure, thus preventing airway collapse.
   (1:291–292)

2. E. A number of potential hazards and adverse patient reactions may occur as a result of IPPB administration. Some of these hazards and reactions warrant the immediate termination of the therapy. Included are (1) diminished patient sensorium, (2) tachycardia, (3) hypotension, (4) hemoptysis, (5) substernal pain, and (6) paresthesia.
   (3:128–129), (4:409–411), (6:546–548), (44:434,448)

3. D. The objective of the concomitant administration of IPPB and aerosol therapy is to provide for maximum penetration of the aerosol particles into a patient's airways. This method of trying to maintain bronchial hygiene is often beneficial for patients with inspissated, retained secretions and maldistribution of ventilation. However, the mode of therapy must be carefully monitored and evaluated.
   (1:533), (6:540–542)

4. A. IPPB, incentive spirometry, periodic PEEP, and periodic CPAP therapy are all considered methods of achieving lung hyperinflation. IPPB provides an increased volume during the inspiratory phase of ventilation. PEEP and CPAP maintain an increased FRC. Incentive spirometry encourages deep inspiratory volumes. The basis for using any of these therapies intermittently is to prevent the occurrence of atelectasis or to reinflate atelectatic areas. The efficacy of these therapeutic modalities for this purpose have been and will most likely continue to be subject to clinical research.
   (1:556–558), (3:144–147), (4:406–412), (44:451)

5. A. IPPB is generally considered more expensive to administer than incentive spirometry (IS). The real distinguishing cost factor is the equipment expense. Most IS equipment is less expensive than IPPB machines, breathing circuits, sa-

line, and other aerosolizing agents. It can be said unequivocally that IS requires the attendance of respiratory care practitioners. A practitioner must be certain that a patient, once initially instructed, could and would reliably self-administer the IS. The time of the practitioner is not necessarily reduced for IS. Appropriate breathing and coughing instruction must occur with IS therapy. Follow-up therapy is always indicated.

(1:557), (3:145), (44:451)

6. B. A constant-flow generator delivers a constant gas flow throughout inspiration. Lung compliance, chest wall compliance, and airway resistance factors have no influence on the pattern of gas flow delivery from a constant-flow generator.

The ventilation time constant is the product of the value for airway resistance times compliance. The time constant value represents the time required for a volume of gas to fill the lungs. For example,

$$\text{Compliance} \times \text{airway resistance} = \text{time constant}$$
$$V/P \times P/\dot{V} = \text{time}$$
$$\text{cc/cm H}_2\text{O} \times \text{cm H}_2\text{O/cc/sec} = \text{sec}$$

Alveolus A:

$$\text{Pulmonary compliance} = 0.2 \text{ cc/cm H}_2\text{O or } 0.0002 \text{ liter/cm H}_2\text{O}$$
$$\text{Airway resistance} = 2 \text{ cm H}_2\text{O/liter/sec}$$
$$0.0002 \text{ liter/cm H}_2\text{O} \times 2 \text{ cm H}_2\text{O/liter/sec}$$
$$= 0.0004 \text{ sec}$$

Alveolus B:

$$\text{Pulmonary compliance} = 0.1 \text{ cc/cm H}_2\text{O or } 0.0001 \text{ liter/cm H}_2\text{O}$$
$$\text{Airway resistance} = 0.8 \text{ cm H}_2\text{O/liter/sec}$$
$$0.0001 \text{ liter/cm H}_2\text{O} \times 0.8 \text{ cm H}_2\text{O/liter/sec}$$
$$= 0.00008 \text{ sec}$$

Alveolus C:

$$\text{Pulmonary compliance} = 0.3 \text{ cc/cm H}_2\text{O or } 0.0003 \text{ liter/cm H}_2\text{O}$$
$$\text{Airway resistance} = 0.8 \text{ cm H}_2\text{O/liter/sec}$$
$$0.0003 \text{ liter/cm H}_2\text{O} \times 0.8 \text{ cm H}_2\text{O/liter/sec}$$
$$= 0.00024 \text{ sec}$$

Alveolus D:

$$\text{Pulmonary compliance} = 0.2 \text{ cc/cm H}_2\text{O or } 0.0002 \text{ liter/cm H}_2\text{O}$$
$$\text{Airway resistance} = 0.8 \text{ cm H}_2\text{O/liter/sec}$$
$$0.0002 \text{ liter/cm H}_2\text{O} \times 0.8 \text{ cm H}_2\text{O/liter/sec}$$
$$= 0.00016 \text{ sec}$$

Alveolus E:

$$\text{Pulmonary compliance} = 0.1 \text{ cc/cm H}_2\text{O or } 0.0001 \text{ liter/cm H}_2\text{O}$$
$$\text{Airway resistance} = 1.0 \text{ cm H}_2\text{O/liter/sec}$$

$$0.0001 \text{ liter/} \cancel{\text{cm H}_2\text{O}} \times 1.0 \cancel{\text{ cm H}_2\text{O}}\text{/liter/sec}$$
$$= 0.0001 \text{ sec}$$

Alveolus D would take longer to fill than alveolus E. Alveolus B would require the shortest time to fill.

(1:181–184), (4:27–32), (3:36–37), (44:187)

7. A. The following patient parameters should be evaluated and monitored *during* the course of an IPPB treatment:

1. Peripheral pulse (assess cardiovascular status)
2. Ventilatory rate (assess work of breathing)
3. Sensorium (assess for oxygen-induced hypoventilation and response to treatment)
4. Chest auscultation (assess distribution of gas)
5. Breathing pattern (assess work of breathing)
6. Patient's position (optimizes diaphragmatic movement)
7. Observation (assess work of breathing and cardiovascular status)
8. Use of accessory muscles (assess work of breathing)

(6:553), (44:436)

8. E. It is generally agreed that incentive spirometry should be performed hourly. Approximately, 10 deep inflations should be taken each hour. According to some studies, shallow tidal volumes without sighs result in gradual alveolar collapse within one hour.

(1:556), (3:145), (4:411)

9. A. CO_2 re-breathing methods, e.g., re-breathing tubes, paper bags, can result in hypercapnia and hypoxia. It is particularly difficult to control the concentration of CO_2. A disadvantage to the use of CO_2 as a means to induce hyperventilation is that the patient usually experiences an increased ventilatory rate more than an increased depth of ventilation.

(4:412), (44:452–453)

10. A. Some of the classic therapeutic goals of IPPB therapy apply to incentive spirometry. These goals include the prevention of postoperative atelectasis by promoting deep breathing and the prevention of postsurgical pneumonia.

(3:144–147), (4:411), (44:452–453)

11. D. Because PEEP elevates intracranial pressure, it is often inadvisable for patients having cerebral hypertension. The effect would be, in that case, to further compromise cerebral circulation. Cor pulmonale results from pulmonary hypertension. Applying PEEP would potentially aggravate this condition and place more strain on the right ventricle. Patients who are in cardiovascular collapse should be stabilized before mechanical ventilation is even given. Administering PEEP in such a condition could possibly accentuate this problem.

(1:626–627), (3:416–417), (44:625)

12. A. Because IPPB purportedly improves the distribution of inspired air and helps nor-

malize $\dot{V}A/\dot{Q}C$, the Pa_{O_2} may be elevated with room air as the source gas. The improved alveolar ventilation should assist in reducing the Pa_{CO_2}. The force exerted by the positive pressure may be useful in inflating atelectatic areas during the administration of IPPB therapy. If atelectatic areas are reinflated and remain so, the intermittent positive pressure would in effect increase the FRC.
(1:529–533), (4:407), (6:532–533)

13. C. The purpose of using negative pressure exhalation is to reduce the mean intrathoracic pressure to an ambient level after a positive pressure inspiration. As a result of the negative pressure, which reduces the mean intrathoracic pressure more completely than passive exhalation, venous return is improved or, at least, less adversely affected.
(1:516,544–545)

14. D. Incentive spirometry is a respiratory maneuver intended to encourage the patient to take deep inspirations through the apparatus used. The main purpose of incentive spirometry is to prevent atelectasis. By inhaling deeply, the patient is mimicking the sigh mechanism. Incentive spirometry is not specifically intended to elevate a patient's Pa_{O_2}; however, attempting to maintain adequate alveolar ventilation may result in elevating the patient's Pa_{O_2} as a consequence.

IPPB has not been scientifically disproved although its once widespread applicability has been drastically reduced. Incentive spirometry provides a more cost-effective, a more individualized, and sometimes a more effective therapeutic modality.
(1:556–557), (4:411), (44:452–453)

15. E. If a pressure-limited, volume-variable device cycles off prematurely, either the flowrate may be reduced to promote laminar flow or the pressure limit may be increased.

Decreasing the flowrate will increase inspiratory time and decrease ventilatory frequency. Increasing the pressure while maintaining a constant flow increases inspiratory time and decreases frequency.
(1:513–514, 519)

16. D. A mixture of 95% O_2 to 5% CO_2 is commonly used for CO_2-induced hyperventilation therapy. Maximum chemoreceptor stimulation is attained with a 10% CO_2 mixture. The use of higher concentrations can depress the respiratory center (CO_2 narcosis) after the initial stimulation.
(1:484), (44:452)

17. B. Aerosol therapy via IPPB is very inefficient. Only about 10% to 20% of the aerosolized medication will be retained in the body.
(6:541)

18. E. Hemoptysis, the coughing up of blood from the respiratory tract, may take place when the patient generates a cough during the treatment. Hemoptysis may occur in bronchiectasis, bronchogenic carcinoma, and pulmonary infarction.

Because the introduction of positive pressure to the respiratory system increases the mean intrathoracic pressure, pressure in other body cavities (i.e., cranial and abdominal) also increases. The drainage of venous blood from the cranium can become impaired.

Elevation of the mean intrathoracic pressure initially increases left ventricular output. However, sustained elevation of this pressure reduces left ventricular output because of coincident reduction of venous return.

An untreated tension pneumothorax is a respiratory emergency. Continued application of positive pressure may result in a buildup of pressure in the intrapleural space. The lung on the affected side will collapse, and venous admixture and hypoxemia may occur if perfusion to the affected lung continues. Mediastinal veins and arteries may kink.

(4:409), (6:546), (44:434)

19. E. When positive pressure is initially applied, left ventricular output is increased because the elevated mean intrathoracic pressure assists in squeezing blood from the pulmonary vasculature to the left side of the heart. After a few breaths of positive pressure ventilation, left ventricular output decreases because of the depletion of the pulmonary vascular reserve and the reduction of venous return.

Even during exhalation when mean intrathoracic pressure decreases, left ventricular output will remain lower than normal because of the reduced blood volume in the pulmonary circulation and the reduced venous return.

Right ventricular output decreases immediately upon the application of positive pressure because venous return is impaired; that is, less blood is available for the right ventricle to pump into the pulmonary vasculature.

(4:406–410), (44:434)

20. D. The expiratory retard cap on the Bird Mark VII allows exhalation to be prolonged, thereby maintaining an elevated intra-alveolar pressure during exhalation. Unlike PEEP, the use of the expiratory retard cap allows the mean intrathoracic pressure to return to ambient.

Pulmonary edema may be treated by applying increased positive pressure throughout exhalation in an attempt to maintain a higher mean intrathoracic pressure, thus reducing venous return. The application of this modality in the treatment of pulmonary emphysema is an attempt to keep the airways open and to prevent airway collapse (air trapping).

(1:555), (4:440,478–479)

21. B. Usually, less than 20% of the aerosol administered via IPPB is retained in the body. Anterior scintiphotos were used to visualize how much aerosol was retained and the anatomic areas of retention. Approximately, 4.4% of the aerosol was deposited in the mouth and pharynx; 7.7% was deposited in the lungs. About 5.4% was retained in the gastrointestinal tract via swallowing.

(6:541, Figure 23-5)

22. D. Preferably, written physician orders for IPPB should be as specific as possible. Ideally, the order should include treatment frequency and duration, treatment objectives, F_{IO_2}, medication dosages, any special limiting instructions, and maximum limiting pressure. It is the physician's responsibility to determine treatment

parameters and not the therapist's discretion. The use of routine standing orders can cause ambiguity and the administration of inappropriate therapy.
(6:84), (44:436)

23. D. The maintenance of bronchial hygiene is essential in postoperative patients. Therefore, IPPB therapy may be useful in the removal of secretions by improving the cough mechanism. Secretion removal is necessary to prevent postoperative atelectasis and pneumonia from developing. Ancillary therapeutic modalities, such as chest physiotherapy and aerosol therapy, should also be used.
(4:406), (6:538–540)

24. B. Careful observation and monitoring must be used when an IPPB treatment is being administered to a comatose patient, because the risk of gastric insufflation is great. Gas administered at pressures of 15 to 20 cm H_2O can enter the stomach. The respiratory care practitioner must be cautious under these clinical conditions.
(3:131), (4:410) (44:434–435)

25. A. The use of IPPB therapy in the treatment of acute cardiogenic (high pressure) pulmonary edema is controversial. If the left side of the heart fails and depends upon the right side for an adequate preload, IPPB therapy may reduce venous return significantly to cause a drastic fall in left ventricular output. If both ventricles are failing, IPPB therapy may reduce the preload to both ventricles; thus, it may relieve pulmonary vascular congestion. In addition to the physiologic effects of IPPB therapy on cardiovascular dynamics, the amelioration of the general hypoxemic condition of the patient is another therapeutic goal of IPPB in this situation.
(1:551), (3:474), (6:542–545)

26. C. IPPB can result in improved minute ventilation by the administration of greater than resting level tidal volumes. If the patient's work of breathing decreases during the treatment, it should be accompanied by a decreased metabolic production of CO_2. The use of positive pressure may recruit low compliance alveolar units to improve gas distribution, thus reducing the Pa_{CO_2}. The use of an increased F_{IO_2} will not *per se* reduce the Pa_{CO_2}.
(6:536–537, Table 23-1, 544–545), (44:433)

27. E. The Puritan-Bennett AP-5 would be an ideal ventilator for home therapy for these patients when the primary objective of IPPB is the delivery of positive pressure to improve $\dot{V}E$ because the AP-5 has a built-in compressor driven unit and does not require an independent pressurized gas source.
(4:441), (5:269,317–347), (44:444–445)

28. D. Having the patient perform an inspiratory hold at end-inspiration allows more time for the inspired gas to be distributed throughout the lungs and, at the same time, permits gas to move across partial airway obstructions. Additionally, if a medication is being administered, more time is allowed for it to settle out in the respiratory tract.
(1:515–516,555), (4:406), (6:561), (44:437)

29. C. Any circumstances causing a rapid development of back pressure from the pa-

tient's lungs toward the positive pressure device can result in premature attainment of the preset pressure. For example, coughing, decreased lung compliance (increased lung elastance), increased airway resistance (decreased airway conductance), spontaneous pneumothorax, breathing against the machine as the machine is in the inspiratory cycle, patient hyperventilation, and airway obstructions can all cause the machine to prematurely cycle off.

A patient who suddenly develops a spontaneous pneumothorax may show a decrease in the peak inspiratory pressure as indicated on the pressure manometer. As air accumulates in the intrathoracic space, back pressure and peak inspiratory pressure increase. At that point a pressure-limited, volume-variable device will cycle off prematurely.

(1:513)

30. D. Both hypotension and evidence of hyperinflation (air trapping) can be described as relative contraindications for IPPB therapy. Hypotension, of course, implies cardiovascular collapse. Because IPPB therapy elevates the mean intrathoracic pressure, its administration to patients with this condition is contraindicated, to prevent a worsening of this presentation. Air trapping may be aggravated by the administration of IPPB therapy.

(3:128), (4:409), (6:542–551), (44:434)

31. A. A respiratory care practitioner should be in attendance to supervise the IPPB therapy of all patients. Because patients, such as home users of IPPB, may be familiar with the therapy, does not ensure appropriate administration. Also, the risk of hazards associated with IPPB is present for nearly every patient. Additionally, the patient must be coached in proper coughing techniques and breathing patterns. Charting patient responses to therapy and the accomplishment or lack of attainment of therapeutic goals necessitates the practitioner's presence during the treatment.

(1:554–556), (4:408), (6:543), (44:449)

32. A. Of the three incentive spirometry devices listed, only the Spirocare is electronically powered.

(44:454–455)

33. B. If a patient cycles on a positive pressure breathing device by exerting a negative 2 cm H_2O pressure, as indicated on the pressure manometer, the patient is assuming some of the work of breathing, that is, initiating inspiration. Actually, the patient need not exert an inspiratory effort of greater than -3 cm H_2O to initiate inspiration. If the patient "pulls" a more negative inspiratory pressure, the sensitivity control should be adjusted. In this instance no change needs to be instituted because -2 cm H_2O is not considered exertional for the patient.

(44:436)

34. D. IPPB therapy (elevated mean intrathoracic pressure) may result in the retention of fluid secondarily to decreasing venous return and increasing venous pressure. Osmoreceptors of the anterior hypothalamus are stimulated by the increased venous vascular pressure. The hypothalamus, in turn, sends impulses to the posterior hypophysis, which then releases antidiuretic hormone (ADH). ADH causes the kid-

neys to retain fluid, thus complicating the pulmonary edema condition.

Hypernatremia (increased blood sodium concentration) can occur as a consequence of having normal saline (0.9% NaCl) nebulized during IPPB therapy. The NaCl may be absorbed into the lung tissue and enter the blood. Lymphatic drainage may be facilitated by the application of positive pressure to the airways and lungs.

(1:547), (4:248,406), (6:535)

35. A. Administering therapy to a patient in strict isolation requires absolute adherence to isolation procedures. The person entering the patient's room should put on a mask, gloves, gown, and cap. Once the therapy is completed, all contaminated equipment should be properly bagged and sterilized. If the equipment is reusable, it should be left in the patient's room. The protective clothing (gown, gloves, cap, and mask) should be removed, folded inside out (so that the outer surface is covered), and immediately discarded outside the patient's room in a designated container.

(6:446), (44:89,106,247)

36. A. The objective of incentive spirometry or sustained maximum inspiration is to encourage the patient to inspire greater than normal V_T breaths. The inspiratory efforts should be sustained for a period of 5 to 15 seconds to generate increased negative transpulmonary pressures. Initially, the incentives set are rather low. With successive breaths, the patient should increase the inspiratory volumes.

(1:556), (4:411), (44:451)

37. C. Generally, the breathing pattern for IPPB treatments is comprised of slow and moderately deep ventilations. Inspiration should be slow and even to accomplish maximum gas distribution and alveolar ventilation. Lower flowrates will increase inspiratory time. COPD patients should be instructed to avoid forced expiratory maneuvers to prevent small airway closure and air trapping. Short breathholding maneuvers are desirable for all patients receiving IPPB to enhance aerosol deposition and even gas distribution.

(1:554–556), (4:406), (44:437)

38. E. If the air-mix plunger is in the pulled-out position, the source gas will be diluted with entrained room air. With the air-mix plunger pushed in, 100% source gas will be delivered to the patient. While delivering 100% source gas, the Bird Mark VII functions as a flow generator.

When this device is operating with the air-mix plunger pulled out, a number of factors cause the F_{IO_2} to increase. These factors include (1) back pressure through the system created by the patient, thus reducing the effectiveness of the Venturi, and (2) the nebulizer operating on 100% source gas.

(5:269–281), (44:448)

39. E. The TRIFLO II incentive deep breathing exerciser consists of three separate chambers arranged in a series. Each chamber contains a light-weight, hollow plastic ball that rises within the chamber when the patient's inspiratory effort generates a subatmospheric pressure above the ball. The overall magnitude of the patient's inspiratory effort will determine the number of balls that rise in the

chambers. An inspiratory flowrate of 600 cc/sec is required to cause the ball to rise in the chamber closest to the tubing.

To elevate the balls in the middle and far-right chamber, the patient must produce inspiratory flowrates of 900 cc/sec to 1,200 cc/sec, respectively.

Inspiratory flowrates of 600 cc/sec and 900 cc/sec are acceptable, and are intended to promote uniform distribution of the inspired air. However, inspiratory flowrates greater than or equal to 1,200 cc/sec are deemed too rapid to enhance uniform air distribution. Therefore, the patient should be instructed to maintain the ball at the bottom of that chamber. Regardless of the prescribed inspiratory flowrate (600 cc/sec or 900 cc/sec), the patient should be instructed to sustain the ball at the top of either or both of those chambers for 3 seconds.

(TRIFLO II℗ Respiratory Exerciser instruction pamphlet, Cheesebrough Pond's, Inc.)

40. E. The Spirocare (models 108B and 108M), Volurex, VOLDYNE®, and the Argyle Tru-Vol incentive spirometers are volume displacement devices. Each one is pictured and labeled below. See Figures 96 through 98, inclusively, on page 374.

(Spirocare instruction pamphlet, Monaghan Medical Corporation), (Volurex instruction pamphlet, DHD Medical Products), (VOLDYNE® instruction pamphlet, Cheesebrough Pond's, Inc.), (Argyle Tru-Vol instruction pamphlet)

41. E. When using incentive spirometers that measure the patient's inspiratory flowrate (e.g., Airlife Air$_X$℗ and TRIFLO II), the respiratory care practitioner can estimate the patient's inspired volume by multiplying the inspiratory flowrate achieved times the time that the flowrate was sustained. Therefore, if a patient achieved an inspiratory flowrate of 400 cc/sec and sustained that flowrate for 3 seconds, her inspired volume would be about 1,200 cc. That is,

$$400 \text{ cc/sec} \times 3 \text{ sec} = 1,200 \text{ cc}$$

(Airlife Air$_X$℗ incentive spirometer instruction pamphlet, Airlife, Inc.,) (TRIFLO II incentive spirometer, Cheesebrough Pond's, Inc.)

42. B. From the responses available, this patient may be an undiagnosed chronic obstructive lung disease (COPD) patient (CO_2 retainer). This type of patient's only stimulus for breathing is his hypoxic drive. If a high concentration of oxygen is administered to this patient, the hypoxic drive will be obliterated. Consequently, hypoventilation will ensue and CO_2 retention may increase to the point of producing CO_2 narcosis.

The Puritan-Bennett PR-2 operating on air-mix will generally deliver an F_{IO_2} of greater than 0.40. This amount of oxygen may be sufficient to produce a loss of sensorium (CO_2 narcosis) in a COPD patient by eliminating the hypoxic drive.

(1:450–451,555), (3:129), (4:409)

43. B. Generally, most patients are anxious during their first IPPB treatment. To ensure maximum benefit and to minimize hazards, it is preferred that the patient be introduced to the therapy gradually. A pressure limit range of 10 to 15 cm H_2O is often initially suggested so the patient can tolerate the first treatment.

(1:554), (44:436)

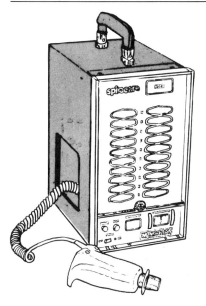

FIGURE 95. Spirocare.

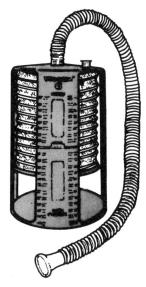

FIGURE 96. Volurex.

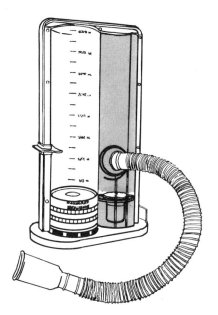

FIGURE 97. Voldyne®.

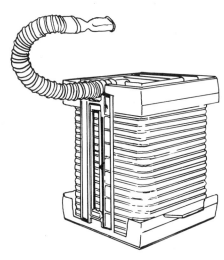

FIGURE 98. Argyle Tru-Vol.

44. B. The application of positive pressure breathing will elevate the mean intrathoracic pressure. As the mean intrathoracic pressure rises, cardiovascular dynamics are influenced. The movement of blood back to the heart is reduced because the venous blood has to flow against a greater amount of pressure than in the case of spontaneous ventilation. By virtue of the reduced venous return, right ventricular output decreases during ventilation and, as a consequence, pulmonary vascular volume is also reduced.

(3:124–130), (4:406)

45. A. For an IPPB treatment, the patient should be placed in a position that least hampers diaphragmatic movement. Most patients should be encouraged to sit upright (Fowler's position is preferable) with the patient's back supported. Variations to this position must be made for those patients incapable of assuming a Fowler's position, e.g., semi-Fowler's. The supine position should be avoided. Ideally, obese patients should stand during the therapy. When an obese patient sits in a chair diaphragmatic movement usually is further limited. A mouthpiece is preferred to a mask. It is more comfortable and can easily be removed for coughing or in the event of vomiting.

(1:554), (44:136)

REFERENCES

1. Spearman, C., and Sheldon, R., *Egan's Fundamentals of Respiratory Therapy,* 4th ed., C.V. Mosby, St. Louis, 1982.

2. Wojciechowski, W., *Respiratory Care Sciences: An Integrated Approach,* John Wiley & Sons, New York, 1985.

3. Shapiro, B., Harrison, R., Kacmarek, R., and Cane, R., *Clinical Application of Respiratory Care,* 3rd ed., Year Book Medical Publishers, Chicago, 1985.

4. Kacmarek, R., Mack, C., and Dimas, S., *The Essentials of Respiratory Therapy,* 2nd ed., Year Book Medical Publishers, Chicago, 1985.

5. McPherson, S., *Respiratory Therapy Equipment,* 3rd ed., C.V. Mosby, St. Louis, 1985.

6. Burton, G., and Hodgkin, J., *Respiratory Care: A Guide to Clinical Practice,* 2nd ed., J.B. Lippincott, Philadelphia, 1985.

7. Frownfelter, D., *Chest Physical Therapy and Cardiopulmonary Rehabilitation, An Interdisciplinary Approach,* Year Book Medical Publishers, Chicago, 1978.

8. Cherniack, R., and Cherniack, L., *Respiration in Health and Disease,* 3rd ed., W. B. Saunders, Philadelphia, 1983.

9. Daily, E., and Schroeder, G., *Techniques in Bedside Hemodynamic Monitoring,* 3rd ed., C.V. Mosby, St. Louis, 1985.

10. Des Jardins, R., *Clinical Manifestations of Respiratory Disease,* Year Book Medical Publishers, Chicago, 1984.

11. Mitchell, R., *Synopsis of Clinical Pulmonary Disease,* 3rd ed., C.V. Mosby, St. Louis, 1982.

12. Comroe, J., *Physiology of Respiration,* 3rd ed., Year Book Medical Publishers, Chicago, 1974.

13. West, J., *Pulmonary Pathophysiology—The Essentials,* 2nd ed., Williams & Wilkins, Baltimore, 1982.

14. West, J., *Respiratory Physiology—The Essentials,* 3rd ed., Williams & Wilkins, Baltimore, 1985.

15. Martz, K., et al., *Management of the Patient-Ventilator System: A Team Approach,* 2nd ed., C.V. Mosby, St. Louis, 1984.

16. Shoup, C., and McHenry, R., *Laboratory Exercises in Respiratory Therapy,* 2nd ed., C.V. Mosby, St. Louis, 1983.

17. Ruppel, G., *Manual of Pulmonary Function Testing,* 3rd ed., C.V. Mosby, St. Louis, 1982.

18. Appelbaum, E., and Bruce, D., *Tracheal Intubation,* W. B. Saunders, Philadelphia, 1976.

19. Rau, J., *Respiratory Therapy Pharmacology,* 2nd ed., Year Book Medical Publishers, Chicago, 1984.

20. United States Department of Health, Education, and Welfare, Public Health Service, *Isolation Techniques for Use in Hospitals,* 2nd ed., Washington, D.C., 1979.

21. Brooks, S., *Integrated Basic Science,* 4th ed., C.V. Mosby, St. Louis, 1979.

22. Comroe, J., *The Lung,* Year Book Medical Publishers, Chicago, 1962.

23. Shibel, E., and Moser, K., *Respiratory Emergencies,* 2nd ed., C.V. Mosby, St. Louis, 1982.

24. Tisi, G., *Pulmonary Physiology in Clinical Medicine,* 2nd ed., Williams & Wilkins, Baltimore, 1985.

25. Cherniack, R., *Pulmonary Function Testing,* W. B. Saunders, Philadelphia, 1977.

26. Altose, M., *The Physiological Basis of Pulmonary Function Testing,* Clinical Symposia-CIBA, Vol. 31, No. 2, Summit, New Jersey, 1979.

27. Shapiro, B., Harrison, R., and Walton, J., *Clinical Application of Arterial Blood Gases,* 3rd ed., Year Book Medical Publishers, Chicago, 1982.

28. West, J., *Ventilation/Blood Flow and Gas Exchange,* 3rd ed., Blackwell Scientific Publications, 1979.

29. Slonim, N., and Hamilton, K., *Respiratory Physiology,* 4th ed., C.V. Mosby, St. Louis, 1981.

30. Rarey, K., and Youtsey, J., *Respiratory Patient Care,* Prentice-Hall, Englewood Cliffs, 1981.

31. Berne, R., and Levy, M., *Physiology,* C.V. Mosby, St. Louis, 1983.

32. Levitzky, M., *Pulmonary Physiology,* 2nd ed., McGraw-Hill, New York, 1986.

33. Wilson, P., Bell, C., and Norton, A., *Rehabilitation of the Heart and Lungs,* SensorMedics, 1980.

34. Clausen, J., and Zarins, L., *Pulmonary Function Testing Guidelines and Controversies,* Academic Press, New York, 1982.

35. Klaus, M., and Fanaroff, A., *Care of the High-Risk Neonate,* 2nd ed., W.B. Saunders, Philadelphia, 1979.

36. Lough, M., et al., *Pediatric Respiratory Therapy,* 3rd ed., Year Book Medical Publishers, Chicago, 1985.

37. Levin, D., et al., *A Practical Guide to Pediatric Intensive Care,* 2nd ed., C.V. Mosby, St. Louis, 1984.

38. O'Ryan, J., and Burns, D., *Pulmonary Rehabilitation from Hospital to Home,* Year Book Medical Publishers, Chicago, 1984.

39. Bell, C., et al., *Home Care and Rehabilitation in Respiratory Medicine,* J.B. Lippincott, Philadelphia, 1984.

40. Wilkins, R., et al., *Clinical Assessment in Respiratory Care,* C.V. Mosby, St. Louis, 1985.

41. Jones, N., and Campbell, E., *Clinical Exercise Testing,* 2nd ed., W.B. Saunders, Philadelphia, 1982.

42. Goldsmith, J., and Karotkin, E., *Assisted Ventilation of the Neonate,* W.B. Saunders, Philadelpia, 1981.

43. Blowers, M., and Sims, R., *How to Read an ECG,* 3rd ed., Medical Economics, New Jersey, 1983.

44. Eubanks, D., and Bone, R., *Comprehensive Respiratory Care,* C.V. Mosby, St. Louis, 1985.

45. Rattenborg, C., *Clinical Use of Mechanical Ventilation,* Year Book Medical Publishers, Chicago, 1981.

46. Witkowski, A. S., *Pulmonary Assessment: A Clinical Guide,* J.B. Lippincott, Philadelphia, 1985.

47. Op't Holt, T. B., *Assessment Based Respiratory Care,* John Wiley & Sons, New York, 1986.

CHEST PHYSIOTHERAPY ASSESSMENT

PURPOSE: The purpose of this 40-item assessment is to evaluate your knowledge of chest physiotherapy (CPT) and clinical ability to position patients for postural drainage, vibrations, and percussion. Aspects concerning breathing re-training, breathing exercises, coughing instructions, and indications and contraindications of CPT are also included.

DIRECTIONS: Each of the questions or incomplete statements is followed by five suggested answers. Select the one which is the best in each case and then blacken the corresponding space on the answer sheet.

Questions 1 and 2 refer to Figure 99.

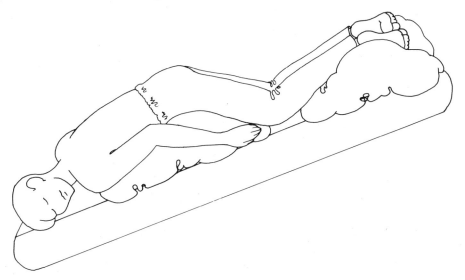

FIGURE 99

1. The patient in the diagram is positioned so that the _____ lobe(s) will be drained.

   I. right lower

  II. left lower

 III. left upper

 IV. right upper

  V. right middle

  A. I, II only   D. I only

  B. III, IV only   E. IV only

  C. V only

2. Which segments of the aforementioned lobe(s) are being drained?

   A. anterior segments   D. lateral segments
   B. lateral segment and lingula   E. superior segments
   C. posterior segments

3. Placing the patient in a flat, prone position with a pillow beneath the abdomen will allow for the postural drainage of which lung segment?

   A. anterior segment of both upper lobes
   B. anterior segment of both lower lobes
   C. posterior segment of both lower lobes
   D. apical-posterior segment of the left upper lobe
   E. superior segment of both lower lobes

4. While overindulging in drink during festivities on December 31, a gentleman, while
   sitting, leaned forward over the bar at the stroke of midnight and began vomiting. All
   the other revelers paid no attention to this bibulous person, who proceeded to aspirate
   a portion of his gastric contents. Which bronchopulmonary segments would most
   likely be involved with the aspirated material?

   A. superior basal   D. posterior basal
   B. apical segments of the upper lobes   E. anterior basal
   C. anterior segments of the upper lobes

5. Vibration of the chest should be applied during which phase of the ventilatory cycle?

   A. inspiration   D. end-expiratory level
   B. end-inspiratory level   E. mid-expiratory level
   C. expiration

6. If a patient aspirated vomitus while lying flat on the right side with the head of the bed
   elevated about 20 in., which lung segment would most likely be the site of involvement?

   A. the medial segment of the right lower lobe
   B. the apical segment of the right upper lobe
   C. the lingula
   D. the lateral segment of the right lower lobe
   E. the anteromedial segment of the left lower lobe

7. Locating a disease process for the purpose of regional postural drainage is achieved
   by which measures?

   I. blood gas analysis
   II. auscultation
   III. pulmonary function studies
   IV. chest radiology

A. I, II, III, IV
B. II, IV only
C. III, IV only

D. II, III only
E. I, II only

8. Which lung segment(s) most often become(s) atelectatic in debilitated patients?

    I. the apical segments of the upper lobes
    II. the posterior segments of the lower lobes
    III. the superior segments of the lower lobes
    IV. the lateral segments of the lower lobes
    V. the segments of the right middle lobe and lingula

    A. I, III only
    B. II, IV only
    C. II, III only

    D. V only
    E. IV, V only

9. In which of the following body positions does the diaphragm move the greatest distance while normal breathing is taking place?

    A. Trendelenburg
    B. sitting upright
    C. lying flat on the left side

    D. semi-Fowler's
    E. supine

10. Which lung segment will be drained by placing a patient flat on the right side with the head tilted downward approximately 45°?

    A. the lateral segment of the right lower lobe
    B. the medial segment of the right middle lobe
    C. the lingula
    D. the posterior segment of the left lower lobe
    E. the cardiac segment of the right lower lobe

11. Which disease conditions generally are indications for postural drainage procedures?

    I. cystic fibrosis
    II. bronchiectasis
    III. empyema
    IV. lung abscess

    A. I, II, III, IV
    B. I, II only
    C. II, III, IV only

    D. I, II, IV only
    E. I, IV only

12. How would you position a patient for the drainage of the superior segment of the lingula?

    A. Place the patient on the right side, one-quarter turn from supine, in a slight head-down position.
    B. Place the patient on the left side in a slight head-down position.

   C. Position the patient on the right side, one-quarter turn from prone, in a slight reverse Trendelenburg position.

   D. Position the patient prone and in Trendelenburg.

   E. Place the patient on the left side, three-quarters turn from supine, in a slight Trendelenburg position.

13. Which statements accurately describe diaphragmatic breathing?

   I. It is the normal breathing pattern.

   II. For patients who are not breathing via their diaphragm, it is best to first instruct them to concentrate on the relaxation of accessory muscles.

   III. During the instructional phase of teaching diaphragmatic breathing, the patient is first encouraged to master the pattern in the supine position, and only then does he practice the pattern in the upright position.

   IV. During diaphragmatic breathing, the patient is instructed to produce prolonged, even exhalations.

   A. II, IV only   D. I, II, III only

   B. II, III, IV only   E. I, II, III, IV

   C. I, III only

14. How should a patient be positioned for effective drainage of the anterior basal segments?

   A. reverse Trendelenburg with 45° elevation

   B. supine with the foot of the bed elevated 45°

   C. lying on the left side, turned three-fourths supine

   D. sitting up and leaning back

   E. flat, prone

15. Which condition(s) may be (a) clinical indication(s) for postural drainage?

   I. prophylactic treatment for a postoperative patient

   II. a patient with a lung abscess

   III. a patient with malfunction of abnormal bronchial hygiene mechanisms

   IV. a patient requiring prolonged bedrest

   A. I, II, III, IV   D. II, III, IV only

   B. I only   E. III, IV only

   C. I, II only

16. Which is the only lung segment that is drained by placing the patient on the same side where the segment is located?

   A. the anteromedial segment of the left lower lobe

   B. the medial segment of the right lower lobe

   C. the apical segment of the left upper lobe

   D. the lateral segment of the left lower lobe

   E. the inferior segment of the right middle lobe

17. Which postural drainage position would allow for the drainage of the apical segment of the right upper lobe?

    A. flat, supine
    B. flat, prone
    C. 30° to 45° reverse Trendelenburg
    D. sitting up with the head of the bed elevated about 45°
    E. lying flat on the right side, turned three-fourths supine

18. Which of the following statements appropriately describe the application of chest percussion?

    I. Hands should be cupped with fingers and thumbs adducted.
    II. The actual percussing of the chest wall should be forcefully performed at a fast rate.
    III. The sternum, clavicles, and areas outside the rib cage boundaries should *not* be percussed.
    IV. A towel may be used to cover the patient's skin, to avoid skin irritation from the percussion.
    V. Thick secretions are best mobilized by postural drainage and percussion as opposed to the sole use of chest vibration.

    A. I, III, V only   D. III, IV only
    B. I, II, V only   E. I, III, IV only
    C. II, III, IV, V only

19. How would you position a patient to drain the superior segment of the right lower lobe?

    A. in reverse Trendelenburg with 45° elevation
    B. in Trendelenburg with 45° elevation
    C. on the left side with feet elevated 45°
    D. in a flat, prone position
    E. in a flat, supine position

20. An order is written: CPT q4h for a bedridden, postoperative, 65-year-old woman. Which statement(s) is(are) true?

    I. CPT is *not* indicated for this type of patient.
    II. CPT should be initiated after the patient is ambulatory.
    III. CPT *cannot* be effective prophylactic treatment for this patient.
    IV. CPT is indicated for this patient.

    A. I, II, III only   D. IV only
    B. I, III only   E. II, IV only
    C. I only

21. Which position will provide for the drainage of the posterior segment of the left lower lobe?

A. flat, supine position
B. flat, prone position
C. lying on the right side with the feet elevated 30°
D. lying prone with the head elevated 30°
E. lying prone with the feet elevated 30°

22. Which of the following statements are true about chest vibration?

 I. It is administered only during inspiration.
 II. Patients may be assisted by a manual resuscitator when taking a deep breath for the maneuver.
 III. Vibration must be performed on every breath during the treatment.
 IV. This procedure is associated with postural drainage.

A. I, II only
B. I, III, IV only
C. III, IV only
D. II, III only
E. II, IV only

23. Which of the segments listed below are individualized on the right lung but *not* on the left lung?

A. apical segment of the upper lobe and the lateral segment of the lower lobe
B. posterior basilar segment and the anterior basilar segment
C. superior segment of the middle lobe and the apical segment of the upper lobe
D. anterior segment of the lower lobe and the apical segment of the upper lobe
E. medial basilar segment and the anterior segment of the upper lobe

24. How would you position a patient for the drainage of the apical-posterior segment of the left upper lobe?

A. Position the patient flat and supine.
B. Place the patient on the right side, one-quarter turn from prone, with the head elevated approximately 30°.
C. Place the patient in a supine position with the feet elevated approximately 45°.
D. Position the patient in a flat, prone position.
E. Have the patient sit up and lean back approximately 45°.

25. What is(are) the precaution(s) asociated with chest physiotherapy (CPT) techniques?

 I. the head-down position for postural drainage, causing decreased intracranial pressure
 II. percussion on a patient with fractured ribs
 III. percussion on a patient with an undrained empyema
 IV. postural drainage for a patient with a lung abscess

A. I, II only
B. II, III, IV only
C. III, IV only
D. II, III only
E. IV only

26. If a patient aspirated vomitus while assuming a flat prone position, which lung segment(s) would most likely become involved?

    A. anterior segments of both upper lobes
    B. posterior segments of both lower lobes
    C. inferior segment of the lingula
    D. apical segments of both upper lobes
    E. posterior segments of both upper lobes

27. How may the effectiveness of postural drainage be evaluated?

    I. patient's subjective assessment
    II. chest auscultation
    III. sputum production assessment
    IV. arterial blood gas analysis

    A. I, II, III only   D. I, III only
    B. II only   E. I, II, III, IV
    C. II, III only

28. What are appropriate instructions to be given to an emphysematous patient for producing an effective cough?

    I. The patient should be instructed to take in the deepest possible breath.
    II. The patient should be instructed to cough from the mid-inspiratory position.
    III. The patient should generate a maximum forceful expulsion of expired air.
    IV. The patient may be instructed to generate a series of rapid, sharp, coughs several times from the end-expiratory position.

    A. I, II, III, IV   D. II, IV only
    B. I, II, IV only   E. I, III, IV only
    C. II, III only

29. How should a patient be positioned for the drainage of the lateral basal segment of the right lung?

    A. prone with the feet elevated approximately 30°
    B. supine with the feet elevated approximately 30°
    C. on the left side with the feet elevated approximately 30°
    D. on the right side with the feet elevated approximately 30°
    E. in a flat, prone position

30. When does the term *splinting* have a negative connotation?

    A. when the patient is taught to support the incision while coughing
    B. when the patient supports the incision during each breath, to avoid pain
    C. if the patient supports the incision during a cough and a therapist is *not* present to assist
    D. when the therapist supports the incision while the patient coughs

    E. when the patient uses a pillow to support the incision, to prevent pain while coughing

31. The term *extraparenchymal* complications includes all the following conditions *except* _____ .

    A. untreated pneumothorax
    B. lung abscess
    C. pleural effusion
    D. empyema
    E. hemothorax

32. The therapist uses cupped hands when performing which therapeutic procedure?

    A. percussion
    B. vibration
    C. postural drainage
    D. palpation
    E. auscultation

33. The patient in the Figure 100 is positioned so that the _____ will be drained.

    A. apical segments of the upper lobes
    B. anterior segment of the right upper lobe
    C. anterior segments of the lower lobes
    D. lateral segments of the right lower lobe
    E. inferior segment of the right middle lobe

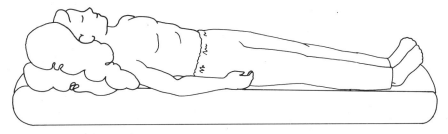

FIGURE 100

34. When a patient is being taught breathing exercises, the therapist's or the patient's hand is sometimes placed upon the patient's _____ to focus on the strengthening of the contractile force of the abdominal musculature.

    A. chest
    B. costophrenic region
    C. epigastrium
    D. gluteus maximus
    E. back

35. Which of the following pediatric/infant disorders or states could be considered indications for CPT?

    I. cystic fibrosis
    II. IRDS
    III. meconium aspiration

IV. preoperative state
V. postoperative state

A. I, II, IV, V only   D. I, IV, V only
B. II, III only   E. I, II, III, IV, V
C. I, III, V only

36. If a patient is lying flat on the right side, which lung is better ventilated?

A. The left lung is ventilated more effectively because it is *not* compressed by the body on the right side.
B. The right lung is better ventilated because the right hemidiaphragm rises higher than that on the left.
C. The right side receives more ventilation because of the angle of the right main-stem bronchus in comparison with the left.
D. The left lung is preferentially ventilated because of the rearranging of the lungs' $\dot{V}/\dot{Q}s$.
E. Both lungs are equally ventilated.

37. Which lung segment(s) represent(s) the most common site(s) for the development of postoperative complications?

I. apical segments of the upper lobes
II. lingular segments
III. posterior basal segments
IV. superior basal segments
V. lateral basal segments

A. I, V only   D. II, III only
B. III, IV only   E. IV, V only
C. II only

38. Which statement(s) is(are) true about the anatomic structure of the lingula?

I. It is a division of the left upper lobe.
II. It is a division of the right lower lobe.
III. It is a division of the left lower lobe.
IV. It is a separate lobe.
V. It has two segments.

A. II only   D. III only
B. II, V only   E. I, V only
C. IV only

39. The anterior segments of the lower lobes are drained when the patient is placed in a _____ position.

A. supine
B. supine Trendelenburg

C. lateral decubitus

D. prone

E. supine, Trendelenburg, lateral decubitus, or prone

40. Which of the following statements are true concerning the lungs?

   I. The left lung has two lobes, and the right lung has three lobes.

   II. There is a total of 18 segments throughout the lungs.

   III. The right lung has 8 segments and the left lung has 10 segments.

   IV. The lingula is part of the left lower lobe.

   A. I, II only   D. III, IV only

   B. I, II, III only   E. I, II, III, IV

   C. II, III, IV only

ASSESSMENT ANSWER SHEET

DIRECTIONS: Darken the space under the selected answer.

	A	B	C	D	E		A	B	C	D	E
1.	[ ]	[ ]	[ ]	[ ]	[ ]	21.	[ ]	[ ]	[ ]	[ ]	[ ]
2.	[ ]	[ ]	[ ]	[ ]	[ ]	22.	[ ]	[ ]	[ ]	[ ]	[ ]
3.	[ ]	[ ]	[ ]	[ ]	[ ]	23.	[ ]	[ ]	[ ]	[ ]	[ ]
4.	[ ]	[ ]	[ ]	[ ]	[ ]	24.	[ ]	[ ]	[ ]	[ ]	[ ]
5.	[ ]	[ ]	[ ]	[ ]	[ ]	25.	[ ]	[ ]	[ ]	[ ]	[ ]
6.	[ ]	[ ]	[ ]	[ ]	[ ]	26.	[ ]	[ ]	[ ]	[ ]	[ ]
7.	[ ]	[ ]	[ ]	[ ]	[ ]	27.	[ ]	[ ]	[ ]	[ ]	[ ]
8.	[ ]	[ ]	[ ]	[ ]	[ ]	28.	[ ]	[ ]	[ ]	[ ]	[ ]
9.	[ ]	[ ]	[ ]	[ ]	[ ]	29.	[ ]	[ ]	[ ]	[ ]	[ ]
10.	[ ]	[ ]	[ ]	[ ]	[ ]	30.	[ ]	[ ]	[ ]	[ ]	[ ]
11.	[ ]	[ ]	[ ]	[ ]	[ ]	31.	[ ]	[ ]	[ ]	[ ]	[ ]
12.	[ ]	[ ]	[ ]	[ ]	[ ]	32.	[ ]	[ ]	[ ]	[ ]	[ ]
13.	[ ]	[ ]	[ ]	[ ]	[ ]	33.	[ ]	[ ]	[ ]	[ ]	[ ]
14.	[ ]	[ ]	[ ]	[ ]	[ ]	34.	[ ]	[ ]	[ ]	[ ]	[ ]
15.	[ ]	[ ]	[ ]	[ ]	[ ]	35.	[ ]	[ ]	[ ]	[ ]	[ ]
16.	[ ]	[ ]	[ ]	[ ]	[ ]	36.	[ ]	[ ]	[ ]	[ ]	[ ]
17.	[ ]	[ ]	[ ]	[ ]	[ ]	37.	[ ]	[ ]	[ ]	[ ]	[ ]
18.	[ ]	[ ]	[ ]	[ ]	[ ]	38.	[ ]	[ ]	[ ]	[.]	[ ]
19.	[ ]	[ ]	[ ]	[ ]	[ ]	39.	[ ]	[ ]	[ ]	[ ]	[ ]
20.	[ ]	[ ]	[ ]	[ ]	[ ]	40.	[ ]	[ ]	[ ]	[ ]	[ ]

CHEST PHYSIOTHERAPY ANALYSES

Note: The references listed after each analysis are numbered and keyed to the reference list located at the end of this section. The first number indicates the text. The second number indicates the page where information about the question can be found. For example, (1:219,384) means that reference number 1 is to be used and that on pages 219 and 384 information about the question will be found. Frequently, it will be necessary to read beyond the page number indicated to obtain complete information. Therefore, reference to the question will be found either on the page indicated or on subsequent pages.

1. A. Placing a patient in the prone position with the foot of the bed/table elevated 18 to 20 in. results in drainage of the posterior segments of the right and left lower lobes.

   (1:657), (6:669), (7:210)

2. C. Placing a patient in the prone position with the foot of the bed/table elevated 18 to 20 in. results in drainage of the posterior segments of the right and left lower lobes.

   (1:657), (6:669), (7:210)

3. E. Placing a patient in a flat, prone position with a pillow beneath the abdomen will provide for the postural drainage of the superior (apical) segments of both lower lobes.

   (6:669), (7:211)

4. C. A person sitting and leaning all the way forward would more than likely aspirate gastric contents into the anterior segments of the upper lobes. Drainage of these segments is accomplished by positioning a patient in a flat, supine manner.

   (6:669), (7:205–206), (8:378), (16:146)

5. C. Chest vibration is accomplished by placing the hands on the chest wall and performing a series of rapid vibratory motions in the arm while gently compressing the chest wall. The therapist instructs the patient to inspire deeply and then performs the chest vibration during the patient's expiratory phase.

   (3:140), (6:665), (7:221), (16:151)

6. D. The lateral segment of the right lower lobe is the most gravity-dependent bronchopulmonary segment when a person is lying flat on the right side with the head of the bed elevated approximately 20 in.

   (1:656), (6:669)

7. B. To determine which lung segments or regions would benefit from postural drainage, the therapist should review the patient's chest radiography reports and auscultate all regions of the lungs to locate the affected sites. Although arterial blood gas analysis and pulmonary function studies may reveal the presence of a disease process, these findings are nonspecific for indentifying the affected lung segments.

   (6:665), (7:203)

8. C. Both the superior (apical) and posterior segments of the right and left lower lobes are the most common sites of atelectasis and pooled secretions because bedridden patients generally assume a flat, supine position (superior segment is gravity dependent) or the semi-Fowler's position (posterior segment is gravity dependent). (1:96), (3:134–137)

9. E. The degree of diaphragmatic movement is influenced by the posture of the patient. In the Trendelenburg position, the abdominal viscera push the diaphragm into the thorax, restricting diaphragmatic excursions. Sitting upright or assuming the semi-Fowler's position results in the downward pull of the diaphragm by the stomach organs. Diaphragmatic movement is least affected by the abdominal contents when the patient is in a supine position. (1:112), (7:9)

10. E. The cardiac (medial) segment of the right lower lobe can be drained by placing the patient flat on the right side in a head-down position with the feet elevated 45°. The medial segment of the right lower lobe is the only bronchopulmonary segment that can be drained by having the patient lie on the same side on which the segment is located. (7:210,215)

11. D. Cystic fibrosis, bronchiectasis, and lung abscess represent general indications for postural drainage. An empyema, pus collecting in the intrapleural space may require surgical removal before postural drainage is instituted. (3:137), (7:201)

12. A. Positioning the patient on the right side one-quarter turn from supine (three-quarters prone) in a slight Trendelenburg (head-down) position will allow for drainage of the lingula. (3:138), (6:668), (7:215)

13. D. Diaphragmatic breathing is the normal breathing pattern. For patients who are primarily accessory muscle breathers, instruction in the relaxation of accessory muscles and proper use of the diaphragm can result in more efficient, less distressful breathing.

During the instructional phase of teaching diaphragmatic breathing, the patient is first encouraged to master the pattern in the supine position, in which it is less difficult to coordinate other movements. Eventually, as the patient masters the breathing pattern, he progresses through sitting, standing, and walking activities that require more coordination. The patient should be discouraged from performing prolonged exhalations. The goal is to move normal lung volumes for the activity involved. For example, sitting requires a lesser tidal volume than lifting objects. If exhalations are prolonged and the patient is "squeezing" out nearly all the air from the lungs, the ensuing inspiratory volume will be quite large. (3:143), (6:660), (8:158–165)

14. B. Placing the patient in a head-down (Trendelenburg), supine position allows for the drainage of the anterior basilar segments. (1:659), (6:669), (7:209), (16:148)

15. A. Postural drainage (PD) involves positioning the patient to use gravity to facilitate the removal of retained secretions. Those patients suffering from retained secretions because of dysfunction of normal bronchial hygiene mechanisms (cough and mucociliary complex) generally benefit from PD.

Assessing patients should include determining whether they may be susceptible to the formation of retained secretions. Essentially, these patients have reduced ambulation; for example, they may require prolonged bedrest or be postsurgical patients. This group of susceptible patients will benefit from the prophylactic implementation of PD to prevent the onset of retained secretions.

Diseases that often require PD to remove secretions include COPD, lung abscess, pneumonia, and cystic fibrosis. Care should be taken to avoid PD on a patient with an undrained empyema (fluid within the pleural space). A lung abscess, on the other hand, is a collection of purulent fluid within the lung parenchyma and may be appropriately drained by PD.

(3:134–137), (7:201)

16. B. The medial segment of the right lower lobe can be drained by positioning the patient on the right side in the head-down position.

(7:210,215)

17. D. When the apical segment of the right upper lobe is to be drained, the patient should be placed in the semi-Fowler's position leaning against the head of the bed elevated 45°.

(6:669), (7:205), (16:146)

18. A. Chest percussion is performed with hands cupped and fingers and thumbs adducted. Cupping the hands provides a cushion of air between the therapist's hands and patient's chest wall, eliminating patient discomfort. The purpose of the procedure is to mechanically loosen retained secretions from the chest wall.

The hands should strike in a rhythmic, alternating fashion. Extreme force should be avoided. Although the rate at which percussion should be performed is questionable, the best approach is to adapt to a rate that is comfortable to the patient.

The therapist should avoid percussing over bony prominences and on areas outside the rib cage boundaries. A layer of thin clothing (T-shirt thickness) should be placed between the patient's skin and the therapist's hand. Heavy material, such as a terry cloth towel, should not be used because the percussion force will dissipate rather than be transmitted through the chest wall.

(1:660), (3:139), (6:665), (7:217–221)

19. D. For the drainage of the superior segments of the right and left lung lower lobes, the patient should be placed in a flat, prone position.

(6:669), (7:215), (16:149)

20. D. Postoperative, bedridden patients are susceptible to accumulating secretions. The implementation of CPT as a prophylactic measure is often used to prevent retained secretions in the patient who is not ambulatory.

(3:137), (6:664), (7:201,220)

21. E. Positioning the patient prone and elevating the foot of the bed 18 to 20 in. (30°)

will allow for the postural drainage of the posterior segment of both the right and left lower lobes.

(1:657), (6:669), (7:210)

22. E. Chest vibration is administered as part of the chest physiotherapy regimen. It is ordinarily administered after percussion. During chest physiotherapy the therapist alternates percussion and chest vibration in an attempt to mechanically loosen secretions from the walls of the airways. Vibration is applied only during the exhalation phase. The patient is instructed to perform a deep inspiration. At the point of end-inspiration the therapist places his hands over the designated area of the chest and tenses his arms to create vibrations that are transmitted to the patient's chest. Gravity is used to assist in these bronchopulmonary drainage procedures.

(1:660), (3:140), (6:665), (7:221)

23. D. The anterior segment of the right lower lobe and the apical segment of the right upper lobe are individualized on the right lung, as opposed to the left lung, where these segments are termed the anteromedial and apical-posterior segments, respectively. Note Table 9 below.

TABLE 9

Right Lung		Left Lung	
Right upper lobe (RUL)	Apical segment Anterior segment Posterior segment	Left upper lobe (LUL)	Apical-posterior segment Anterior segment Inferior ⟶ lingula Superior ⟶
Right middle lobe (RML)	Medial segment Lateral segment		
Right lower lobe (RLL)	Posterior basal segment Anterior basal segment Lateral basal segment Medial basal segment Superior basal segment	Left lower lobe (LLL)	Anteromedial basal segment Posterior basal segment Lateral basal segment Superior basal segment

(6:666), (7:25,29)

24. B. Placing the patient on the right side, one-quarter turn from prone position, with the head elevated 30°, will drain the apical-posterior segment of the left upper lobe.

(6:666), (7:207)

25. D. In evaluating a patient's readiness for CPT, the practitioner should consider whether any precautions against such therapy exist, so as to avoid the therapy or to modify the therapeutic approach.

A full postural drainage (PD) rotation may be contraindicated for certain patients. Of particular concern is the head-down PD position, which may cause a reduction in venous return from the head and a resultant increased intracranial pressure. The head-down position should be avoided for postoperative neurosurgical patients and for patients with intracranial disease. In patients who have an unstable cardio-vascular condition, position changing may add significantly to their distress. PD and percussion should be avoided in patients suffering from extraparenchymal complications, (e.g., pleural effusion, undrained empyema).

Most of the same precautions exist for percussion (e.g., unstable cardiovascular condition, untreated tension pneumothorax, and pulmonary embolism). In addi-tion, particular precautions against percussion include flail chest or fractured ribs, brittle bones, recent skin grafts, and surgical incision areas. The general condition and age of the patient should always be taken into consideration before CPT is ad-ministered.

(1:656–660), (3:137–140), (664–667), (7:203,220)

26. A. The anterior segments of both upper lobes are gravity dependent when a person assumes a flat, prone position.
(6:668–669), (16:148–149)

27. A. Evaluating the effectiveness of postural drainage should be performed consistent with the goals and indications for the therapy. If the indications included secretion removal, secretion characteristics (amount, consistency, color, etc.) would be one criterion for evaluating therapeutic effectiveness. Chest auscultation should be performed to check for improved lung aeration. The patient's subjective assess-ment as to whether breathing has improved is always a helpful indicator in assess-ment.
(16:152)

28. D. Essentially, there are five steps involved in the cough mechanism (1) an inspira-tory effort approximately equal to two-thirds of one's vital capacity, (2) closure of the glottis, (3) contraction of the abdominal and chest wall muscles, (4) opening of the glottis, and (5) a rapid, expulsive exhalation.

However, the type of cough instructions given to a patient will vary according to the patient's clinical problem. An emphysematous patient, for example, runs the risk of experiencing airway closure if high intrathoracic pressures develop when a cough is generated from a deep, end-inspiratory position. Therefore, this type of patient should be instructed to cough from the mid-inspiratory position to prevent the development of high intrathoracic pressure. Alternatively, an emphysematous patient may be told to take a deep inspiration and generate a series of rapid stac-cato-like coughs originating from the end-inspiratory position.

Cough instructions for other types of patients, for example, postoperative thoraco-tomy or laparotomy, include (1) splinting the surgical site with a pillow, (2) as-suming an appropriate posture, (3) inspiring a maximum volume of air, and (4) exhaling as rapidly and forcefully as possible.
(1:660), (3:83,141), (6:667), (7:179–184), (8:149)

29. C. Drainage of the right lateral basal segment is accomplished by placing the patient on the left side with the feet elevated approximately 30°.
(6:669), (16:149)

30. B. If a patient experiences pain upon movement of the chest wall, a reflex response

may be elicited, resulting in contraction of thoracic musculature to avoid painful chest wall movement. This response is referred to as *chest wall splinting* and is a restrictive condition opposing an effective cough.

For patients who experience pain when coughing, supporting the painful area or incision site during the forceful expiratory phase helps minimize the pain. Splinting can be performed with the hands firmly supporting a pillow or blanket over the affected area. The patient should be instructed to perform this procedure without the therapist's assistance so that even when the patient is alone, he can cough effectively.

(3:141), (7:182–183)

31. B. Extraparenchymal complications are those situated outside the lung parenchyma. Pleural effusion, pneumothorax, empyema, and hemothorax are complications involving the pleura and thoracic cavity. A lung abscess, however, is an intraparenchymal complication, that is, a collection of purulent fluid within the lung itself.

(3:137–140), (8:341–351)

32. A. When performing percussion, the therapist's hand must be formed in a cupped manner. Therefore, when percussions are applied to the patient's thorax, air is compressed between the therapist's hands and the patient's thorax, setting up vibrations. These vibrations are transmitted from the thoracic surface to the airways, where they are effective in loosening secretions adhering to the airway walls.

(1:660), (3:139), (6:665), (7:217), (16:151)

33. B. Placing the patient in a flat, supine position (head and knees supported by pillows for comfort) allows for the drainage of the anterior segment of the right upper lobe. The drainage of the anterior segment of the left upper lobe can also be accomplished in this position.

(6:668), (7:205), (16:147)

34. C. The placing of the practitioner's or the patient's hand on the patient's epigastrium helps the patient focus attention on this area while inhaling and exhaling. The purpose of this maneuver is to strengthen the contractile force of the abdominal musculature.

(1:663), (3:143), (7:158)

35. E. Prophylactic implementation of CPT may prevent the accumulation of secretions in postoperative pediatric patients, in patients with cystic fibrosis, and in infants with respiratory distress syndrome (RDS).

Preoperative CPT will most likely vary with the age of the child. Involving the parents in the instructional process may aid in gaining the child's cooperation.

CPT may be effective in removing the residue of meconium aspirate. Although immediate aspiration from the airways is performed, the residue in the distal airways may be difficult to drain.

(3:137), (7:371–388)

36. B. The right lung receives more ventilation than the left because the right hemidi-

aphragm moves farther into the thorax than that on the left side. As the diaphragm contracts, a greater negative pressure will develop on the right (lower) side. (7:10)

37. B. Hospitalized patients generally assume a flat, supine position or the Flower's position (head of the bed raised approximately 30° to 45°). The flat, supine position makes the superior (apical) basal segments gravity dependent, while the Fowler's position leads to the accumulation of secretions in the posterior basal segments. (3:135)

38. E. The lingula is actually the lower division of the left upper lobe rather than a separate lung lobe. The lingula is composed of two segments: superior and inferior. (6:666), (7:24–71)

39. B. The anterior segments of the lower lobes are drained when the patient is placed in the supine Trendelenburg position. This position requires that the patient be placed supine on a table or bed, head downward, with the foot of the bed/table elevated 18 to 20 in. (6:669), (7:209), (16:148)

40. A. The right lung includes the following anatomic features.

> Upper lobe
> apical segment
> anterior segment
> posterior segment
>
> Middle lobe
> medial segment
> lateral segment
>
> Lower lobe
> posterior basal segment
> anterior basal segment
> lateral basal segment
> medial basal segment
> superior basal segment

The left lung includes the following anatomic features.

> Upper lobe
> apical-posterior segment
> anterior segment
> inferior ⟩ lingula
> superior ⟩ lingula
>
> Lower lobe
> anteromedial basal segment
> posterior basal segment
> lateral basal segment
> superior basal segment

(4:63–65), (6:666), (7:24,29)

REFERENCES

1. Spearman, C., and Sheldon, R., *Egan's Fundamentals of Respiratory Therapy,* 4th ed., C.V. Mosby, St. Louis, 1982.

2. Wojciechowski, W., *Respiratory Care Sciences: An Integrated Approach,* John Wiley & Sons, New York, 1985.

3. Shapiro, B., Harrison, R., Kacmarek, R., and Cane, R., *Clinical Application of Respiratory Care,* 3rd ed., Year Book Medical Publishers, Chicago, 1985.

4. Kacmarek, R., Mack, C., and Dimas, S., *The Essentials of Respiratory Therapy,* 2nd ed., Year Book Medical Publishers, Chicago, 1985.

5. McPherson, S., *Respiratory Therapy Equipment,* 3rd ed., C.V. Mosby, St. Louis, 1985.

6. Burton, G., and Hodgkin, J., *Respiratory Care: A Guide to Clinical Practice,* 2nd ed., J.B. Lippincott, Philadelphia, 1985.

7. Frownfelter, D., *Chest Physical Therapy and Cardiopulmonary Rehabilitation, An Interdisciplinary Approach,* Year Book Medical Publishers, Chicago, 1978.

8. Cherniack, R., and Cherniack, L., *Respiration in Health and Disease,* 3rd ed., W. B. Saunders, Philadelphia, 1983.

9. Daily, E., and Schroeder, G., *Techniques in Bedside Hemodynamic Monitoring,* 3rd ed., C.V. Mosby, St. Louis, 1985.

10. Des Jardins, R., *Clinical Manifestations of Respiratory Disease,* Year Book Medical Publishers, Chicago, 1984.

11. Mitchell, R., *Synopsis of Clinical Pulmonary Disease,* 3rd ed., C.V. Mosby, St. Louis, 1982.

12. Comroe, J., *Physiology of Respiration,* 3rd ed., Year Book Medical Publishers, Chicago, 1974.

13. West, J., *Pulmonary Pathophysiology—The Essentials,* 2nd ed., Williams & Wilkins, Baltimore, 1982.

14. West, J., *Respiratory Physiology—The Essentials,* 3rd ed., Williams & Wilkins Company, Baltimore, 1985.

15. Martz, K., et al., *Management of the Patient-Ventilator System: A Team Approach,* 2nd ed., C.V. Mosby, St. Louis, 1984.

16. Shoup, C., and McHenry, R., *Laboratory Exercises in Respiratory Therapy,* 2nd ed., C.V. Mosby, St. Louis, 1983.

17. Ruppel, G., *Manual of Pulmonary Function Testing,* 3rd ed., C.V. Mosby, St. Louis, 1982.

18. Appelbaum, E., and Bruce, D., *Tracheal Intubation,* W. B. Saunders, Philadelphia, 1976.

19. Rau, J., *Respiratory Therapy Pharmacology,* 2nd ed., Year Book Medical Publishers, Chicago, 1984.

20. United States Department of Health, Education, and Welfare, Public Health Service, *Isolation Techniques for Use in Hospitals,* 2nd ed., Washington, D.C., 1975.

21. Brooks, S., *Integrated Basic Science,* 4th ed., C. V. Mosby, St. Louis, 1979.

22. Comroe, J., *The Lung,* Year Book Medical Publishers, Chicago, 1962.

23. Shibel, E., and Moser, K., *Respiratory Emergencies,* 2nd ed., C. V. Mosby, St. Louis, 1982.

24. Tisi, G., *Pulmonary Physiology in Clinical Medicine,* 2nd ed., Williams & Wilkins, Baltimore, 1985.

25. Cherniack, R., *Pulmonary Function Testing,* W. B. Saunders, Philadelphia, 1977.

26. Altose, M., *The Physiological Basis of Pulmonary Function Testing,* Clinical Symposia-CIBA, Vol. 31, No. 2, Summit, New Jersey, 1979.

27. Shapiro, B., Harrison, R., Walton, J., *Clinical Application of Arterial Blood Gases,* 3rd ed., Year Book Medical Publishers, Chicago, 1982.

28. West, J., *Ventilation/Blood Flow and Gas Exchange,* 3rd ed., Blackwell Scientific Publications, 1979.

29. Slonim, N., and Hamilton, K., *Respiratory Physiology*, 4th ed., C. V. Mosby, St. Louis, 1981.

30. Rarey, K., and Youtsey, J., *Respiratory Patient Care*, Prentice-Hall, Englewood Cliffs, 1981.

31. Berne, R., and Levy, M., *Physiology*, C. V. Mosby, St. Louis, 1983.

32. Levitzky, M., *Pulmonary Physiology*, 2nd ed., McGraw-Hill, New York, 1986.

33. Wilson, P., Bell, C., and Norton, A., *Rehabilitation of the Heart and Lungs*, SensorMedics, 1980.

34. Clausen, J., and Zarins, L., *Pulmonary Function Testing Guidelines and Controversies*, Academic Press, New York, 1982.

35. Klaus, M., and Fanaroff, A., *Care of the High-Risk Neonate*, 2nd ed., W. B. Saunders, Philadelphia, 1979.

36. Lough, M., et al., *Pediatric Respiratory Therapy*, 3rd ed., Year Book Medical Publishers, Chicago, 1984.

37. Levin, D., et al., *A Practical Guide to Pediatric Intensive Care*, 2nd ed., C. V. Mosby, St. Louis, 1984.

38. O'Ryan, J., and Burns, D., *Pulmonary Rehabilitation from Hospital to Home*, Year Book Medical Publishers, Chicago, 1984.

39. Bell, C., et al., *Home Care and Rehabilitation in Respiratory Medicine*, J. B. Lippincott, Philadelphia, 1984.

40. Wilkins, R., et al., *Clinical Assessment in Respiratory Care*, C. V. Mosby, St. Louis, 1985.

41. Jones, N., and Campbell, E., *Clinical Exercise Testing*, 2nd ed., W. B. Saunders, Philadelphia, 1982.

42. Goldsmith, J., and Karotkin, E., *Assisted Ventilation of the Neonate*, W. B. Saunders, Philadelphia, 1981.

43. Blowers, M., and Sims, R., *How to Read an ECG*, 3rd ed., Medical Economics, New Jersey, 1983.

44. Eubanks, D., and Bone, R., *Comprehensive Respiratory Care*, C. V. Mosby, St. Louis, 1985.

45. Rattenborg, C., *Clinical Use of Mechanical Ventilation*, Year Book Medical Publishers, Chicago, 1981.

46. Witkowski, A. S., *Pulmonary Assessment: A Clinical Guide*, J. B. Lippincott, Philadelphia, 1985.

47. Op't Holt, T. B., *Assessment Based Respiratory Care*, John Wiley & Sons, New York, 1986.

CARDIOPULMONARY RESUSCITATION ASSESSMENT

PURPOSE: The purpose of this 50-item assessment is to determine the extent of your knowledge, comprehension, and decision-making capabilities related to the theory and clinical application of cardiopulmonary resuscitation (CPR). Included in this assessment are questions pertaining to artificial ventilation, cardiac compressions, patient evaluation, ECG interpretation, pharmacologic intervention, and basic cardiac life support (BCLS) and advanced cardiac life support (ACLS) procedures.

DIRECTIONS: Each of the questions or incomplete statements is followed by five suggested answers. Select the one which is the best choice in each case and then blacken the corresponding space on the answer sheet.

1. Which positioning maneuver of the head and neck will provide an optimal condition for endotracheal intubation?

A. hyperextension
B. flexion
C. sniffing

D. neutral
E. hypoextension

2. Select the types of compression movements that enhance effective closed-chest compression during CPR efforts?

  I. regular
  II. quick jabs to produce quick bursts of cardiac output
  III. smooth
  IV. uninterrupted

A. I, II, III, IV
B. I, III, IV only
C. II, IV only

D. III, IV only
E. I, III only

3. What is the most reliable indication that rescue breathing is inflating the patient's lungs?

A. observing that the patient has lost much of his blue color
B. observing the rise and fall of the patient's chest
C. perceiving little resistance as inflation is performed
D. observing responsive pupils
E. feeling a palpable carotid pulse

4. When is it appropriate to perform endotracheal intubation during cardiopulmonary resuscitation?

A. Intubation should be attempted as soon as possible during the resuscitative effort.
B. Intubation should be delayed until the victim has been ventilated by bag-mask for at least 15 minutes.
C. Intubation should be delayed until a physician determines that an endotracheal tube can be safely passed.
D. There is no guideline regarding the decision of when to intubate.
E. Intubation should be performed after the initial ventilation of the victim has been accomplished via bag-mask or mouth-to-mouth and when the procedure can be performed unhurriedly.

5. Which conditions can be considered complications of closed-chest cardiac massage?

  I. fat embolization
  II. pneumoperitoneum
  III. fractured ribs
  IV. hepatic laceration
  V. cardiac contusions

A. III, IV, V only
B. II, III, V only
C. III, V only

D. I, IV only
E. I, II, III, IV, V

6. Which statements relate to the administration of sodium bicarbonate during cardiopulmonary resuscitation?

   I. Excessive administration of this drug can lead to iatrogenic metabolic alkalosis.
   II. It decreases cardiac contractility as well as corrects acidemia by supplying more sodium ions to the sodium pump in the myocardium.
   III. The use of this drug in correcting the metabolic acidosis is associated with increased arterial carbon dioxide tension.
   IV. It also inhibits the occurrence of cardiac dysrhythmias.

   A. I, III only   D. II, IV only
   B. I, IV only   E. I, III, IV only
   C. II, III only

7. What are the advantages associated with mouth-to-nose ventilation during CPR?

   I. reduced incidence of aspiration
   II. reduced incidence of gastric insufflation
   III. increased $\dot{V}A$
   IV. reduced occurrence of gastric regurgitation

   A. I, II, III, IV   D. II, III only
   B. I, II, IV only   E. I, II, III only
   C. II, IV only

8. Which condition(s) may preclude effective closed-chest cardiac massage?

   I. mediastinal shift
   II. vertebral abnormalities
   III. crushed chest injury
   IV. tension pneumothorax

   A. I, II, IV only   D. I, III only
   B. II only   E. I, II, III, IV
   C. II, IV only

9. You walk into the room to administer an aerosol treatment to an adult patient, and find the patient apparently comatose. You immediately notice that the ECG monitor indicates cardiac standstill. What should your first response be in this situation?

   A. Administer a precordial thump in an attempt to get the heart pumping again.
   B. Perform bag-mask ventilation.
   C. Try to awaken the patient.
   D. Begin one-rescuer resuscitation measures.
   E. Call the hospital operator to alert the cardiac arrest team.

10. Where on an adult victim's sternum should rescuer's hands be positioned for external cardiac massage?

A. lower half of the sternum
B. middle third of the sternum
C. upper half of the sternum
D. lower third of the sternum
E. middle of the sternum

11. Recognition of ventricular fibrillation can occur through _____ .

   I. palpation of an abnormal, racing, thready pulse
   II. observation of consistently wide QRS complexes on the ECG monitor
   III. palpation of a rapid pulse
   IV. observation of distorted and irregular complexes on the ECG tracing

A. I, II, III, IV
B. I only
C. IV only
D. II, III only
E. I, IV only

12. When mouth-to-mouth ventilation is performed on a neonate, what is the potential $P_{I_{O_2}}$ under standard pressure conditions?

A. 159 mm Hg
B. 152 mm Hg
C. 136 mm Hg
D. 128 mm Hg
E. 100 mm Hg

13. What manipulative activities can cause stimulation of the vagus nerve?

   I. intravenous administration of atropine
   II. carotid sinus massage
   III. mechanical stimulation of the pharynx
   IV. an artificial pacemaker

A. II, III only
B. I, II, III only
C. II, III, IV only
D. I, II, III only
E. I, IV only

14. Which statement is *most* accurate regarding the depth of external cardiac compressions?

A. Initially, compress the sternum $1\frac{1}{2}$ to 2 in. and maintain that pattern.
B. Initially, compress the sternum less than $1\frac{1}{2}$ in. and gradually increase the depth $1\frac{1}{2}$ to 2 in.
C. The depth of compressions should be maintained at 2 in. to achieve an effective cardiac output.
D. Initially, compress to a depth of 2 to $2\frac{1}{2}$ in.; then increase the depth by one-third during resuscitation.
E. Maintain the depth of compressions to 1 in. maximum.

15. Which medications are useful in treating cardiac arrest?

   I. epinephrine
   II. calcium chloride

III. lidocaine
IV. isoproterenol

A. I, III, IV only
B. II, III only
C. III, IV only

D. I, II only
E. I, II, III, IV

16. Which statement is correct regarding the use of epinephrine during CPR?

A. If an intravenous line cannot be established, epinephrine can be instilled into the tracheobronchial tree via the ET tube.
B. Intracardiac injection of epinephrine is the preferred route of administration.
C. Absorption of epinephrine after tracheobronchial instillation occurs rather slowly and unpredictably; therefore, this route is *not* acceptable.
D. Epinephrine should *never* be instilled through an ET tube during resuscitation.
E. If tracheobronchial instillation of epinephrine is to occur, the recommended dosage is 5 mg.

17. When is it appropriate to administer a precordial thump?

A. In any cardiac arrest situation.
B. Situations in which the rescuer has witnessed a cardiac arrest.
C. Situations in which the rescuer has witnessed a cardiac arrest on an ECG-monitored patient.
D. It should never be performed.
E. When a patient has a foreign object lodged in a large airway.

18. Which conditions would indicate the performance of a cricothyroidotomy on a cardiac arrest victim?

 I. obstructive laryngeal edema
 II. a noticeable inability to provide adequate ventilation via mouth-to-mouth or mouth-to-nose ventilation
III. deviated nasal septum
IV. diffuse bronchospasm

A. I, II, III, IV
B. I, III only
C. I, II only

D. II, III only
E. III, IV only

19. Under what circumstance is the Heimlich maneuver indicated?

A. When a victim is coughing and breathing with a rapid, shallow pattern.
B. For all respiratory arrest victims.
C. For all forms of airway obstruction.
D. When a victim aspirates a foreign object and loses her ability to breathe.
E. When foreign body airway obstruction is thought to exist in the distal airways.

20. What may be indicators evidencing complete airway obstruction?

    I. gurgling
    II. wheezing
    III. marked use of supraclavicular muscles
    IV. marked use of intercostal muscles

    A. I, II, III IV   D. I, II only
    B. I, IV only   E. III, IV only
    C. II, III, only

21. How many breaths per minute should be administered to an adult respiratory arrest victim?

    A. 60   D. 12
    B. 20   E. 10
    C. 16

22. How should the head of an infant be positioned during mouth-to-nose ventilation?

    A. The infant's head and neck should be maintained in the same position used for an adult.
    B. The head of the infant should *not* be tilted back to the same degree used in the adult maneuver.
    C. The sniffing position should be assumed.
    D. The head of the infant should be completely flexed.
    E. The head of the infant can be placed in either a completely flexed or hyperextended position.

23. What is a disadvantage associated with the use of propranolol during CPR?

    A. It stimulates beta-1 receptors, thereby increasing myocardial irritability.
    B. It can increase the permeability of the pulmonary capillaries.
    C. It can induce hypotension.
    D. It can cause rapid diuresis.
    E. It can rapidly induce a metabolic alkalosis.

24. The increased blood [H^+] associated with cardiac arrest caused by which factor(s)?

    I. hypoxemia
    II. intracardiac medications
    III. iatrogenic intervention
    IV. metabolic acidosis

    A. IV only   D. I, IV only
    B. II, III only   E. II, IV only
    C. I, III, IV only

Questions 25 and 26 refer to Figure 101.

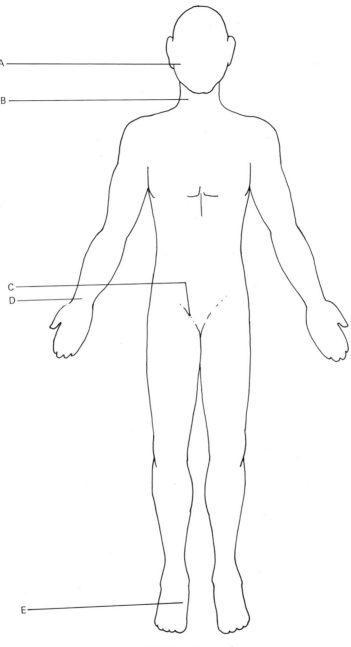

FIGURE 101

25. Which letter in Figure 101 represents the preferred site for pulse palpation when one is assessing for cardiac arrest during one-rescuer CPR?

   A. A   D. D
   B. B   E. E
   C. C

26. Which letter in Figure 101 represents the best site for drawing an arterial blood gas sample during cardiopulmonary resuscitation.

   A. A   D. D
   B. B   E. E
   C. C

27. Which clinical situation(s) might benefit from the application of external cardiac compressions?

   I. sinus arrhythmia
   II. ventricular fibrillation
   III. premature ventricular contractions
   IV. sinus bradycardia

   A. II only   D. I, II, IV only
   B. II, IV only   E. I, III, IV only
   C. II, III, IV only

28. If a monitored CCU patient displayed the ECG shown in Figure 102, what course of action should be taken?

   A. Do nothing at this time, but closely monitor the patient.
   B. Defibrillate the patient.
   C. Commence external cardiac compressions.
   D. Administer isoproterenol to increase the heart rate.
   E. Administer calcium chloride to increase the force of myocardial contractility.

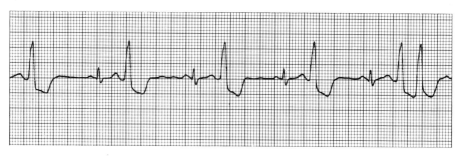

FIGURE 102

29. As a guideline, how much time generally elapses before complete dilatation of the pupils occurs after a cardiac arrest?

A. 10 to 15 seconds

B. 15 to 20 seconds

C. 20 to 30 seconds

D. 30 to 40 seconds

E. 50 to 60 seconds

30. Which of the following cardiac dysrhythmias (Figures 103–106) may cause a decreased cardiac output?

   I.

   II.

   III.

   IV.

A. I, II, III, IV

B. I, IV only

C. I, II, III only

D. III, IV only

E. I, III, IV only

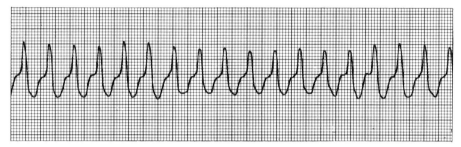

FIGURE 103

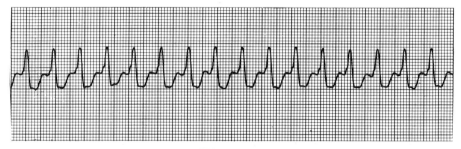

FIGURE 104

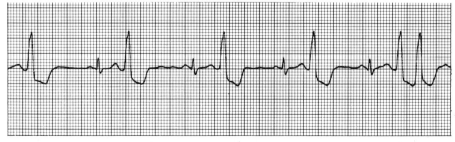

FIGURE 105

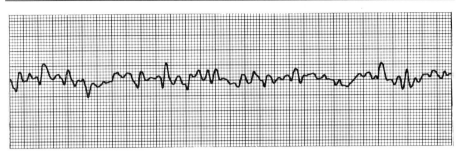

FIGURE 106

31. The respiratory care practitioner enters the room of a 54-year-old patient in the neuro-logic ICU. She observes that the patient, whose neck is in traction, resulting from an automobile accident, is not breathing. Which of the following actions is most appropriate in this case?

A. Place the patient on a partial re-breathing mask operating at 6 liters/min.
B. Establish an airway by hyperextending the patient's head and neck and perform mouth-to-mouth ventilation.
C. Insert an oropharyngeal airway and apply bag-mask ventilation with 100% O_2.
D. Employ the modified jaw thrust maneuver to establish an airway.
E. Release the patient from traction and forwardly displace the patient's mandible.

32. What is the approximate maximum P_{IO_2} that can be administered to a respiratory arrest victim via mouth-to-mouth ventilation?

A. 106 torr   D. 152 torr
B. 135 torr   E. 160 torr
C. 143 torr

33. The respiatory care practitioner has just given an apneic adult victim four rapid, mouth-to-mouth ventilations. He immediately palpates the carotid artery and per-ceives a pulse. What would be the most appropriate action taken by the practitioner at this time?

A. Perform 15 external cardiac compressions.
B. Administer a precordial thump and assess the pulse once again.
C. Continue performing mouth-to-mouth ventilations at a rate of 12 breaths/min.
D. Assess cerebral circulation by noting pupil status.
E. Check the airway for the presence of a foreign object.

34. Ordinarily, CPR should *not* be interrupted for more than 5 seconds. What are the ex-ceptions to this guideline?

I. To evaluate cerebral circulation by observing pupil status.
II. To perform endotracheal intubation.
III. To transport the patient to a more convenient site if the present one is *not* condu-cive to effective CPR procedures.

IV. To align the head, neck, and chest when the victim is suspected of having spinal cord damage.

A. III, IV only

B. II, III only

C. II, III, IV only

D. I, IV only

E. I, II only

35. What is the purpose of performing the Heimlich maneuver?

A. It reestablishes circulation.

B. It is a technique devised to relieve gastric distention.

C. It is a procedure to relieve large-airway obstruction.

D. It prevents aspiration of stomach contents.

E. It is used to get the heart beating again, much like defibrillation.

36. What blood pressure can usually be achieved by properly applied external cardiac compressions on an adult victim?

A. systolic pressure: 100 mm Hg; diastolic pressure: 0 mm Hg

B. systolic pressure: 70 mm Hg; diastolic pressure: 10 mm Hg

C. systolic pressure: 60 mm Hg; diastolic pressure: 10 mm Hg

D. systolic pressure: 50 mm Hg; diastolic pressure: 30 mm Hg

E. systolic pressure: 40 mm Hg; diastolic pressure: 40 mm Hg

37. Which cardiac condition or dysrhythmia is represented by the electrocardiogram shown in Figure 107?

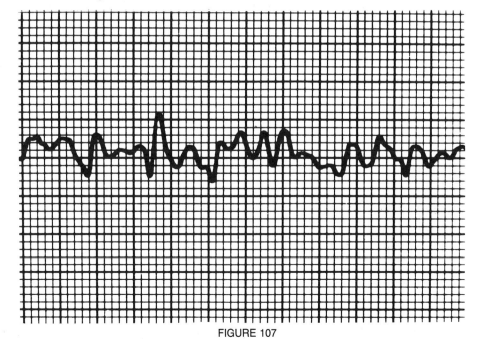

FIGURE 107

A. ventricular tachycardia

B. atrial fibrillation

C. right ventricular hypertrophy

D. premature ventricular contractions

E. ventricular fibrillation

38. If a cardiac arrest victim had a 5 liter/min cardiac output before his arrest, what cardiac output would be reasonable to expect from properly performed external cardiac compressions?

A. 5.00 liters/min

B. 3.00 to 3.75 liters/min

C. 2.50 to 3.00 liters/min

D. 1.75 to 2.50 liters/min

E. 1.25 to 1.75 liters/min

39. Upon entering a patient's room to perform chest physiotherapy, a respiratory care practitioner discovers that the patient is unconscious. What should be the correct sequence of actions conducted by the practitioner?

A. Call for help, establish the airway, establish unresponsiveness, establish breathlessness, and begin ventilation.

B. Establish unresponsiveness, establish breathlessness, call for help, establish the airway, and begin ventilation.

C. Establish breathlessness, establish unresponsiveness, call for help, establish the airway, and begin ventilation.

D. Establish unresponsiveness, call for help, establish the airway, establish breathlessness, and begin ventilation.

E. Establish unresponsiveness, establish the airway, establish breathlessness, call for help, and begin ventilation.

40. An orally intubated cardiac arrest victim is being manually resuscitated at a rate of 22 inflations/min via a 1200-cc resuscitation bag with an F_{IO_2} of 0.95. An arterial blood gas is drawn 30 minutes into the procedure. The data reveal a Pa_{CO_2} of 50 torr. What is a possible cause of this high Pa_{CO_2}?

A. More $NaHCO_3$ needs to be given.

B. The number of cardiac compressions may need to be increased.

C. The ventilation rate may have been inadequate.

D. The volume provided by the manual resuscitator may have been inadequate.

E. The high F_{IO_2} may be causing ventilatory depression.

41. Which of the following statements are true concerning two-rescuer CPR?

I. The person performing the compressions initiates the command to switch.

II. Immediately before ventilating, the person who was previously compressing should feel for a carotid pulse for no more than 5 seconds.

III. Before switching to do compressions, the person ventilating should evaluate pupil status and establish breathlessness.

IV. If a pulse is perceived before the switch, the two persons performing CPR should *not* switch and continue their respective duties.

A. II, III, IV only
B. I, III only
C. II, IV only

D. I, II, IV only
E. I, II only

42. Which of the following situations warrant the termination of CPR?

   I. When the victim becomes clinically dead.
   II. When the rescuer becomes exhausted and is unable to continue.
   III. When the victim's pupils remain fixed and dilated.
   IV. When spontaneous ventilation and circulation are restored.

A. II, IV only
B. II, III, IV only
C. II, III only

D. I, II, IV only
E. I, III only

43. An ECG-monitored, 10-month-old girl weighing 13 lb is in ventricular fibrillation. Medical personnel are about to defibrillate the infant for the first time. What energy level on the defibrillator would you recommend in this situation?

A. 2 joules
B. 4 joules
C. 12 joules

D. 18 joules
E. 20 joules

44. While assessing for the presence of a cardiac arrest on a one year-old boy, the respiratory care practitioner experiences difficulty attempting to palpate the carotid pulse because the infant has a short, fat neck. Which is the *most* appropriate action for the practitioner to take at this time?

A. Palpate the brachial pulse to assess circulatory status.
B. Listen over the precordium to evaluate cardiac activity.
C. Palpate the dorsalis pedis to assess the infant's circulatory status.
D. Assume the presence of a cardiac arrest, and begin ventilations and compressions.
E. Examine the pupils to determine circulatory status.

45. For neonates, external cardiac compressions are indicated when _____ .

A. the 1-minute Apgar score is 9.
B. the 1-minute Apgar score is 5, and the 5-minute Apgar score is 8.
C. the 1-minute Apgar score is 7.
D. the 1-minute Apgar score is 1, and the 5-minute Apgar score is 2.
E. the 1 minute Apgar score is 4, and the 5-minute Apgar score is 9.

46. A respiratory care practitioner is babysitting his 20-month-old niece. Being the good uncle that he is, he hands her a bag of peanuts that he bought for her at the circus that day. While eating the peanuts, the girl suddenly begins forcefully coughing and wheezing. What should uncle respiratory therapist do at this time?

A. He should *not* attempt to remove the peanut because his niece is still gas exchanging.

B. He should pick her up and deliver four blows with his hand to her back to dislodge the peanut.

C. He should insert his first and index fingers into his niece's airway to extract the peanut.

D. He should perform a modified Heimlich maneuver since the victim is a baby.

E. He should immediately begin mouth-to-nose ventilation.

47. Which statement(s) is(are) true concerning basic life support of a near drowning victim?

   I. *No* resuscitation efforts should be attempted while both the rescuer and victim are in the water.
   II. External chest compressions should always be initiated as soon as possible, even while the victim is still in the water.
   III. Artificial ventilation should always be initiated as soon as possible, even while the victim is still in the water.
   IV. The rescuer should *not* place himself at great risk to get to the victim.

   A. I only
   B. I, IV only
   C. II, III, IV only
   D. III only
   E. III, IV only

48. Which of the following statements are potential advantages of an esophageal obturator?

   I. It can be easily inserted by untrained personnel.
   II. Direct visualization of the upper airway is usually *not* necessary.
   III. A tight seal is easily obtained when a mask is placed over the face when an esophageal obturator is present.
   IV. It is easier to insert than an endotracheal tube.

   A. I, IV only
   B. II, IV only
   C. I, III only
   D. II, III only
   E. II, III, IV only

49. Which statement best describes the universal sign of choking?

   A. The victim will exhibit peripheral cyanosis.
   B. The victim will have an aimless look in his eyes and be diaphoretic.
   C. The victim will grasp his neck in the laryngeal area.
   D. The victim will cough forcefully and begin wheezing.
   E. The victim's voice will become hoarse or raspy.

50. Which electrocardiogram (Figures 108–112) reflects a dysrhythmia indicating a need for immediate defibrillation?

A.

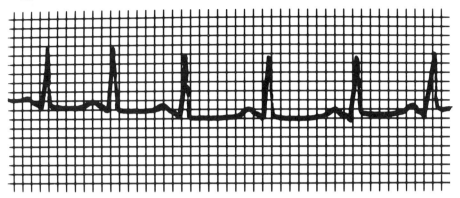

FIGURE 108

B.

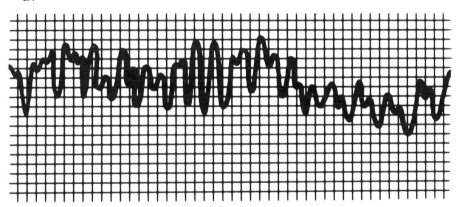

FIGURE 109

C.

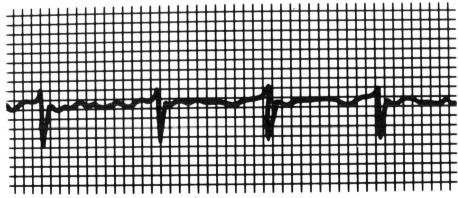

FIGURE 110

D.

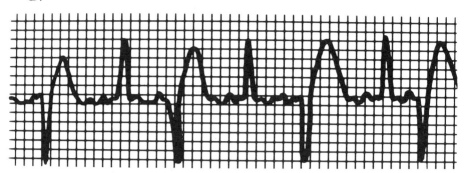

FIGURE 111

E.

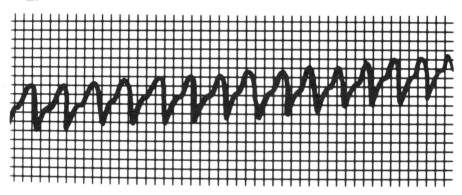

FIGURE 112

ASSESSMENT ANSWER SHEET

DIRECTIONS: Darken the space under the selected answer.

	A	B	C	D	E		A	B	C	D	E
1.	[ ]	[ ]	[ ]	[ ]	[ ]	26.	[ ]	[ ]	[ ]	[ ]	[ ]
2.	[ ]	[ ]	[ ]	[ ]	[ ]	27.	[ ]	[ ]	[ ]	[ ]	[ ]
3.	[ ]	[ ]	[ ]	[ ]	[ ]	28.	[ ]	[ ]	[ ]	[ ]	[ ]
4.	[ ]	[ ]	[ ]	[ ]	[ ]	29.	[ ]	[ ]	[ ]	[ ]	[ ]
5.	[ ]	[ ]	[ ]	[ ]	[ ]	30.	[ ]	[ ]	[ ]	[ ]	[ ]
6.	[ ]	[ ]	[ ]	[ ]	[ ]	31.	[ ]	[ ]	[ ]	[ ]	[ ]
7.	[ ]	[ ]	[ ]	[ ]	[ ]	32.	[ ]	[ ]	[ ]	[ ]	[ ]
8.	[ ]	[ ]	[ ]	[ ]	[ ]	33.	[ ]	[ ]	[ ]	[ ]	[ ]
9.	[ ]	[ ]	[ ]	[ ]	[ ]	34.	[ ]	[ ]	[ ]	[ ]	[ ]
10.	[ ]	[ ]	[ ]	[ ]	[ ]	35.	[ ]	[ ]	[ ]	[ ]	[ ]
11.	[ ]	[ ]	[ ]	[ ]	[ ]	36.	[ ]	[ ]	[ ]	[ ]	[ ]
12.	[ ]	[ ]	[ ]	[ ]	[ ]	37.	[ ]	[ ]	[ ]	[ ]	[ ]
13.	[ ]	[ ]	[ ]	[ ]	[.]	38.	[ ]	[ ]	[ ]	[ ]	[ ]
14.	[ ]	[ ]	[ ]	[ ]	[ ]	39.	[ ]	[ ]	[ ]	[ ]	[ ]
15.	[ ]	[ ]	[ ]	[ ]	[ ]	40.	[ ]	[ ]	[ ]	[ ]	[ ]
16.	[ ]	[ ]	[ ]	[ ]	[ ]	41.	[ ]	[ ]	[ ]	[ ]	[ ]
17.	[ ]	[ ]	[ ]	[ ]	[ ]	42.	[ ]	[ ]	[ ]	[ ]	[ ]
18.	[ ]	[ ]	[ ]	[ ]	[ ]	43.	[ ]	[ ]	[ ]	[ ]	[ ]
19.	[ ]	[ ]	[ ]	[ ]	[ ]	44.	[ ]	[ ]	[ ]	[ ]	[ ]
20.	[ ]	[ ]	[ ]	[ ]	[ ]	45.	[ ]	[ ]	[ ]	[ ]	[ ]
21.	[ ]	[ ]	[ ]	[ ]	[ ]	46.	[ ]	[ ]	[ ]	[ ]	[ ]
22.	[ ]	[ ]	[ ]	[ ]	[ ]	47.	[ ]	[ ]	[ ]	[ ]	[ ]
23.	[ ]	[ ]	[ ]	[ ]	[ ]	48.	[ ]	[ ]	[ ]	[ ]	[ ]
24.	[ ]	[ ]	[ ]	[ ]	[ ]	49	[ ]	[ ]	[ ]	[ ]	[ ]
25.	[ ]	[ ]	[ ]	[ ]	[ ]	50.	[ ]	[ ]	[ ]	[ ]	[ ]

CARDIOPULMONARY RESUSCITATION ANALYSES

Note: The references listed after each analysis are numbered and keyed to the reference list located at the end of this section. The first number indicates the text. The second number indicates the page where information about the question will be found. For example, (1:219,384) means that reference number 1 is to be used and that on pages 219 and 384 information about the question will be found. Frequently, it will be necessary to read beyond the page number indicated to obtain complete information. Therefore, reference to the question will be found either on the page indicated or on subsequent pages.

1. C. The sniffing position, or modified Jackson position, provides the optimal condition for endotracheal intubation because of the minimal angulation between the pharyngeal and tracheal planes. The application of finger pressure on the thyroid cartilage may further serve to optimize the angle for easier intubation.
   (3:223), (6:906–909)

2. B. The effectiveness of external cardiac compressions is the presence of a palpable carotid or femoral pulse. The presence of a pulse results from an adequate stroke volume and rate producing effective cardiac output. Quick jabs increase the possibility of injury and do not enhance stroke volume. The compression movements should be regular, smooth, and uninterrupted.
   (6:922), (30:244)

3. B. The most reliable indication that rescue breathing (e.g., mouth-to-mouth) is inflating the patient's lungs is to observe the rise and fall of the victim's chest. Chest excursions can only be the result of increased lung volume. Although the resistance characteristics of the lungs as they expand are a useful indicator, they are not the most reliable. Inflation of the lungs may still be achieved even in the presence of increased resistance.
   (6:906,913), (30:245)

4. E. The first concern when ventilating during CPR is to provide oxygenated air to the victim as quickly as possible. Mouth-to-mouth or bag-mask ventilation can accomplish this end more quickly than ET intubation in most circumstances. Consuming time to intubate upon finding a victim is contrary to basic principles of ventilating during CPR. Once the early stages of CPR have passed and intubation can be accomplished in a controlled manner, maintenance of a patent airway is best accomplished with the insertion of an ET tube.
   (3:230), (6:905,911,914), (30:244–245)

5. E. Perhaps the greatest number of complications results from external cardiac compression. Failure to locate the proper compression site or applying pressure with the fingers and palm of the hand may produce rib fractures. The broken ends of the fractured ribs may penetrate lung tissue or lacerate the liver. The compressions of the rib cage may result in small fractures of the ribs and sternum allowing fat from the bone marrow to enter venous circulation. If the esophageal or gastric wall ruptures, air is allowed to enter the peritoneal cavity (pneumoperitoneum). This condition elevates abdominal pressure, creating further resistance to ventila-

tion. Too much pressure exerted on the sternum and the application of chest compressions for too long a period may cause cardiac contusions.
(6:928), (30:249)

6. A. When the salt of a weak acid and the weak acid itself are dissolved in the same solution, the solution has the ability to react with both bases and acids. Small additions of either acids or bases produce little change in the pH of a buffer solution. Physiologically, the body has such a buffer system. Sodium bicarbonate ($NaHCO_3$) is a salt of a weak acid, and carbonic acid (H_2CO_3) is a weak acid. When a cardiac arrest occurs, biologic death does not immediately ensue. The cells of the body continue to metabolize. However, they do so via the anaerobic route, producing lactic acid as one of their metabolites. The CO_2 levels increase because ventilation and gas exchange have ceased. The accumulation of CO_2 ($H_2CO_3 \leftrightharpoons CO_2 + H_2O$) and lactic acid depletes the body's store of $NaHCO_3$ essential for effective physiologic buffering. In this clinical condition exogenous $NaHCO_3$ must be administered to alleviate the acidosis by replenishing the body's buffer stores.

Excessive administration of $NaHCO_3$ can result in medically induced (iatrogenic) metabolic alkalosis. During CPR, ventilation must be adequate, of course, to eliminate the increased CO_2 from $NaHCO_3$ administration.

$$HCO_3^- + H^+ \rightleftharpoons H_2CO_3 \rightleftharpoons H_2O + CO_2$$

The law of mass action favors this reaction to the right in this situation.
(1:216), (2:80–81,84–85), (6:934)

7. B. The occurrence of gastric inflation depends on the pressure in the upper airways. When this pressure exceeds 25 cm H_2O, gastric inflation is uniformly produced. Gastric insufflation rarely occurs with inflation pressures less than 15 cm H_2O. Ventilating via the nasal route produces an increased resistance to airflow, thereby generating a reduction of the pressure in the pharynx and at the gastric cardia. If gastric insufflation is reduced, gastric regurgitation and aspiration will also be reduced. Improvement in $\dot{V}A$ is not an expected outcome of nasal insufflation.
(6:914)

8. E. The effectiveness of closed-chest cardiac massage is largely associated with the ability to adequately compress the heart between the sternum and the vertebrae. Conditions, such as marked scoliosis, kyphosis, pectus excavatum, and pectus carinatum, may preclude external massage because adequate compression cannot occur between these structures. Pathologic states causing a shift of the mediastinum cause similar difficulties.
(6:930–933), (30:247)

9. D. Assuming that all ECG leads are intact and that the monitor is functioning properly, there is no need to attempt to arouse the patient. Once pulselessness and the absence of spontaneous ventilations have been determined, the first step is to begin one-rescuer CPR. A precordial thump is inappropriate in this case because the rescuer did not witness the arrest. Upon initiating CPR, the rescuer should attempt to call for help.
(6:912,926), (11:94)

10. D. To perform external cardiac massage, the rescuer places the base of the palm of the hand on the lower third of the victim's sternum.
(6:922), (11:94–95), (30:244)

11. C. An ECG tracing (Figure 113) indicating ventricular fibrillation demonstrates complete distortion and irregularity of the complexes. No palpable pulse is present during ventricular fibrillation. During ventricular tachycardia the ECG displays a rapid rate and wide QRS complexes.
(1:255–256), (30:250,377), (33:35–36)

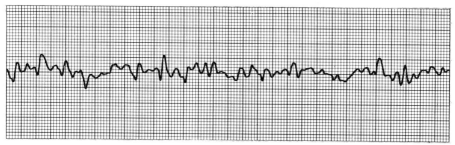

FIGURE 113

12. B. When mouth-to-mouth ventilation is performed on a neonate, the person performing the ventilation does not exhale a large tidal volume into the neonate's lungs. Rather, air from the rescuer's mouth and nose usually is adequate for ventilation of the neonate.

Air in the rescuer's oral and nasal cavities is approximately 80% humidified at body temperature.

STEP 1: Calculate the partial pressure of water vapor (P_{H_2O}) in the rescuer's expirate (content) by using the formula

$$content = \frac{(relative\ humidity)(capacity)}{100}$$
$$= \frac{(80\%)(47\ mm\ Hg)}{100}$$
$$= (0.80)(47\ mm\ Hg)$$
$$= 37\ mm\ Hg$$

STEP 2: Determine the corrected barometric pressure.

$$corrected\ P_B = P_B - P_{H_2O}$$
$$= 760\ mm\ Hg - 37\ mm\ Hg$$
$$= 723\ mm\ Hg$$

STEP 3: Calculate the partial pressure of the inspired oxygen ($P_{I_{O_2}}$).

$$P_{I_{O_2}} = (corrected\ P_B)(F_{I_{O_2}})$$
$$= (723\ mm\ Hg)(0.21)$$
$$= 152\ mm\ Hg$$

(4:22–23), (6:912)

13. A. Activation of vagal reflexes may lead to cardiac arrest. Intravenous administration of atropine inhibits the vagus nerve, thus increasing the heart rate. An artificial pacemaker can do the same. Carotid massage, used for persistent paroxysmal atrial tachycardia (PAT), stimulates the vagus nerve, thereby slowing the heart rate. Vagal stimulation may result from pharyngeal initiation, e.g., excessive movement of the ET tube within the pharynx and trachea.
   (1:258), (3:232), (4:382), (33:21–24)

14. B. Beginning with shallow depressions of the sternum and gradually increasing the depth of compressions allows the sternum and rib cage to become slightly more mobile and elastic. This approach may reduce the incidence of complications associated with closed-chest compression, e.g., rib fractures, soft tissue injuries. The sternum should eventually be depressed $1\frac{1}{2}$ to 2 in. for effective compression.
   (6:922–923)

15. E. The objectives governing the selection of pharmacologic agents for use during cardiac arrest are (1) to increase cardiac output, (2) to strengthen myocardial contractility, and (3) to provide effective circulatory volume.
   Epinephrine, a sympathomimetic catecholamine, increases myocardial contractility (positive inotropism). Isuprel (isoproterenol hydrochloride) is a potent cardiac stimulant, increasing heart rate and stroke volume producing an overall increase in the cardiac output (positive chronotropism). Isuprel is also effective in correcting bradycardia and hypotension. Calcium chloride effectively increases myocardial contractility. Calcium gluconate also may be administered alternatively to increase cardiac output. Because the myocardium is especially irritable during a cardiac arrest, it is important to reduce ventricular irritablity. Lidocaine is a commonly used antiarrhythmic drug.
   (4:536–537,556), (6:933–937)

16. A. Epinephrine increases myocardial contractility and perfusion pressures. Epinephrine is promptly absorbed after tracheobronchial instillation via the ET tube. The recommended dose is 1 mg (10 ml of the 1:10,000 solution). If an intravenous route cannot be established and an ET tube is in place (or can be quickly inserted), the tracheobronchial administration route should be used. Intracardiac injection should only be used when other routes are unavailable.
   (6:935–936)

17. C. While the precordial thump is no longer recommended for use as a basic life support technique, it has been shown to be effective in evoking ventricular depolarization with associated myocardial contraction in asystole. When the thump is delivered early after the onset of ventricular tachycardia and ventricular fibrillation, it has been demonstrated to restore a sinus rhythm. It is recommended for use exclusively in the setting of ECG-monitored patients and is not recommended in pediatric patients.
   (6:926), (30:244)

18. C. Any situation that does not allow for ventilation to occur (e.g., laryngeal edema, extensive facial trauma) is an indication for the use of the cricothyroidotomy procedure on cardiac arrest victims. Similarly, conditions preventing the passage

and/or insertion of ancillary airway equipment warrant consideration of this emergency airway procedure.

(3:227), (4:385–386), (6:919)

19. D. The Heimlich maneuver is indicated when one witnesses a victim experiencing sudden airway obstruction caused by the aspiration of a foreign object which results in the absence of the victim's ability to cough, breathe, or speak. The victim also displays the universal sign of choking, and frequently becomes cyanotic and collapses. Two to four back blows should be quickly delivered, and if ineffective, followed by a series of four to six compressions to the victim's upper abdomen (epigastrium).

(6:911–912)

20. E. The absence of any sounds of air flow is a primary indication of complete airway obstruction. If the airway obstruction is partial, the intensity of air flow sounds will vary with the degree (severity) of the obstruction. Victims may demonstrate marked efforts to breathe, e.g., the use of accessory muscles of ventilation.

(6:907)

21. D. Twelve breaths per minute is considered adequate for adults in respiratory arrest. This rate averages one breath every 5 seconds.

(6:913)

22. B. Because an infant's neck and upper airway structures are more pliable than those of an adult, an infant's head should not be tilted back as far when positioning an infant victim for mouth-to-nose ventilation. Hyperextension of an infant's neck can produce airway obstruction or make ventilation less effective.

(6:914)

23. C. Propranolol (Indural) is a beta-blocker. It has a negative inotropic and negative chronotropic effect on the myocardium. Problems associated with its use during CPR include bronchoconstriction (potentially problematic for COPD patients) and hypotension caused by a decreased cardiac output. Its intended purpose during CPR is to reduce the occurence of dysrhythmias.

(6:937)

24. D. The increased [H^+] associated with cardiac arrest is caused by accumulating arterial CO_2 and lactic acidosis. Inadequate alveolar ventilation produces hypoxemia and hypercarbia (respiratory acidosis). Metabolism continues even though adequate tissue oxygen is unavailable. The result is that the anaerobic pathway is followed. The products of anaerobic metabolism are lactate ions and H^+ ions that enter the blood and form lactic acid (metabolic acidosis). Therefore, decreased arterial pH, associated with cardiac arrest, results from increased arterial CO_2 levels (respiratory acidosis), decreased arterial O_2 tensions, and lactic acidosis (metabolic acidosis).

(27:95,246,266)

25. B. The location of the carotid arteries makes them the most reasonable choice for palpation of the pulse when one is assessing a cardiac arrest victim. While the

evaluator palpates the carotid site, he can rapidly and easily assess the victim's ventilatory status at the same time. With the ear directly over the victim's nose and mouth area, the evaluator can listen for breathing while directing his vision to the victim's chest to observe the chest movement. Furthermore, the carotid site is generally accessible immediately. Palpating peripheral pulse may not accurately allow for assessment because a feeble cardiac output may not create a palpable peripheral pulse.

(6:912), (11:94–95)

26. C. The femoral artery is a large artery relatively close to the heart. Blood flow generated by external chest massage usually provides a palpable femoral pulse. At the same time, an arterial blood sample can usually be obtained from that site. The cardiac compressions may not generate an adequate flow peripherally to produce a palpable peripheral pulse.

(JAMA, August 1, 1980, VOl. 244, No. 5, p. 467)

27. A. Ventricular fibrillation and asystole are indications for external cardiac compressions. During ventricular fibrillation the ventricles are depolarizing in a rapid, chaotic manner. Consequently, stroke volume and cardiac output are inadequate to maintain a sufficient perfusion pressure.

Sinus arrythima and sinus bradycardia are dysrhythmias originating from the sinoatrial (SA) node. During the former the heart rate is ordinarily normal. However, normal QRS complexes occur irregularly. Cardiac output is usually adequate. In the case of sinus bradycardia, all ECG aspects are normal except that a heart rate of less than 60 beats/min exists.

Premature ventricular contractions (PVC) interrupt the normal succession and rate of ventricular depolarizations (QRS complexes). After a PVC, there is a long interval before another atrial depolarization (P-wave) occurs. The presence of PVCs may or may not pose an immediate threat to the patient. Their frequency of occurrence will ultimately reflect the degree of danger.

(30:368,369,375,377)

28. A. The patient is displaying premature ventricular contractions (PVCs). Without additional clinical data it is difficult to assess the hazard these PVCs are posing to the patient. Therefore, it is reasonable to assume that the patient is not in any imminent danger. However, the presence of PVCs indicates that the ventricles are more irritable and are more prone to the development of a lethal dysrhythmia.

Lidocaine administration to reduce myocardial irritability may be considered.

(6:934), (30:375–376)

29. D. Pupil status reflects cerebral oxygenation. It takes approximately 30 to 40 seconds for the pupils to completely dilate after the cessation of blood flow to the head.

(6:905)

30. A.   I = ventricular tachycardia (Figure 103)
              II = nodal tachycardia (Figure 104)
              III = premature ventricular contractions (PVCs) (Figure 105)
              IV = ventricular fibrillation (Figure 106)

Each of the dysrhythmias shown can cause a decreased cardiac output. During ventricular tachycardia, nodal tachycardia, and ventricular fibrillation, ventricular diastole may be insufficient to provide an adequate preload, thereby reducing stroke volume and ultimately cardiac output. The presence of PVCs can, if they occur frequenty, adversely influence cardiac output. PVCs can cause the heart pattern to degenerate to ventricular fibrillation.
(30:372,375–377)

31. D. The patient described here has a spinal cord injury. Such patients should not have their head and neck hyperextended because this maneuver can further injure the patient. Instead, the rescuer should use the modified jaw thrust method to establish an airway.
(6:910)

32. B. Exhaled air has an oxygen percentage of approximately 16% to 19% (FE_{O_2}). To obtain the approximate partial pressure of the inspired oxygen (PI_{O_2}) that the arrest victim will receive,

$$(\text{atmospheric pressure } - \text{ water vapor pressure}) FE_{O_2} = PI_{O_2}$$
$$(760 \text{ torr } - 47 \text{ torr})0.19 = 135 \text{ torr}$$

(6:912), (30:245)

33. C. This person is experiencing a respiratory arrest because she is apneic, but has a palpable carotid pulse. Therefore, the most appropriate action for the respiratory care practitioner to take is to continue ventilating the victim at the prescribed adult rate (12 breaths/min), unless spontaneous ventilation is re-established. Cardiac compressions are inappropriate in this case because cardiac activity exists. All the other responses available were, likewise, inappropriate.
(6:906), (11:94–95)

34. B. Cardiopulmonary resuscitation should not ordinarily be interrupted. However, CPR can be interrupted up to 30 seconds for endotracheal intubation and for repositioning or transporting the victim to a site that is conducive to more effective resuscitation efforts.
Repositioning or transportation should not be undertaken until the victim has been stabilized and all preparations have been made.
(JAMA, August 1, 1980, Vol. 244, No. 5, pp 469,481)

35. C. The purpose of the Heimlich maneuver is to expel objects or foreign matter that obstruct the airway when aspirated. The airway obstruction is relieved by manually compressing the epigastrium (upper abdomen). This action will force the diaphragm upward, thereby increasing intrathoracic pressure and compressing air behind the obstruction. The obstruction is often alleviated by the compression of air behind it.
(6:911–912)

36. A. When external cardiac compressions are properly performed, a systolic pressure of 100 mm Hg can usually be attained. Diastolic pressure drops to 0 mm Hg.
(30:247)

37. E. Ventricular fibrillation is usually characterized by (1) an unsynchronized rate of over 150 beats/min; (2) an irregular rhythm; (3) nondiscernible waves, intervals, and complexes; and (4) multiple ventricular ectopic foci. Causes of such a dysrhythmia include tissue hypoxia, hypokalemia, congestive heart failure, and acidosis.
(30:250,377)

38. E. The maximum cardiac output that is said to be attainable when external cardiac compressions are properly performed is 25% to 35% of normal. Therefore, if someone has a normal cardiac output of 5 liters/min, the best cardiac output that ordinarily can be expected during CPR is 1.25 to 1.75 liters/min.
(30:244,247)

39. D. If a victim is found unconscious and the cause is not known, the practitioner should (1) establish unresponsiveness, (2) call for help, (3) establish the airway, (4) establish breathlessness, and (5) begin ventilation.
(JAMA, August 1, 1980, Vol. 224, No. 5, p. 466)

40. B. From the data given, it is reasonable to conclude that the ventilation aspect of the resuscitation effort is, at least, adequate. Although no information was given about the arrest victim's size or weight, a $\dot{V}E$ of 26.4 liters/min (22 breaths/min $\times$ 1.2 liters VT) over a 30-minute period would certainly produce a Pa_{CO_2} less than 50 torr. More specifically, this clinical picture does not represent a ventilation problem; rather it poses a perfusion problem. A possible cause of the high Pa_{CO_2} may be $\dot{V}A/\dot{Q}C$ mismatching. Increased perfusion may provide a more normal $\dot{V}A/\dot{Q}C$ ratio. Cardiac massage may not be adequate. Therefore, the rescuer may not be applying sufficient force or may need to increase the number of compressions.
(1:306–307), (3:53–54), (8:51–53)

41. E. During two-rescuer CPR, the two rescuers assume positions on opposite sides of the victim. The person performing the compressions initiates the command to switch. The switch is made after the fifth compression is administered. After the switch, the person previously doing compressions assumes a position near the victim's head, and evaluates the carotid pulse for no more than 5 seconds. If pulselessness is ascertained, the person now ventilating administers a breath, and directs the other person to perform compression.
(JAMA, August 1, 1980, Vol. 244, No. 5, p. 468)

42. A. Cardiopulmonary resuscitation warrants termination in each of the following circumstances: (1) when the rescuer becomes too exhausted to continue efforts, (2) if the rescuer is a nonphysician and a physician assumes responsibility, (3) when the victim begins breathing and circulating spontaneously, (4) when another trained person assumes CPR responsibilities, and (5) when the victim comes under the care of personnel who have EMS responsibilities.
(JAMA, August 1, 1980, Vol. 244, No. 5, p. 470)

43. C. According to American Heart Association Standards and Guidelines for Cardiopulmonary Resuscitation (CPR) and Emergency Cardiac Care (ECC), the rec-

ommendation is that infants and children about to be defibrillated be given an initial dose of 2 joules/kg of body weight. Therefore, an infant weighing 13 lb is suggested to receive about 12 joules of energy via initial defibrillation.

STEP 1: 13 lb = _____ kg

$$\frac{13 \text{ lb}}{2.2 \text{ lb/kg}} = 5.9 \text{ kg}$$

STEP 2: 2 joules/kg applied on initial defibrillation.

$$(5.9 \text{ kg})(2 \text{ joules/kg}) = 11.8 \text{ joules}$$

(JAMA, August 1, 1980, Vol. 244, No. 5, p. 490), (2:29–30)

44. A. Some infants have short, fat necks which make palpating their carotid artery difficult. In such a situation the respiratory care practitioner should, alternatively, palpate the infant's brachial pulse. Listening over the precordial area is not recommended because precordial activity represents an impulse instead of a pulse.

(JAMA, August 1, 1980, Vol. 244, No. 5, p. 476)

45. D. The Apgar scoring system is useful for evaluating the need for neonatal resuscitation. The Apgar score is taken at 1 and 5 minutes after birth. Table 10 outlines the clinical signs that are assessed and the rating attributed to each sign depending on the neonate's clinical condition. Infants who have a 1-minute Apgar score ranging from 0 to 2 require immediate resuscitation. Infants having a 1-minute Apgar score of 3 to 6 are classified as having mild to moderate asphyxia. If the infant's 5-minute Apgar score falls, resuscitation is also indicated.

TABLE 10

Sign	Rating		
	0	1	2
Heart Rate	Absent	< 100/min	> 100/min
Ventilatory effort	Absent	Slow, irregular	Good, crying
Muscle tone	Limp	Some flexion	Active, motion
Reflex irritability	No response	Grimace	Cough or sneeze
Color	Central and peripheral cyanosis	Peripheral cyanosis	Completely pink

(JAMA, August 1, 1980, Vol. 244, No. 5, pp 495,496), (6:709–710), (35:31–34), (36:53–54)

46. A. The respiratory care practitioner should encourage his niece to continue coughing. Because the presence of wheezing and coughing implies that she is still moving air into and out of her lungs, he should not intervene to physically or mechanically remove the lodged peanut.

The presence of an ineffective cough, dyspnea, and cyanosis would warrant immediate intervention to remove or alleviate airway obstruction. In such a situation the infant should be turned backside up and head down. The rescuer should then deliver four back flows (between the infant's shoulder blades) with the heel of his hand. Chest thrusts are also recommended.

Abdominal thrusts (Heimlich maneuver) are not recommended for the relief of airway obstruction in infants and children. Injury to abdominal viscera is a potential hazard.

(JAMA, August 1, 1980, Vol. 244, No. 5, p. 475)

47. E. Persons attempting to remove victims from the water should not place themselves at great risk of danger. Because external chest compressions cannot be effectively given while both the rescuer and victim are in the water, they should not be attempted. Artificial (mouth-to-mouth or mouth-to-nose) ventilation should be attempted as soon as possible even if both the victim and rescuer are in the water.

(JAMA, August 1, 1980, Vol. 244, No. 5, p. 469)

48. B. An esophageal obturator (EOA) generally requires no direct visualization for insertion. Ordinarily, it is easier to insert than an endotracheal tube. When an EOA is in place, it is difficult to create a tight seal if a mask is also used. Trained personnel are required for the proper insertion and maintenance of an EOA.

(JAMA, August 1, 1980, Vol. 244, No. 5, p. 480)

49. C. The universal sign of choking (Figure 114) consists of the victim grasping his neck in the area of the larynx between his thumb and index finger.

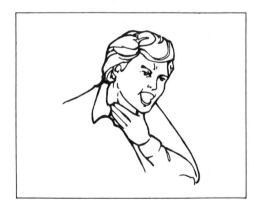

FIGURE 114. Universal distress signal for choking.

(JAMA, August 1, 1980, Vol. 244, No.5, p. 464)

50. B. Ventricular fibrillation indicates numerous ectopic foci, resulting in inadequate cardiac output. No pulse can be palpated when this dysrhythmia occurs. It may be considered a form of cardiac arrest. Defibrillation is immediately indicated.
(30:377)

REFERENCES

1. Spearman, C., and Sheldon, R., *Egan's Fundamentals of Respiratory Therapy*, 4th ed., C.V. Mosby, St. Louis, 1982.
2. Wojciechowski, W., *Respiratory Care Sciences: An Integrated Approach*, John Wiley & Sons, New York, 1985.
3. Shapiro, B., Harrison R., Kacmarek, R., and Cane, R., *Clinical Application of Respiratory Care*, 3rd ed., Year Book Medical Publishers, Chicago, 1985.
4. Kacmarek, R., Mack, C., and Dimas, S., *The Essentials of Respiratory Therapy*, 2nd ed., Year Book Medical Publishers, Chicago, 1985.
5. McPherson, S., *Respiratory Therapy Equipment*, 3rd ed., C.V. Mosby, St. Louis, 1985.
6. Burton, G., and Hodgkin, J., *Respiratory Care: A Guide to Clinical Practice*, 2nd ed., J.B. Lippincott, Philadelphia, 1985.
7. Frownfelter, D., *Chest Physical Therapy and Cardiopulmonary Rehabilitation, An Interdisciplinary Approach*, Year Book Medical Publishers, Chicago, 1978.
8. Cherniack, R., and Cherniack, L., *Respiration in Health and Disease*, 3rd ed., W.B. Saunders, Philadelphia, 1983.
9. Daily, E., and Schroeder, G., *Techniques in Bedside Hemodynamic Monitoring*, 3rd ed., C.V. Mosby, St. Louis, 1985.
10. Des Jardins, R., *Clinical Manifestations of Respiratory Disease*, Year Book Medical Publishers, Chicago, 1984.
11. Mitchell, R., *Synopsis of Clinical Pulmonary Disease*, 3rd ed., C.V. Mosby, St. Louis, 1982.
12. Comroe, J., *Physiology of Respiration*, 3rd ed., Year Book Medical Publishers, Chicago, 1974.
13. West, J., *Pulmonary Pathophysiology—The Essentials*, 2nd ed., Williams & Wilkins, Baltimore, 1982.
14. West, J., *Respiratory Physiology—The Essentials*, 3rd ed., Williams & Wilkins, Baltimore, 1985.
15. Martz, K., et al. *Management of the Patient-Ventilator System: A Team Approach*, 2nd ed., C.V. Mosby, St. Louis, 1984.
16. Shoup, C., and McHenry, R., *Laboratory Exercises in Respiratory Therapy*, 2nd ed., C.V. Mosby, St. Louis, 1983.
17. Ruppel, G., *Manual of Pulmonary Function Testing*, 3rd ed., C.V. Mosby, St. Louis, 1982.
18. Appelbaum, E., and Bruce, D., *Tracheal Intubation*, W.B. Saunders, Philadelphia, 1976.
19. Rau, J., *Respiratory Therapy Pharmacology*, 2nd ed., Year Book Medical Publishers, Chicago, 1984.
20. United States Department of Health, Education, and Welfare, Public Health Service, *Isolation Techniques for Use in Hospitals*, 2nd ed., Washington, D.C., 1975.
21. Brooks, S., *Integrated Basic Science*, 4th ed., C.V. Mosby, St. Louis, 1979.
22. Comroe, J., *The Lung*, Year Book Medical Publishers, Chicago, 1962.
23. Shibel, E., and Moser, K., *Respiratory Emergencies*, 2nd ed., C.V. Mosby, St. Louis, 1982.
24. Tisi, G., *Pulmonary Physiology in Clinical Medicine*, 2nd ed., Williams & Wilkins, Baltimore, 1985.
25. Cherniack, R., *Pulmonary Function Testing*, W.B. Saunders, Philadelphia, 1977.
26. Altose M., *The Physiological Basis of Pulmonary Function Testing*, Clinical Symposia-CIBA, Vol. 31, No. 2, Summit, New Jersey, 1979.
27. Shapiro, B., Harrison, R., and Walton, J., *Clinical Application of Arterial Blood Gases*, 3rd ed., Year Book Medical Publishers, Chicago, 1982.
28. West, J., *Ventilation/Blood Flow and Gas Exchange*, 3rd ed., Blackwell Scientific Publications, 1979.

29. Slonim, N., and Hamilton, K., *Respiratory Physiology,* 4th ed., C.V. Mosby, St. Louis, 1981.
30. Rarey, K., and Youtsey, J., *Respiratory Patient Care,* Prentice-Hall, Englewood Cliffs, 1981.
31. Berne, R., and Levy, M., *Physiology,* C.V. Mosby, St. Louis, 1983.
32. Levitzky, M., *Pulmonary Physiology,* 2nd ed., McGraw-Hill, New York, 1986.
33. Wilson, P., Bell, C., and Norton, A., *Rehabilitation of the Heart and Lungs,* SensorMedics, 1980.
34. Clausen, J., and Zarins, L., *Pulmonary Function Testing Guidelines and Controversies,* Academic Press, New York, 1982.
35. Klaus, M., and Fanaroff, A., *Care of the High-Risk Neonate,* 2nd ed., W.B. Saunders, Philadelphia, 1979.
36. Lough, M., et al., *Pediatric Respiratory Therapy,* 3rd ed., Year Book Medical Publishers, Chicago, 1985.
37. Levin, D., et al., *A Practical Guide to Pediatric Intensive Care,* 2nd ed., C.V. Mosby, St. Louis, 1984.
38. O'Ryan, J., and Burns, D., *Pulmonary Rehabilitation from Hospital to Home,* Year Book Medical Publishers, Chicago, 1984.
39. Bell, C., et al., *Home Care and Rehabilitation in Respiratory Medicine,* J. B. Lippincott, Philadelphia, 1984.
40. Wilkins, R., et al., *Clinical Assessment in Respiratory Care,* C. V. Mosby, St. Louis, 1985.
41. Jones, N., and Campbell, E., *Clinical Exercise Testing,* 2nd ed., W. B. Saunders, Philadelphia, 1982.
42. Goldsmith, J., and Karotkin, E., *Assisted Ventilation of the Neonate,* W. B. Saunders, Philadelpia, 1981.
43. Blowers, M., and Sims, R., *How to Read an ECG,* 3rd ed., Medical Economics, New Jersey, 1983.
44. Eubanks, D., and Bone, R., *Comprehensive Respiratory Care,* C. V. Mosby, St. Louis, 1985.
45. Rattenborg, C., *Clinical Use of Mechanical Ventilation,* Year Book Medical Publishers, Chicago, 1981.
46. Witkowski, A. S., *Pulmonary Assessment: A Clinical Guide,* J. B. Lippincott, Philadelphia, 1985.
47. Op't Holt, T. B., *Assessment Based Respiratory Care,* John Wiley & Sons, New York, 1986.

AIRWAY MANAGEMENT ASSESSMENT

PURPOSE: The purpose of this section is to provide you the opportunity to review your understanding and knowledge in the area of airway management. In this 50-item section you will be asked to make clinical judgments and decisions about suctioning, intubation, cuff inflation and deflation, extubation, pharmacologic agents, and airway care equipment. You will also be challenged with mathematical problems, for example, endotracheal tube and suction catheter sizes. Questions pertaining to anatomic structures of the airway also are included.

DIRECTIONS: Each of the questions or incomplete statements is followed by five suggested answers. Select the one which is the best in each case and then blacken the corresponding space on the answer sheet.

1. An adult female ventilator patient is nasally intubated with an endotracheal tube hav-

ing an internal diameter of 8.0 mm. What size suction catheter would be the most appropriate to use when performing tracheobronchial suctioning on this patient?

A. 8 Fr   D. 14 Fr
B. 10 Fr   E. 16 Fr
C. 12 Fr

2. Which statements describe the use of an esophageal obturator?

I. It has the versatility to provide for either nasal or oral insertion.
II. As with oral and nasal ET and tracheostomy tubes, the minimal leak technique should be used.
III. It is useful in reducing the risk of tracheobronchial aspiration of vomitus.
IV. A manual resuscitator may be the source of positive pressure ventilation when this device is in place.

A. III only   D. II, III only
B. I, II, III only   E. III, IV only
C. II only

3. Which of the following statements are true concerning endotracheal tube suctioning?

I. In some instances suctioning should be ordered on a predetermined basis.
II. Endotracheal tube suctioning routinely may be performed as long as 25 seconds.
III. Vagal nerve stimulation is a possible complication of tracheal suctioning.
IV. It is acceptable if the suction catheter occupies as much as 50% of the internal diameter of the ET tube.

A. I, II, III, IV   D. II, III only
B. III, IV only   E. I, IV only
C. I, II, IV only

4. Which of the following statements represent potential hazards associated with the use of an oropharyngeal airway that is too large for the patient?

I. It may result in laryngeal obstruction.
II. Tracheobronchial aspiration may occur.
III. Gastric insufflation may result.
IV. Effective ventilation may be prevented.

A. I, II, III, IV   D. I, IV only
B. I, III, IV only   E. III, IV only
C. II, III only

5. Sputum is usually made up of which component(s)?

I. mucus
II. saliva
III. lacrimae
IV. cellular debris

A. I, II, III, IV
B. I, II only
C. II, IV only

D. I, II, IV only
E. II, III, IV only

6. Which anatomic structure(s) serve(s) the respiratory system by functioning to prevent tracheobronchial aspiration?

    I. aryepiglottic folds
    II. false vocal cords
    III. epiglottis
    IV. true vocal cords

A. I, II, III, IV
B. I, II, IV only
C. III only

D. I, III, IV only
E. II, III only

7. When a patient's trachea is being intubated using a Macintosh laryngoscope blade, where should the blade be positioned for exposing the glottis?

A. under the epiglottis
B. either above or below the epiglottis
C. against the roof of the mouth

D. into the vallecula
E. against the uvula

8. After tracheal intubation, proper tube placement should be assessed by which procedures?

    I. auscultation of the chest
    II. observation for equal bilateral chest expansion
    III. observation for adequate cough mechanism
    IV. portable chest x-ray

A. I, II, III, IV
B. I, IV only
C. II, III only

D. I, II, IV only
E. IV only

9. Mucoid sputum usually is associated with which disease(s)?

    I. cystic fibrosis
    II. lung abscess
    III. bronchial asthma
    IV. bronchogenic carcinoma
    V. chronic bronchitis

A. III only
B. I only
C. III, IV only

D. III, V only
E. II, V only

10. Which anatomic sites generally serve as landmarks during the oral intubation procedure?

I. epiglottis

II. hyoid bone

III. esophagus

IV. uvula

V. arytenoid cartilages

A. II, IV only

B. I, V only

C. III, IV only

D. II, III, IV only

E. I, IV, V only

11. Which statements refer to a fenestrated tracheostomy tube?

I. Such a device does *not* use a cuff.

II. It allows the patient to become an upper-airway breather.

III. The inner cannula should be reinserted during tracheobronchial suctioning.

IV. The cuff should always be inflated when the patient is eating.

A. I, III only

B. II, III only

C. I, II, III only

D. II, IV only

E. II, III, IV only

12. Which statement represents one of the criteria of a suction catheter for suctioning through an ET tube?

A. The catheter's external diameter should *not* exceed one-half of the internal diameter of the ET tube.

B. As long as the suction catheter will pass through the ET tube, it can be used.

C. The suction catheter having the largest internal diameter should be used so that laminar flow through the catheter will be maintained.

D. During intubation the largest ET tube should be chosen so that the largest suction catheter possible can be used when suctioning will be performed.

E. The length of the suction catheter need *not* be considered.

13. Which factors characterize a low-pressure cuff?

I. low residual volume

Ii. high residual volume

III. cuff-to-tracheal wall pressure of approximately 20 cm H_2O

IV. cuff constructed of latex

A. I, III only

B. II, III only

C. II, IV only

D. II, III, IV only

E. I, III, IV only

14. What is the purpose of using phenylephrine during nasotracheal intubation?

A. to elicit an alpha-adrenergic response throughout the nasal mucosa

B. to act as a topical anesthetic to eliminate the gag reflex

C. to create a beta-1 response in the upper airways so that the patient can move more air during the procedure
D. to serve as a lubricant facilitating tube insertion through the nasal cavity
E. to test for nasal patency

15. Which condition(s) is(are) (a) potential complication(s) associated only with a patient having a nasotracheal tube in place as opposed to an oral ET tube?

   I. otitis media
   II. acute sinusitis
   III. epiglottitis
   IV. tracheitis

A. II only
B. I, III, IV only
C. II, IV only
D. I, III only
E. I, II only

16. Which statements refer to the procedure of inserting an oropharyngeal airway?

   I. The patient is placed in a supine position.
   II. The patient is placed in the Trendelenburg position.
   III. The buccal end of the airway is inserted and positioned between the base of the tongue and the posterior pharyngeal wall.
   IV. The patient's mouth may need to be forced open with the thumb and index fingers crossed.

A. I, III, IV only
B. II, III, IV only
C. I, IV only
D. II, III only
E. I, III only

17. Which technique(s) is(are) useful for obtaining sputum specimens *not* contaminated by upper airway microorganisms?

   I. passing a suction catheter through a nasal or oral ET tube
   II. fiberoptic bronchoscopy
   III. passing a suction catheter through a tracheostomy tube
   IV. performing transtracheal aspiration

A. I, III only
B. II, III, IV only
C. II only
D. II, IV only
E. I, II, III, IV

18. Which conditions represent major complications of tracheobronchial suctioning?

   I. tachycardia
   II. cardiac dysrhythmia
   III. bradycardia
   IV. hyperventilation
   V. aphonia

A. II, III only

B. I, II, IV, V only

C. II, III, IV only

D. I, IV only

E. IV, V only

19. Which conditions can be considered complications of a tracheotomy procedure?

   I. hemorrhage

   II. subcutaneous emphysema

   III. pneumothorax

   IV. mediastinal emphysema

A. I, II, III, IV

B. II, IV only

C. I, II, III only

D. I, III only

E. III, IV only

20. Which statements refer to a cricothyroidotomy?

   I. The incision is made through the cricothyroid membrane, which lies immediately above the thyroid cartilage.

   II. Extreme caution must be exercised when cutting the cricothyroid membrane because the brachiocephalic artery lies directly behind it.

   III. The incision is made below the level of the vocal cords.

   IV. Once the airway is established by this method, it should *not* be maintained in this manner longer than 24 hours.

A. I, II, III, IV

B. I, II only

C. III, IV only

D. I, III, IV only

E. II, III, IV only

21. Which statement refers to the minimal leak technique?

A. The cuff is inflated just to the point where *no* leak occurs.

B. A minimal leak is allowed to occur around the cuff during exhalation.

C. A minimal leak is allowed to occur around the cuff during inhalation.

D. The cuff is inflated until 15 mm Hg cuff-to-tracheal wall pressure exists.

E. A patient undergoes a reduction in the administration of a diuretic.

22. Which manufacturer produces an ET tube having a cuff inflated with air at atmospheric pressure?

A. Kamen-Wilkinson

B. Lanz

C. Shiley

D. Portex

E. Foregger

23. Copious, foul smelling, bloody, and purulent sputum that separates into three distinct layers upon standing is characteristic of which disease condition?

A. chronic bronchitis

B. asthma

C. bronchiectasis

D. cystic fibrosis

E. tuberculosis

24. If subglottic edema develops after endotracheal extubation, what alternative procedures could be beneficially implemented?

    I. Nebulized racemic epinephrine could be administered.
    II. The patient might need to be reintubated.
    III. Instituting mist tent therapy would be helpful.
    IV. A tracheotomy may be required.

    A. I, IV only   D. I, III only
    B. II, IV only   E. II, III only
    C. I, II, IV only

25. Which statements correctly compare/contrast nasal and oral ET tubes?

    I. All nasal tubes have a beveled angle of 45°.
    II. Only oral tubes are available with the Murphy eye.
    III. Both tubes usually have a pilot balloon.
    IV. Both tubes have approximately the same radius of curvature.
    V. Nasal tubes may display their beveled end (opening) in either direction.

    A. I, II, III, IV, V   D. I, II, III, V only
    B. I, III, IV, V only   E. I, IV only
    C. III, IV, V only

26. Which of the following statements accurately refer to airway obstruction?

    I. Small airway obstruction is generally less symptomatic than large airway obstruction.
    II. Under resting ventilatory conditions, a partial airway obstruction may lead to hyperinflation distal to the point of obstruction.
    III. Flaring of the alae nasi and the use of accessory muscles of ventilation may indicate airway obstruction.
    IV. The use of a nasopharyngeal airway is one of a few means of establishing a patent airway.

    A. I, II, III, IV   D. II, IV only
    B. I, IV only   E. II, III only
    C. I, II, III only

27. At what level along the trachea should a tracheotomy incision be made?

    A. at the cricothyroid membrane
    B. just above the Adam's apple
    C. at the seventh or eighth tracheal ring
    D. just above the larynx
    E. at the second, third, or fourth tracheal ring

28. When oral endotracheal intubation is being performed, how should the patient's head and neck be positioned?

A. maximally hyperextended

B. moderately flexed

C. in neutral position

D. maximally flexed

E. in the sniffing position

29. Which of the following statements describe uses of an artificial airway?

    I. for relief of airway obstruction

    II. for protection of the airway

    III. for facilitation of tracheobronchial suctioning

    IV. for prolonged artificial ventilation

A. I, II, III, IV

B. I, II, IV only

C. II, IV only

D. I, III only

E. I, III, IV only

30. When a patient is nasally or orally intubated, generally, how much time should elapse before a tracheotomy is considered?

    A. If the patient is comatose, a tracheotomy should be done 24 hours after the patient is intubated.

    B. A tracheotomy should be done immediately if tracheobronchial secretions are thick.

    C. If the patient appears to be in further need of the artificial airway, a tracheotomy should be done 72 hours after intubation.

    D. Because each clinical condition and situation is different, the decision to perform a tracheotomy is an individualized medical determination.

    E. The usual time to switch to a tracheotomy is after 48 hours.

31. Which statement(s) represent(s) the proper procedure(s) concerning ET tube cuff care?

    I. Before the cuff is to be deflated, the trachea should be suctioned.

    II. The oropharynx should be thoroughly suctioned before cuff deflation.

    III. Once the minimal leak has been established, it requires no further attention.

    IV. A minimal leak established with the ventilator delivering low airway pressures would inadequately seal the trachea if system pressure suddenly increased.

A. I, III only

B. II, IV only

C. I, II, IV only

D. III only

E. II only

32. Generally, which intracuff pressure range will prevent arterial blood flow from entering that portion of the trachea in an intubated patient?

A. 5 to 10 torr

B. 10 to 15 torr

C. 15 to 20 torr

D. 20 to 25 torr

E. 30 to 35 torr

33. The usual range for suction pressure for nasal, oral, pharyngeal, and tracheobronchial suctioning is _____ mm Hg.

    A. −10 to −50   D. −130 to −170
    B. −20 to −60   E. −160 to −200
    C. −80 to −120

34. When is the use of an oropharyngeal airway indicated?

    A. in all bag-mask ventilation situations
    B. when tracheobronchial suctioning is difficult
    C. when performing bag-mask ventilation on a comatose patient
    D. only in respiratory arrest cases
    E. only in cardiac arrest cases

35. Which statements can be considered advantages of nasal ET tubes as compared with oral ET tubes?

    I. Nasal ET tubes are of a larger diameter, providing for more laminar flow.
    II. Nasal tubes are considered to be better tolerated by the patient.
    III. Once inserted, nasal tubes present fewer chances of kinking.
    IV. Nasal tubes provide a better and more secure attachment for respiratory care equipment.

    A. II, III, IV only   D. III, IV only
    B. I, III only   E. I, II, III, IV
    C. II, III only

36. An 18 Fr. ET tube is equivalent to which of the following sizes?

    A. 6.0 mm I.D.   D. 9.0 mm O.D.
    B. 6.0 mm O.D.   E. 6.0 cm I.D.
    C. 9.0 mm I.D.

37. Purulent sputum is often associated with which disease condition(s)?

    I. bronchiectasis
    II. cystic fibrosis
    III. pneumonia
    IV. chronic bronchitis

    A. I, II, IV only   D. IV only
    B. I, IV only   E. I, II, III, IV
    C. II, III only

38. Magill forceps are generally used in which procedure?

A. cricothyroidotomy

B. tracheotomy

C. nasotracheal intubation

D. oral intubation

E. extubation

39. A patient with a tracheostomy tube in place has his anatomic dead space reduced by approximately what percent?

A. 20%

B. 30%

C. 40%

D. 50%

E. 60%

40. Which endotracheal and tracheostomy tubes can be safely autoclaved?

I. those composed of polyvinylchloride

II. silicone tubes

III. tubes containing Teflon

IV. metal tubes

A. II, III, IV only

B. II, III only

C. I, II, IV only

D. IV only

E. I, II, III, IV

41. Which conditions can result from inadequate humidification in a patient with a tracheostomy tube in place?

I. pneumonia

II. otitis media

III. tracheitis

IV. tracheoesophageal fistula

A. I, II, III, IV

B. I, III only

C. I, IV only

D. II, III only

E. I, II, III only

42. The letters IT printed on an ET tube indicate that the tube has been _____ .

A. implantation tested

B. treated by irradiation (presterilized)

C. intubation tested

D. thermally impregnable

E. internally treated

43. An eccentrically inflated cuff causing the tip of an ET tube to impinge against the anterior tracheal wall may cause _____ .

A. a tracheoesophageal fistula

B. brachiocephalic artery erosion

C. ventilation of the right mainstem bronchus

D. otitis media

E. tracheitis

44. The French system of tracheal tube sizing refers to which dimension?

    A. the angle of the bevel   D. the tube's outer circumference
    B. the internal diameter of the tube   E. the external diameter of the tube
    C. the tube's length

45. Which ET tube would offer the greatest airway resistance for a given flowrate?

    A. 24 French (Fr)   D. 34 Fr
    B. 36 Fr   E. 10 mm O.D.
    C. 12 mm O.D.

46. A _____ tracheostomy tube allows the patient to inspire through the tube
    but closes during exhalation.

    A. fenestrated   D. Reusch
    B. Kistner   E. Geudel
    C. Lanz

47. What is the function of an obturator associated with a tracheostomy tube?

    A. It is used as a decannulation cannula.
    B. It is used for pushing any dried secretions back down the tube.
    C. It often replaces the need for cuff inflation.
    D. It facilitates tube insertion.
    E. It should be in use to prevent aspiration when the patient is eating.

48. Which upper airway reflex(es) is(are) stimulated when an orally intubated patient on
    IMV is deep suctioned?

      I. laryngeal reflex
     II. pharyngeal reflex
    III. carinal reflex
     IV. sneeze reflex

    A. I, II, III only   D. I, II only
    B. III only   E. IV only
    C. I, III only

49. Which mathematical relationship(s) best represent(s) the influence of the internal di-
    ameter of an ET tube on the nature of the gas flow through the tube?

      I. $P_1 - P_2 = v_2^2 - v_1^2$

     II. $\dfrac{\Delta P}{\dot{V}} = \dfrac{8L}{\pi r^4 \eta}$

    III. $P_1 V_1 = P_2 V_2$

     IV. $\dfrac{r_1}{r_2} = \dfrac{\sqrt{density_2}}{\sqrt{density_1}}$

$$\text{V.} \quad \frac{V}{P} = \frac{1}{\text{elastance}}$$

A. III only

B. II only

C. I, II only

D. I, V only

E. III, IV only

50. Which material is used most widely in artificial airways?

A. polyethylene

B. polyvinylchloride

C. polypropylene

D. Teflon

E. silicone

ASSESSMENT ANSWER SHEET

DIRECTIONS: Darken the space under the selected answer.

	A	B	C	D	E		A	B	C	D	E
1.	[ ]	[ ]	[ ]	[ ]	[ ]	26.	[ ]	[ ]	[ ]	[ ]	[ ]
2.	[ ]	[ ]	[ ]	[ ]	[ ]	27.	[ ]	[ ]	[ ]	[ ]	[ ]
3.	[ ]	[ ]	[ ]	[ ]	[ ]	28.	[ ]	[ ]	[ ]	[ ]	[ ]
4.	[ ]	[ ]	[ ]	[ ]	[ ]	29.	[ ]	[ ]	[ ]	[ ]	[ ]
5.	[ ]	[ ]	[ ]	[ ]	[ ]	30.	[ ]	[ ]	[ ]	[ ]	[ ]
6.	[ ]	[ ]	[ ]	[ ]	[ ]	31.	[ ]	[ ]	[ ]	[ ]	[ ]
7.	[ ]	[ ]	[ ]	[ ]	[ ]	32.	[ ]	[ ]	[ ]	[ ]	[ ]
8.	[ ]	[ ]	[ ]	[ ]	[ ]	33.	[ ]	[ ]	[ ]	[ ]	[ ]
9.	[ ]	[ ]	[ ]	[ ]	[ ]	34.	[ ]	[ ]	[ ]	[ ]	[ ]
10.	[ ]	[ ]	[ ]	[ ]	[ ]	35.	[ ]	[ ]	[ ]	[ ]	[ ]
11.	[ ]	[ ]	[ ]	[ ]	[ ]	36.	[ ]	[ ]	[ ]	[ ]	[ ]
12.	[ ]	[ ]	[ ]	[ ]	[ ]	37.	[ ]	[ ]	[ ]	[ ]	[ ]
13.	[ ]	[ ]	[ ]	[ ]	[ ]	38.	[ ]	[ ]	[ ]	[ ]	[ ]
14.	[ ]	[ ]	[ ]	[ ]	[ ]	39.	[ ]	[ ]	[ ]	[ ]	[ ]
15.	[ ]	[ ]	[ ]	[ ]	[ ]	40.	[ ]	[ ]	[ ]	[ ]	[ ]
16.	[ ]	[ ]	[ ]	[ ]	[ ]	41.	[ ]	[ ]	[ ]	[ ]	[ ]
17.	[ ]	[ ]	[ ]	[ ]	[ ]	42.	[ ]	[ ]	[ ]	[ ]	[ ]
18.	[ ]	[ ]	[ ]	[ ]	[ ]	43.	[ ]	[ ]	[ ]	[ ]	[ ]
19.	[ ]	[ ]	[ ]	[ ]	[ ]	44.	[ ]	[ ]	[ ]	[ ]	[ ]
20.	[ ]	[ ]	[ ]	[ ]	[ ]	45.	[ ]	[ ]	[ ]	[ ]	[ ]
21.	[ ]	[ ]	[ ]	[ ]	[ ]	46.	[ ]	[ ]	[ ]	[ ]	[ ]
22.	[ ]	[ ]	[ ]	[ ]	[ ]	47.	[ ]	[ ]	[ ]	[ ]	[ ]
23.	[ ]	[ ]	[ ]	[ ]	[ ]	48.	[ ]	[ ]	[ ]	[ ]	[ ]
24.	[ ]	[ ]	[ ]	[ ]	[ ]	49.	[ ]	[ ]	[ ]	[ ]	[ ]
25.	[ ]	[ ]	[ ]	[ ]	[ ]	50.	[ ]	[ ]	[ ]	[ ]	[ ]

AIRWAY MANAGEMENT ANALYSES

Note: The references listed after each analysis are numbered and keyed to the reference list located at the end of this section. The first number indicates the text. The second number indicates the page where information about the question will be found. For example, (1:219,384) means that reference number 1 is to used and that on pages 219 and 384 information about the question will be found. Frequently, it will be necessary to read beyond the page number indicated to obtain complete information. Therefore, reference to the question will be found either on the page indicated or on subsequent pages.

1. C. French sizes actually represent the outer circumference of a suction catheter (or atificial airway) in millimeters (mm). The relationship of circumference to diameter is given by the formula

$$C = \pi d$$

where

$$C = \text{circumference}$$
$$\pi = 3.14$$
$$d = \text{diameter (outer)}$$

The following expression can be conveniently used to obtain the French size

$$\text{French gauge} = 3 \times \text{outer diameter}$$

The outer diameter (O.D.) of a suction catheter should not exceed one-half the inner diameter (I.D.) of the endotracheal tube (ET). The ET tube in this problem is 8.0 mm I.D. Therefore,

STEP 1: Use the formula that converts French size to the metric system.

$$\frac{\text{French gauge}}{3.0} = \text{external diameter (mm)}$$

STEP 2: Insert the known values and determine the external diameter in millimeters.

$$\frac{12 \text{ Fr}}{3.0} = \text{external diameter (mm)}$$

$$4.0 \text{ mm} = \text{external diameter}$$

For optimum secretion removal it is desirable to use the largest suction catheter possible without violating the rule stated above. The appropriate French gauge would be determined by solving the equation previously given (Fr gauge = 3 × outer diameter). Therefore,

$$\text{Fr gauge} = 3 \times 4.00 \text{ mm (O.D.)}$$
$$= 12 \text{ Fr}$$

The most appropriate suction catheter to use for suctioning an 8.0 mm I.D. endotracheal tube is a 12 Fr size.
(4:389), (6:510), (7:34)

2. E. Generally used by emergency medical personnel for the quick, easy establishment of a patent airway, the esophageal obturator intubates the esophagus instead of the trachea. The face area is sealed by a mask that has an opening for the movement of air into and out of the tube. On the tube in the oropharyngeal area there are 16 holes through which air can move. Because the face area is sealed and the tracheal site is open, the patient can be ventilated. A manual resuscitator may serve as the source of positive pressure ventilation. The chances of tracheobronchial aspiration are reduced.

(3:230), (4:384–385), (5:165), (6:494)

3. B. Suctioning should be performed only when necessary. Establishing a specific time schedule for suctioning may be detrimental to the patient. Tracheobronchial suctioning generally should not exceed 15 seconds. The risk of removing too much tidal volume and oxygen increases beyond this time interval.

When the suction catheter impinges on the carina, the vagal reflex can be stimulated, causing bradycardia and hypotension. The external diameter of the suction catheter must not exceed 50% of the ET tube's internal diameter.

(1:292,586), (3:248–252), (4:388–389), (6:515–520)

4. A. Oropharyngeal airways that are too long for the patient may impinge on the epiglottis, forcing it down so that it obstructs the larynx. During bag-mask ventilation air may enter the stomach and gastric distention may occur. Both of these occurrences would prevent effective alveolar ventilation. If a comatose person with an oropharyngeal airway in place becomes conscious, stimulation of the oropharynx may cause gagging, vomiting, or laryngospasm.

(3:215), (4:381), (5:163), (6:493)

5. A. Sputum is composed of an array of substances, including salivary, nasal, tracheobronchial, and lacrimal secretions; cellular debris; alveolar lining substances; etc.

(6:458), (12:224)

6. A. Among other functions, the larynx serves to protect the lower airway by closing the glottis, thus preventing food, drink, and so on from entering the trachea. The structures responsible for this action are the (1) epiglottis, (2) aryepiglottic folds, (3) false vocal cords, and (4) true vocal cords.

(3:7), (4:47,52), (18:16–18)

7. D. The curved (e.g., Macintosh) laryngoscope blade should be placed between the base of the tongue and above the epiglottis. This region is termed the *vallecula*. The straight blade (e.g., Miller) is placed under the anterior portion of the epiglottis, to expose the glottis.

(3:221), (16:98), (18:33,46,49)

8. D. Both lungs should be auscultated after tracheal intubation, to determine if ventilation is going to both lungs and to rule out inadvertant intubation of the esophagus. Visual inspection of the chest wall helps determine air movement within the lungs. The portable chest x-ray film indicates the position of the tube in relation-

ship to the carina. The radiopaque line that extends down to the distal tip assists in locating the tube's position.

(3:226), (16:99), (18:50)

9. D. In chronic bronchitis, the sputum may range from mucoid to mucopurulent. In asthma the sputum is usually mucoid unless the patient has an underlying infection or a complicating disease state.

(4:307,311), (6:752,792), (8:281,284–285)

10. B. During oral intubation, one generally looks for the epiglottis and the arytenoid cartilages to indicate the glottic site. The glottis is sometimes thought of as resembling an inverted triangle or an inverted "V."

(3:221), (4:52)

11. B. A fenestrated tracheostomy tube is used to help wean a tracheotomized patient. An opening is present on the shoulder of the tube. This opening allows for air to move through the tube and into the upper airway when the inner cannula has been removed. The stoma is decannulated, and the cuff is deflated when the patient breathes through the upper airway. The quality of the patient's upper-airway reflexes will determine whether the cuff is to be inflated or not. If the patient exhibits an adequate cough, cuff inflation may not be necessary.

(3:261), (4:383), (6:499,655)

12. A. The following list represents suction catheter criteria. A suction catheter must:

1. offer little resistance to insertion through an artificial airway
2. have a smooth, rounded tip to prevent mucosal damage
3. be of adequate length to extend below an artificial airway
4. have side holes at the distal end to prevent mucosal damage
5. not occlude the airway when inserted (less than $\frac{1}{2}$ internal diameter of airway)

(1:586), (3:250), (4:389), (6:515–519), (12:12)

13.   B. A low-pressure cuff is one that exerts low pressure against the tracheal wall, thereby potentially allowing arterial and venous blood flow to continue throughout the tracheal wall. Generally, 20 cm H_2O preserves blood flow in the trachea. Low-pressure cuffs are characterized by high compliance and high residual volume. As volume is added during cuff inflation, only small increases in pressure occur. Low-pressure cuffs are constructed of soft, durable plastics or silicone, *not* latex.

(1:568), (3:273–276), (4:386–387), (5:170), (6:506), (18:34)

14. A. Phenylephrine (Neo-Synephrine) is a vasoconstrictor (alpha-adrenergic response). This drug or a similar medication should be sprayed down both nares before nasal intubation to minimize any nasal bleeding that may occur during tube insertion.

(1:573), (3:233), (4:537), (6:502)

15. E. The auditory (eustachian) tube opening into the nasopharynx is sometimes blocked by the presence of a nasotracheal tube. Otitis media (middle-ear infec-

tion) can result from this blockage. Sinus drainage is often blocked as well, leading to acute sinusitis. Tracheitis is a late complication of a tracheotomy. Epiglottitis is not a complication of any form of tracheal intubation; in fact, it often is an indication.

(3:234), (4:381–382), (6:502), (7:84), (18:84)

16. C. With the patient supine, the pharyngeal end of the oropharyngeal airway is inserted and positioned between the base of the tongue and the posterior pharyngeal wall. The buccal end's insertion is limited by the gingiva or teeth. At times, the patient's mouth needs to be forced open.

(1:571–572), (3:215), (4:381), (5:163), (6:493)

17. D. Fiberoptic bronchoscopy and transtracheal aspiration are two methods of obtaining anaerobic sputum specimens. Oral, nasal, and tracheostomy suctioning and expectorated samples are not useful techniques for obtaining such specimens.

(6:439), (11:46)

18. A. The following conditions are complications of tracheobronchial suctioning: (1) hypoxemia, (2) dysrhythmia, (3) hypotension, (4) bradycardia, and (5) lung collapse .

(3:249), (4:388–389), (6:519)

19. A. Hemorrhage from the tracheotomy procedure usually comes from the anterior jugular venous system, brachiocephalic (innominate) artery, or inferior thyroid veins. Air can be drawn through the cut tissue by negative intrathoracic pressure or forced into body tissues by positive pressure (misplaced tracheotomy tube). Both situations can result in subcutaneous and mediastinal emphysema. If the pneumomediastinum is extensive, it can result in a pneumothorax.

(1:575), (3:237), (4:382–383), (6:501,789), (7:429), (18:18,88)

20. C. The cricothyroidotomy is an emergency procedure to establish a patent airway in situations in which endotracheal (oral or nasal) intubation is impossible or a tracheotomy cannot be performed. A midline incision along the cricothyroid membrane, which lies immediately below the thyroid cartilage, provides laryngeal entry below the vocal cord level.

The cricothyroid membrane is located between the thyroid and cricoid cartilages. This membrane is approximately located at the C-5 level.

Ordinarily, the membrane lies well above major blood vessels, thus reducing the risk of hemorrhage considerably.

(3:7,227), (4:385–386), (6:493), (7:26,54,75), (18:26,54,75)

21. C. After the tube (nasal, oral, or tracheostomy) is in position, the cuff is inflated. The volume placed into the cuff should be just enough to create a complete seal. A slight amount of air should be aspirated out to establish a slight leak during the inspiratory phase. This technique serves to reduce the hazard of pressure damage to the tracheal mucosa.

(1:579), (3:255,273), (4:387–388), (5:170), (6:506,514), (16:100)

22. A. Before endotracheal tube insertion, air is evacuated from the cuff by a syringe and the pilot balloon is closed. However, once the tube is in position, the pilot balloon is opened to atmospheric air, which allows the foam material inside the cuff to expand (self-inflating), thereby creating a low-pressure seal against the trachea.
(3:278), (4:387), (5:171), (6:507)

23. C. Bronchiectasis is characterized by sputum that is copious, bloody, and foul smelling and that separates into three layers when allowed to stand in the sputum collection cup. Cystic fibrosis is often complicated by bronchiectasis.
(4:308–309), (6:286,802), (8:293), (11:178)

24. C. Glottic edema is commonly treated by applying a topical alpha-adrenergic medication (nebulized racemic epinephrine) or by steriod therapy. Subglottic edema, on the other hand, poses a much more serious problem. It generally requires reintubation and may sometimes require a tracheotomy.
(3:266–268), (18:83–84)

25. C. Nasal tubes less than 6.0 mm (I.D.) have a 45° bevel, whereas those larger than 6.0 mm have a 30° bevel. All oral tubes have a 45° bevel. The Murphy eye is the opening (Murphy tip) at the distal end of the tube. The eye serves the purpose of providing a potential point for air movement in the event that the beveled edge becomes occluded. The beveled end, by the way, facilitates insertion during intubation and provides a larger cross-sectional area for air movement, as opposed to an opening similar to that on a tracheostomy tube. All cuffed ET tubes have a pilot balloon. Generally, oral tubes have the bevel on the left when the tube is concavely viewed from the adapter end, in the vertical plane, with the beveled end directed upward. Nasal tubes have the bevel in either direction.
(6:494,496,509–512)

26. C. Because of the vast cross-sectional area provided by the small airways (< 2 mm in diameter), a small airway obstruction generally does not prove as symptomatic as an obstruction in a large airway (> 2 mm in diameter) unless, of course, the small airway obstruction is diffuse and complete. An upper-airway obstruction can be more immediately life threatening if no air can reach any of the gas exchange units.

Overdistention (air trapping) may occur during normal resting ventilaton in the presence of a partial airway obstruction. During inspiration the airways elongate and widen; on exhalation they contract and narrow. Consequently, air may move beyond an obstruction during inspiration and get trapped on exhalation.

When airway obstruction (small or large) becomes symptomatic, the work of breathing increases. This situation may be clinically illustrated when the patient displays nasal flaring (alae nasi) and accessory ventilatory muscle use.
(2:154–155), (3:217), (8:270–276), (13:59)

27. E. Usually, the incision is made halfway between the cricoid cartilage and the suprasternal notch (second to fourth tracheal ring).
(1:574), (3:236), (18:60)

28. E. A straight route from the mouth to the glottis should be achieved. The head and neck should be extended and raised to a plane above shoulder level. This position is called the sniffing position.

(3:223), (7:40), (10:95)

29. A. Artificial airways are indicated in all four conditions. These represent general indications. Specific diseases requiring the use of an artificial airway can be placed under one or more of these indication categories.

(3:217), (4:381), (6:500)

30. D. The decision to perform a tracheotomy or to continue with endotracheal intubation is not a clear one. Much controversy has centered on this dilemma. The duration of intubation has expanded in recent years. Certain references adhere to a policy of ". . . if on the third day of intubation there is a reasonable chance for the patient *not* to need an artificial airway for an additional 72 hours, leave the endotracheal tube in place." If it is determined that the patient will definitely need an artificial airway, then a tracheotomy should be performed. This "guideline," however, is very much based on the patient's medical condition. The respiratory care practitioner should be cautious in forming absolute statements relative to this clinical question. Studies attempting to answer this question have shown that an absolute criterion cannot be established regarding when to perform a tracheotomy on an intubated patient.

(1:572), (3:242), (6:495), (18:28)

31. C. The trachea should be suctioned before cuff deflation, to make the airway as clear as possible. Also, the oropharynx should be thoroughly suctioned before cuff deflation, to prevent the aspiration of pooled secretions when the cuff is evacuated. Once the minimal leak has been used, continuous monitoring is required to maintain this cuff inflation technique. Regarding ventilator patients, as peak system pressure changes, adjustments of cuff volume are needed. If the minimal leak was instituted when peak system pressure was high, the volume in the cuff would be too large in the event of a decrease in delivery pressure. The opposite situation is likewise true.

(1:578–585), (3:255), (4:387–388), (6:506), (7:75), (12:110)

32. E. Intracuff pressures exceeding 18 mm Hg restrict the flow of tracheal venous blood in that region. Intracuff pressures exceeding 30 mm Hg cause tracheal arterial blood flow to be obstructed.

Ideally, intracuff pressure should seal the airway by means of the least amount of pressure possible.

(1:587), (3:255), (4:387–388), (5:170), (6:501,506)

33. C. For routine suctioning, the negative pressure should be set within the range of −80 to −120 mm Hg. Of course, when secretions are copious and tenacious, the pressure setting may need to be changed accordingly. However, other factors such as the internal diameter and the length of the suction catheter influence the resulting flow. Once flow through the catheter becomes turbulent, the negative pressure in the suction jar must be increased greatly before the flow through the catheter is

appreciably increased. The range -80 to -120 mm Hg generally maintains adequate flow for suctioning.

(3:251), (4:389), (6:516)

34. C. Oropharyngeal airways are indicated only for comatose patients. Otherwise, the laryngeal reflexes will be activated, e.g., gagging, vomiting, and laryngospasm.

(3:216), (4:381), (5:163), (6:493)

35. A. Nasal ET tubes are said to be (1) better suited for long-term airway management, (2) better tolerated by the patient, and (3) less prone to kinking because they are more stable within the nasal cavity. Subsequently, respiratory care equipment can be attached more comfortably and securely.

(1:573), (3:233), (4:381), (18:27–29)

36. E. The French scale is based upon tube circumference ($\pi \times$ external diameter). Usually, π is rounded off to 3.0; therefore, an 18 Fr tube is equivalent to a tube with an external diameter of approximately 6.0 mm.

1. French size $= \pi \times$ external diameter

2. $\dfrac{18 \text{ Fr}}{3.0} = 6.0$ mm (O.D.)

(4:389), (6:511), (18:35)

37. E. Chronic bronchitis, cystic fibrosis, bronchiectasis, and pneumonia are diseases associated with the production of purulent sputum. Each of these pulmonary pathologies is associated with bacterial infections. Bacterial infections generally involve the presence of white blood cells (WBCs), or leukocytes, to the area of the infection. Sputum resulting from the presence of WBCs is termed purulent.

(1:290), (3:244), (4:301–312), (6:286)

38. C. Magill forceps are used to direct the nasal tracheal tube into the trachea.

(3:233), (16:96), (18:32,52)

39. D. Anatomic dead space is reduced as much as 50% when a tracheostomy tube is in place. The use of an ET tube reduces the anatomic dead space by approximately 30%.

(12:14)

40. A. Silicone, Teflon, and metal tubes can be autoclaved, but Nylon, polyethylene, and polyvinylchloride should not.

(3:239–241), (6:505), (18:37)

41. B. Tracheitis can result from inadequate humidification of the upper airway, usually when a tracheostomy tube is in place. As a sequela, pneumonia may develop.

(3:106,253), (6:501), (18:91)

42. A. The letters IT printed on an endotracheal tube designate the fact that the tube has been implantation tested. This procedure is meant to ensure against tissue toxicity.

(3:239), (5:167), (6:510)

43. B. The brachiocephalic (innominate) artery lies anterior to the trachea. Erosion of the anterior tracheal wall may cause eventual erosion of the brachiocephalic artery although such an occurrence is uncommon.
    (10:181), (18:91)

44. D. The French system refers to the circumference of the tube given by the formula $\pi \times$ O.D. ($\pi = 3.14$ and O.D. = external diameter in millimeters). The external diameter in millimeters multiplied by 3.14 will give the corresponding French size. The value of π is rounded off to 3 during the calculation.
    (4:389), (6:509–513), (18:35–36)

45. A. A 24 Fr size is equivalent to 8.0 mm outer (external) diameter.

$$\frac{24 \text{ Fr}}{3} = 8.0 \text{ mm (O.D.)}$$

    This tube would have the smallest internal diameter (5.5 mm) hence, the airway resistance through it for any given flowrate (compared with the other tube sizes given) would be the highest.
    (4:389), (6:513), (18:34,35)

46. B. Certain tracheostomy tubes, such as the Kistner tube, prevent the immediate closure of the stoma. If the patient experiences copious secretions, this type of tube is used until he can generate an effective cough. The Kistner tube allows the patient to breathe through the upper airway.
    (3:263), (4:384), (6:499)

47. D. An obturator, which fits into the outer cannula, facilitates insertion of a tracheostomy tube. The conically shaped tip of the obturator protrudes from the distal end of the tube. With the obturator in place, chances of lacerating the posterior tracheal wall during the insertion are minimized. It also minimizes chances of blood or mucus entering the tube during insertion.
    (1:577), (5:172), (6:496), (18:59)

48. B. Because an oral ET tube bypasses the upper airway, the upper airway reflexes, that is, laryngeal and pharyngeal, are not stimulated. However, the tracheal reflex may be stimulated because the tip of the ET tube ends before the trachea does. Therefore, the suction catheter can stimulate the trachea, initiating the tracheal reflex. The carinal reflex will be stimulated if the suction catheter is inserted to that point, which it generally is.
    (3:249), (4:388–389), (6:519)

49. B. As the internal diameter of an ET tube decreases, the airway resistance through that tube increases, assuming all other factors remain constant. This phenomenon is explained by Poiseuille's law of laminar flow.
    (1:146), (2:160–164), (4:36–37), (6:512,1018)

50. B. Each of the substances listed, except polypropylene, is commonly found in ET

tubes. However, polyvinylchloride is the most widely used of these synthetic materials.

(3:240), (6:504), (7:431)

REFERENCES

1. Spearman, C., and Sheldon, R., *Egan's Fundamentals of Respiratory Therapy,* 4th ed., C.V. Mosby, St. Louis, 1982.
2. Wojciechowski, W., *Respiratory Care Sciences: An Integrated Approach,* John Wiley & Sons, New York, 1985.
3. Shapiro, B., Harrison R., Kacmarek, R., and Cane, R., *Clinical Application of Respiratory Care,* 3rd ed., Year Book Medical Publishers, Chicago, 1985.
4. Kacmarek, R., Mack, C., and Dimas, S., *The Essentials of Respiratory Therapy,* 2nd ed., Year Book Medical Publishers, Chicago, 1985.
5. McPherson, S., *Respiratory Therapy Equipment,* 3rd ed., ed., C.V. Mosby, St. Louis, 1985.
6. Burton, G., and Hodgkin, J., *Respiratory Care: A Guide to Clinical Practice,* 2nd ed., J.B. Lippincott, Philadelphia, 1985.
7. Frownfelter, D., *Chest Physical Therapy and Cardiopulmonary Rehabilitation, An Interdisciplinary Approach,* Year Book Medical Publishers, Chicago, 1978.
8. Cherniack, R., and Cherniack, L., *Respiration in Health and Disease,* 3rd ed., W.B. Saunders, Philadelphia, 1983.
9. Daily, E., and Schroeder, G., *Techniques in Bedside Hemodynamic Monitoring,* 3rd ed., C.V. Mosby, St. Louis, 1985.
10. Des Jardins, R., *Clinical Manifestations of Respiratory Disease,* Year Book Medical Publishers, Chicago, 1984.
11. Mitchell, R., *Synopsis of Clinical Pulmonary Disease,* 3rd ed.,C. B. Mosby, St. Louis, 1982.
12. Comroe, J., *Physiology of Respiration,* 3rd ed., Year Book Medical Publishers, Chicago, 1974.
13. West, J., *Pulmonary Pathophysiology—The Essentials,* 2nd ed., Wiliams & Wilkins, Baltimore, 1982.
14. West, J., *Respiratory Physiology—The Essentials,* 3rd ed., Wiliams & Wilkins, Baltimore, 1985.
15. Martz, K., et al. *Management of the Patient-Ventilator System: A Team Approach,* 2nd ed., C.V. Mosby, St. Louis, 1984.
16. Shoup, C., and McHenry, R., *Laboratory Exercises in Respiratory Therapy,* 2nd ed., C.V. Mosby, St. Louis, 1983.
17. Ruppel, G., *Manual of Pulmonary Function Testing,* 3rd ed., C.V. Mosby, St. Louis, 1982.
18. Appelbaum, E., and Bruce, D., *Tracheal Intubation,* W.B. Saunders, Philadelphia, 1976.
19. Rau, J., *Respiratory Therapy Pharmacology,* 2nd ed., Year Book Medical Publishers, Chicago, 1984.
20. United States Department of Health, Education, and Welfare, Public Health Service, *Isolation Techniques for Use in Hospitals,* 2nd ed., Washington, D.C., 1975.
21. Brooks, S., *Integrated Basic Science,* 4th ed., C.V. Mosby, St. Louis, 1979.
22. Comroe, J., *The Lung,* Year Book Medical Publishers, Chicago, 1962.
23. Shibel, E., and Moser, K., *Respiratory Emergencies,* 2nd ed., C.V. Mosby, St. Louis, 1982.
24. Tisi, G., *Pulmonary Physiology in Clinical Medicine,* 2nd ed., Williams & Wilkins, Baltimore, 1985.
25. Cherniack, R., *Pulmonary Function Testing,* W.B. Saunders, Philadelphia, 1977.

26. Altose M., *The Physiological Basis of Pulmonary Function Testing,* Clinical Symposia-CIBA, Vol. 31, No. 2, Summit, New Jersey, 1979.

27. Shapiro, B., Harrison, R., and Walton, J., *Clinical Application of Arterial Blood Gases,* 3rd ed., Year Book Medical Publishers, Chicago, 1982.

28. West, J., *Ventilation/Blood Flow and Gas Exchange,* 3rd ed., Blackwell Scientific Publications, 1979.

29. Slonim, N., and Hamilton, K., *Respiratory Physiology,* 4th ed., C.V. Mosby, St. Louis, 1981.

30. Rarey, K., and Youtsey, J., *Respiratory Patient Care,* Prentice-Hall, Englewood Cliffs, 1981.

31. Berne, R., and Levy, M., *Physiology,* C.V. Mosby, St. Louis, 1983.

32. Levitzky, M., *Pulmonary Physiology,* 2nd ed., McGraw-Hill, New York, 1986.

33. Wilson, P., Bell, C., and Norton, A., *Rehabilitation of the Heart and Lungs,* SensorMedics, 1980.

34. Clausen, J., and Zarins, L., *Pulmonary Function Testing Guidelines and Controversies,* Academic Press, New York, 1982.

35. Klaus, M., and Fanaroff, A., *Care of the High-Risk Neonate,* 2nd ed., W.B. Saunders, Philadelphia, 1979.

36. Lough, M., et al., *Pediatric Respiratory Therapy,* 3rd ed., Year Book Medical Publishers, Chicago, 1985.

37. Levin, D., et al., *A Practical Guide to Pediatric Intensive Care,* 2nd ed., C.V. Mosby, St. Louis, 1984.

38. O'Ryan, J., and Burns, D., *Pulmonary Rehabilitation from Hospital to Home,* Year Book Medical Publishers, Chicago, 1984.

39. Bell, C., et al., *Home Care and Rehabilitation in Respiratory Medicine,* J. B. Lippincott, Philadelphia, 1984.

40. Wilkins, R., et al., *Clinical Assessment in Respiratory Care,* C. V. Mosby, St. Louis, 1985.

41. Jones, N., and Campbell, E., *Clinical Exercise Testing,* 2nd ed., W. B. Saunders, Philadelphia, 1982.

42. Goldsmith, J., and Karotkin, E., *Assisted Ventilation of the Neonate,* W. B. Saunders, Philadelpia, 1981.

43. Blowers, M., and Sims, R., *How to Read an ECG,* 3rd ed., Medical Economics, New Jersey, 1983.

44. Eubanks, D., and Bone, R., *Comprehensive Respiratory Care,* C. V. Mosby, St. Louis, 1985.

45. Rattenborg, C., *Clinical Use of Mechanical Ventilation,* Year Book Medical Publishers, Chicago, 1981.

46. Witkowski, A. S., *Pulmonary Assessment: A Clinical Guide,* J. B. Lippincott, Philadelphia, 1985.

47. Op't Holt, T. B., *Assessment Based Respiratory Care,* John Wiley & Sons, New York, 1986.

MECHANICAL VENTILATION ASSESSMENT

PURPOSE: The purpose of this 50-item section is to afford you the opportunity to evaluate your knowledge and comprehension of mechanical ventilation. Items included in this section pertain to (1) establishing ventilatory parameters for various clinical conditions, (2) indications and contraindications for mechanical ventilation, (3) modes of ventilation, (4) ventilator management and weaning procedures, (5) mechanical ventilation equipment, (6) ventilator classification, and (7) fluidics. Calculations concerning tidal volume, anatomic dead space volume, effective static compliance, airway resistance, and inspiratory/expiratory (I/E) ratios are also included.

DIRECTIONS: Each of the questions or incomplete statements is followed by five suggested answers. Select the one which is the best in each case and then blacken the corresponding space on the answer sheet.

1. Which statement(s) correctly describe(s) the I/E ratio as it applies to a patient on a controlled mechanical ventilator?

   I. The mean airway pressure will increase as expiratory time is lengthened, while inspiratory time, $\dot{V}$, and V_T remain constant.

   II. Keeping all other parameters constant while lengthening the inspiratory time lowers the mean intrathoracic pressure.

   III. A large ratio tends to decrease venous return.

   A. I only   D. III only
   B. II, III only   E. I, II, III
   C. II only

Questions 2 and 3 refer to the same patient.

2. An average-sized 90-kg (ideal body weight) patient is receiving controlled volume cycled ventilation with the following settings:

   $$
   \begin{array}{rl}
   V_T: & 800 \text{ cc} \\
   \text{ventilatory rate:} & 15 \text{ breaths/min} \\
   \dot{V}: & 50 \text{ liters/min} \\
   F_{IO_2}: & 0.60 \\
   \text{Peak inspiratory pressure:} & 30 \text{ cm H}_2\text{O} \\
   \text{static pressure:} & 20 \text{ cm H}_2\text{O}
   \end{array}
   $$

   Calculate this patient's $\dot{V}_A$.

   A. 120 cc/min   D. 7.56 liters/min
   B. 198 cc/sec   E. 9.03 liters/min
   C. 2.97 liters/min

3. If this patient had the following arterial blood gas values: Pa_{O_2} 50 torr; Pa_{CO_2} 45 torr; pH 7.37. What therapeutic intervention would be most appropriate for this situation?

   A. Decrease the ventilatory rate.
   B. Increase the F_{IO_2}.
   C. Add positive end-expiratory pressure (PEEP).
   D. Add mechanical dead space.
   E. Decrease the tidal volume.

4. Consider the operation of volume-cycled ventilators and pressure-cycled ventilators in terms of their respective responses to obstructions or leaks in the patient-ventilator system. Which statements are correct?

   I. Volume-cycled ventilators will deliver the preset V_T to the patient despite encountering a mild obstruction.

   II. Pressure-cycled ventilators compensate for minimal leaks.

   III. Volume-cycled ventilators compensate for leaks and indicate a decrease in the peak inspiratory pressure.

IV. Pressure-cycled ventilators *cannot* compensate for mild obstructions and deliver a decreased V_T.

V. Volume ventilators indicate an increase in the peak inspiratory pressure when a mild obstruction is encountered.

A. I, II only

B. IV, V only

C. I, II, III only

D. I, II, IV, V only

E. III, IV, V only

5. A Bennett PR-2 is functioning in the control mode as a short-term mechanical ventilator in the Recovery Room. The therapist increases the preset pressure limit from 30 cm H_2O to 35 cm H_2O. What will be the effect on the ventilatory rate and inspiratory time? Neither the peak flow nor the sensitivity was changed.

A. inspiratory time ↑ ; ventilatory rate ↓

B. inspiratory time ↓ ; ventilatory rate ↑

C. inspiratory time ↓ ; ventilatory rate ↓

D. inspiratory time ↑ ; ventilatory rate ↑

E. Neither the inspiratory time nor the ventilatory rate will change.

6. Consider the ventilator management of a postoperative patient who has undergone a "routine," uneventful thoracotomy (coronary bypass surgery) and that of a patient in acute pulmonary edema. What differences and/or similarities might exist? Assume that all patient factors and variables, for example, age, weight, and sex, are equal except the clinical condition of these two persons.

I. Both patients would probably be maintained on a high $F_{I_{O_2}}$, that is, 0.60.

II. Peak inspiratory pressure for the pulmonary edema patient would be greater than that for the postoperative thoracotomy patient.

III. Both patients would probably be candidates for PEEP.

IV. The acute pulmonary edema patient should be placed on IMV immediately, whereas the other patient should *not*.

V. The postoperative thoracotomy patient may benefit more from the sigh mechanism than the pulmonary edema patient.

A. I, II, III, IV, V

B. II, IV, V only

C. I, II, IV only

D. II, IV only

E. II, V only

7. A teenage drug overdose victim was admitted through the Emergency Room. Blood gas data revealed:

Pa_{O_2}:   59 torr
Pa_{CO_2}:   82 torr
pH: 7.13
HCO_3^-:   27 mEq/liter
B.E: 0
Sa_{O_2}:   70%

Which acid-base interpretation(s) and/or therapeutic intervention(s) would be acceptable?

    I. This patient has an uncompensated respiratory acidosis.

    II. Acute ventilatory failure is present.

    III. The patient should probably be placed on a mechanical ventilator.

    IV. Intermittent mandatory ventilation (IMV) with PEEP may be useful.

A. I, II, III only   D. I, II, V only

B. I, II only   E. I only

C. IV, V only

8. An 83-kg (ideal body weight) patient is receiving controlled mechanical ventilation on a volume ventilator with the following settings:

$$
\begin{aligned}
V_T: &\quad 900 \text{ cc} \\
\text{Ventilatory rate}: &\quad 16 \text{ breaths/min} \\
\dot{V}: &\quad 50 \text{ liters/min} \\
F_{I_{O_2}}: &\quad 0.40 \\
\text{Peak inspiratory pressure}: &\quad 44 \text{ cm } H_2O \\
\text{Static pressure}: &\quad 36 \text{ cm } H_2O
\end{aligned}
$$

Calculate this patient's $\dot{V}_D$.

A. 1.44 liters/min   D. 3.20 liters/min

B. 1.66 liters/min   E. 8.30 liters/min

C. 2.93 liters/min

9. A 25-year-old football player incurred a flail chest injury in an automobile accident while en route to his home after practice. While on a volume ventilator with an $F_{I_{O_2}}$ of 0.30, he displayed the following blood gases: Pa_{O_2} 120 mm Hg; Pa_{CO_2} 44 mm Hg; pH 7.38. A PEEP of 5 cm H_2O has been ordered by the physician. What is the probable rationale for this decision? This person has never had a pleural effusion or pneumothorax.

A. To increase the patient's Pa_{O_2} without having to increase the $F_{I_{O_2}}$.

B. To overcome the patient's severe shunting problem.

C. To assist in stabilizing the chest wall.

D. To overcome the patient's lung parenchymal problem.

E. To help absorb air that might be trapped in the pleural space resulting from this accident.

10. Which calculation(s) often prove(s) sufficient when one establishes an initial ventilator V_T for an adult patient?

    I. multiplying the patient's ideal body weight in kilograms by 1 ml/kg

    II. dividing the patient's ideal body surface area by the Pa_{CO_2}

    III. using the Fick equation

    IV. multiplying the patient's ideal body weight in kilograms by approximately 10 ml/kg

    V. multiplying the patient's ventilatory rate by 50

A. I only   D. IV only

B. II, IV only   E. III, IV only

C. I, II only

11. Which ventilatory rate and tidal volume most closely describe those associated with IMV used for weaning? (Assume a 65-kg adult male patient.)

    A. Ventilator rate of 12 breaths/min; V_T of 12 cc/kg.

    B. Ventilator rate of 8 breaths/min with the patient triggering the machine an additional 6 times/min, delivering a V_T of 10 cc/kg on each cycle.

    C. Ventilator rate of 2 breaths/min accompained by a spontaneous ventilatory rate for the patient of 12 breaths/min; 10 cc/kg V_T delivered by the machine; 8 cc/kg V_T spontaneously breathed.

    D. Ventilator rate of 5 breaths/min phased with a patient spontaneously breathing at 12 breaths/min; none of the 5 machine breaths will interfere with any of the patient's spontaneous efforts; both machine and patient V_T are at 10 cc/kg.

    E. Ventilator rate of 0 breaths/min; with the patient spontaneously breathing at 14 breaths/min, generating a V_T of <8 cc/kg.

12. Which of the following statements accurately refer to PEEP.

    I. Applying PEEP to a patient may decrease the pulmonary compliance.

    II. PEEP is often effective in relieving hypoxemia produced by increased intrapulmonary shunting when the FRC is bilaterally decreased.

    III. Physiologic PEEP can be defined as the application of greater than 10 cm H_2O PEEP to a patient's airways.

    IV. PEEP may increase intrapulmonary shunting.

    A. I, II, IV only   D. II, III only

    B. I, III only   E. I, II, III, IV

    C. II, IV only

13. Intermittent mandatory ventilation (IMV) is useful in which situation(s)?

    I. while a patient is sedated

    II. for an assisting patient receiving an $F_{I_{O_2}}$ of 0.30, and having the following blood gases: Pa_{O_2} 93 mm Hg; Pa_{CO_2} 29 mm Hg; pH 7.47

    III. while a patient is on intermittent demand ventilation (IDV)

    IV. for a patient in status asthmaticus

    A. II only   D. II, III only

    B. II, IV only   E. I, IV only

    C. I, III only

14. For a patient on a mechanical ventilator, which I/E ratio would *most* adversely influence the cardiac output?

    A. 1:2   D. 2:1

    B. 1:4   E. 2:4

    C. 2:3

15. Which physiologic event(s) does(do) *not* generally occur during the inspiratory phase when continuous mechanical positive pressure breathing is administered?

I. Compression of major blood vessels occurs.

II. Decreased venous return occurs.

III. Decreased output of the left side of the heart occurs as mean intrathoracic pressure increases.

IV. Intrathoracic pressure remains subambient.

V. Bronchodilatation occurs.

A. IV only
B. V only
C. III, IV only
D. I only
E. II, III only

16. When positive pressure is applied on expiration, a potential complication that must be carefully monitored is:

A. The patient may become unconscious.
B. Systolic blood pressure may fall.
C. Marked tachycardia may occur.
D. Irregular ventilatory movements may occur.
E. Convulsions may occur.

17. If a patient on a volume ventilator in the control mode receiving a 0.60 F_{IO_2} displayed the following gases: Pa_{O_2} 80 mm Hg; Pa_{CO_2} 28 mm Hg; pH 7.46, which setting change would be most appropriate?

A. increasing the F_{IO_2}
B. decreasing V_T
C. increasing the ventilatory rate
D. adding mechanical dead space
E. increasing the flowrate

18. If the flowrate were to be decreased on a pressure preset ventilator while all the other parameters remained the same, what would be the result?

A. The V_T would increase.
B. The ventilatory rate would increase.
C. The inspiratory time would decrease
D. The inspiratory pressure would increase.
E. The expiratory time would increase.

19. A patient is being maintained on controlled mechanical ventilation via a volume ventilator, with the following parameters:

Ventilatory rate: 12 breaths/min
Inspiratory flowrate: 40 liters/min
V_T: 800 cc

Determine the approximate I/E ratio.

A. 1:2
B. 2:1
C. 1:4
D. 1:1.5
E. 1:3

20. Which conditions might cause an increase in the peak inspiratory pressure reading?

    I. adding 4 cm H_2O PEEP
   II. reducing the F_{IO_2}
  III. a spontaneous pneumothorax developed by the patient
  IV. eliminating expiratory resistance to the system
   V. decreasing the sensitivity control

    A. I, II, III, IV, V
    B. II, IV only
    C. I, III, IV only
    D. II, V only
    E. I, III only

Questions 21, 22, and 23 refer to the same patient.

A 70-kg patient is about to be mechanically ventilated by a Puritan-Bennett 7200 microprocessor ventilator. Before setting the initial ventilation parameters, the respiratory care practitioner wishes to determine the system compliance for this ventilator. She sets the tidal volume to 200 ml and allows the machine to cycle to inspiration while occluding the patient connector. She then notes that the peak inspiratory pressure is 65 cm H_2O.

21. What is the system compliance in this situation?

    A. 1.00 ml/cm H_2O D. 3.08 ml/cm H_2O
    B. 2.35 ml/cm H_2O E. 3.49 ml/cm H_2O
    C. 2.65 ml/cm H_2O

22. The respiratory care practitioner then establishes the following initial ventilation parameters:

               V_T: 900 cc
               f: 12 breaths/min
            F_{IO_2}: 0.50
    Peak flowrate: 45 liters/min
         PEEP: 10 cm H_2O
  Plateau duration: 0.2 sec

    The patient is then placed on the ventilator, and it is noted that the peak inspiratory pressure achieved is 45 cm H_2O. Calculate the patient's actual tidal volume.

    A. 808 cc   D. 762 cc
    B. 792 cc   E. 743 cc
    C. 781 cc

23. When the exhalation valve line is occluded, the pressure noted is 35 cm H_2O. Determine the patient's static compliance.

    A. 21.77 cc/cm H_2O
    B. 22.65 cc/cm H_2O

   C. 30.48 cc/cm H_2O

   D. 31.24 cc/cm H_2O

   E. 31.68 cc/cm H_2O

24. The use of PEEP in conjunction with mechanical ventilation may produce which of the following effects?

   I. increase the FRC

   II. increase intracranial pressure

   III. reduce the $P(A - a)O_2$

   IV. prevent atelectasis

   V. impede venous return

   A. I, II, III, IV, V   D. II, IV only

   B. I, III, IV, V only   E. I, V only

   C. I, IV, V only

25. An accumulation of secretions in the airway of a patient on a pressure-cycled ventilator operating as a continuous mechanical ventilator will result in which situation?

   A. an increase in the peak system pressure

   B. an increase in the delivered flowrate

   C. an increase in tidal volume

   D. an alteration of the I/E ratio

   E. a decrease in the ventilatory rate

26. What may indicate that the pulmonary compliance of a patient on a controlled volume-cycled ventilator has decreased?

   A. a minute volume decrease

   B. a decrease in the delivered tidal volume

   C. an increase in the flowrate

   D. an increase in the system pressure

   E. an increase in the ventilatory rate

27. Which of the following fluidic logic devices (Figures 115–119 located on pages 458–460) is termed AND/NAND?

28. A patient undergoing controlled volume ventilation (tubing compliance = 2 cc/cm H_2O) at a rate of 14 breaths/min has a tidal volume of 1,100 cc and a peak flow setting of 40 liters/min. The peak inspiratory pressure is 51 cm H_2O and the plateau pressure is 39 cm H_2O. The airway resistance is _____ cm H_2O/liter/sec.

   A. 20.00   D. 7.57

   B. 17.91   E. 2.25

   C. 8.89

A.

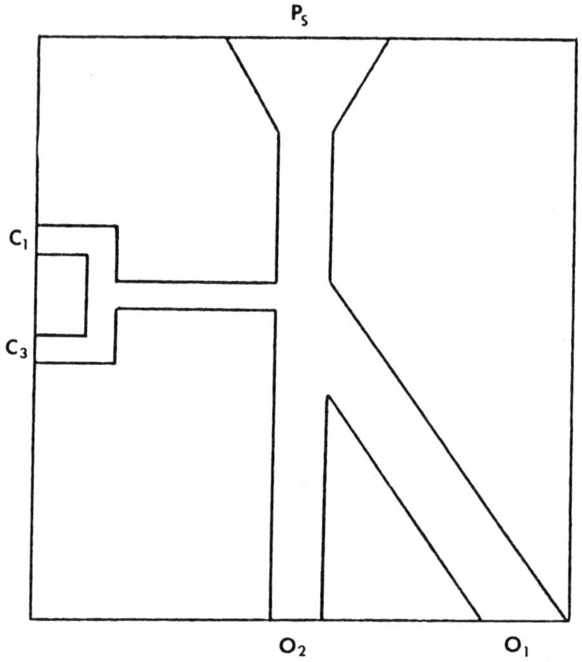

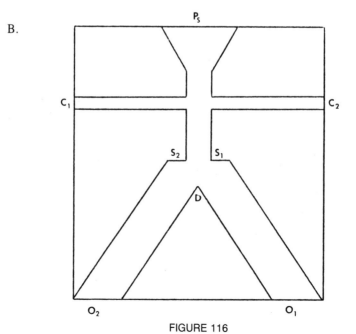

FIGURE 115

B.

FIGURE 116

C.

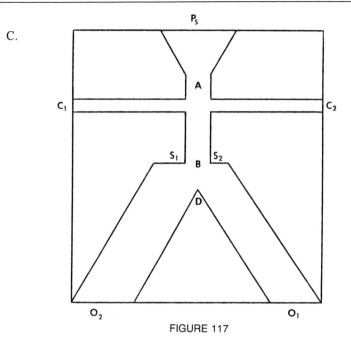

FIGURE 117

D.

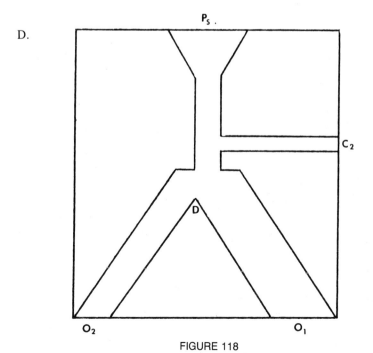

FIGURE 118

E.

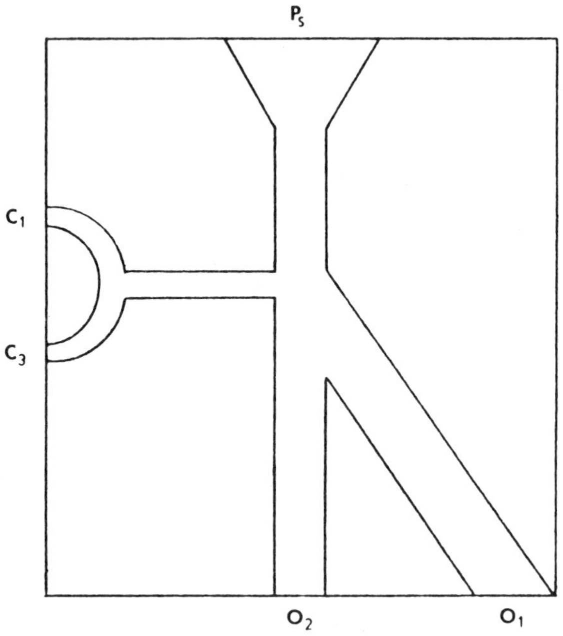

FIGURE 119

29. Which statement(s) refer(s) to the function of a constant-flow pressure ventilator?

    I. Inspiratory time will increase if the patient's lung compliance decreases.
    II. As the patient's airway resistance increases, the delivered flowrate will adjust accordingly.
    III. Increasing back pressure in the system reduces the machine's flowrate.
    IV. Neither a change in the patient's lung compliance nor a change in airway resistance will result in a change in the machine's flowrate.

    A. II, III only
    B. IV only
    C. I only

    D. I, III only
    E. II only

30. Which statement correctly refers to Figure 120?

    A. The diagram represents flow patterns in an endotracheal tube associated with positive pressure ventilation.
    B. The diagram represents coaxial flow as seen with positive pressure ventilation.
    C. The diagram depicts airway flow patterns associated with the application of PEEP.
    D. The diagram depicts bidirectional flow associated with high-frequency ventilation.
    E. The diagram represents the changing flow patterns associated with continuous distending airway pressure.

31. After a patient is placed on a PEEP of 10 cm H_2O, what settings may require changing to accommodate the PEEP? (Assume volume ventilation.)

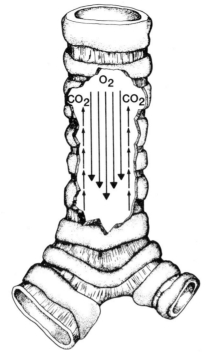

FIGURE 120

I. sensitivity
II. pressure limit
III. V$_T$
IV. peak flow
V. sigh controls

A. I, II, III, IV
B. I, II, V only
C. II, III only

D. I, III, IV only
E. III, V only

32. When considering the assist/control mode for mechanically ventilating a patient, the respiratory care practitioner should be cognizant of which of the following potential conditions and/or changes, as the patient is managed on the ventilator?

I. changes in acid-base status caused by fluctuations in the patient's ventilatory rate
II. decreased venous return as the patient's ventilatory rate increases
III. failure to ventilate if the patient ceases spontaneous breathing
IV. increased demand valve sensitivity causing increased work of breathing

A. I, II only
B. II, III only
C. I, II, IV only

D. III, IV only
E. I, III, IV only

33. Which V_D/V_T ratio range is acceptable when evaluating a mechanically ventilated patient for weaning?

    A. >0.40   D. <0.40
    B. >0.30   E. <0.25
    C. <0.60

34. Determine an appropriate flowrate needed to deliver a 40-ml V_T to an infant breathing 45 breaths/min while on a mechanical ventilator. The desired I/E ratio is 1:2.

    A. 150 ml/sec   D. 100 ml/sec
    B. 126 ml/sec   E. 90 ml/sec
    C. 120 ml/sec

35. The following information refers to a 150-lb (ideal body weight) middle-aged man. What procedure(s) would be acceptable after attempting to normalize the blood gas data shown below?

    Pa_{O_2}:   88 torr
    Pa_{CO_2}: 26 torr
    pH: 7.50
    HCO_3^-: 22 mEq/liter

    The patient is on controlled ventilation with the following parameters: V_T 700 cc; ventilatory rate 14 breaths/min; $F_{I_{O_2}}$ 0.40.

    A. Administer NH_4Cl and add mechanical dead space.
    B. Increase the $F_{I_{O_2}}$ and increase the $\dot{V}_E$.
    C. Decrease the ventilatory rate.
    D. Add mechanical dead space and increase the $F_{I_{O_2}}$.
    E. Administer NH_4Cl, decrease the ventilatory rate, and increase the $F_{I_{O_2}}$.

36. What is(are) the expected advantage(s) of using the method illustrated in Figure 121 for patient extubation and/or discontinuance from mechanical ventilation?

BRIGGS ADAPTER SETUP

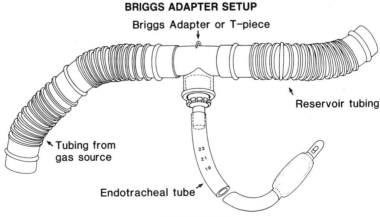

FIGURE 121

    I. It increases the mechanical dead space, thereby challenging the patient to breathe spontaneously.

II. The reservoir tubing serves to maintain a consistent F_{IO_2}.

III. The system provides continuous distending airway pressure, as the patient breathes without mechanical assistance.

IV. It allows for fluctuations in the F_{IO_2} and challenges the peripheral chemoreceptors.

A. I, IV only

B. I, II only

C. II, III only

D. II only

E. I, III, IV only

37. A patient placed on a mechanical ventilator has experienced a $\dot{V}_A/\dot{Q}_C$ ratio increase as a consequence. What might be a reason for this phenomenon?

A. re-established circulation

B. impeded venous return

C. increased ventilatory rate

D. increased dead space volume

E. absorption atelectasis caused by an increased F_{IO_2}

38. Which pressure-time tracing (Figures 122–126 located on page 464) represents intermittent mandatory ventilation (IMV)?

39. What actions should be taken to reduce the incidence of nosocomial infections for patients receiving mechanical ventilation?

I. Frequently drain breathing circuit condensate into the humidifier reservoir.

II. Replace the breathing circuit every 8 hours.

III. Handwash before and after handling the patient and/or equipment.

IV. Before refilling the humidifier reservoir, discard the unused water.

A. I, III, IV only

B. II, III only

C. I, II only

D. III, IV only

E. I, II, III only

40. If the pressure needed to deliver a 1-liter tidal volume to a patient is 30 cm H_2O (peak pressure manometer reading), calculate the effective static compliance.

A. 0.033 liter/cm H_2O

B. 0.04 liter/cm H_2O

C. 0.20 liter/cm H_2O

D. 30 cm H_2O/liter

E. Calculation is impossible because insufficient data are given.

41. A 5 ft 7 in., 33-year-old woman weighing 450 lb is brought into the Emergency Room requiring mechanical ventilation. What tidal volume would be most appropriate initially?

A. 450 cc

B. 900 cc

C. 1,200 cc

D. 2,000 cc

E. 2,250 cc

A.

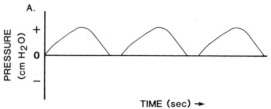

FIGURE 122

B.

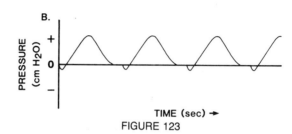

FIGURE 123

C.

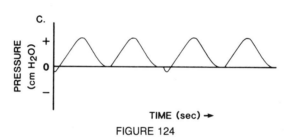

FIGURE 124

D.

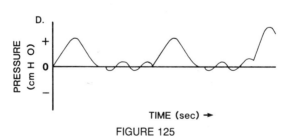

FIGURE 125

E.

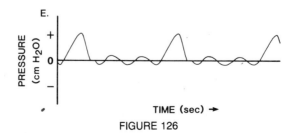

FIGURE 126

42. You are working in a CCU and suspect that a ventilator malfunction is occurring with a patient who is on controlled mechanical ventilation. What procedures should you *sequentially* perform?

    I. Disconnect the patient from the ventilator and provide ventilation via a manual resuscitator.
    II. Clinically, assess the patient for level of consciousness, breathing activity, changes in system pressure, unusual patient and/or machine sounds.
    III. Check all tubing connections, humidifier seal, IMV/PEEP valves, etc.
    IV. Replace the ventilator.

    A. I, II, III, IV   D. I, IV, II, III
    B. II, I, III, IV   E. III, I, II, IV
    C. III, II, I, IV

43. Calculate the time constant given the following data:

Peak inspiratory pressure:	40 cm H_2O
Plateau pressure:	20 cm H_2O
Tidal volume:	800 cc
PEEP:	5 cm H_2O
Inspiratory flowrate:	50 liters/min
Inspiratory time:	1 second

    A. 1.27 sec   D. 0.33 sec
    B. 0.95 sec   E. 0.02 sec
    C. 0.79 sec

44. Which of the following clinical parameters are criteria for deciding discontinuance of mechanical ventilation?

    I. a maximum inspiratory pressure of -25 cm H_2O
    II. a vital capacity greater than or equal to 10 to 15 ml/kg of the patient's ideal body weight
    III. $V_D/V_T = 0.85$
    IV. $\dot{Q}s/\dot{Q}_T = 0.40$

    A. III, IV only   D. I, III only
    B. I, III, IV only   E. I, II only
    C. II, IV only

45. Having observed a patient on a mechanical ventilator, you determine that the patient is "fighting the ventilator." What situations that caused the patient to "fight the ventilator" might be occurring?

    I. increased flowrate
    II. insensitive demand valves
    III. decreased inspiratory time
    IV. patient irritability and agitation

A. I, II, III, IV
B. I, III only
C. II, IV only
D. I, II, IV only
E. II, III, IV only

46. Identify desirable characteristics associated with infant mechanical ventilators.

   I. low compressibility factor for the breathing circuit
   II. rapid response time to patient-initiated breaths
   III. PEEP and CPAP capabilities
   IV. use of a pressure-controlled, time-cycled machine for infants with noncompliant lungs

A. I, II, III, IV
B. III only
C. I, II, III only
D. II, IV only
E. I, III only

47. Assuming a patient on controlled mechanical ventilation with the following settings:

$$V_T: \quad 850 \text{ cc}$$
Inspiratory time: 1 second
Peak inspiratory pressure: 43 cm H_2O
Static pressure: 25 cm H_2O

Calculate the airway resistance.

A. 18 cm H_2O/liter/sec
B. 21 cm H_2O/liter/sec
C. 31 cm H_2O/liter/sec
D. 50 cm H_2O/liter/sec
E. 76 cm H_2O/liter/sec

Questions 48, 49, and 50 refer to the same patient.

An automobile accident victim is admitted to the Emergency Room. Clinical examination of the victim reveals massive head injury with cerebral hemorrhage. The victim presents comatose with an irregular ventilatory pattern, a spontaneous rate of 7 breaths/min, and V_T of 270 cc. The victim weighs approximately 72 kg and is 52 years of age.

48. What therapeutic intervention is immediately recommended for this patient?

A. CPAP
B. mechanical ventilation with 5 cm H_2O of PEEP
C. assist/control mechanical ventilation
D. mechanical ventilation with an IMV rate of 10
E. controlled mechanical ventilation maintaining a low Pa_{CO_2}

49. How should intracranial pressure be managed for this patient?

   I. Maintain adequate Pa_{O_2} to reduce cerebral vasodilation.
   II. Maintain a low Pa_{CO_2}.
   III. Reduce the resistance of the cerebral vasculature to enhance cerebral blood flow.
   IV. Avoid inducing coughing, gagging, and excessive peak inspiratory pressures.

A. I, II, III, IV
B. I, II only
C. III, IV only
D. I, IV only
E. II, III only

50. The patient's Pa_{CO_2} should be maintained in the range of _____ .

A. 10 to 15 mm Hg
B. 20 to 25 mm Hg
C. 30 to 50 mm Hg
D. 35 to 45 mm Hg
E. 50 to 60 mm Hg

ASSESSMENT ANSWER SHEET

DIRECTIONS: Darken the space under the selected answer.

	A	B	C	D	E		A	B	C	D	E
1.	[ ]	[ ]	[ ]	[ ]	[ ]	26.	[ ]	[ ]	[ ]	[ ]	[ ]
2.	[ ]	[ ]	[ ]	[ ]	[ ]	27.	[ ]	[ ]	[ ]	[ ]	[ ]
3.	[ ]	[ ]	[ ]	[ ]	[ ]	28.	[ ]	[ ]	[ ]	[ ]	[ ]
4.	[ ]	[ ]	[ ]	[ ]	[ ]	29.	[ ]	[ ]	[ ]	[ ]	[ ]
5.	[ ]	[ ]	[ ]	[ ]	[ ]	30.	[ ]	[ ]	[ ]	[ ]	[ ]
6.	[ ]	[ ]	[ ]	[ ]	[ ]	31.	[ ]	[ ]	[ ]	[ ]	[ ]
7.	[ ]	[ ]	[ ]	[ ]	[ ]	32.	[ ]	[ ]	[ ]	[ ]	[ ]
8.	[ ]	[ ]	[ ]	[ ]	[ ]	33.	[ ]	[ ]	[ ]	[ ]	[ ]
9.	[ ]	[ ]	[ ]	[ ]	[ ]	34.	[ ]	[ ]	[ ]	[ ]	[ ]
10.	[ ]	[ ]	[ ]	[ ]	[ ]	35.	[ ]	[ ]	[ ]	[ ]	[ ]
11.	[ ]	[ ]	[ ]	[ ]	[ ]	36.	[ ]	[ ]	[ ]	[ ]	[ ]
12.	[ ]	[ ]	[ ]	[ ]	[ ]	37.	[ ]	[ ]	[ ]	[ ]	[ ]
13.	[ ]	[ ]	[ ]	[ ]	[ ]	38.	[ ]	[ ]	[ ]	[ ]	[ ]
14.	[ ]	[ ]	[ ]	[ ]	[ ]	39.	[ ]	[ ]	[ ]	[ ]	[ ]
15.	[ ]	[ ]	[ ]	[ ]	[ ]	40.	[ ]	[ ]	[ ]	[ ]	[ ]
16.	[ ]	[ ]	[ ]	[ ]	[ ]	41.	[ ]	[ ]	[ ]	[ ]	[ ]
17.	[ ]	[ ]	[ ]	[ ]	[ ]	42.	[ ]	[ ]	[ ]	[ ]	[ ]
18.	[ ]	[ ]	[ ]	[ ]	[ ]	43.	[ ]	[ ]	[ ]	[ ]	[ ]
19.	[ ]	[ ]	[ ]	[ ]	[ ]	44.	[ ]	[ ]	[ ]	[ ]	[ ]
20.	[ ]	[ ]	[ ]	[ ]	[ ]	45.	[ ]	[ ]	[ ]	[ ]	[ ]
21.	[ ]	[ ]	[ ]	[ ]	[ ]	46.	[ ]	[ ]	[ ]	[ ]	[ ]
22.	[ ]	[ ]	[ ]	[ ]	[ ]	47.	[ ]	[ ]	[ ]	[ ]	[ ]
23.	[ ]	[ ]	[ ]	[ ]	[ ]	48.	[ ]	[ ]	[ ]	[ ]	[ ]
24.	[ ]	[ ]	[ ]	[ ]	[ ]	49.	[ ]	[ ]	[ ]	[ ]	[ ]
25.	[ ]	[ ]	[ ]	[ ]	[ ]	50.	[ ]	[ ]	[ ]	[ ]	[ ]

MECHANICAL VENTILATION ANALYSES

Note: The references listed after each analysis are numbered and keyed to the reference list located at the end of this section. The first number indicates the text. The second number indicates the page where information about the question can be found. For example, (1:219,384) means that reference number 1 is to be used and that on pages 219 and 384 information about the question will be found. Frequently, it will be necessary to read beyond the page number indicated to obtain complete information. Therefore, reference to the question will be found either on the page indicated or on subsequent pages.

1. D. A large I/E ratio (inspiratory time greater than expiratory time) would maintain a higher-than-normal mean intrathoracic pressure for a longer time. As a consequence, the potential for a decreased venous return is greater than with a lower I/E ratio. Generally, the I/E ratio should be about 1:2; that is, inspiratory time should be approximately half as long as expiratory time. This ratio more closely approximates that associated with spontaneous ventilation.

   (1:544), (2:8–9), (3:129–130,346,347,363,366,383), (4:406–409), (5:242)

2. E. STEP 1: Convert kg to lb.

   1. 1 kg = 2.2 lb
   2. 90 kg × 2.2 lb/kg = 198 lb

   STEP 2: Estimate the amount of anatomic dead space. Guideline: one cubic centimeter (cc) of anatomic dead space (V_D) per pound (lb) of ideal body weight. Therefore,

   198 lb × 1 cc/lb of ideal body weight = 198 cc (V_D)

   STEP 3: Calculate the alveolar volume (V_A).

   800 cc V_T − 198 cc V_D = 602 cc V_A

   STEP 4: Calculate the minute alveolar ventilation ($\dot{V}_A$).

   ($\dot{V}_A$) (ventilatory rate) = $\dot{V}_A$
   (602 cc)(15 breaths/min) = 9,030 cc/min, or 9.03 liters/min ($\dot{V}_A$)

   (1:118), (2:29,151), (3:53), (4:225), (12:13)

3. C. The pH is within the normal range, that is, 7.35 to 7.45. Therefore, no intervention is indicated to alter the pH. Likewise, the Pa_{CO_2} value lies within normal limits (Pa_{CO_2} 35 mm Hg to 45 mm Hg). Consequently, no corrective measures are required for this parameter either. The Pa_{O_2} value, however, is low. The $F_{I_{O_2}}$ of 0.60 is already in the high range. Applying PEEP may serve to increase the Pa_{O_2}. Because no cardiovascular problem is mentioned in this situation, it may be assumed that the application of PEEP would not be contraindicated.

   (1:517–519,621–633), (3:431–433,409–414), (4:498–514), (6:264,565–566)

4. D. Volume ventilators generally can overcome small or mild obstructions in the patient-ventilator system, with a concomitant rise in system delivery pressure.

Therefore, the preset V_T can still be delivered. In terms of encountering leaks of any discernible size, volume ventilators will not deliver the preset volume and will display a lower delivery pressure on inspiration. Pressure ventilators, on the other hand, can compensate for minor leaks in the patient-ventilator system so long as the leak is not large enough to prevent achievement of the preset pressure. When pressure ventilators encounter obstructions, the preset pressure is prematurely reached, resulting in volume loss, decreased inspiratory time, and increased ventilatory rate.

(1:519–523), (3:380), (4:433), (6:563)

5. A. Increasing the preset pressure on the Bennett PR-2 will increase the inspiratory time and decrease the ventilatory rate, assuming that all the other controls remain constant. More volume can be delivered as a result of increasing the preset pressure.

(1:599)

6. E. A "routine" thoracotomy (e.g., coronary bypass surgery) patient would be expected to be extubated approximately after 24 hours of mechanical ventilation. An F_{IO_2} near 0.40 is usually sufficient. High inspiratory pressure and PEEP usually are not needed nor recommended for fear of potential cardiovascular compromise. IMV may be tolerated. Because high inspiratory pressures and PEEP generally are not used here, the sigh mode may be useful in the prevention of microatelectasis. However, some clinicians believe that *low* levels of PEEP may benefit the post-thoracotomy patient by preventing post surgical atelectasis. These patients are prone to shallow breathing because of incisional pain and lower chest wall compliance. It is thought that low levels of PEEP may help maintain the FRC, without causing cardiovascular embarrassment.

In acute pulmonary edema management, high F_{IO_2}s, high delivery pressures, and PEEP are commonly used. IMV is usually not considered because that mode of ventilation is associated with lower mean intrathoracic pressures (as are IDV and SIMV). Sighs would not be necessary because PEEP and larger tidal volumes tend to hyperinflate the lungs.

(3:476–478), (4:512), (6:545,878)

7. A. This condition can be deceiving. The absorption of more drug may worsen the situation quickly. Therefore, mechanical ventilation is indicated. Arterial blood gases reveal that this patient is experiencing uncompensated respiratory acidosis; that is, acute ventilatory failure. The blood gas and acid-base condition resulted from CNS depression caused by the drug abuse. Ventilatory support would be expected to improve the patient's oxygenation status.

(1:592, (12:275)

8. C. STEP 1: Convert 83 kg to lb.

       1. 1 kg = 2.2 lb/kg
       2. 83 kg × 2.2 lb/kg = 182.6 lb

STEP 2: Estimate the amount of anatomic dead space.
       Guideline: each pound of ideal body weight equals 1 cc of anatomic dead space.

$$183 \text{ lb} \times 1 \text{ cc/lb} = 183 \text{ cc } V_D$$

STEP 3: Determine the dead space ventilation ($\dot{V}_D$).

$$(V_D)(f) = \dot{V}_D$$
$$(183 \text{ cc})(16 \text{ breaths/min}) = 2{,}928 \text{ cc/min}$$
$$= 2.93 \text{ liters/min}$$

(1:116–120), (3:59–60), (4:224), (12:13)

9. C. This patient's Pa_{O_2} of 120 mm Hg is more than adequate. In fact, it should be reduced because it is at least 20 mm Hg greater than the upper limit of normal. This patient is not exhibiting a great degree of shunting. In flail chest it may be useful to further stabilize the chest wall. It does not necessarily mean that the patient has oxygenation problems. This patient has no lung parenchymal problem that can be helped by PEEP. If a pneumothorax is diagnosed, chest tubes should be used to evacuate air from the intrapleural space.
(3:461–462), (6:335)

10. D. Generally, a patient's tidal volume can be estimated by multiplying his ideal body weight in kilograms by 10 ml/kg. The key word here is *ideal*. For example, a Pickwickian syndrome patient would not be correctly ventilated if his actual body weight in kg was multiplied by 10 ml/kg when establishing an initial ventilator tidal volume setting. Rather, the patient's ideal body weight in kilograms, that is, what the patient's weight should be for his height and sex, is multiplied by 10 ml/kg.
(1:595–597, Appendix 718), (4:75)

11. C. A = controlled mechanical ventilation

B = assisted mechanical ventilation

C = intermittent mandatory ventilation

D = synchronized intermittent demand ventilation

E = spontaneous ventilation

IMV is a mode of ventilation that combines controlled (mandatory) mechanical breaths with the patient's spontaneous breaths.
(1:504,609–612,645) (3:384)

12. A. Hyperinflation of alveoli leads to decreased pulmonary compliance. One means of ascertaining optimal positive end-expiratory pressure (PEEP) is by applying small increments of PEEP and performing serial compliance checks. The point at which total compliance begins to decrease is the point at which the optimum PEEP level has been surpassed. The PEEP level should be set where the total compliance is the greatest.

Overdistention of normal alveoli may reduce pulmonary capillary perfusion as a result of decreasing venous return. Such a situation results in increased intrapulmonary shunting. Although PEEP is often instituted to reduce intrapulmonary shunting, PEEP may also increase the amount of shunting if it is carelessly applied and poorly monitored.

When the FRC is reduced, PEEP is often effective in reversing any associated hypoxemia because it reinflates collapsed alveoli. The FRC may be reduced by dis-

ease or clinical conditions that are unresponsive to PEEP therapy, e.g., pneumonia, pleural effusion, and pneumothorax.
(1:627–628), (3:425), (4:498–502)

13. A. A sedated patient (one with a depressed ventilatory drive) would not benefit from IMV. A patient receiving IDV ventilation is being administered a similar mode of ventilation; therefore, there would be no apparent reason to convert to IMV. A patient in status asthmaticus will generally require sedation and controlled mechanical ventilatory support because of his anxiety and the diffuse bronchospasm. The assisting patient who appears to be hyperventilating (Pa_{CO_2} 29 mm Hg) seems to be a reasonable IMV candidate because the Pa_{O_2} is adequate (93 mm Hg), while breathing a moderate Fi_{O_2} (0.30). The IMV may reduce the patient's $\dot{V}E$, thus increase the Pa_{CO_2} and lower the pH.
(1:611–612), (3:390–392), (4:468–474)

14. D. An I/E ratio of 2:1 represents an inspiratory time twice that of exhalation. Cardiac output is impaired during positive pressure mechanical ventilation, as a result of the elevated mean intrathoracic pressure. Consequently, if inspiratory time is allowed to exceed expiratory time, mean intrathoracic pressures will remain elevated longer. Usually, an I/E ratio of 1:2 or less is preferred.
(1:598–600), (3:347)

15. A. The elevation of the mean intrathoracic pressure is associated with (1) reducing venous return by physically compressing the vasculature, (2) decreasing left ventricular output as a consequence of reducing right ventricular output and venous return, and (3) promoting mechanical bronchodilatation. During inspiration, bronchi expand and elongate. This phenomenon is more pronounced during positive pressure ventilation.
(1:529–548), (3:362), (4:462), (6:531,546–549,574)

16. B. PEEP elevates the mean intrathoracic pressure, which reduces ventricular output. Hypotension is a possible complication.
(1:529–548), (3:362), (4:462), (6:531,546–549,574)

17. D. A pH of 7.46 and a Pa_{O_2} of 80 mm Hg both lie within approximately normal limits although a pH of 7.46 is 0.01 pH unit above the upper limit of normal. Because reducing the V_T or ventilatory rate might lower the Pa_{O_2}, neither one should be reduced. The best approach here is to add some mechanical dead space to elevate the Pa_{CO_2}. Because the patient is in the control mode, elevating the Pa_{CO_2} in this manner would not be difficult.
(4:488)

18. A. The tidal volume would increase as the flowrate was decreased because less volume/time ($\dot{V}$) would be delivered to the system. As a consequence, inspiratory time would increase. The longer time provided for inspiration allows for a better distribution of inhaled gas.
(1:513,522,599), (5:242–245)

19. E. STEP 1: Determine the length of the ventilatory cycle.

$$\frac{60 \text{ sec/min}}{\text{ventilatory rate}} = \text{length of ventilatory cycle}$$

$$\frac{60 \text{ sec/min}}{12 \text{ breath/min}} = 5 \text{ sec/breath}$$

STEP 2: Convert the inspiratory flowrate to liters/sec.

$$\frac{40 \text{ liters/min}}{60 \text{ sec/min}} = 0.66 \text{ liter/sec}$$

STEP 3: Convert 800 cc to _____ liter.

$$800 \text{ cc} = 0.8 \text{ liter}$$

STEP 4: Compute the inspiratory flowrate.

$$\frac{V_T}{\dot{V}} = \frac{0.8 \text{ liter}}{0.66 \text{ liter/sec}} = 1.21 \text{ sec I}_T$$

STEP 5: Obtain the expiratory time.

$$
\begin{array}{l}
5.00 \text{ sec (length of ventilatory cycle)} \\
\underline{- 1.21 \text{ sec I}_T} \\
3.79 \text{ sec E}_T
\end{array}
$$

$$\frac{1.21 \text{ sec (I}_T)}{3.79 \text{ sec (E}_T)} = \frac{1}{3} = 1{:}3$$

(5:242–245), (34:628)

20. E. Adding 4 cm H_2O PEEP will elevate the ventilatory baseline above ambient pressure, thus increasing the mean intrathoracic pressure throughout the entire ventilatory cycle. Rather than starting each inspiration at 0 cm H_2O, each inspiration will begin at 4 cm H_2O. A spontaneous pneumothorax would result in air being continuously deposited in the intrapleural space with each successive inspiration. The compression effect of the intrapleural air would make ensuing volumes difficult to deliver. Marked elevations of inspiratory pressure would be noted.
(3:410–441), (6:501,565–566,574,851), (16:177,194)

21. D. The term *system compliance* refers to the compliance (volume/pressure) of the ventilator-tubing system. The patient's pulmonary, chest wall, and total compliance measurements are *not* included in this value. Knowing the system compliance allows the respiratory care practitioner to determine the actual tidal volume the patient is receiving. System compliance is obtained as follows.

STEP 1: Set a tidal volume, e.g., 200 cc.

STEP 2: Set the pressure limit to its maximum limit.

STEP 3: Cycle the ventilator on to inspiration, occlude the patient wye, and note the peak inspiratory pressure (PIP). In this example the PIP is 65 cm H_2O.

STEP 4: Divide the V_T (200 cc) by the PIP (65 cm H_2O) to calculate the system compliance factor.

$$\frac{200 \text{ cc}}{65 \text{ cm } H_2O} = 3.08 \text{ cc/cm } H_2O$$

This value means that for each cm H_2O indicated on the pressure manometer during the patient's inspiration, 3.08 ml of gas are compressed ("lost") in the ventilator-tubing system.

22. B. By multiplying the difference between the peak inspiratory pressure (PIP) and PEEP by the system compliance factor, the respiratory care practitioner can compute the amount of the preset tidal volume lost in the ventilator-tubing system. The patient's actual tidal volume can then be obtained by subtracting the compressed volume from the preset tidal volume.

   STEP 1: Subtract the amount of PEEP from the PIP to determine the pressure generated to deliver the preset V_T.

   $$\text{PIP} - \text{PEEP} = \text{pressure generated to deliver the preset } V_T$$
   $$45 \text{ cm } H_2O - 10 \text{ cm } H_2O = 35 \text{ cm } H_2O$$

   STEP 2: Multiply the pressure generated to deliver the preset V_T by the system compliance factor to compute the volume compressed in the ventilator-tubing system.

   $$(35 \text{ cm } H_2O)(3.08 \text{ cc/cm } H_2O) = 107.8 \text{ cc}$$

   STEP 3: Subtract the compressed volume from the V_T set on the ventilator to calculate the patient's actual tidal volume.

   $$900 \text{ cc} - 108 \text{ cc} = 792 \text{ cc}$$

(4:482), (6:1002)

23. E. The PIP registered on the pressure manometer has two components. One is a static component and the other is a dynamic one. The static component refers to the pressure caused by the compliance of the patient-ventilator system. It represents the pressure generated to effect the volume change in that system.

   The dynamic component reflects the pressure generated to overcome airway resistance. It refers to the pressure resulting from the interaction of the molecules of the flowing gas, and the molecules and the walls (tubing and airways) of the patient-ventilator system.

   Again, the PIP incorporates both these components. However, each one can be obtained by occluding the tubing leading to the exhalation valve when the PIP has been achieved. When the exhalation valve tubing is occluded at end inspiration, the pressure manometer needle will fall to a reading termed the *plateau pressure* or *static pressure*. It is from this point that the static and dynamic components of the PIP can be isolated. Note the diagram of a pressure manometer shown in Figure 127.

   The static pressure is the pressure that is required to effect the volume change in the patient's lungs during inspiration. It is the pressure being exerted by the 792 ml of gas residing in the lungs at end-inspiration.

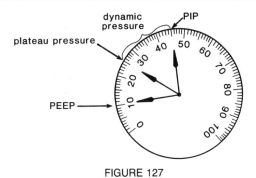

FIGURE 127

The dynamic pressure is the pressure that was generated to overcome the resistance of the patient-ventilator system while the volume was being delivered to the lungs. The static compliance can be calculated as follows.

STEP 1: Subtract the PEEP from the plateau pressure.

$$plateau\ pressure\ -\ PEEP\ =\ \Delta P$$
$$35\ cm\ H_2O\ -\ 10\ cm\ H_2O\ =\ 25\ cm\ H_2O$$

STEP 2: Calculate the static compliance by dividing the patient's actual tidal volume by the ΔP, or plateau pressure minus PEEP.

$$\frac{tidal\ volume}{\Delta P}\ =\ static\ compliance$$

$$\frac{792\ cc}{25\ cm\ H_2O}\ =\ 31.68\ cc/cm\ H_2O$$

(4:482), (6:247–249, 1002)

24. A. Therapeutically, PEEP often has the effect of increasing the FRC, reducing the alveolar-arterial oxygen tension difference, and preventing atelectasis by keeping the lungs hyperinflated during exhalation. PEEP is known to impede venous return, decrease cardiac output, and increase intracranial pressure.

(1:516–519,621–630), (3:408–441), (4:498–516), 12:121)

25. D. Because pressure ventilators are pressure preset, secretions or any obstruction, for that matter, would not elevate the inspiratory pressure. However, the inspiratory pressure limit would be met before an adequate amount of time elapsed. The result would be a decreased inspiratory time, an increased ventilatory rate, a decreased I/E ratio, and a decreased tidal volume.

(1:513,597–599), (3:81), (4:407–408,437)

26. D. A decrease in lung compliance indicates that the lungs are more difficult to inflate. A greater pressure is required to deliver the same volume. On a controlled volume-cycled ventilator, reduced compliance may be discernible by a higher peak inspiratory pressure indicated on the pressure manometer. The manometer reflects system pressure which includes the pressure characteristics of the lungs.

(1:593,601,633–636), (3:380,337,482–486), (4:314)

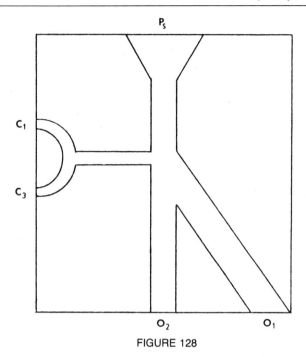

FIGURE 128

27. E. The AND/NAND fluidic logic device is shown in Figure 128. A constantly stable gas flow enters at P_s and flows out at O_2. Flow will only exit from O_1 if simultaneous amplification occurs from both C_1 and C_3. Gas flow through C_1 alone or C_3 alone will not deflect the main gas to exist O_1. When amplification from C_1 and C_3 terminates, flow will once again exit O_2. The AND/NAND device is, therefore, monostable. The other fluidic logic devices shown in the question are as follows

$$A = OR/NOR$$

$$B = symmetric\ bistable$$

$$C = asymmetric\ bistable$$

$$D = asymmetric\ monostable$$

(4:428–429)

28. B. The pressure difference (dynamic pressure) between the peak inspiratory pressure and the plateau (static) pressure represents the pressure generated in the patient-ventilator system needed to overcome airway resistance.

STEP 1: Subtract the plateau pressure from the peak inspiratory pressure (PIP) to compute the dynamic pressure.

$$PIP - plateau\ pressure = dynamic\ pressure$$
$$51\ cm\ H_2O - 39\ cm\ H_2O = 12\ cm\ H_2O$$

STEP 2: Convert the inspiratory flowrate from liters/min to liters/sec.

$$\frac{40\ liters/\cancel{min}}{60\ sec/\cancel{min}} = 0.67\ liter/sec$$

STEP 3: Calculate the airway resistance from the following relationship.

$$\frac{\text{transairway pressure}}{\text{flowrate}} = \frac{\Delta P}{\dot{V}} = R_{aw}$$

$$\frac{12 \text{ cm } H_2O}{0.67 \text{ liter/sec}} = 17.91 \text{ cm } H_2O/\text{liter/sec}$$

(1:144–148), (2:148,156,159), (4:80–82,483), (6:249–251,1002), (8:30–39)

29. B. Constant-flow pressure ventilators maintain the maximum flowrate throughout the inspiratory phase until the preset pressure is attained. As a result, the machine will not compensate nor adjust its flow automatically in the face of increased airway resistance or decreased lung compliance.
(1:505–512), (3:381), (4:434), (6:558–560)

30. D. Figure 120 illustrates a theoretical depiction of coaxial flow. Coaxial flow occurs with high frequency ventilation. Inspiration purportedly occurs through the center of the airway, whereas exhalation takes place simultaneously along the walls of the airway.
(2:149–152)(44:684–689)

31. B. If the patient has been assisting before the PEEP was added, the sensitivity should be adjusted so that the machine cycles on at about +8 cm H_2O, assuming the patient continues to assist. If the original pressure limit is reached or closely approached, the setting should be somewhat increased. A difference of 10 cm H_2O between peak inspiratory pressure and the pressure limit is generally safe. If the patient was receiving sigh volumes before PEEP was instituted, this mode should probably be discontinued because the sigh volumes may generate dangerously high intrathoracic pressures. Also, its function of preventing atelectasis is now taken over by the PEEP.
(1:627–629), (16:194)

32. A. The assist/control mode of mechanical ventilation allows the patient to control the ventilatory rate as long as his spontaneous rate is greater than the machine's rate. If not, the mode switches to control. As the ventilatory rate fluctuates, changes in the Pa_{CO_2} and acid-base status occur. As the patient's ventilatory rate increases, mean intrapulmonary pressures increase, which may, in turn, increase the mean intrathoracic pressure and decrease venous return.
(4:468–469), (6:566), (45:48)

33. C. The dead space/tidal volume ratio (V_D/V_T) represents the portion of the tidal volume that does not participate in gas exchange, i.e., wasted ventilation. As intrapulmonary gas exchange improves, the V_D/V_T ratio is generally reduced. Dead space volume is approximately equal to 1 cc/lb of ideal body weight, and comprises about 20% to 40% of the V_T.

The V_D/V_T ratio is a useful measurement for evaluating the effectiveness of ventilation. Consequently, it is often determined when a patient is being weaned from mechanical ventilation. A V_D/V_T ratio <0.60 is considered acceptable for supporting spontaneous breathing.
(4:227), (6:651), (44:632)

34. B. STEP 1: Determine the length of the ventilatory cycle by using the following relationship.

$$\frac{\text{\# of sec/min}}{\text{ventilatory rate}} = \text{length of ventilatory cycle}$$

$$\frac{60 \text{ sec/min}}{45 \text{ breaths/min}} = 1.33 \text{ sec/breath}$$

STEP 2: Determine the number of time segments comprising the desired I/E ratio. The desired I/E ratio of 1:2 has 3 time segments, i.e., $1 + 2 = 3$.

STEP 3: Compute the inspiratory time by dividing the length of the ventilatory cycle by the number of time segments comprising the I/E ratio.

$$\frac{1.33 \text{ sec}}{3} = 0.443 \text{ sec (I}_T)$$

STEP 4: Calculate the inspiratory flowrate by dividing the tidal volume by the inspiratory time.

$$\frac{V_T}{I_T} = \dot{V}$$

$$\frac{40 \text{ ml}}{0.443 \text{ sec}} = 90 \text{ ml/sec}$$

(4:474–476)

35. C. The patient's blood gas data indicate an uncompensated respiratory alkalosis. His Pa_{O_2} is in the normal range, although with an $F_{I_{O_2}}$ of 0.40, one would expect it to be higher. Because, according to the alveolar air equation, the PA_{O_2} is 255.3 torr. That is,

$$PA_{O_2} = (760 \text{ torr} - 47 \text{ torr})0.4 - 26 \text{ torr}\left(0.4 + \frac{1 - 0.4}{0.8}\right)$$

$$= (713 \text{ torr})0.4 - 29.9 \text{ torr}$$

$$= 255.3 \text{ torr}$$

Nonetheless, this patient's hypoxemia has been corrected.

The patient weighs 150 lb (68 kg); therefore, his V_T (700 cc) appears adequate for his size (60 kg × 10 cc/kg = 680 cc). His ventilatory rate could be reduced to 12 and still provide the patient with a $\dot{V}_E$ of 8.4 liters/min (700 cc × 12 breaths/min).

(1:595), (4:475)

36. D. The T-piece or Briggs adapter allows for trial periods of spontaneous ventilation. It acts as a weaning technique before the decision to extubate the patient and discontinue mechanical ventilatory support. The reservoir tubing serves to maintain a constant $F_{I_{O_2}}$. A liter flow of approximately 10 liters/min and reservoir tubing of 120 cc can generally maintain an $F_{I_{O_2}}$ of 0.50 without much difficulty.

Another advantage of this system is that it is easily adaptable to re-instituting mechanical ventilatory support if the patient requires it. However, the system is free from all the effects of positive airway pressure. During these trials the patient may experience hypoventilation, atelectasis, and increased intrapulmonary shunting. Consequently, an F_{IO_2} greater than that set on the mechanical ventilator should be provided by this mode of gas delivery.

(4:492–496), (6:652), (44:311–319)

37. B. The increased mean intrathoracic pressure impedes venous return which ultimately reduces left ventricular output. Mechanically assisted ventilation generally increases $\dot{V}_A$. Therefore, a decrease in cardiac output (decreased $\dot{Q}_C$) and an increase in $\dot{V}_A$ results in an increased $\dot{V}_A/\dot{Q}_C$.

(3:363,370–371), (12:273)

38. D. Intermittent mandatory ventilation (IMV) is depicted by tracing D (Figure 125). Positive pressure breaths are available via the control mode, while the patient is capable of breathing spontaneously in between these mandatory ventilations. The mandatory (controlled) ventilations are depicted by the tracing below the baseline. The spontaneous breaths are represented by those below the baseline. The other forms of ventilation shown are

> A = controlled mechanical ventilation (Figure 122)
>
> B = assisted mechanical ventilation (Figure 123)
>
> C = assist/control mechanical ventilation (Figure 124)
>
> E = synchronized intermittent mandatory ventilation (Figure 126)

Figure 129 depicts the pressure-time tracings of each of these five forms of mechanical ventilation. The letter *I* indicates the length of the inspiratory phase, and the letter *E* represents the duration of the expiratory phase. Tracings located below the baseline depict subambient or negative pressure generated by the patient during inspiration.

(1:503,505), (4:468–473), (6:570–573), (45:62–63)

39. D. No harm would come from more frequently changing tubing circuits, humidifier reservoir water, etc. However, the promulgated guidelines for practice to reduce the incidence of nosocomial infections of ventilator patients advise that: (1) the patient breathing circuit should be changed every 24 hours, (2) the humidifier reservoir should be completely emptied before refilling with fresh water, (3) the patient breathing circuit should be drained frequently and the condensate should not be allowed to drain back into the humidifier reservoir, and (4) the personnel in contact with the patient and/or equipment should handwash frequently.

(4:480), (38:289), (44:710)

40. E. If the pressure line leading to the exhalation valve is occluded when the peak inspiratory pressure has been achieved, the static or plateau pressure can be obtained. The static pressure approximates the pressure needed to expand the lungs. Dividing the static pressure into the tidal volume setting on the machine results in the static compliance. The term *effective static compliance* is often used to account for the presence of slight airflow between and within the lungs. The static compliance of the patient in this question cannot be calculated because the static pressure is not given.

(1:620), (4:482), (6:249), (7:51), (16:259)

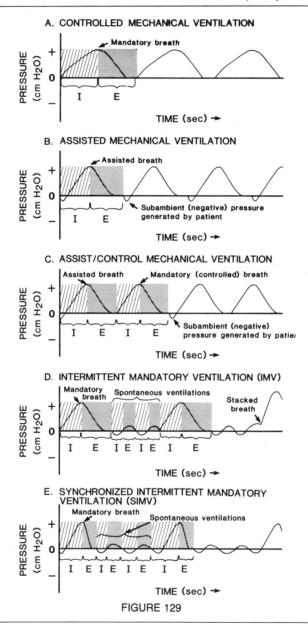

A. CONTROLLED MECHANICAL VENTILATION

B. ASSISTED MECHANICAL VENTILATION

C. ASSIST/CONTROL MECHANICAL VENTILATION

D. INTERMITTENT MANDATORY VENTILATION (IMV)

E. SYNCHRONIZED INTERMITTENT MANDATORY VENTILATION (SIMV)

FIGURE 129

41. B. A 5 ft 7 in. woman should weigh approximately 135 lb, which converts to approximately 61 kg. Using 10 cc/kg of ideal body weight as the rule of thumb, a VT of 610 cc would be appropriate. However, because of the obesity, a higher VT should be used to adequately ventilate the patient in the presence of this restrictive condition. A VT of 900 cc initially seems reasonable. Blood gas data are needed to ultimately determine the most suitable VT for this patient.

(1:595–597), (3:346,382), (4:475)

42. B. When a respiratory care practitioner suspects that a ventilator is malfunctioning, the first appropriate response is to evaluate the patient's level of consciousness, color, breathing activity, etc. Any unusual patient and/or machine sounds should be noted. The system pressure manometer also should be observed. Increasing peak inspiratory pressure is indicative of an obstruction. Decreasing pressure indicates a volume leak or a disconnection. If it is believed that the equipment is malfunctioning, disconnect the ventilator from the patient and provide ventilation via a manual resuscitator, which should be kept in close proximity to the ventilator at all times. A thorough check of all tubing connections should then be performed along with equipment functions. If the malfunction cannot be corrected, replace the ventilator. During this process the patient should be reassured and comforted. (38:710)

43. A. STEP 1: Calculate the effective static compliance according to the following formula.

$$\text{effective static compliance} = \frac{\text{tidal volume}}{\text{plateau pressure} - \text{PEEP}}$$

$$= \frac{0.8 \text{ liter}}{20 \text{ cm } H_2O - 5 \text{ cm } H_2O}$$

$$= 0.053 \text{ liter/cm } H_2O$$

STEP 2: Compute the airway resistance (R_{aw}) according to the following relationship.

$$R_{aw} = \frac{\text{pressure gradient}}{\text{gas flowrate}}$$

1. Convert the inspiratory flowrate ($\dot{V}$) of 50 liters/min to liters/sec. Because 1 min = 60 sec,

$$\frac{50 \text{ liters/min}}{60 \text{ sec/min}} = 0.83 \text{ liter/sec}$$

2. Obtain the pressure gradient or dynamic pressure (ΔP) by subtracting the plateau pressure from the peak inspiratory pressure (PIP).

$$\Delta P = \text{PIP} - \text{plateau pressure}$$
$$= 40 \text{ cm } H_2O - 20 \text{ cm } H_2O$$
$$= 20 \text{ cm } H_2O$$

3. $R_{aw} = \dfrac{\Delta P}{\dot{V}}$

$$= \frac{20 \text{ cm } H_2O}{0.83 \text{ liter/sec}}$$
$$= 24 \text{ cm } H_2O/\text{liter/sec}$$

STEP 3: Calculate the time constant by multiplying the compliance (C) by the airway resistance (R_{aw}).

$$\text{time constant} = C \times R_{aw}$$
$$= 0.053 \text{ liter/cm } H_2O \times 24 \text{ cm } H_2O \text{ liter/sec}$$
$$= 1.27 \text{ sec}$$

The time constant represents the length of time required to fill the lungs.
(4:82,482–483), (6:560–561), (45:12–14)

44. E. If a ventilator patient exhibits a maximum inspiratory pressure (MIP) of -25 cm H_2O, and a vital capacity greater than or equal to 10 to 15 ml/kg of the patient's ideal body weight, discontinuance of mechanical ventilation should be considered. Of course, other criteria should be assessed, for example, arterial blood gases, ventilatory rate, F_{IO_2}, vital signs, V_D/V_T, and $\dot{Q}_S/\dot{Q}_T$. The V_D/V_T ratio should be less than 0.6, whereas the $\dot{Q}_S/\dot{Q}_T$ should be less than 0.2.
(1:640), (3:75,348,373), (4:492), (6:650–651)

45. C. Patients may "fight the ventilator," or breath asynchronously, because of technical errors in setting machine parameters. If the patient does not "feel" like he is getting enough air, he may try to buck the machine. Inadequate flowrates from the ventilator or an IMV gas source causes lengthy inspiratory times unable to satisfy the need for volume in an expected time period. The flowrates must be sufficiently high and the inspiratory time sufficiently short, with adequate volume delivery to satisfy a person's inspiratory needs. It is also possible for clinically related conditions, such as patient anxiety, irritability, acid-base disturbances, to be reasons for "fighting" the ventilator.
(1:613), (4:476,485), (44:630,708)

46. A. Because of the small V_T used to ventilate infants it is especially important to minimize volume lost to tubing compressibility. A low compressibility factor for the breathing circuit is critical. The normally high infant ventilatory rate requires a machine capable of rapidly responding to patient-initiated breaths for SIMV or assist/control modes. Many infants requiring mechanical ventilatory support have low pulmonary compliance; PEEP or CPAP is often used. Thus, these capabilities are desirable characteristics of infant ventilators. For the care of infants with noncompliant lungs, a pressure controlled ventilator is preferred.
(5:536), (6:721)

47. B. STEP 1: Determine the transairway or dynamic pressure by subtracting the static (plateau) pressure from the peak inspiratory pressure (PIP).

$$\begin{array}{r} 43 \text{ cm } H_2O \text{ PIP} \\ -25 \text{ cm } H_2O \text{ static pressure} \\ \hline 18 \text{ cm } H_2O \text{ transairway pressure } (\Delta P) \end{array}$$

STEP 2: Calculate the flowrate ($\dot{V}$) by dividing the inspiratory time (I_T) into the tidal volume (V_T).

$$\frac{V_T}{I_T} = \dot{V}$$

$$\frac{850 \text{ cc}}{1 \text{ sec}} = 850 \text{ cc/sec or } 0.85 \text{ liter/sec}$$

STEP 3: Calculate the airway resistance (R_{aw}) by dividing the $\dot{V}$ into the ΔP.

$$\frac{\Delta P}{\dot{V}} = R_{aw}$$

$$\frac{18 \text{ cm } H_2O}{0.85 \text{ liter/sec}} = 21.1 \text{ cm } H_2O/\text{liter/sec}$$

(1:144–148), (2:148,156,159), (4:80–82,483), (6:249–251)

48. E. The primary concerns for this patient with massive cerebral hemorrhage are to provide an adequate alveolar ventilation and to reduce the intracranial pressure (ICP). The ICP can be lowered by reducing cerebral vascular resistance and providing adequate cerebral blood flow.

    The patient's inability to maintain adequate spontaneous minute ventilation requires that he be mechanically ventilated. A V_T of 270 cc and ventilatory rate of 7 breaths/min is insufficient to meet metabolic demands. It is important to precisely control the Pa_{CO_2}, as an increased Pa_{CO_2} causes cerebral vasodilatation, thereby increasing the intracranial pressure. Controlled ventilation is indicated.

    (6:838–840), (38:120–126)

49. A. Intracranial pressure can be monitored continuously. Hypoxia and hypercapnia produce cerebral vasodilatation increasing cerebral blood volume and increasing the ICP. An increased ICP will reduce cerebral perfusion pressure and cause a decrease in cerebral blood flow. It is necessary to control the ICP while continuing to maintain cerebral blood flow above critically low levels to avoid cerebral infarction.

    (6:838–840), (38:120–126)

50. B. In cases of severe intracranial hypertension, the Pa_{CO_2} should be maintained in a range of 20 to 25 mm Hg.

    (6:838–840), (38:120–126)

REFERENCES

1. Spearman, C., and Sheldon, R., *Egan's Fundamentals of Respiratory Therapy,* 4th ed., C.V. Mosby, St. Louis, 1982.
2. Wojciechowski, W., *Respiratory Care Sciences: An Integrated Approach,* John Wiley & Sons, New York, 1985.
3. Shapiro, B., Harrison, R., Kacmarek, R., and Cane, R., *Clinical Application of Respiratory Care,* 3rd ed., Year Book Medical Publishers, Chicago, 1985.
4. Kacmarek, R., Mack, C., and Dimas, S., *The Essentials of Respiratory Therapy,* 2nd ed., Year Book Medical Publishers, Chicago, 1985.
5. McPherson, S., *Respiratory Therapy Equipment,* 3rd ed., ed., C.V. Mosby, St. Louis, 1985.
6. Burton, G., and Hodgkin, J., *Respiratory Care: A Guide to Clinical Practice,* 2nd ed. J.B. Lippincott, Philadelphia, 1985.
7. Frownfelter, D., *Chest Physical Therapy and Cardiopulmonary Rehabilitation, An Interdisciplinary Approach,* Year Book Medical Publishers, Chicago, 1978.
8. Cherniack, R., and Cherniack, L., *Respiration in Health and Disease,* 3rd ed., W.B. Saunders, Philadelphia, 1983.

9. Daily, E., and Schroeder, G., *Techniques in Bedside Hemodynamic Monitoring,* 3rd ed., C.V. Mosby, St. Louis, 1985.

10. Des Jardins, R., *Clinical Manifestations of Respiratory Disease,* Year Book Medical Publishers, Chicago, 1984.

11. Mitchell, R., *Synopsis of Clinical Pulmonary Disease,* 3rd ed., C.V. Mosby, St. Louis, 1982.

12. Comroe, J., *Physiology of Respiration,* 3rd ed., Year Book Medical Publishers, Chicago, 1974.

13. West, J., *Pulmonary Pathophysiology—The Essentials,* 2nd ed., Wiliams & Wilkins, Baltimore, 1982.

14. West, J., *Respiratory Physiology—The Essentials,* 3rd ed., Williams & Wilkins, Baltimore, 1985.

15. Martz, K., et al. *Management of the Patient-Ventilator System: A Team Approach,* 2nd ed., C.V. Mosby, St. Louis, 1984.

16. Shoup, C., and McHenry, R., *Laboratory Exercises in Respiratory Therapy,* 2nd ed., C.V. Mosby, St. Louis, 1983.

17. Ruppel, G., *Manual of Pulmonary Function Testing,* 3rd ed., C.V. Mosby, St. Louis, 1982.

18. Appelbaum, E., and Bruce, D., *Tracheal Intubation,* W.B. Saunders, Philadelphia, 1976.

19. Rau, J., *Respiratory Therapy Pharmacology,* 2nd ed., Year Book Medical Publishers, Chicago, 1984.

20. United States Department of Health, Education, and Welfare, Public Health Service, *Isolation Techniques for Use in Hospitals,* 2nd ed., Washington, D.C., 1975.

21. Brooks, S., *Integrated Basic Science,* 4th ed., C.V. Mosby, St. Louis, 1979.

22. Comroe, J., *The Lung,* Year Book Medical Publishers, Chicago, 1962.

23. Shibel, E., and Moser, K., *Respiratory Emergencies,* 2nd ed., C.V. Mosby, St. Louis, 1982.

24. Tisi, G., *Pulmonary Physiology in Clinical Medicine,* 2nd ed., Williams & Wilkins, Baltimore, 1985.

25. Cherniack, R., *Pulmonary Function Testing,* W.B. Saunders, Philadelphia, 1977.

26. Altose M., *The Physiological Basis of Pulmonary Function Testing,* Clinical Symposia-CIBA, Vol. 31, No. 2, Summit, New Jersey, 1979.

27. Shapiro, B., Harrison, R., and Walton, J., *Clinical Application of Arterial Blood Gases,* 3rd ed., Year Book Medical Publishers, Chicago, 1982.

28. West, J., *Ventilation/Blood Flow and Gas Exchange,* 3rd ed., Blackwell Scientific Publications, 1979.

29. Slonim, N., and Hamilton, K., *Respiratory Physiology,* 4th ed., C.V. Mosby, St. Louis, 1981.

30. Rarey, K., and Youtsey, J., *Respiratory Patient Care,* Prentice-Hall, Englewood Cliffs, 1981.

31. Berne, R., and Levy, M., *Physiology,* C.V. Mosby, St. Louis, 1983.

32. Levitzky, M., *Pulmonary Physiology,* 2nd ed., McGraw-Hill, New York, 1986.

33. Wilson, P., Bell, C., and Norton, A., *Rehabilitation of the Heart and Lungs,* SensorMedics, 1980.

34. Clausen, J., and Zarins, L., *Pulmonary Function Testing Guidelines and Controversies,* Academic Press, New York, 1982.

35. Klaus, M., and Fanaroff, A., *Care of the High-Risk Neonate,* 2nd ed., W.B. Saunders, Philadelphia, 1979.

36. Lough, M., et al., *Pediatric Respiratory Therapy,* 3rd ed., Year Book Medical Publishers, Chicago, 1985.

37. Levin, D., et al., *A Practical Guide to Pediatric Intensive Care,* 2nd ed., C.V. Mosby, St. Louis, 1984.

38. O'Ryan, J., and Burns, D., *Pulmonary Rehabilitation from Hospital to Home,* Year Book Medical Publishers, Chicago, 1984.

39. Bell, C., et al., *Home Care and Rehabilitation in Respiratory Medicine,* J.B. Lippincott, Philadelphia, 1984.

40. Wilkins, R., et al., *Clinical Assessment in Respiratory Care,* C.V. Mosby, St. Louis, 1985.

41. Jones, N., and Campbell, E., *Clinical Exercise Testing,* 2nd ed., W.B. Saunders, Philadelphia, 1982.

42. Goldsmith, J., and Karotkin, E., *Assisted Ventilation of the Neonate,* W.B. Saunders, Philadelpia, 1981.

43. Blowers, M., and Sims, R., *How to Read an ECG,* 3rd ed., Medical Economics, New Jersey, 1983.

44. Eubanks, D., and Bone, R., *Comprehensive Respiratory Care,* C.V. Mosby, St. Louis, 1985.

45. Rattenborg, C., *Clinical Use of Mechanical Ventilation,* Year Book Medical Publishers, Chicago, 1981.

46. Witkowski, A. S., *Pulmonary Assessment: A Clinical Guide,* J.B. Lippincott, Philadelphia, 1985.

47. Op't Holt, T. B., *Assessment Based Respiratory Care,* John Wiley & Sons, New York, 1986.

CARDIOPULMONARY EVALUATION/CARDIOPULMONARY MONITORING AND INTERPRETATION ASSESSMENT

PURPOSE: The purpose of this 55-item section is to afford you the opportunity to evaluate your knowledge, comprehension, and clinical judgment in the following two areas (1) assessment of patient cardiopulmonary status, and (2) cardiopulmonary monitoring and interpretation. In this section you will be asked to (1) review signs and symptoms of patients with a variety of cardiopulmonary disorders; (2) perform radiographic evaluations; (3) assess data derived from inspection, palpation, percussion, and auscultation of the chest; and (4) evaluate pulmonary mechanics. Aspects of hemodynamic and transcutaneous monitoring, electrocardiography, ear oximetry, and umbilical artery catheterization also are included.

DIRECTIONS: Each of the questions or incomplete statements is followed by five suggested answers. Select the one which is the best in each case and then blacken the corresponding space on the answer sheet.

Questions 1 and 2 refer to the same patient.

A 5 ft 10 in., 210-lb, 63-year-old male factory worker is admitted to the General Medicine Ward. He displays the following physical features and signs:

1. stocky body build
2. dusky skin color
3. accessory ventilatory muscle usage
4. wheezing audible via auscultation
5. intercostal retractions
6. distended neck veins
7. peripheral edema
8. Pa_{O_2} 59 mm Hg, Pa_{CO_2} 68 mm Hg; pH 7.31
9. copious mucopurulent secretions

1. Which disease process is this patient most likely exhibiting?

   A. bronchial asthma   D. status asthmaticus
   B. pulmonary emphysema   E. bronchiectasis
   C. chronic bronchitis

2. What therapeutic interventions should be instituted on this patient?

   I. Venturi mask at an oxygen flowrate of 3 liters/min
   II. rotating tourniquets to reduce the strain on the heart
   III. ultrasonic nebulization as necessary to facilitate the removal of secretions
   IV. bronchodilator therapy

   A. I, II, III, IV   D. II, IV only
   B. I, IV only   E. I, III only
   C. I, II, III only

3. Which radiographic technique provides the best method for studying diaphragmatic activity?

   A. the standard chest roentgenogram   D. tomography
   B. bronchography   E. scintiscanning
   C. fluoroscopy

4. If it is suspected that a patient has a pulmonary embolism, what is the usual *sequence* of diagnostic procedures used for making a diagnosis?

   I. laboratory tests including chest x-ray, electrocardiogram, complete blood count, and arterial blood gases
   II. observation of the patient for the presence of clinical signs and symptoms, e.g., breathlessness and substernal pain
   III. pulmonary angiography
   IV. radioisotope lung scans

   A. I, II, III, IV   D. II, I, III, IV
   B. II, I, IV, III   E. II, IV, III, I
   C. II, IV, I, III

5. What diagnostic procedures would confirm the presence of pulmonary thromboembolism?

   I. pulmonary angiography
   II. chest x-ray
   III. radioisotope lung scan
   IV. bronchoscopy

   A. I, II, III only   D. I, III only
   B. II, IV only   E. I, II, III, IV
   C. I, III, IV only

6. Which breath sounds may sometimes disappear as a result of an effective cough generated by the patient?

   A. rales
   B. bronchovesicular
   C. vesicular
   D. amphoric
   E. rhonchi

7. What is the amount of inspiratory pressure that is generally sufficient to produce a vital capacity approximately equivalent to 15 ml/kg?

   A. 20 cm H_2O
   B. 15 mm Hg
   C. -10 mm Hg
   D. -20 cm H_2O
   E. -35 cm H_2O

8. Which clinical manifestations would represent the presence of a primary respiratory alkalosis?

   I. paresthesia
   II. tetany
   III. somnolence
   IV. decreased cerebral blood flow

   A. I, II only
   B. II, III only
   C. I, III, IV only
   D. III, IV only
   E. I, II, III, IV

9. Which clinical manifestations can be classified as symptoms of respiratory disease?

   I. dyspnea
   II. the degree of movement of the chest wall during ventilation
   III. breath sounds
   IV. the position of the trachea
   V. shortness of breath

   A. I, II, III, IV, V
   B. I, V only
   C. II, III, V only
   D. III, IV only
   E. I, III, V only

10. What is capnography?

    I. It is a means of measuring the carbon dioxide concentration in exhaled gas.
    II. It is the process of comparing the carbon dioxide concentration to the hemoglobin saturation.
    III. It is a carbon dioxide measurement process based on the principle of carbon dioxide absorption of infrared light.
    IV. It is a process whereby the exhaled carbon dioxide, oxygen, and nitrogen concentrations can be measured.

    A. I, II, III, IV
    B. II, IV only
    C. II, III only
    D. I, II, III only
    E. I, III only

11. Which of the following types of hemoglobin can be measured by a Co-Oximeter?

    I. carboxyhemoglobin
    II. oxyhemoglobin
    III. reduced hemoglobin
    IV. methemoglobin

    A. I, II, III, IV   D. I, II, III only
    B. I only   E. II, III only
    C. II only

12. Which patient would tend to exhibit cyanosis sooner?

    A. an anemic patient
    B. a patient with a hemoglobin concentration ranging from 12 g% to 15 g%
    C. a patient with polycythemia
    D. a patient having a reduced hematocrit
    E. a patient with a decreased P_{50}

13. Which statement(s) are true about radiographs?

    I. The closer the object is to the film, the larger the object will appear on the film.
    II. The black portions of an x-ray film are made by the most radiolucent objects exposed to the beam.
    III. A radiograph is named from the source of the x-rays to the film; for example, a recumbent or supine patient is between the photographic plate and the x-ray source on an anteroposterior film.
    IV. Standard x-ray films are more difficult to read than portable x-ray films.

    A. III, IV only   D. I, II, III only
    B. II, III only   E. I, II, III, IV
    C. II, III, IV only

14. Which statements relate to palpation of the thorax?

    I. The intensity of the sound is normally the lowest over the right upper lobe as compared with the rest of the lung.
    II. The vibrations felt above consolidated lung areas are more intense than those felt above air-filled areas.
    III. Palpation can be performed either by a stethoscope or by hand.
    IV. Symmetry of chest expansion is best evaluated by this means.

    A. I, II, III, IV   D. II, IV only
    B. I, III, IV only   E. I, III only
    C. II, III, IV only

15. Which of the following clinical manifestations are assessed as part of the Apgar score?

    I. heart rate
    II. reflex irritability

III. ventilatory rate

IV. color

V. xiphoid retractions

A. I, II, IV only   D. I, III, IV only

B. I, II, III only   E. I, II, III, IV only

C. II, IV, V only

16. What clinical monitoring should be performed on a post-operative pulmonary patient?

    I. a chest roentgenogram to rule out atelectasis

    II. arterial blood gases to rule out hypoxemia

    III. bedside spirometry to determine V_T and FVC

    IV. chest physical assessment

    A. I, II, III, IV   D. II only

    B. II, IV only   E. I, II only

    C. II, III, IV only

17. Anatomically, where should a pulmonary artery catheter be placed to measure pulmonary capillary wedge pressure?

    A. right atrium

    B. superior vena cava

    C. right ventricle

    D. inferior vena cava

    E. branch of the right or left pulmonary artery

18. Which procedures should be performed during a physical examination of the chest?

    I. percussion

    II. vibration

    III. auscultation

    IV. palpation

    A. I, III, IV only   D. II, IV only

    B. III, IV only   E. I, II, III, IV

    C. I, II only

19. What breathing pattern is characterized by cyclic increases and decreases in ventilation accompanied by apneic intervals?

    A. Cheyne-Stokes breathing   D. Biot's breathing

    B. apneustic breathing   E. paroxysmal breathing

    C. Kussmaul's breathing

20. Which of the following sounds can be considered abnormal breath sounds heard via auscultation?

    I. rales

    II. bronchovesicular

    III. vesicular
    IV. rhonchi
     V. vocal fremitus

   A. I, IV only   D. I, IV, V only
   B. II, V only   E. I, III, IV only
   C. II, III only

21. What are the components of the Silverman score used to evaluate newborns?

     I. ventilatory rate
    II. xiphoid retractions
   III. expiratory grunt
   IV. color
    V. dilation of the nares

   A. I, II, III, IV, V   D. II, IV, V only
   B. I, II, III only   E. II, IV only
   C. II, III, V only

22. Which of the following statements are true about an electrocardiogram?

     I. It is useful for calculating the cardiac output.
    II. It reflects the status of electrical conduction through the heart.
   III. It traces only ventricular repolarization and depolarization.
   IV. It measures an electric current moving from the heart to the body's surface.

   A. I, IV only   D. II, III, IV only
   B. I, II, III only   E. I, III only
   C. II, IV only

23. Which breath sounds are ordinarily more pronounced during exhalation?

   A. rales   D. crepitant
   B. bronchovesicular   E. rhonchi
   C. vocal fremitus

24. Which of the following statements are true regarding transcutaneous P_{O_2} (TcP_{O_2}) monitoring?

     I. The TcP_{O_2} and Pa_{O_2} measurements are equal when peripheral perfusion is low.
    II. TcP_{O_2} measures oxygen that diffuses through the skin.
   III. It is necessary to warm the skin surface at the measuring electrode to 43°C to 45°C.
   IV. The Clark electrode position should be changed every 3 to 4 hours.

   A. I, II, III, IV   D. II, III only
   B. II, III, IV only   E. I, III, IV only
   C. I, IV only

25. Which pulmonary function parameter *most* reflects a patient's ability to cough?

    A. IC

    B. SVC

    C. FVC

    D. $\dot{V}_E$

    E. TLC

26. How will mechanical ventilation affect central venous pressure (CVP) measurements obtained while the patient remains connected to a ventilator?

    A. If the patient is on the control mode, the CVP reading will be higher than if he were assisting the machine.

    B. If the patient is assisting the ventilator, the CVP measurement will be higher than it would be if the patient were controlled.

    C. In either the assist or control mode, CVP readings will be lower than if the patient were breathing spontaneously.

    D. CVP measurements will be higher in either the control or assist mode compared with CVP readings taken during spontaneous breathing.

    E. There is essentially no difference between CVP measurements taken during mechanical ventilation and those taken during spontaneous breathing.

27. How should the respiratory care practitioner position her hand for palpation of a patient during physical assessment of the chest?

    I. The ulnar surface may be used.

    II. The heel may be used.

    III. The fingertips may be used.

    IV. The palm may be used.

    A. II, III, IV only

    B. I, III only

    C. II, IV only

    D. I, III, IV only

    E. I, II, III, IV

28. Increased ventilatory rate, deviated trachea, unilaterally decreased vocal and tactile fremitus, and unilaterally decreased breath sounds may all be signs of which respiratory condtion?

    A. pneumonia

    B. pulmonary emphysema

    C. consolidation

    D. herniation

    E. pneumothorax

29. Which clinical feature represents the earliest sign of hypoxemia?

    A. tachycardia

    B. tachypnea

    C. cyanosis

    D. polycythemia

    E. dilated pupils

30. What is generally the sequence of performing a physical assessment of the chest?

    A. (1) auscultation, (2) inspection, (3) percussion (4) palpation

    B. (1) inspection, (2) percussion, (3) palpation, (4) auscultation

C. (1) palpation, (2) percussion, (3) inspection, (4) auscultation
D. (1) inspection, (2) palpation, (3) percussion, (4) auscultation
E. (1) percussion, (2) palpation, (3) inspection, (4) auscultation

31. Which of the following statements are true of the tracing shown in Figure 130?

   I. The tracing shows a pattern consistent with left ventricular failure.
   II. Point A on the tracing represents systolic pressure.
   III. Point B coincides with the sudden closure of the aortic valve.
   IV. Point C depicts diastolic pressure.

   A. I, II, III, IV   D. II, IV only
   B. II, III, IV only   E. I, II, III only
   C. I, III only

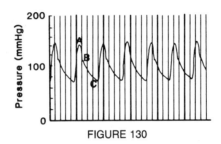

FIGURE 130

32. Which of the following breath sounds are considered abnormal?

   I. bronchovesicular
   II. vesicular
   III. rhonchi
   IV. amphoric

   A. II, III, IV only   D. I, II only
   B. III, IV only   E. II, IV only
   C. I, III only

33. On an electrocardiogram the T wave represents _____ .

   A. atrial depolarization   D. atrial repolarization
   B. ventricular depolarization   E. SA node to AV node conduction
   C. ventricular repolarization

34. Upon visually inspecting the chest of a 59-year-old factory worker who has smoked
    two packs of cigarettes a day for 40 years, you notice that his chest appears to be in a
    permanent state of inspiration while his ribs are held in a horizontal position. Further
    inspection reveals that the transverse chest diameter is almost equal to its anteroposte-
    rior diameter. While he breathes, you notice that his thorax moves up and down verti-
    cally as a whole. Which word or phase best describes this physical appearance of his
    chest?

A. scoliosis

B. bucket-handle movement

C. Pendelluft breathing

D. barrel chest

E. pectus carinatum

35. Which of the following statments are correct regarding the technique of transillumination?

    I. A bright light is placed against the chest wall while the patient is in a dark room.

    II. The technique is successfully used with infants and adults.

    III. The normal effect of transillumination is to "light up" the entire thorax.

    IV. The technique is useful in identifying a pneumothorax or a pneumomediastinum.

A. I, IV only

B. I, II, III only

C. II, III only

D. I, III, IV only

E. I, II, III, IV

36. Which pathologic conditions would cause a decrease in tactile fremitus?

    I. atelectasis

    II. pneumothorax

    III. thickened pleura

    IV. pleural effusion

A. II, IV only

B. I, II only

C. II, III, IV only

D. I, III only

E. I, II, III, IV

37. Letter A on the electrocardiogram in Figure 131 represents which cardiac activity?

A. the absolute refractory period

B. atrial depolarization

C. ventricular repolarization

D. atrial repolarization

E. ventricular depolarization

38. Regarding the use of ear oximetry for adults, which statement is true?

A. Ear oximetry is *not* a suitable monitoring technique for long-term use.

B. The device warms the ear upon placement from 45°C to 50°C.

C. It can be a useful technique for monitoring sleep apnea.

D. Ear oximetry is an equally effective monitoring technique for hemodynamically stable and unstable patients.

E. The device is easily maintained on the patient's ear and requires only occasional checking for proper placement.

39. What are indications for umbilical artery catheterization?

    I. central venous pressure monitoring

    II. frequent arterial blood gas sampling

    III. continuous blood pressure monitoring

    IV. large scale blood replacement

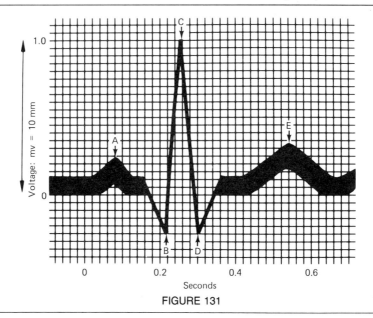

FIGURE 131

A. I, II, III, IV
B. II, III, IV only
C. I, II, III only

D. II, IV only
E. I, III only

40. Radiographically, what thoracic abnormalities would be associated with pulmonary emphysema?

   I. Bronchi and bronchioles appear dilated (enlarged).
   II. The heart presents itself as being elongated.
   III. The hemidiaphragms have a flattened appearance.
   IV. The lungs are shown to be hyperinflated.

A. I, II, IV only
B. II, III, IV only
C. II, III only

D. I, IV only
E. I, II, III, IV

41. The waveform depicted in Figure 132 was generated as a pulmonary artery catheter was floated into position. What does section B represent?

A. pulmonary capillary wedge pressure
B. pulmonary artery pressure
C. right atrium pressure

D. superior vena cava pressure
E. right ventricle pressure

42. Which of the following clinical conditions would cause a mediastinal shift toward the involved lungs?

   I. pleural effusion
   II. pulmonary consolidation
   III. atelectasis

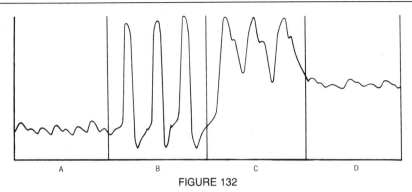

FIGURE 132

IV. pulmonary fibrosis
V. pneumothorax

A. II, III, IV only   D. II, IV only
B. I, II, V only   E. III, IV only
C. I, III, IV, V only

43. What are the expected physiologic effects of the intra-aortic ballon pump?

    I. The device pumps when the heart is in diastole, forcing blood back into the aortic root.
    II. The device increases coronary perfusion.
    III. Systolic pressure usually decreases.
    IV. It increases the cardiac output.

    A. I, II, III, IV   D. I, II only
    B. II, IV only   E. II, III only
    C. I, IV only

44. What safety considerations should be kept in mind when operating electrical equipment?

    I. Nearly all electrical equipment has some current leakage.
    II. When using multiple electrical devices on a patient, each device should be attached to a common ground.
    III. The detection of minor electrical tactile sensations should *not* interfere with equipment use.
    IV. Proper grounding of electrical equipment allows the current to flow from the patient to the ground.

    A. I, II, III, IV   D. I, II only
    B. I, III, IV only   E. II, IV only
    C. III, IV only

45. Which of the following intrathoracic features or conditions may be observed from a portable anteroposterior chest radiograph?

I. mediastinal shift

II. tension pneumothorax

III. cardiomegaly

IV. atelectasis

A. I, II, III, IV

B. III, IV only

C. II, III only

D. I, II only

E. I, II, IV only

46. Identify the ECG pattern demonstrated on the strip in Figure 133.

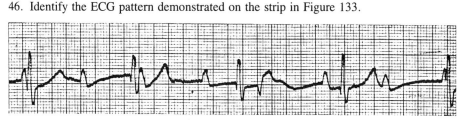

FIGURE 133

A. Mobitz II

B. Wenckebach

C. first-degree AV block

D. third-degree AV block

E. premature ventricular contractions

47. Which of the following clinical manifestations may be classified as symptoms of respiratory disease?

I. abnormal breath sounds

II. dyspnea

III. tachypnea

IV. chest pain

A. I, II, III, IV

B. II, III, IV only

C. II, III only

D. I, IV only

E. II, IV only

Questions 48 through 50 refer to the same patient.

48. A patient's cardiac rate is 110 beats/min and his cardiac output is 5 liters/min. Calculate the ventricular stroke volume.

A. 20.1 ml

B. 45.5 cc

C. 95.7 ml

D. 105.6 cc

E. 550.0 ml

49. Which statement(s) might describe this patient's cardiac status?

I. He has bradycardia.

II. He has suffered an acute myocardial infarction.

III. He has tachycardia.

IV. His ventricular contractility has decreased.

V. His ventricular contractility has increased.

A. II only

B. I only

C. III, IV only

D. III, V only

E. III only

50. Further studies reveal that this patient's $\dot{V}_A/\dot{Q}_C$ is 0.6:1. What would his $\dot{V}_A$ be?

A. 0.012 liter/min

B. 0.6 liter/min

C. 3.0 liters/min

D. 12.0 liters/min

E. 30.0 liters/min

The normal chest radiograph shown in Figure 134 refers to questions 51 and 52.

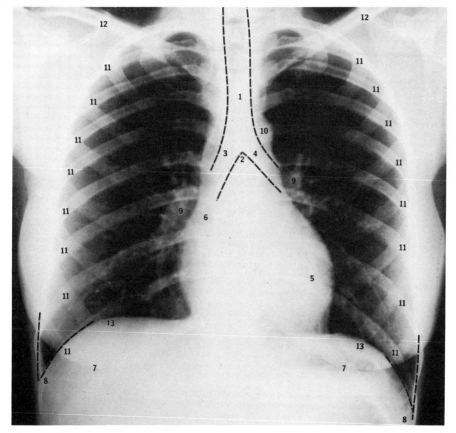

FIGURE 134

51. Which number identifies the costophrenic angle?

A. 2

B. 5

C. 8

D. 11

E. 12

52. Which number represents vascular markings?

    A. 6   D. 11
    B. 7   E. 13
    C. 9

53. Which of the following statements are accurate concerning air bronchograms?

    I. Air bronchograms are usually present in pulmonary emphysema.

    II. Air bronchograms are air-filled bronchi surrounded by atelectatic lung tissue.

    III. If a lesion occupies space within a bronchi and adjacent alveoli, an air bronchogram will be apparent.

    IV. Air bronchograms present as radiolucent shadows contrasted by radiopaque lung parenchyma.

    A. I, II, IV only   D. I, IV only
    B. II, III only   E. II, IV only
    C. I, II, III only

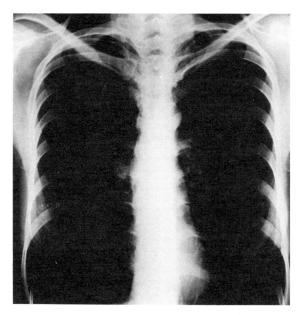

FIGURE 135

54. The chest roentgenogram shown in Figure 135 is most consistent with which of the following lung pathologies?

    A. pulmonary edema   D. massive pleural effusion
    B. pulmonary emphysema   E. diffuse infiltrates
    C. bilateral pneumothorax

55. Which of the following laws describes the principle of operation of the Fleisch pneumotach?

    A. Poiseuille's law of laminar flow
    B. Boyle's law
    C. Ohm's law

    D. Dalton's law of partial pressure
    E. Fick's law

ASSESSMENT ANSWER SHEET

DIRECTIONS: Darken the space under the selected answer.

	A	B	C	D	E		A	B	C	D	E
1.	[ ]	[ ]	[ ]	[ ]	[ ]	29.	[ ]	[ ]	[ ]	[ ]	[ ]
2.	[ ]	[ ]	[ ]	[ ]	[ ]	30.	[ ]	[ ]	[ ]	[ ]	[ ]
3.	[ ]	[ ]	[ ]	[ ]	[ ]	31.	[ ]	[ ]	[ ]	[ ]	[ ]
4.	[ ]	[ ]	[ ]	[ ]	[ ]	32.	[ ]	[ ]	[ ]	[ ]	[ ]
5.	[ ]	[ ]	[ ]	[ ]	[ ]	33.	[ ]	[ ]	[ ]	[ ]	[ ]
6.	[ ]	[ ]	[ ]	[ ]	[ ]	34.	[ ]	[ ]	[ ]	[ ]	[ ]
7.	[ ]	[ ]	[ ]	[ ]	[ ]	35.	[ ]	[ ]	[ ]	[ ]	[ ]
8.	[ ]	[ ]	[ ]	[ ]	[ ]	36.	[ ]	[ ]	[ ]	[ ]	[ ]
9.	[ ]	[ ]	[ ]	[ ]	[ ]	37.	[ ]	[ ]	[ ]	[ ]	[ ]
10.	[ ]	[ ]	[ ]	[ ]	[ ]	38.	[ ]	[ ]	[ ]	[ ]	[ ]
11.	[ ]	[ ]	[ ]	[ ]	[ ]	39.	[ ]	[ ]	[ ]	[ ]	[ ]
12.	[ ]	[ ]	[ ]	[ ]	[ ]	40.	[ ]	[ ]	[ ]	[ ]	[ ]
13.	[ ]	[ ]	[ ]	[ ]	[ ]	41.	[ ]	[ ]	[ ]	[ ]	[ ]
14.	[ ]	[ ]	[ ]	[ ]	[ ]	42.	[ ]	[ ]	[ ]	[ ]	[ ]
15.	[ ]	[ ]	[ ]	[ ]	[ ]	43.	[ ]	[ ]	[ ]	[ ]	[ ]
16.	[ ]	[ ]	[ ]	[ ]	[ ]	44.	[ ]	[ ]	[ ]	[ ]	[ ]
17.	[ ]	[ ]	[ ]	[ ]	[ ]	45.	[ ]	[ ]	[ ]	[ ]	[ ]
18.	[ ]	[ ]	[ ]	[ ]	[ ]	46.	[ ]	[ ]	[ ]	[ ]	[ ]
19.	[ ]	[ ]	[ ]	[ ]	[ ]	47.	[ ]	[ ]	[ ]	[ ]	[ ]
20.	[ ]	[ ]	[ ]	[ ]	[ ]	48.	[ ]	[ ]	[ ]	[ ]	[ ]
21.	[ ]	[ ]	[ ]	[ ]	[ ]	49.	[ ]	[ ]	[ ]	[ ]	[ ]
22.	[ ]	[ ]	[ ]	[ ]	[ ]	50.	[ ]	[ ]	[ ]	[ ]	[ ]
23.	[ ]	[ ]	[ ]	[ ]	[ ]	51.	[ ]	[ ]	[ ]	[ ]	[ ]
24.	[ ]	[ ]	[ ]	[ ]	[ ]	52.	[ ]	[ ]	[ ]	[ ]	[ ]
25.	[ ]	[ ]	[ ]	[ ]	[ ]	53.	[ ]	[ ]	[ ]	[ ]	[ ]
26.	[ ]	[ ]	[ ]	[ ]	[ ]	54.	[ ]	[ ]	[ ]	[ ]	[ ]
27.	[ ]	[ ]	[ ]	[ ]	[ ]	55.	[ ]	[ ]	[ ]	[ ]	[ ]
28.	[ ]	[ ]	[ ]	[ ]	[ ]						

CARDIOPULMONARY EVALUATION/CARDIOPULMONARY MONITORING AND INTERPRETATION ANALYSES

Note: The references listed after each analysis are numbered and keyed to the reference list located at the end of this section. The first number indicates the text. The second number indicates the page where information about the questions will be found. For example, (1:219,384) means that reference number 1 is to be used and that on pages 219 and 384 information about the question will be found. Frequently, it will be necessary to read beyond the page number indicated to obtain complete information. Therefore, reference to the question will be found either on the page indicated or on subsequent pages.

1. C. Chronic bronchitics generally are of stocky body build. They are often referred to as "blue bloaters," a term which describes the ashen, dusky skin color (cyanosis) produced by their chronic hypoxemia. During exacerbations of chronic bronchitis the following signs are often present: (1) the accessory ventilatory muscles are used, producing (a) increased work of breathing and increased oxygen consumption, (b) hypoxemia resulting from the inefficiency of the ventilatory system, and (c) depending on the degree of ventilatory distress, intercostal retractions; (2) wheezing revealed upon auscultation; and (3) peripheral edema, particularly associated with the decompensated cor pulmonale (later stages). The hypersecretive condition normally present in chronic bronchitis often advances to a greater amount of mucopurulent sputum productions during exacerbations associated with pulmonary infections. Patients at this point usually have a great deal of difficulty expectorating these secretions.
    (4:306–308), (6:790–792), (7:70), (8:282–286), (44:215–217)

2. B. The therapeutic interventions most commonly used during an exacerbation of chronic bronchitis include oxygen administration and bronchodilator therapy. When specific pathogens are identified, the appropriate antibiotic therapy should be implemented. Careful attention should be given to adequate humidification of secretions and secretion removal, that is, chest physiotherapy. Although ultrasonic therapy is one approach to providing adequate humidification, ultrasonic aerosols are often aggravating and may induce bronchospasm. The patient is usually instructed to consume large amounts of water to thin out these secretions and facilitate expectorations. However, this latter recommendation has no empirical basis.
    (4:306–308), (6:790–792), (7:70), (8:282–286), (44:215–217)

3. C. Fluoroscopy provides dynamic pictures of the thorax during inspiration and exhalation. It is, therefore, the best radiographic technique for studying diaphragmatic activity.
    (6:303–305), (8:239)

4. B. To substantiate the suspicion of the presence of a pulmonary embolism, the patient should first be carefully observed for signs and symptoms. Clinical manifestations commonly include breathlessness. In patients in whom the embolic obstruction is 50% or more, substernal chest pain, not unlike the pain associated with myocardial ischemia, also may be present. If pulmonary blood flow is

severely impeded causing a reduction in cardiac output, the patient may experience syncope. The second step in the assessment process is to perform routine laboratory tests. These include an ECG, ABGs, a CBC, and a chest x-ray. Most often the results of these tests will be abnormal in both pulmonary embolism and nonembolic patients. The third step involves performing lung scans, necessary in most patients to differentiate embolic from nonembolic conditions. Pulmonary angiography may be required when results of the lung scan are not definitive.
(4:227,324–326), (6:821–826), (8:329–332)

5. D. To differentiate the presence of pulmonary thromboembolism from other diseases with similar clinical findings, it may be necessary to perform lung scanning and in some cases pulmonary angiography. The radioisotope lung scans visualize the distribution of pulmonary blood flow. Pulmonary angiography provides anatomic information and may be required if the lung scan is not definitive. The performance of a chest x-ray is an intermediary procedure and not conclusive.
(4:227,324–326), (6:821–826), (8:241–242,329–332)

6. E. The narrowing of any portion of the tracheobronchial tree increases airway resistance and promotes the presence of turbulent flow in that area. This narrowing can be caused by secretions, fluid, a foreign body, etc. If the obstruction can be cleared by the generation of an effective cough, the characteristic breath sound (rhonchi) associated with such a situation can disappear. In some instances, bronchodilator therapy may eliminate rhonchi.
(3:67,156), (4:293), (6:294,296), (30:68,70), (44:26,389)

7. D. A maximum inspiratory pressure (MIP) of approximately −20 cm H_2O ordinarily is sufficient to produce a vital capacity of about 15 ml/kg of ideal body weight.
(3:75,348), (4:297), (17:112), (40:245)

8. E. Some of the expected clinical manifestations of primary respiratory alkalosis include (1) paresthesia (tingling of the extremities), (2) tetany, (3) somnolence, and (4) decreased cerebral blood flow. Hypocarbia may reach dangerous levels, leading to cardiac dysrhythmias.
(1:233–234), (44:197)

9. B. Clinical manifestations of respiratory distress include objective evaluation of whether the patient is short of breath, as well as the patient's complaint (subjective evaluation) of difficulty of ventilation (dyspnea). Signs refer to what the practitioner can objectively observe, whereas symptoms refer to the patient's subjective complaints.
(8:195–204)

10. E. Capnography is a process whereby the carbon dioxide concentration in a sample of exhaled gas is measured. The measurement usually occurs based on the amount of infrared absorption. CO_2 absorbs infrared light, whereas O_2 and N_2 do not.
(4:421–422), (5:215–216)

11. A. The Co-Oximeter uses light wave spectra specific to carboxyhemoglobin, oxy-

hemoglobin, reduced hemoglobin, and methemoglobin.
(4:421), (6:982–983), (17:138–140)

12. C. Normal hemoglobin concentration ranges from 12 g% to 16 g%. Cyanosis is a clinical sign related to the degree of unsaturated hemoglobin in total circulation. Generally, it is accepted that cyanosis does not occur until the oxygen saturation of arterial blood falls to approximately 80% (Pa_{O_2} 50 torr). As the amount of hemoglobin in the blood increases (e.g., polycythemia secondary to COPD), cyanosis is more likely to occur because more oxygen will be needed to saturate the increased amount of hemoglobin. Because oxygenation is a problem in COPD, this type of patient has a greater chance of having 5 g% of unsaturated (reduced) hemoglobin than someone who is anemic. Someone who is anemic (<12 g% Hb) would need to be extremely hypoxemic (much more than someone with polycythemia) before exhibiting cyanosis.
(1:281), (8:184), (30:120–121), (44:21,203–206)

13. B. The shades of gray to black appearing on an x-ray film depend on the density of the object through which the x-rays pass. More dense objects absorb more x-rays, thus appear a lighter shade on film. Conversely, less dense structures absorb fewer x-rays; consequently, more x-rays pass through to the film, creating a darker shade to black color on the film. Objects that allow x-rays to pass through them are termed *radiolucent,* and objects that hinder or prevent the passage of x-rays are said to be *radiopaque.*

The farther away the photographic plate is from the object to be x-rayed, the larger the object will appear on the film. A radiograph is named from the source of the x-rays to the x-ray film.

Portable chest films are usually taken with the patient lying supine. The film cassette is placed behind the patient and the machine in front. The result is an AP film and not the usual PA film. Frequently, the film is off center, either over or under exposed, or is not taken with the patient in full inspiration. It may, therefore, be more difficult to read a portable chest film, as compared with standard chest x-rays.

Other problems associated with portable AP films include (1) the presence of a larger heart shadow obscuring more of the lung field, (2) a shorter focal distance resulting in a less clear picture, and (3) an inability to determine air-liquid interfaces.
(3:69–73), (6:298–302), (7:441), (8:231–238), (40:163–166)

14. D. The process of placing the hands on the patient's chest to assess (1) the quality of chest movement, (2) vibrations produced by the vocal cords during phonation, and (3) formation of the thorax is called *palpation.* Symmetry of chest expansion is best evaluated by palpation. Palpation may be performed using the heel of the hand with the ulnar surface of the hand, or with the fingers flat against the patient's back.

The vibrations produced over the chest wall by vocal sounds are called *vocal fremitus.* Generally, the intensity of fremitus is nearly equal over both lungs; however, it is increased over the right lung because of the location there of the large bronchi, which are situated in close proximity to the chest wall.

Vibrations perceived via a stethoscope during auscultation are termed *auditory fremitus,* whereas those perceived by the hand during palpation are called *tactile fremitus.*

(3:64), (4:290–293), (7:132), (8:180,215–220), (40:59–61)

15. A. The Apgar score, performed 1 and 5 minutes after birth, involves the assessment of the following clinical signs:

    1. heart rate
    2. ventilatory effort
    3. muscle tone
    4. reflex irritability
    5. color

    The score ranges from 0 to 10. Ten is the best possible score.
    (4:171), (6:709), (40:195), (44:285–287)

16. A. Thoracic surgery is often associated with postoperative pulmonary complications, e.g., atelectasis and pneumonia. The patient should be properly monitored in anticipation of these possible complications. The extent and duration of postoperative pulmonary complications depend on the surgical procedure performed, the length of the operation, and the anesthesia. Surgical procedures performed on the thorax and upper abdomen pose the greatest threat to pulmonary function. Knowledge of whether or not the patient had any pre-existing pulmonary compromise helps the therapists and physicians develop an appropriate plan to monitor the patient. Chest physical assessment provides for the evaluation of the character of breath sounds, muscle use, and ventilatory pattern. Beside spirometry for V_T and FVC measurements quantify the degree of volume exchange, and aid in determining whether hypoxemia and hypercapnia may be anticipated with underventilation. Detecting atelectasis is best assessed by a chest roentgenogram. ABGs reveal the patient's status in terms of hypoxemia and hypercapnia.
    (3:521–527), (6:876–880)

17. E. When properly placed, the pulmonary artery catheter tip should be positioned in a branch of the pulmonary artery. The balloon should be inflated to completely occlude the proximal blood flow through that branch as shown in Figure 135A. The recorded pressure measurement is referred to as the pulmonary capillary wedge pressure (PCWP) or pulmonary artery occluding pressure (PAOP). The normal mean range of the PCWP is 4 to 12 mm Hg.
    (1:271–273), (3:304), (4:234–235), (9:86,283), (45:222)

18. A. Chest physical assessment includes the following procedures (1) inspection, (2) palpation, (3) percussion, and (4) auscultation. Inspection affords the clinician the opportunity to observe any changes in the normal contour of the thorax, e.g., kyphosis and barrel chest. Other aspects noted during inspection are patient position, ventilatory pattern, and accessory muscle usage.

    Palpation is a means of assessing chest movement, expansion, and symmetry by placement of the examiner's hands on the patient's thorax.

    Percussion allows for the assessment of the lung via the quality of sound transmission through the thorax. The sound is produced by the examiner's fingers.

    Auscultation provides the means of assessing via a stethoscope the nature of

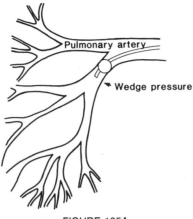

FIGURE 135A

breath sounds as air moves in and out of the respiratory tract.

Vibration is a part of the chest physiotherapy regimen to help promote bronchial hygiene.

(3:62–68), (4:290–293), (6:286,292), (7:132), (8:214–222), (40:55–73)

19. A. Cheyne-Stokes breathing is characterized by periods of hyperventilation and hypoventilation followed by periods of apnea. Physiologists suggest that the cause of this ventilatory aberration is both circulatory and neurologic. The volume-time tracing shown in Figure 136 illustrates Cheyne-Stokes ventilation. Kussmaul's breathing is manifested by deep and rapid ventilations. It is associated with ketoacidosis occurring in patients who have diabetes mellitus. Kussmaul's breathing is shown in Figure 137. Biot's breathing is irregular breathing followed by periods of apnea, as shown in Figure 138. (See page 510 for Figures 136–138.)

(6:834), (8:105–106), (12:30), (40:59), (44:21,113–114), (47:58–59)

20. A. Abnormal breath sounds heard during auscultation include rales, rhonchi, wheezes, stridor, amphoric sounds, and an absence of sounds. Normal breath sounds heard during chest auscultation include tracheal, bronchial, vesicular, and bronchovesicular sounds.

Vocal fremitus represents sounds that are produced by the vocal cords. There are two types of fremitus, tactile and auditory. These sounds are *not* created by air moving through a person's lungs. They represent vibrations throughout the chest caused by vocal cord vibrations during phonation.

(3:67), (4:292,293), (7:136), (8:178–182,219,221–222), (40:66–73)

21. C. The Silverman score is an assessment process used to evaluate the degree of neonatal respiratory distress. It is based on a scale of 0 to 10. The lower the score, the more positive is the outlook or prognosis regarding respiratory distress. Scores 0 to 3 are indicative of no respiratory distress to mild respiratory distress. Scores 4 to 6 correlate with moderate respiratory distress. Scores of 7 to 10 indicate severe respiratory distress. There are five scoring components: (1) upper chest movement, (2) lower chest movement, (3) xiphoid retractions, (4) dilation of the nares, and (5) expiratory grunt.

(4:171), (43:786–787)

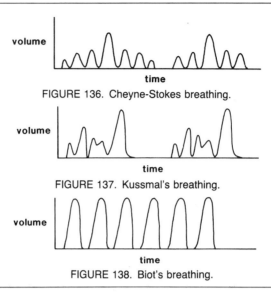

FIGURE 136. Cheyne-Stokes breathing.

FIGURE 137. Kussmal's breathing.

FIGURE 138. Biot's breathing.

22. C. An ECG measures the electrical activity of the myocardium. As the current moves through the heart, it radiates to the body surface, where it can be measured. Cardiac events can be monitored, namely atrial depolarization, ventricular depolarization, and ventricular repolarization.

(1:246–250), (4:259–262), (7:60), (43:1)

23. E. Rhonchi are produced when the lumen of the airway is obstructed, causing an increased resistance to airflow. Rhonchi are more pronounced during the expiratory phase because the bronchi normally become shorter and narrower during expiration.

(3:67), (6:294,296), (8:178–182), (40:68,70), (44:26,389)

24. B. The principle of TcP_{O_2} monitoring is based on the measurable capability of oxygen diffusion through the skin. Heating the skin to 43°C to 45°C improves capillary flow through the dermis and enhances O_2 diffusion through the skin. The position of the measuring electrode should be changed every 3 to 6 hours to reduce the incidence of skin burns or blisters. Transcutaneous monitoring is a useful noninvasive measuring technique. It often eliminates the need for frequent arterial punctures. The TcP_{O_2} may fall well below the Pa_{O_2} value in times of hypoperfusion. In fact, during such times it may even drop below the $P\overline{v}_{O_2}$ value.

(4:177), (5:213–214), (6:946), (9:143), (27:39), (40:210), (44:418), (Respiratory Therapy, "Practical, Noninvasive Monitoring of Oxygenation," Vol. 16, No. 1, Jan/Feb 1986)

25. C. The ability to generate a sufficient forced vital capacity is essential to producing an effective cough. The inhalation of an adequate volume is necessary along with the ability to rapidly exhale.

(3:43,154), (12:230)

26. D. Central venous pressure (CVP) measurements will appear higher when a patient is on mechanical ventilation. Any patient on mechanical ventilation with a CVP line in place may remain connected to the ventilator while CVP readings are taken. Personnel should note the circumstances in their charting concerning any CVP measurements.

   (3:301), (9:55–66)

27. D. The fingertips, the ulnar surface, or the palm of the hand may be used for palpation for vocal fremitus (tactile fremitus).

   (7:132), (8:219), (40:59–62)

28. E. A pneumothorax takes on a variety of clinical forms (1) tension pneumothorax, (2) spontaneous pneumothorax, (3) iatrogenic pneumothorax, and (4) traumatic pneumothorax. A tension pneumothorax exists if air trapped in the intrapleural space rises above atmospheric pressure. A spontaneous pneumothorax is often seen in young, tall, otherwise healthy persons. This form of pneumothorax is usually associated with a subpleural bleb rupture. An iatrogenic pneumothorax is either intentionally or accidentally induced for or during medical treatment. Before antituberculosis medications, a pneumothorax was frequently induced to treat pulmonary tuberculosis. Inadvertent creation of a pneumothorax can occur in conjunction with thoracentesis, Swan-Ganz catheter insertion, mechanical ventilation (barotrauma), etc. A traumatic pneumothorax can result from a penetrating or nonpenetrating chest wall injury.

   The presence of a pneumothorax may be asymptomatic if the amount of air in the intrapleural space is small. However, if a pneumothorax is symptomatic, the patient is usually dyspneic and expresses chest pain. Chest wall movement on the affected side is decreased. Tactile and vocal fremitus and breath sounds, likewise, decrease in that lung region. Percussion over a pneumothorax produces hyperresonance. The trachea is deviated from midline.

   (4:317–318), (8:348–351), (47:245–246)

29. A. The earliest sign of hypoxemia is tachycardia. Other signs may also be present (e.g., tachypnea and cyanosis). However, tachycardia is considered, by most clinicians, to be the earliest sign of hypoxemia.

   (4:371–372)

30. D. Inspecting the physical appearance of the chest (thorax) is the first step in the overall physical chest assessment. The second phase involves chest palpation to discern the degree of thoracic wall movement and the status of lung tissue, that is, the presence of pleural fluid or lung secretions. The third step entails assessing the sounds produced by the examiner's fingers over the lung area. This process is termed *percussion* and reveals information about tissue density. Auscultation involves the use of the stethoscope to evaluate the quality of breath sounds.

   (3:62), (4:290–293), (6:286–292), (7:130–137), (8:214–222)

31. B. Figure 139 represents a normal intra-arterial pressure tracing. The highest point of the pressure waveform is the systolic pressure (point A). As the pressure in the ventricle drops below the aortic pressure, the aortic valve closes. This sudden clo-

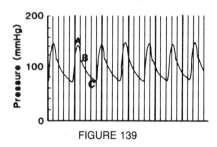

FIGURE 139

sure of the aortic valve produces a notch on the downslope of the tracing and is called the dicrotic notch (point B). Diastole appears as the lowest point of pressure on the tracing (point C).

(4:229–230), (6:941–943), (9:104–109)

32. B. Rhonchi are caused by partial airway obstruction during exhalation. During exhalation, airways contract and narrow. The sound produced is generally described as a whistling sound.

Amphoric breath sounds characteristically occur during exhalation as air moves over lung cavities. The sound produced is similar to that produced as one blows air across the open mouth of an empty bottle.

Vesicular sounds are normal breath sounds taking place during inspiration and represent the movement of air over normal lung tissue.

Bronchovesicular sounds are also normal breath sounds. They are louder and higher pitched than vesicular and represent air moving through large airways close to the chest wall.

(3:67), (4:293), (6:289–297), (7:136), (8:221–222)

33. C. The T wave follows the QRS complex and represents ventricular repolarization. The QRS complex represents ventricular depolarization. Note Figure 140, which depicts the various electrophysiologic events of the normal cardiac cycle.

(1:246–250), (4:259–262), (43:15)

34. D. The barrel chest appearance is sometimes associated with pulmonary emphysema. Both chest diameters, transverse and anteroposterior (AP), are approximately equal. The chest assumes the appearance of permanent inspiration. During the ventilatory cycle the thorax moves up and down as a whole.

(1:295), (4:301), (6:284–292,797–800), (7:6), (8:353), (40:82)

35. A. Transillumination is a technique frequently used on infants to identify a pneumothorax or a pneumomediastinum. It is successfully used on infants because the chest wall is sufficiently thin to allow light to shine through. The usual light source is a bright fiberoptic light placed against the chest wall in a dark room. The normal configuration produced is a lighted "halo" around the point of contact with the skin. In the presence of a pneumothorax or pneumomediastinum the entire area "lights up." Transillumination has been used to help visualize an artery to facilitate arterial puncture. The artery appears as a line lighter than surrounding tissue. Transillumination is a quick, safe method of identification of structures.

(4:177), (40:203)

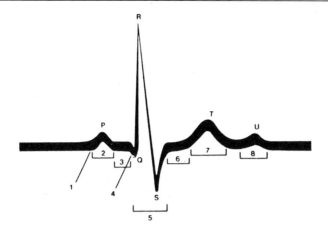

Electrical Event	ECG Representation
1. Impulse from sinus node	Not visible
2. Depolarization of atria	P wave
3. Depolarization of A–V node	Isoelectric
4. Repolarization of atria	Obscured by QRS complex
5. Depolarization of ventricles	QRS complex
a. Intraventricular septum	a. Initial portion
b. Right & left ventricles	b. Central & terminal portions
6. Activated state of ventricles immediately after depolarization	ST segment: isoelectric
7. Repolarization of ventricles	T wave
8. After-potentials following repolarization of ventricles	U wave

FIGURE 140

36. C. Fluid, air, or solid tissue in the pleural space slows the transmission of sound waves from the larynx to the chest wall, resulting in a decreased tactile fremitus. (3:62–65), (4:292), (6:295–297), (7:132), (8:219)

37. B. The letter A in Figure 131 designates atrial depolarization, that is, atrial contraction. The letters BCD represent ventricular depolarization. The letter E signifies ventricular repolarization. (1:246,250), (4:259–262), (43:13–16), (44:548)

38. C. Ear oximetry is a noninvasive means of monitoring oxygen saturation. The oximeter is positioned on the ear lobe or the flat superior surface of the ear. To improve blood flow to the measurement area, the skin is warmed to 40°C. Monitoring can be conducted both intermittently and continuously. Thus, long-term monitoring is possible. Ear oximetry has been used in monitoring ventilator maintenance, sleep apnea, sleep studies, exercise studies, and in rehabilitation programs. Therapists must take care to verify that the device is well positioned. Ear oximetry is best

suited for hemodynamically stable patients.
(4:421), (6:946), (17:140–141), (40:312–315)

39. B. Cannulation of the umbilical artery and vein is relatively easy. The indications for umbilical artery catheterization include: (1) frequent blood gas sampling, (2) continuous blood pressure monitoring, and (3) large scale blood replacement. The indications for umbilical venous catheterization include central venous pressure (CVP) monitoring and large scale blood replacement.
(4:175), (9:159), (40:213–215)

40. B. Chest roentgenograms taken of pulmonary emphysema patients usually reveal a depressed and flattened diaphragm. Usually, the heart is elongated and narrow, having been drawn downward by the descending diaphragm. The lungs are hyperlucent because of hyperinflation and generalized destruction of lung parenchyma and vessels.
(4:302), (6:318f,321,800–801,801f), (7:74), (8:238,290–291)

41. E. The diagram depicting the waveforms generated from floating a Swan-Ganz catheter into position corresponds to the anatomic structures through which the catheter passes. Figure 141 shows the location of the tip of a Swan-Ganz catheter and its corresponding waveform, as the catheter is being advanced to the wedged position.
Section A represents pressures in the right atrium; section B represents pressures in the right ventricle; section C represents pressures in the pulmonary artery; and section D represents pressure in the pulmonary capillary with the catheter "wedged."
(4:232–234), (6:944), (9:98), (40:286)

42. E. The end-expiratory intrapleural pressure determines the side toward which the mediastinum will shift. If the end-expiratory intrapleural pressure is decreased on the affected side, the mediastinum shifts toward the affected side, as in atelectasis and pulmonary fibrosis. If fluid or air collects in the intrapleural space, end-expiratory pressure is increased on that side; therefore, the mediastinum shifts to the uninvolved lung, as in a pleural effusion and pneumothorax.
(3:72–73), (6:316–317), (8:175,216,276,314,315,347)

43. A. The intra-aortic balloon pump operates on the principle of counterpulsation. The device pumps (intra-aortic balloon fills) when the ventricles are in diastole and relaxes (intra-aortic balloon empties) when the ventricles are in systole. When the intra-aortic balloon fills, blood is displaced and forced back into the aortic root which produces an increase in diastolic pressure. Approximately, 70% of arterial perfusion to the myocardium occurs during the diastolic phase. Thus, coronary perfusion is improved without increasing oxygen demands or myocardial work. Systolic pressure usually decreases with the use of the intra-aortic balloon pump. The heart can eject more blood per beat because of the decreased resistance to forward flow, facilitated by the rapid deflation of the intra-aortic balloon immediately before systole. Stroke volume and cardiac output increase.
(9:246)

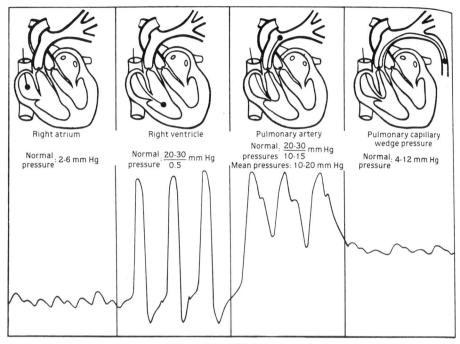

Right atrium

Normal pressure: 2-6 mm Hg

Right ventricle

Normal pressure: 20-30 / 0.5 mm Hg

Pulmonary artery

Normal pressures: 20-30 / 10-15 mm Hg

Mean pressures: 10-20 mm Hg

Pulmonary capillary wedge pressure

Normal pressure: 4-12 mm Hg

FIGURE 141

44. D. Almost every piece of electrical equipment has some leakage of current from the circuitry to the equipment frame. Maximal leakage of current should be 100 μA for exposed metal surfaces and 10 μA for patient connections. Proper grounding allows the current to flow from the equipment frame to the ground wire. A three-pronged electrical outlet and plug are necessary for grounding. Many are monitored simultaneously by multiple devices. Each device should be attached to a common ground wire to drain all current leakage to a single ground point. (9:51–54)

45. A. A normal chest x-ray film presents the lungs as black areas with white vascular markings radiating from the hilus of each lung. Atelectasis appears as a density. Under normal conditions the cardiac shadow is clearly perceived. Cardiomegaly can be easily determined from having knowledge of the normal heart size and configuration. The trachea appears as a translucent shadow. Any deviation of it from midline usually can be easily observed. (3:69–73), (6:298–302), (7:441–451), (8:231–237)

46. D. The ECG depicts a third-degree atrioventricular (AV) block, or complete heart block. No atrial impulses, represented by the P waves, activate the ventricles. The P waves and QRS complexes occur independently. The QRS complex originates from a junctional or ventricular pacemaker site.

An AV block occurs when the AV node is diseased and has difficulty conducting atrial impulses (P waves) to the ventricles. Common causes are myocardial infarc-

tion and arteriosclerosis. Atrioventricular blocks are classified as first-, second-, and third-degree blocks. In first-degree AV blocks, the PR-interval is increased over 0.20 second. Wenckebach (Mobitz I) and Mobitz II are both types of second-degree AV blocks. The Mobitz II pattern shows a progressively strengthening PR interval from one beat to the next until, finally, the AV node cannot conduct the impulse and a beat fails. The rested AV node then is able to fire on the next beat but the cycle repeats. In Mobitz II some beats are conducted and others are not. The PR interval is consistent for conducted beats. Failed beats are identified by the presence of a P wave without an ensuing QRS complex.
(4:266–268), (30:373–375)

47. E. Symptoms are those clinical manifestations that the patient expresses, whereas signs are those aspects of disease that the examiner can ascertain. Symptoms are subjective; signs are objective.

Dyspnea and chest pain are classified as disease symptoms because they must be expressed by the patient to the examiner. The examiner cannot objectively discern those clinical manifestations.
(8:163,166–168), (9:14–15), (40:4–6,7–8)

48. B. STEP 1: Convert 5 liters/min to cc/min.

$$(5 \text{ liters/min})(1,000 \text{ cc/liter}) = 5,000 \text{ cc/min}$$

STEP 2: Because the cardiac output is the product of the stroke volume times the heart rate (cardiac output = stroke volume × heart rate), rearrange the expression to solve for the stroke volume. Therefore,

$$\text{stroke volume} = \frac{\text{cardiac output}}{\text{cardiac rate}}$$
$$= \frac{5,000 \text{ cc/min}}{110 \text{ beats/min}}$$
$$= 45.5 \text{ cc/beat}$$

(1:246), (4:127)

49. C. With a cardiac rate of 110 beats/min, the patient can be considered as having tachycardia. A stroke volume of 45.5 cc is considered low. A normal stroke volume is within the range of 60 to 130 cc.
(1:246), (4:127), (9:124,126,283)

50. C. STEP 1: Use the expression representing the relationship between alveolar ventilation and pulmonary capillary perfusion.

$$\dot{V}_A/\dot{Q}_C = \frac{\text{alveolar ventilation}}{\text{pulmonary capillary perfusion}}$$

STEP 2: Express this relationship as a proportion and solve for X.

$$\frac{0.6}{1} = \frac{X}{5}$$
$$\frac{0.6 \times 5}{1} = 3 \text{ liters/min}$$

(1:118), (3:56–59), (8:66–69)

51. C. The costophrenic angle is identified by the number 8 (Figure 134) on the normal chest radiograph. The costophrenic angle is defined as the junction of the diaphragm and the lungs. A pleural effusion, fluid in the intrapleural space, causes blunting of the costophrenic angle.

(40:170–171,188–190), (47:100–103,107–108)

52. C. In the normal chest radiograph presented, vascular markings can be observed near the hilum. These vascular markings represent the major vessels entering (pulmonary artery) and leaving (pulmonary veins) the lungs. Vascular markings may be present elsewhere on the chest x-ray in pathologic conditions, such as pulmonary edema and cor pulmonale.

(40:185–186), (47:100–102,247)

53. E. Air bronchograms are useful in locating areas of atelectasis. Normally, bronchi and surrounding alveoli are air filled; consequently, the bronchi cannot be seen. However, when the surrounding alveoli collapse and become airless (atelectasis), the underlying bronchi can be viewed if they remain patent to the movement of air. Air bronchograms will then present as radiolucent shadows against radiopaque lung parenchyma. Air bronchograms are frequently observed in pneumonia and pulmonary edema. Air bronchograms are normal when seen in contrast to the heart shadow.

(40:174,185), (47:155)

54. B. The chest radiograph presented depicts that of a patient with pulmonary emphysema. A number of radiographic findings are characteristic of this lung pathology. They include:

1. flattened, low-lying diaphragms
2. hyperlucent lung fields caused by hyperinflation
3. enlarged intercostal spaces
4. midline, narrowed heart
5. decreased vascular markings

(8:238,290–291), (40:178–180,361), (47:106–107,221)

55. A. A pneumotach (anemometer, pneumotachograph, or pneumotachometer) is a device that measures gas flow by acting as a linear resistance to respiratory gas flow. Gas flow through a pneumotach is directly proportional to the pressure drop across its resistive elements. The Fleisch pneumotach consists of fixed resistance comprised of a capillary mesh. The capillary mesh represents resistance connected in parallel; therefore, the total resistance to gas flow is low. The narrow capillary tubes effectively lower Reynold's number in the system so that laminar flow occurs across the resistance even at high gas velocities. In this case, the pressure drop across the capillary mesh is proportional to the gas flow moving through it (Figure 142). Therefore, the Fleisch pneumotach, shown in Figure 142, operates in accordance with Poiseuille's law of laminar flow. Poiseuille's law is expressed as follows:

$$\eta = \frac{\Delta P \pi r^4}{8 L \dot{V}}$$

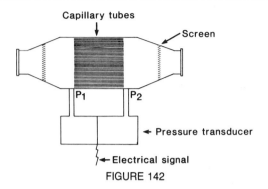

FIGURE 142

where

η = viscosity index of the gas
ΔP = driving pressure (pressure gradient)
$\pi/8$ = mathematical constant
r = radius of the conducting tube
L = length of the conducting tube
$\dot{V}$ = gas flowrate

Rearranging this expression in terms of the pressure drop across a given resistance, as measured by this device, the equation becomes

$$\Delta P = \frac{8L\dot{V}\eta}{\pi r^4}$$

(2:160–164), (5:225–226), (17:182–183), (30:345), (34:91), (Respiratory Care, "Pneumotachs: Theory and Clinical Application," Vol. 29, No. 7, July 1984).

REFERENCES

1. Spearman, C., and Sheldon, R., *Egan's Fundamentals of Respiratory Therapy,* 4th ed., C.V. Mosby, St. Louis, 1982.

2. Wojciechowski, W., *Respiratory Care Sciences: An Integrated Approach,* John Wiley & Sons, New York, 1985.

3. Shapiro, B., Harrison, R., Kacmarek, R., and Cane, R., *Clinical Application of Respiratory Care,* 3rd ed., Year Book Medical Publishers, Chicago, 1985.

4. Kacmarek, R., Mack, C., and Dimas, S., *The Essentials of Respiratory Therapy,* 2nd ed., Year Book Medical Publishers, Chicago, 1985.

5. McPherson, S., *Respiratory Therapy Equipment,* 3rd ed., C.V. Mosby, St. Louis, 1985.

6. Burton, G., and Hodgkin, J., *Respiratory Care: A Guide to Clinical Practice,* 2nd ed., J.B. Lippincott, Philadelphia, 1985.

7. Frownfelter, D., *Chest Physical Therapy and Cardiopulmonary Rehabilitation, An Interdisciplinary Approach,* Year Book Medical Publishers, Chicago, 1978.

8. Cherniack, R., and Cherniack, L., *Respiration in Health and Disease,* 3rd ed., W.B. Saunders, Philadelphia, 1983.

9. Daily, E., and Schroeder, G., *Techniques in Bedside Hemodynamic Monitoring,* 3rd ed., C.V. Mosby, St. Louis, 1985.

10. Des Jardins, R., *Clinical Manifestations of Respiratory Disease,* Year Book Medical Publishers, Chicago, 1984.

11. Mitchell, R., *Synopsis of Clinical Pulmonary Disease,* 3rd ed., C.V. Mosby, St. Louis, 1982.

12. Comroe, J., *Physiology of Respiration,* 3rd ed., Year Book Medical Publishers, Chicago, 1974.

13. West, J., *Pulmonary Pathophysiology—The Essentials,* 2nd ed., Williams & Wilkins, Baltimore, 1982.

14. West, J., *Respiratory Physiology—The Essentials,* 3rd ed., Williams & Wilkins, Baltimore, 1985.

15. Martz, K., et al., *Management of the Patient-Ventilator System: A Team Approach,* 2nd ed., C.V. Mosby, St. Louis, 1984.

16. Shoup, C., and McHenry, R., *Laboratory Exercises in Respiratory Therapy,* 2nd ed., C.V. Mosby, St. Louis, 1983.

17. Ruppel, G., *Manual of Pulmonary Function Testing,* 3rd ed., C.V. Mosby, St. Louis, 1982.

18. Appelbaum, E., and Bruce, D., *Tracheal Intubation,* W.B. Saunders, Philadelphia, 1976.

19. Rau, J., *Respiratory Therapy Pharmacology,* 2nd ed., Year Book Medical Publishers, Chicago, 1984.

20. United States Department of Health, Education, and Welfare, Public Health Service, *Isolation Techniques for Use in Hospitals,* 2nd ed., Washington, D.C., 1975.

21. Brooks, S., *Integrated Basic Science,* 4th ed., C.V. Mosby, St. Louis, 1979.

22. Comroe, J., *The Lung,* Year Book Medical Publishers, Chicago, 1962.

23. Shibel, E., and Moser, K., *Respiratory Emergencies,* 2nd ed., C.V. Mosby, St. Louis, 1982.

24. Tisi, G., *Pulmonary Physiology in Clinical Medicine,* 2nd ed., Williams & Wilkins, Baltimore, 1985.

25. Cherniack, R., *Pulmonary Function Testing,* W.B. Saunders, Philadelphia, 1977.

26. Altose, M., *The Physiological Basis of Pulmonary Function Testing,* Clinical Symposia-CIBA, Vol. 31, No. 2, Summit, New Jersey, 1979.

27. Shapiro, B., Harrison, R., and Walton, J., *Clinical Application of Arterial Blood Gases,* 3rd ed., Year Book Medical Publishers, Chicago, 1982.

28. West, J., *Ventilation/Blood Flow and Gas Exchange,* 3rd ed., Blackwell Scientific Publications, 1979.

29. Slonim, N., and Hamilton, K., *Respiratory Physiology,* 4th ed., C.V. Mosby, St. Louis, 1981.

30. Rarey, K., and Youtsey, J., *Respiratory Patient Care,* Prentice-Hall, Englewood Cliffs, 1981.

31. Berne, R., and Levy, M., *Physiology,* C.V. Mosby, St. Louis, 1983.

32. Levitzky, M., *Pulmonary Physiology,* 2nd ed., McGraw-Hill, New York, 1986.

33. Wilson, P., Bell, C., and Norton, A., *Rehabilitation of the Heart and Lungs,* SensorMedics, 1980.

34. Clausen, J., and Zarins, L., *Pulmonary Function Testing Guidelines and Controversies,* Academic Press, New York, 1982.

35. Klaus, M., and Fanaroff, A., *Care of the High-Risk Neonate,* 2nd ed., W.B. Saunders, Philadelphia, 1979.

36. Lough, M., et al., *Pediatric Respiratory Therapy,* 3rd ed., Year Book Medical Publishers, Chicago, 1985.

37. Levin, D., et al., *A Practical Guide to Pediatric Intensive Care,* 2nd ed., C.V. Mosby, St. Louis, 1984.

38. O'Ryan, J., and Burns, D., *Pulmonary Rehabilitation from Hospital to Home,* Year Book Medical Publishers, Chicago, 1984.

39. Bell, C., et al., *Home Care and Rehabilitation in Respiratory Medicine,* J.B. Lippincott, Philadelphia, 1984.

40. Wilkins, R., et al., *Clinical Assessment in Respiratory Care,* C.V. Mosby, St. Louis, 1985.

41. Jones, N., and Campbell, E., *Clinical Exercise Testing,* 2nd ed., W.B. Saunders, Philadelphia, 1982.
42. Goldsmith, J., and Karotkin, E., *Assisted Ventilation of the Neonate,* W.B. Saunders, Philadelphia, 1981.
43. Blowers, M., and Sims, R., *How to Read an ECG,* 3rd ed., Medical Economics, New Jersey, 1983.
44. Eubanks, D., and Bone, R., *Comprehensive Respiratory Care,* C.V. Mosby, St. Louis, 1985.
45. Rattenborg, C., *Clinical Use of Mechanical Ventilation,* Year Book Medical Publishers, Chicago, 1981.
46. Witkowski, A. S., *Pulmonary Assessment: A Clinical Guide,* J.B. Lippincott, Philadelphia, 1985.
47. Op't Holt, T. B., *Assessment Based Respiratory Care,* John Wiley & Sons, New York, 1986.

CARDIOPULMONARY DIAGNOSTICS AND INTERPRETATION ASSESSMENT

PURPOSE: The purpose of this 80-item assessment is to afford you the opportunity to determine the extent of your understanding and comprehension of cardiopulmonary diagnostic testing procedures. The diagnostic procedures included in this assessment are arterial and venous punctures, pulmonary function tests, hemodynamic monitoring, instrumentation, and bronchial provocation testing. A number of mathematical problems related to data gathering are included. Data interpretation and clinical application of these procedures also are presented.

DIRECTIONS: Each of the questions or incomplete statements is followed by five suggested answers. Select the one which is the best in each case and then blacken the corresponding space on the answer sheet.

1. What are the potential hazards of an iatrogenically induced respiratory alkalosis to a patient in acute ventilatory failure?

   I. a rightward shift in $Hb-O_2$ dissociation curve
   II. cardiac dysrhythmias
   III. hyperkalemia
   IV. tetany
   V. cerebral vasoconstriction

   A. I, II, III, IV, V
   B. I, III, IV only
   C. II, III, IV only
   D. II, IV, V only
   E. II, III, IV, V only

2. Which of the following breathing tests provides data about closing volumes?

   A. closed-circuit helium equilibration
   B. forced vital capacity
   C. single-breath nitrogen elimination
   D. 7-minute nitrogen washout
   E. body plethysmography

3. A combined CO_2 to dissolved CO_2 ratio of 12 mEq/liter:0.6 mEq/liter can be described by which acid-base interpretation(s)?

     I. uncompensated respiratory alkalosis
    II. compensated metabolic acidosis
   III. compensated respiratory alkalosis
   IV. uncompensated metabolic acidosis

A. I only   D. II, IV only
B. I, II only   E. II, III only
C. IV only

4. Pulmonary function studies were performed on a 55-year-old woman who has had a
   two-year history of dyspnea. Which diagnosis(es) would be compatible with the following data?

	ACTUAL	PREDICTED	% PREDICTED
TLC	6.90 liters	6.30 liters	110
VC	5.04 liters	5.04 liters	100
FVC	3.52 liters	5.04 liters	69
RV	1.86 liters	1.26 liters	147
FRC	4.39 liters	2.52 liters	174
FEV_1	3.07 liters	4.33 liters	70
PEF	310 liters/min	485 liters/min	64

     I. myasthenia gravis
    II. pulmonary emphysema
   III. pulmonary embolism
   IV. postoperative thoractomy
    V. kyphoscoliosis

A. II only   D. IV only
B. I, V only   E. II, IV only
C. III, V only

5. An uncompensated respiratory alkalosis is associated with a(n) _____ in
   arterial blood pH and a(n) _____ in CSF pH.

A. decrease; increase   D. increase; increase
B. increase; decrease   E. increase; normal status
C. decrease; decrease

6. Which of the following measurements can be directly obtained from a forced vital capacity recording?

     I. peak expiratory flowrate
    II. $FEF_{200-1200}$
   III. FEV_1
   IV. $\dot{V}_E$
    V. FRC

A. II, III, IV only

B. I, II, III only

C. II, III, IV, V only

D. I, IV, V only

E. I, III only

7. Figure 143 represents a maximum expiratory flow-volume curve. The dotted line represents the maneuver performed using a helium-oxygen mixture. The heavy line is the tracing obtained using room air. Which letter represents the volume of isoflow?

A. A

B. B

C. C

D. D

E. E

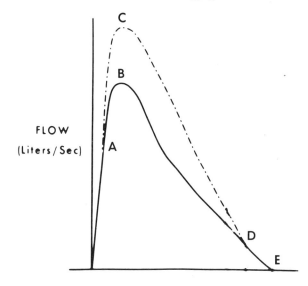

VOLUME (Liters)

FIGURE 143

8. What is the utility of the ^{133}Xe elimination study?

A. It allows for the determination of alveolar dead space as well as anatomic dead space.

B. It is useful when the $\dot{Q}s/\dot{Q}T$ ratio needs to be determined.

C. It provides data for the calculation of the airway resistance in the small airways.

D. It indicates the distribution of ventilation and perfusion in the lungs.

E. It renders information needed for the computation of the closing capacity.

9. Which of the following clinical conditions or situations can cause a metabolic alkalosis?

I. therapy

II. diarrhea

III. hypokalemia

IV. hypochloremia

A. II, IV only   D. I, II only

B. I, II, III only   E. I, II, III, IV

C. III, IV only

Questions 10, 11, and 12 refer to the same patient.

After a recent OPEC meeting, Mr. P. Troleum, a 50-year-old Standard Oil executive, was admitted through the Emergency Room of King Faisal's Hospital in Saudi Arabia, complaining of severe chest pains and dyspnea.

Clinically, he exhibited tachypnea, cyanosis around the lips, and diffuse gurgling breath sounds. Lasix and 100% oxygen via a non-rebreathing mask were immediately administered.

Historically, this patient has suffered from heart ailments for 7 years. This history includes two myocardial infarctions and coronary bypass surgery.

After Mr. Troleum's second day of convalescence, while he was still on O_2 and Lasix, the lab reports indicated that he had a total CO_2 content of 84.00 vol% and a Pa_{CO_2} of 49 torr.

10. Determine this patient's plasma HCO_3^- in millimoles of CO_2/liter.

A. 1.47 mM CO_2/liter   D. 36.20 mM CO_2/liter

B. 5.62 mM CO_2/liter   E. 37.66 mM CO_2/liter

C. 25.40 mM CO_2/liter

11. What is this patient's HCO_3^-/P_{CO_2} ratio?

A. 27.3:1   D. 18.6:1

B. 24.6:1   E. 15.4:1

C. 20.0:1

12. Which interpretation(s) represent(s) this patient's acid-base status?

   I. chronic ventilatory failure

  II. chronic alveolar hyperventilation

 III. compensated respiratory acidosis

 IV. compensated metabolic alkalosis

  V. compensated metabolic acidosis

A. IV only   D. I, III, IV only

B. II, V only   E. I, III only

C. III only

13. Calculate the $FEV_{3\%}$ given the pulmonary function data shown in Table 11.

A. 69.0%   D. 80.9%

B. 74.2%   E. 95.9%

C. 77.3%

14. How is the $FEV_{1\%}$ calculated?

A. $\dfrac{FEV_1}{FVC} \times 100$

B. $\dfrac{\text{actual FEV}_1}{\text{predicted FEV}_1} \times 100$

C. $\dfrac{\text{predicted FEV}_1}{\text{actual FEV}_1} \times 100$

D. $\dfrac{\text{actual FEV}_1 - \text{predicted FEV}_1}{\text{actual FVC}} \times 100$

E. $\dfrac{\text{predicted FEV}_1 - \text{actual FEV}_1}{\text{predicted FVC}} \times 100$

TABLE 11

Parameter	Predicted Normal	Actual
TLC	7.31 liters	10.12 liters
FVC	5.26 liters	7.60 liters
FEV$_1$	4.26 liters	5.64 liters
FEV$_3$	5.10 liters	7.29 liters
PEF	9.00 liters/sec	13.54 liters/sec

15. Which statements accurately refer to a flow-volume loop?

    I. The curve is obtained by having the patient perform an FVC immediately followed by a forced maximum inspiration.
    II. The exhaled volume is plotted on the ordinate, and the flowrate is represented on the abscissa.
    III. V$_T$, ERV, and IC can be obtained from flow-volume loop tracings.
    IV. Expiratory and inspiratory flows at 25%, 50%, and 75% of the vital capacity can be obtained.

    A. I, II, III, IV   D. I, II only
    B. I, III, IV only   E. III, IV only
    C. I, IV only

16. Which pH would be associated with the largest arterial-venous difference, assuming all other physiologic factors are equal?

    A. 7.31   D. 7.45
    B. 7.35   E. 7.49
    C. 7.40

17. When the 7-minute N$_2$ washout test is performed, what should the %N$_2$ be in the remaining alveolar gas in order for the results to be considered normal?

    A. < 1.5%   D. > 5.0%
    B. < 2.5%   E. ≈ 79%
    C. > 2.5%

18. Which statements are true about the Severinghaus electrode?

I. It incorporates a platinum cathode and a Ag/AgCl anode.

II. It measures the P_{CO_2} potentiometrically.

III. When CO_2 diffuses across the Teflon membrane, the reaction in the electrode buffer solution becomes

$$CO_2 + H_2O \rightleftharpoons H_2CO_3 \rightleftharpoons H^+ + HCO_3^-$$

IV. The CO_2 electrode also incorporates pH-sensitive glass.

A. I, II, III, IV
B. II, IV only
C. I, II, III only
D. I, III, IV only
E. II, III, IV only

19. Which statement(s) correctly refer(s) to the carbon monoxide diffusing capacity test?

I. Carbon dioxide can be used as an alternate gas when one is performing this study.

II. An inverse relationship exists between the diffusion capacity and the subject's alveolar volume. That is, as the diffusion capacity increases, alveolar volume decreases.

III. The gas mixture breathed in the single-breath test usually has the following constituents and concentrations: 0.3% CO, 10% He, and remainder air.

IV. Smokers may provide inaccurate results when performing this test.

A. I, II only
B. III, IV only
C. III only
D. II, III, IV only
E. II only

20. Which of the following statements are true about flexible fiberoptic bronchoscopy?

I. One main disadvantage of the flexible fiberoptic bronchoscope is that it must be used with a fluoroscope.

II. Ventilator patients may have this procedure performed without much interference with their ventilation.

III. This procedure provides a means of obtaining anaerobic specimens from the lower respiratory tract.

IV. This procedure may be performed with the patient under either local or general anesthesia.

A. I, II, III only
B. II, III only
C. II, III, IV only
D. I, III only
E. I, II, III, IV

Questions 21, 22, and 23 refer to the same patient.

The pulmonary function data shown in Table 12 were obtained from a 35-year-old white male:

Data from the open-circuit 7-minute N_2 washout procedure are shown below:

Expired volume collected in Tissot spirometer: 27,000 cc
Alveolar %N_2: approximately 75%
Final %N_2: 9%

TABLE 12

Parameter	Predicted	Actual	% Predicted
FVC	5.45 liters	6.44 liters	118
FEV$_1$	4.43 liters	5.02 liters	113
FEV$_{1\%}$	81.5%	77.9%	
ERV	1.00 liter	1.22 liters	122
TLC	7.41 liters	9.56 liters	129

21. Calculate this person's residual volume from the data available.

    A. 1.04 liters   D. 3.24 liters
    B. 1.31 liters   E. 6.32 liters
    C. 2.02 liters

22. Calculate this person's RV/TLC ratio from the data available.

    A. 10.5%   D. 46.6%
    B. 13.7%   E. 66.1%
    C. 21.1%

23. What interpretation would you place on the patient's condition from the data obtained?

    A. The patient's breathing is mildly obstructed, based upon the air trapping reflected in the increased TLC and ERV values.
    B. The patient's breathing is moderately restricted, based upon the decreased FEV$_{1\%}$, the small RV, and the low RV/TLC ratio.
    C. The patient's breathing is normal, based upon the large TLC accompanied by good flowrates, and a normal RV/TLC ratio.
    D. Bronchiectasis may be present, reflected in the increased lung volumes and capacities, and an extremely high RV/TLC ratio.
    E. Insufficient data are available for interpretation.

24. Which of the following statements accurately describe the Sanz electrode?

    I. It is used to measure P$_{CO_2}$.
    II. It contains glass sensitive to H$^+$.
    III. This electrode contains a Ag/AgCl calomel reference electrode.
    IV. It consists, in part, of a Ag/AgCl anode that is in communication with the electrolyte solution.

    A. I, II, III only   D. I, IV only
    B. II, IV only   E. II, III only
    C. II, III, IV only

25. A 40-year-old patient exhibits the following blood gas data while breathing room air: Pa$_{O_2}$ 50 torr; Pa$_{CO_2}$ 49 torr; pH 7.32. Calculate this patient's PA$_{O_2}$ after the F$_{I_{O_2}}$ was elevated 0.10. Assume a normal $\dot{V}_{CO_2}/\dot{V}_{O_2}$ ratio and atmospheric conditions at this instant.

A. 11 torr
B. 114 torr
C. 124 torr

D. 164 torr
E. 181 torr

26. Restrictive pulmonary disorders generally tend to influence which of the following pulmonary function measurements?

    I. peak expiratory flowrate
    II. total lung capacity
    III. inspiratory reserve volume
    IV. percent of forced expiratory volume after 1 second

A. I, III, IV only
B. I, IV only
C. II, IV only

D. I, II only
E. II, III only

27. Calculate the $FEV_{2\%}$ for a person with the pulmonary function data shown in Table 13.

TABLE 13

Parameter	Actual	Predicted
FVC	7.48 liters	7.83 liters
$FEV_{0.5}$	4.11 liters	4.30 liters
$FEV_{1.0}$	5.98 liters	6.26 liters
$FEV_{2.0}$	7.03 liters	7.36 liters
$FEV_{3.0}$	7.25 liters	7.59 liters

A. 97%
B. 95%
C. 94%

D. 90%
E. 79%

28. A metabolic alkalosis would be associated with a(n) _____ in _____ .

    I. normal P_{50}; arterial and venous blood
    II. decrease; P_{50}
    III. decrease; $Hb\text{-}O_2$ affinity
    IV. increase; $Hb\text{-}O_2$ affinity
    V. increase; P_{50}

A. I only
B. III, V only
C. IV only

D. V only
E. II, IV only

29. What condition(s) may be responsible for the configuration of the flow-volume tracing shown in Figure 144?

    I. pulmonary fibrosis

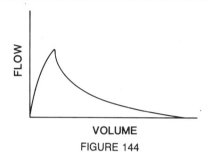

FIGURE 144

II. chronic bronchitis

III. pulmonary emphysema

IV. normal representation

A. IV only

B. I only

C. II only

D. II, III only

E. I, II, III only

30. What is the approximate normal FRC in a healthy adult male?

A. 20% of the TLC

B. 30% of the TLC

C. 60% of the TLC

D. 2,400 ml

E. 3,400 ml

31. Which statement(s) describe(s) the appropriate use of the Wright respirometer?

I. It can be directly attached to a 50 psig source to accurately measure the flowrate.

II. Its range for measuring flows is between 3 liters/min and 300 liters/min.

III. A major disadvantage of using this device is that a large degree of inaccuracy results because of the mechanical resistance offered by the instrument's gears.

IV. This device can be used to measure tidal volume, minute volume, and VC.

A. I, II, III, IV

B. II only

C. II, IV only

D. III, IV only

E. II, III, IV only

32. What is the purpose of performing the single-breath carbon dioxide elimination test?

A. The purpose is to determine the peripheral chemoreceptor response to acute arterial CO_2 increases.

B. The purpose is to investigate the response of the central chemoreceptors to abrupt changes in CSF CO_2.

C. This test indicates the degree to which pulmonary perfusion and ventilation match.

D. This maneuver establishes the amount of buffer in the blood.

E. It is useful in determining the closing volume; however, it is not as accurate as the conventional method.

33. What is considered to be the approximate normal $FEV_{1\%}$ for a healthy young adult?

A. 64%   D. 92%
B. 70%   E. 97%
C. 83%

34. Which of the following measurements *cannot* be directly obtained from a forced vital capacity tracing?
    I. $FEF_{25\%-75\%}$
    II. FEV_3
    III. MVV
    IV. RV
    V. MBC

    A. III, IV only   D. III, IV, V only
    B. I, II only   E. I, IV only
    C. II, IV, V only

35. Which arterial blood gas and/or acid-base status is(are) typical of a person having an acute asthmatic attack?
    I. hypoxemia
    II. increased arterial carbon dioxide tension
    III. metabolic and respiratory acidosis
    IV. respiratory alkalosis

    A. I, II, III only   D. III only
    B. I, IV only   E. IV only
    C. II, III only

36. Which expression correctly depicts the calculation of ERV?
    A. TLC − VC   D. VC − RV
    B. (IRV + V_T + FRC) − (RV)   E. (IC + FRC) − (IRV + RV)
    C. TLC − (IC + RV)

37. Which pulmonary function parameter *most* reflects a patient's ability to cough?
    A. IC   D. $\dot{V}_E$
    B. VC   E. TLC
    C. FVC

38. Which statement(s) is(are) true about the closing capacity?
    I. It is usually presented as a percentage of the TLC.
    II. Closing capacity reflects the status of small airways.
    III. It increases in value with increasing age.
    IV. The 7-minute N_2 washout test provides this measurement.

    A. II only   D. III, IV only
    B. I, II, III only   E. I, II, III, IV
    C. I, III only

39. Which disease condition(s) increase(s) TLC?

    I. pulmonary edema
    II. atelectasis
    III. pulmonary emphysema
    IV. kyphoscoliosis

    A. II only
    B. I, IV only
    C. III, IV only

    D. II, III, IV only
    E. III only

40. What is the normal range of variance for the RV/TLC ratio among healthy young adults?

    A. 2% to 5%
    B. 5% to 15%
    C. 15% to 20%

    D. 20% to 35%
    E. 35% to 40%

41. Which pulmonary function parameter is the *best* indicator of small-airway obstructive disease?

    A. $FEF_{25\%-75\%}$
    B. $FEF_{200-1200}$
    C. $FEV_{1\%}$

    D. PEF
    E. FVC

42. What does II on Figure 145 represent?

    A. expired gas from the oral and nasal cavities and the trachea
    B. expired gas from the lung apices
    C. mixed expired bronchial and alveolar gas
    D. expired alveolar gas
    E. gas expired from the lower zones of the lungs

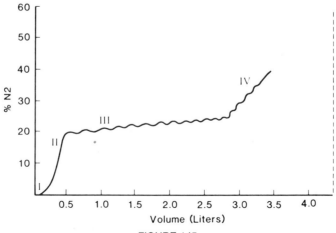

FIGURE 145

43. Which statements correctly describe $\Delta\%N_2$?

    I. It is obtained from the single-breath N_2 elimination procedure.

    II. The normal $\Delta\%N_2$ value for healthy young adults is 2.5%.

    III. It records the $\%N_2$ difference between the first 750 cc and 1,250 cc expired.

    IV. $\Delta\%N_2$ values increase with increasing degrees of airway obstruction.

    A. I, II, III, IV   D. I, II, IV only

    B. II, III, IV only   E. I, III, IV only

    C. III, IV only

44. Which method of determining the functional residual capacity of a pulmonary emphysema patient will render the largest FRC value?

    A. 7-minute nitrogen washout   D. single-breath nitrogen elimination

    B. diffusion capacity   E. body plethysmography

    C. spirometry

45. Which statement *best* describes the correct inspiratory breathing maneuver for performing the single-breath nitrogen elimination test?

    A. The person inspires as much 100% O_2 as possible from the FRC level.

    B. The person maximally inspires 100% O_2 from the FRC level and breath-holds for 15 seconds.

    C. After performing an MVV for 15 seconds, the subject maximally inspires 100% O_2 from the RV level.

    D. The person maximally inspires 100% O_2 from the RV level.

    E. The subject is instructed to hyperventilate for approximately 10 seconds, then maximally inspire 100% O_2 from the end-inspiratory level.

46. Which statements are true regarding the use of mass spectrometry?

    I. It allows for continuous analysis of oxygen.

    II. A latent response time prevents its use for breath-by-breath analysis of exhaled gases.

    III. The principle of mass spectrometry monitoring is based on the ionization property of gases.

    IV. Only oxygen gas mixtures can be monitored.

    A. I, II, III, IV   D. II, III, IV only

    B. I, II, III only   E. III, IV only

    C. I, III only

47. Identify letter E in Figure 146.

    A. expiratory reserve volume   D. inspiratory capacity

    B. functional residual capacity   E. inspiratory reserve volume

    C. residual volume

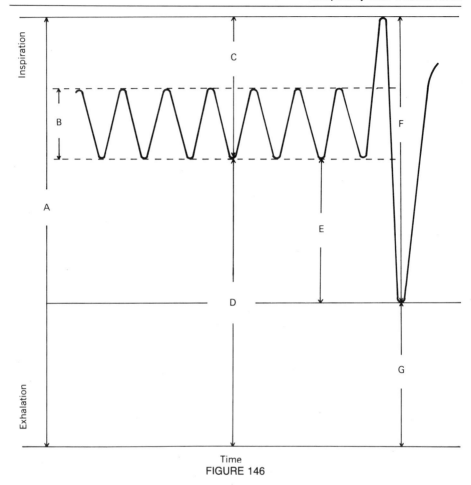

Time
FIGURE 146

48. What is the diagnostic value of the methacholine challenge test?

   A. It is a test to determine the effectiveness of beta-2 adrenergic drugs.
   B. It is a drug administered to determine pre- and post-bronchodilator spirometry functions.
   C. The methacholine challenge test is a skin test used to identify specific antigens responsible for allergic reactions.
   D. It is a bronchial provocation test in which hyperactive airways respond with bronchoconstriction to methacholine.
   E. When administered, methacholine measures specific IgE antibodies in the patient's serum.

49. Compute the $FEF_{25-75\%}$ using the volume-time tracing shown in Figure 147 obtained from the Med Science 570 Wedge Spirometer at BTPS.

   A. 0.65 liter/sec
   B. 1.80 liters/sec
   C. 2.77 liters/sec
   D. 3.60 liters/sec
   E. 3.83 liters/sec

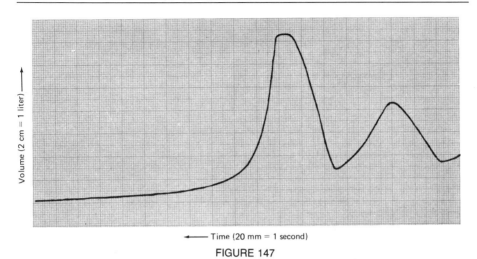

Time (20 mm = 1 second)

FIGURE 147

50. Which of the following pulmonary function findings characterize kyphoscoliosis?

  I. reduced TLC
  II. significant increase in flow resistance
  III. reduction in minute ventilation
  IV. reduction in FEV$_1$/FVC ratio
  V. reduced VC

  A. I, II, III, IV, V   D. II, V only
  B. I, II, IV, V only   E. I, V only
  C. II, III, IV only

51. Identify the dysrhythmia shown in Figure 148.

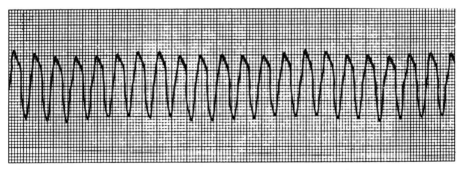

FIGURE 148

  A. atrial flutter   D. ventricular fibrillation
  B. ventricular tachycardia   E. sinus bradycardia
  C. atrial fibrillation

52. Identify letter D in the pressure tracings shown in Figure 149.

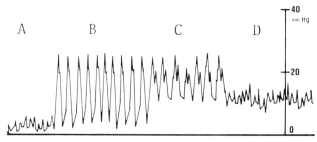

FIGURE 149

A. pulmonary capillary wedge pressure   D. pulmonary artery pressure
B. left atrial pressure   E. right ventricular pressure
C. right atrial pressure

53. Which of the following complications is most likely to be associated with arterial cannulation?

A. hypotension   D. thrombosis
B. venous stasis   E. bradycardia
C. polycythemia

54. What is the normal time interval on an electrocardiogram for ventricular depolarization?

A. 0.01 to 0.03 second   D. 0.14 to 0.26 second
B. 0.03 to 0.12 second   E. > 0.24 second
C. 0.12 to 0.20 second

55. Which of the following statements are true concerning the determinations of airway resistance via body plethysmography?

I. The shutter remains open when alveolar pressure and plethysmograph pressure are obtained.
II. The shutter closes when air flowrate and plethysmograph pressure are obtained.
III. The shutter remains open when air flowrate and plethysmograph pressure are obtained.
IV. The shutter closes when alveolar pressure and plethysmograph pressure are obtained.

A. I, III only   D. III, IV only
B. I, II only   E. II, III only
C. II, IV only

56. What are the common sites for insertion of an indwelling arterial catheter during exercise testing?

I. femoral artery
II. brachial artery

III. ulnar artery

IV. radial artery

A. III, IV only
B. II, III only
C. I, IV only
D. I, II only
E. II, IV only

57. Interpret the following arterial blood gas data:

Pa_{O_2}: 95 mm Hg
Pa_{CO_2}: 20 mm Hg
pH: 7.32
HCO_3^-: 10 mEq/liter

A. partially compensated metabolic acidosis
B. uncompensated respiratory alkalosis
C. uncompensated metabolic alkalosis
D. partially compensated respiratory acidosis
E. compensated metabolic acidosis

58. Which of the following physiologic components influence the DL_{CO} value derived from either the steady-state or the single-breath lung diffusion study?

I. ventilatory rate
II. pulmonary capillary blood volume
III. rate of reaction between carbon monoxide and hemoglobin
IV. diffusion capacity of the alveolar-capillary membrane

A. I, II, III, IV
B. II, III only
C. I, IV only
D. II, III, IV only
E. II, IV only

59. The spirometric data shown in Table 14 were obtained during a pre- and post-bronchodilator study. What interpretation can be made from this study?

TABLE 14

Variable	Prebronchodilator	Postbronchodilator
FVC	3.24 liters	3.29 liters
FEV_1	2.25 liters	2.34 liters
FEV_1/FVC	69%	71%
$FEF_{25\%-75\%}$	1.65 liters/sec	1.72 liters/sec

A. Insufficient data are available for an interpretation to be made.
B. Significant bronchodilator response is present.
C. Insignificant bronchodilator response is present.
D. Restrictive lung disease is present.
E. The two patient efforts are inconsistent and should be repeated.

60. The arterial blood gas data shown below are most characteristic of which of the following clinical conditions? (Assume that the patient is breathing room air.)

    Pa_{O_2}: 52 mm Hg
    Pa_{CO_2}: 68 mm Hg
    pH: 7.32
    HCO_3^-: 36 mEq/liter

    I. asbestosis
    II. sarcoidosis
    III. COPD
    IV. kyphoscoliosis

    A. I, II only   D. II, III, IV only
    B. II, IV only   E. I, III only
    C. III, IV only

61. Identify letter D in the arterial pressure tracing shown in Figure 150.

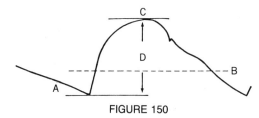

FIGURE 150

    A. dicrotic notch   D. systolic pressure
    B. pulse pressure   E. diastolic pressure
    C. mean arterial pressure

62. Which of the following statements accurately describe central venous pressure (CVP)?

    I. The CVP is a good indicator of right ventricular preload.
    II. The normal adult CVP range is 0 to 8 cm H_2O.
    III. Vasodilatation of the venous vasculature will increase the CVP.
    IV. Infarction of the right ventricle causes the CVP reading to increase.

    A. I, II, IV only   D. I, II only
    B. II, III only   E. I, II, III, IV
    C. I, III, IV only

63. What is the purpose of performing an Allen test before an arterial puncture procedure?

    A. to assess capillary refill
    B. to establish the presence of collateral circulation
    C. to obtain a baseline for the oxygen pulse
    D. to determine the adequacy of the radial pulse
    E. to determine the pulse pressure.

64. What would be an appropriate time interval between a before and after bronchodilator study? [Assume Alupent (metaproterenol sulfate) is used.]

    A. 30 to 40 minutes   D. 5 to 10 minutes

    B. 20 to 30 minutes   E. 2 to 3 minutes

    C. 15 to 20 minutes

65. Calculate the pulmonary vascular resistance from the cardiovascular data presented below.

    Pa_{O_2}: 95 mm Hg
    Pa_{CO_2}: 38 mm Hg
    pH: 7.37
    HCO_3^-: 22 mEq/liter
    Cardiac output: 5 liters/min
    Cardiac index: 2.5 liters/min/m²
    Mean pulmonary artery pressure: 15 mm Hg
    Pulmonary capillary wedge pressure: 5 mm Hg
    Mean arterial pressure: 80 mm Hg

    A. 2 mm Hg/liter/min   D. 10 mm Hg/liter/min

    B. 4 mm Hg/liter/min   E. 12 mm Hg/liter/min

    C. 8 mm Hg/liter/min

66. Which Pa_{CO_2} value is compatible with an uncompensated respiratory alkalosis?

    A. 55 mm Hg   D. 35 mm Hg

    B. 50 mm Hg   E. 30 mm Hg

    C. 45 mm Hg

67. Which of the following measures would be useful in preventing the balloon of a Swan-Ganz catheter in the pulmonary artery from rupturing?

    I. By inserting 3 to 4 cc of air using a small volume syringe.

    II. By pulling back on the syringe plunger to deflate the balloon after a wedge pressure reading has been obtained.

    III. By inflating the balloon slowly with the minimum amount of air to obtain a wedge pressure measurement.

    IV. By allowing the balloon to passively deflate through the stopcock after obtaining a wedge pressure reading.

    A. I, IV only   D. I, III, IV only

    B. II, III only   E. I, II, III only

    C. III, IV only

68. Which of the following parameters are *directly* measured during arterial blood gas analysis via a blood gas analyzer?

    I. P_{O_2}

    II. HCO_3^-

    III. P_{CO_2}

    IV. S_{O_2}

A. I, III only
B. I, III, IV only
C. II, IV only

D. I, II, III only
E. I, II, III, IV

69. Which of the following pulmonary measurements are obtained and evaluated during exercise testing?

   I. respiratory exchange ratio
   II. forced expiratory volume in one second
   III. minute ventilation
   IV. frequency dependence of compliance

A. I, II, III only
B. II, IV only
C. I, III only

D. I, III, IV only
E. I, II, III, IV

70. Which arterial pH measurement represents an uncompensated metabolic alkalosis?

A. 7.20
B. 7.30
C. 7.40

D. 7.45
E. 7.50

71. Which of the following pathophysiologic conditions will cause the pulmonary capillary wedge pressure to be greater than normal?

   I. mitral valve stenosis
   II. right ventricular failure
   III. myocardial infarction of posterior left ventricular wall
   IV. tricuspid valve stenosis

A. I, II, III, IV
B. I, II, III only
C. I, III only

D. III, IV only
E. II, IV only

72. Arterial blood gas analysis is required for which of the following pulmonary function tests?

A. volume of isoflow
B. steady-state carbon monoxide lung diffusion capacity study
C. body plethysmography
D. single-breath nitrogen elimination study
E. 7-minute nitrogen washout test

Questions 73 and 74 refer to the same patient.

73. Calculate a patient's FRC (ATPS) based on the following data obtained from the closed-circuit helium dilution technique.

   helium added: 0.70 liter
   initial helium concentration: 10%

final helium concentration: 7.5%
temperature: 25°C
helium-blood absorption factor: 0.10 liter
atmospheric pressure: standard

A. 0.80 liter
B. 1.98 liters
C. 2.23 liters

D. 2.50 liters
E. 3.03 liters

74. Convert the FRC calculated at ATPS to BTPS. (See Appendix III.)

A. 2.68 liters
B. 2.39 liters
C. 2.13 liters

D. 1.98 liters
E. 0.86 liter

75. Which of the following factors influence stroke volume?

I. ventricular afterload
II. the state of myocardial contractility
III. ventricular end-diastolic volume
IV. ventricular preload

A. I, II, III, IV
B. II, III, IV only
C. I, II only

D. I, II, IV only
E. III, IV only

76. A before-and-after bronchodilator spirometry study was conducted on a 48-year-old female. The volume-time tracings for the two forced vital capacity maneuvers are shown in Figure 151. Which of the following pulmonary disorders does this patient most likely have?

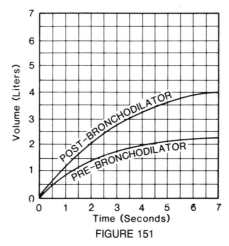

FIGURE 151

A. pulmonary emphysema
B. bronchial asthma
C. pneumoconiosis

D. Pickwickian syndrome
E. pneumonia

77. Determine the $\Delta N_{2_{750-1,250}}$ from the tracing of the single-breath nitrogen elimination curve shown in Figure 152.

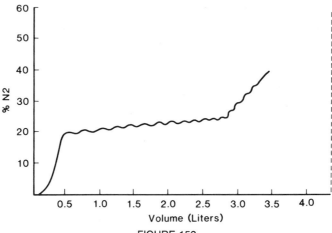

FIGURE 152

A. 42%   D. 5%

B. 20%   E. 2%

C. 10%

78. Calculate the P_{O_2} calibration factor for a blood gas analyzer given the following data.

PB: 760 torr
Temperature: 37°C
P_{H_2O}: 47 torr
F_{O_2}: 0.12

A. 91.2 torr   D. 12.0 torr

B. 85.6 torr   E. 5.6 torr

C. 20.9 torr

79. If a blood sample of pH 6.840 is introduced into a calibrated pH electrode, the potential difference measured by this instrument should be _____ millivolt(s).

A. −0.01   D. 1.00

B. 0.00   E. 1.01

C. 0.01

80. Based on the quality control record and data shown in Figure 153, what percentage of the data reside within the range of ±2 SDs from the mean?

A. 33%   D. 95%

B. 50%   E. 99%

C. 68%

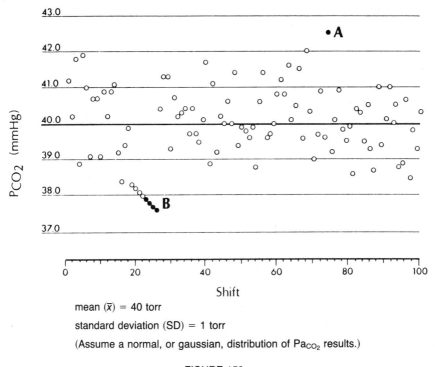

mean ($\bar{x}$) = 40 torr

standard deviation (SD) = 1 torr

(Assume a normal, or gaussian, distribution of Pa_{CO_2} results.)

FIGURE 153

ASSESSMENT ANSWER SHEET

DIRECTIONS: Darken the space under the selected answer.

	A	B	C	D	E		A	B	C	D	E
1.	[ ]	[ ]	[ ]	[ ]	[ ]	28.	[ ]	[ ]	[ ]	[ ]	[ ]
2.	[ ]	[ ]	[ ]	[ ]	[ ]	29.	[ ]	[ ]	[ ]	[ ]	[ ]
3.	[ ]	[ ]	[ ]	[ ]	[ ]	30.	[ ]	[ ]	[ ]	[ ]	[ ]
4.	[ ]	[ ]	[ ]	[ ]	[ ]	31.	[ ]	[ ]	[ ]	[ ]	[ ]
5.	[ ]	[ ]	[ ]	[ ]	[ ]	32.	[ ]	[ ]	[ ]	[ ]	[ ]
6.	[ ]	[ ]	[ ]	[ ]	[ ]	33.	[ ]	[ ]	[ ]	[ ]	[ ]
7.	[ ]	[ ]	[ ]	[ ]	[ ]	34.	[ ]	[ ]	[ ]	[ ]	[ ]
8.	[ ]	[ ]	[ ]	[ ]	[ ]	35.	[ ]	[ ]	[ ]	[ ]	[ ]
9.	[ ]	[ ]	[ ]	[ ]	[ ]	36.	[ ]	[ ]	[ ]	[ ]	[ ]
10.	[ ]	[ ]	[ ]	[ ]	[ ]	37.	[ ]	[ ]	[ ]	[ ]	[ ]
11.	[ ]	[ ]	[ ]	[ ]	[ ]	38.	[ ]	[ ]	[ ]	[ ]	[ ]
12.	[ ]	[ ]	[ ]	[ ]	[ ]	39.	[ ]	[ ]	[ ]	[ ]	[ ]
13.	[ ]	[ ]	[ ]	[ ]	[ ]	40.	[ ]	[ ]	[ ]	[ ]	[ ]
14.	[ ]	[ ]	[ ]	[ ]	[ ]	41.	[ ]	[ ]	[ ]	[ ]	[ ]
15.	[ ]	[ ]	[ ]	[ ]	[ ]	42.	[ ]	[ ]	[ ]	[ ]	[ ]
16.	[ ]	[ ]	[ ]	[ ]	[ ]	43.	[ ]	[ ]	[ ]	[ ]	[ ]
17.	[ ]	[ ]	[ ]	[ ]	[ ]	44.	[ ]	[ ]	[ ]	[ ]	[ ]
18.	[ ]	[ ]	[ ]	[ ]	[ ]	45.	[ ]	[ ]	[ ]	[ ]	[ ]
19.	[ ]	[ ]	[ ]	[ ]	[ ]	46.	[ ]	[ ]	[ ]	[ ]	[ ]
20.	[ ]	[ ]	[ ]	[ ]	[ ]	47.	[ ]	[ ]	[ ]	[ ]	[ ]
21.	[ ]	[ ]	[ ]	[ ]	[ ]	48.	[ ]	[ ]	[ ]	[ ]	[ ]
22.	[ ]	[ ]	[ ]	[ ]	[ ]	49.	[ ]	[ ]	[ ]	[ ]	[ ]
23.	[ ]	[ ]	[ ]	[ ]	[ ]	50.	[ ]	[ ]	[ ]	[ ]	[ ]
24.	[ ]	[ ]	[ ]	[ ]	[ ]	51.	[ ]	[ ]	[ ]	[ ]	[ ]
25.	[ ]	[ ]	[ ]	[ ]	[ ]	52.	[ ]	[ ]	[ ]	[ ]	[ ]
26.	[ ]	[ ]	[ ]	[ ]	[ ]	53.	[ ]	[ ]	[ ]	[ ]	[ ]
27.	[ ]	[ ]	[ ]	[ ]	[ ]	54.	[ ]	[ ]	[ ]	[ ]	[ ]

	A	B	C	D	E		A	B	C	D	E
55.	[ ]	[ ]	[ ]	[ ]	[ ]	73.	[ ]	[ ]	[ ]	[ ]	[ ]
56.	[ ]	[ ]	[ ]	[ ]	[ ]	74.	[ ]	[ ]	[ ]	[ ]	[ ]
57.	[ ]	[ ]	[ ]	[ ]	[ ]	75.	[ ]	[ ]	[ ]	[ ]	[ ]
58.	[ ]	[ ]	[ ]	[ ]	[ ]	76.	[ ]	[ ]	[ ]	[ ]	[ ]
59.	[ ]	[ ]	[ ]	[ ]	[ ]	77.	[ ]	[ ]	[ ]	[ ]	[ ]
60.	[ ]	[ ]	[ ]	[ ]	[ ]	78.	[ ]	[ ]	[ ]	[ ]	[ ]
71.	[ ]	[ ]	[ ]	[ ]	[ ]	79.	[ ]	[ ]	[ ]	[ ]	[ ]
72.	[ ]	[ ]	[ ]	[ ]	[ ]	80.	[ ]	[ ]	[ ]	[ ]	[ ]

CARDIOPULMONARY DIAGNOSTICS AND INTERPRETATION ANALYSES

Note: The references listed after each analysis are numbered and keyed to the reference list located at the end of this section. The first number indicates the text. The second number indicates the page on which information about the questions will be found. For example, (1:219,384) means that reference number 1 is to be used and that on pages 219 and 384 information about the question will be found. Frequently, it will be necessary to read beyond the page number indicated to obtain complete information. Therefore, reference to the question will be found either on the page indicated or on subsequent pages.

1. D. Ventilating a patient from a respiratory acidosis to a respiratory alkalosis can produce a variety of negative physiologic consequences; for example, cardiac dysrhythmias caused by hypokalemia and/or digitalis toxicity (if the patient is receiving digitalis), convulsive spasms (tetany), cerebrovascular constriction, and a leftward shift in Hb-O_2 dissociation curve. A deleterious consequence of a leftward shift of the Hb-O_2 dissociation curve is an increased affinity between Hb and O_2. The release of oxygen to the tissues is then impaired.
(1:602), (6:535)

2. C. The single-breath N_2 elimination technique is used to determine the closing volume (Figure 154). A straight line superimposed on the phase III and phase IV tracings is drawn. The point at which the upward deviation, phase IV, begins indicates the closing volume.

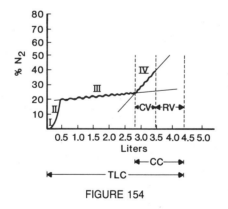

FIGURE 154

CV = closing volume
RV = residual volume
CC = closing capacity
TLC = total lung capacity

(6:242,251), (7:24), (10:48), (11:156), (17:50)

3. E. Because a 20:1 ratio is preserved despite abnormal values, compensation can be assumed. The denominator in the ratio represents the respiratory component. If it

was the primary cause for the acid-base imbalance presented, the ratio would be interpreted as a compensated respiratory alkalosis because the renal component became acidotic to compensate for the respiratory parameter. On the other hand, if the numerator, which reflects the renal component, was the primary cause of the acid-base disturbance, a compensated metabolic acidosis would be represented. The respiratory component would indicate that compensation (hyperventilation) has taken place.

(1:228), (6:276), (8:84), (10:159), (12:211)

4. A. The reduced flowrates accompanied by increased lung volumes and capacities indicate the presence of an obstructive process and air trapping, respectively. The flowrates decrease in obstructive diseases because airway mechanics prohibit effective forced exhalation. Air trapping during exhalation accounts for the increased lung volumes and capacities. In pulmonary emphysema, for example, air trapping generally results from airway collapse caused by loss of lung elastic recoil. The difference between the VC and FVC values indicates that the patient's airways collapsed (air trapping) during the forced maneuver. Sometimes a COPD patient will display a normal slow vital capacity (SVC) but, when the patient is performing an FVC, airway obstruction becomes apparent.

(6:235), (7:21), (8:131), (10:91–98), (12:134), (17:149), (25:199–201)

5. D. An uncompensated respiratory alkalosis represents acute alveolar hyperventilation. As the carbon dioxide tension in the blood decreases, the CO_2 tension in the CSF also decreases. The blood-brain barrier that separates the blood from the CSF is passively permeable to carbon dioxide. Consequently, blood CO_2 changes will reflect CSF$_{CO_2}$ changes.

(1:228), (6:276–280), (10:134), (12:59), (27:107)

6. B. A forced vital capacity (FVC) maneuver is obtained by spirometry. Such a maneuver is performed by achieving TLC and rapidly and forcefully exhaling from TLC to RV.

The following measurements can be obtained from an FVC tracing:

1. FEV_1: forced expired volume in 1 second
2. $FEV_{1\%}$: the FEV_1 divided by the FVC multiplied by 100
3. $FEV_{200-1200}$: forced expiratory flow between the first 200 ml and 1,200 ml of exhaled volume
4. $FEF_{25\%-75\%}$: maximum mid-expiratory flowrate between 25% and 75% of the exhaled volume (the middle 50% of the FVC)
5. PEF: peak expiratory flowrate, or the maximum flowrate attainable at any point during the FVC

(3:42), (6:232), (8:128), (10:84–87,102), (12:131), (17:27–37), (25:198) (26:20–21)

7. D. To determine the volume of isoflow (Viso$\dot{V}$), which reflects the lung volume at which gas flow becomes density independent, an FVC maneuver while breathing air and an FVC maneuver while breathing a He-O_2 (80%-20%) mixture must be performed. The tracing obtained from one of these two maneuvers is superim-

posed on the other tracing. The point (D) at which both tracings intersect represents the volume of isoflow (Figure 143).

(17:37), (25:141), (26:22,38)

8. D. Radioactive xenon^{133} (^{133}Xe) is injected intravenously after it is dissolved in normal saline. The uniformity of ventilation and pulmonary perfusion can be assessed by means of a scintillation camera as the ^{133}Xe gas enters the alveoli. The advantage of this maneuver is that it indicates only the alveoli that are ventilated and perfused.

(6:252), (10:87), (12:182), (17:56)

9. E. Diuretics generally are associated with a loss of K^+ and H^+ ions. The excretion of these two cations will eventually disrupt normal acid-base balance and produce a metabolic alkalosis.

Normally, the Na^+ ion is reabsorbed 80% of the time accompanied by the Cl^- ion; the remaining 20% of the Na^+ is reabsorbed in exchange for either K^+ or H^+. If hypochloremia exists, Na^+ will be reabsorbed more frequently in exchange for K^+ or H^+. Consequently, hypochloremia can lead to hypokalemia and/or a depletion of H^+ ions. The ultimate result is a metabolic alkalosis.

Diarrhea, especially in infants may produce a metabolic alkalosis because upper gastrointestinal (GI) contents are lost because an infant's GI tract is not very large. Diarrhea in an adult is usually associated with a metabolic acidosis. However, extensive diarrhea in an adult may result in the removal of upper GI tract contents and produce a metabolic alkalosis.

(1:236), (3:246), (6:277), (8:90–91), (12:211)

10. D. The combined CO_2, that is, the amount carried as HCO_3^-, is obtained in terms of vol% and is converted to mM CO_2/liter. The dissolved CO_2, obtained as torr or mm Hg, is converted to mM CO_2/liter.

Volumes percent (vol%) can be converted to mM/liter as shown in the following seven steps.

STEP 1: Determine the conversion factor needed to convert vol% to millimoles of CO_2 per liter.

$$1 \text{ m}M \text{ } CO_2/\text{liter} = X \text{ vol\%}$$

STEP 2: Under standard conditions 1 g molecular weight (mole) of CO_2 occupies a volume of 22.3 liters.*

$$1 \text{ mole } CO_2 \text{ @ STP} = 22.3 \text{ liters, or } 22,300 \text{ ml}$$

STEP 3: If a mole of CO_2 occupies 22,300 ml at STP, then a millimole (one one-thousandth of a mole) of CO_2 will occupy 22.3 ml.

$$\text{m}M \text{ } CO_2 = \frac{22,300 \text{ ml}}{1,000} = 22.3 \text{ ml}$$

---

*Carbon dioxide is not an ideal gas. Therefore, it deviates slightly from the volume (22.4 liters) occupied by an ideal gas at standard temperature (0°C) and standard pressure (760 torr). STP represents standard temperature and standard pressure.

STEP 4: Now that a millimole of CO_2 has been defined, it is necessary to apply this unit physiologically (i.e., in terms of one liter of plasma). Therefore,

$$1 \text{ m}M \text{ } CO_2/\text{liter plasma} = \frac{22.3 \text{ ml } CO_2}{1 \text{ liter plasma}} = \frac{22.3 \text{ ml } CO_2}{1,000 \text{ ml plasma}}$$

Recall from Step 3 that the volume 22.3 ml represents that volume occupied by a millimole of CO_2 at STP.

STEP 5: Ordinarily, gas volumes in plasma are expressed as vol% (ml/100 ml plasma) and *not* as ml/1,000 ml plasma. Therefore,

$$22.3 \text{ ml } CO_2/1,000 \text{ ml plasma} = 2.23 \text{ ml } CO_2/100 \text{ ml plasma}$$

Note the difference in the placement of the decimal point.

STEP 6: Recall that the expression *volumes percent,* which represents some volume of gas dissolved in 100 ml of plasma, is abbreviated as *vol%.* Hence,

$$2.23 \text{ ml } CO_2/100 \text{ ml plasma} = 2.23 \text{ vol\%}$$

STEP 7: Therefore, 2.23 vol% CO_2 equals 1 mM CO_2 per liter of plasma. Consequently,

$$\text{m}M \text{ } CO_2/\text{liter} = \frac{\text{vol\%}}{2.23 \text{ vol\%/m}M \text{ } CO_2/\text{liter}}$$

Therefore, there are 2.23 vol% of CO_2 per mM CO_2/liter. When dividing this factor into the amount of combined CO_2 (HCO_3^-), the units vol% cancel and the answer is expressed as mM CO_2/liter.

The following three steps show how to determine the plasma HCO_3^- in mM CO_2/liter, as asked for in question 10.

STEP 1: Convert the total CO_2 content expressed in vol% to mM/liter.

$$\frac{84.00 \text{ vol\%}}{2.23 \text{ vol\%/m}M/\text{liter}} = 37.67 \text{ m}M/\text{liter}$$

STEP 2: Convert the Pa_{CO_2} expressed in mm Hg to mM/liter.*

$$(49 \text{ mm Hg})(0.03 \text{ m}M/\text{liter/mm Hg}) = 1.47 \text{ m}M/\text{liter}$$

STEP 3: Determine the combined CO_2, i.e., HCO_3^-.

$$
\begin{array}{r}
37.67 \text{ m}M/\text{liter (total } CO_2 \text{ content)} \\
-1.47 \text{ m}M/\text{liter (dissolved } CO_2) \\
\hline
36.20 \text{ m}M/\text{liter (combined } CO_2)
\end{array}
$$

(1:216–222), (2:65–66), (4:192)

---

*Refer to Wojciechowski, W., *Respiratory Care Sciences: An Integrated Approach* (pp 64 and 66) for the derivation of the conversion factor 0.03 mM/liter/mm Hg.

11. B. STEP 1: $\dfrac{HCO_3^-}{P_{CO_2}} = \dfrac{\text{combined } CO_2}{\text{dissolved } CO_2} = \dfrac{36.20 \text{ mM/liter}}{1.47 \text{ mM/liter}} = 24.6$

STEP 2: $\dfrac{24.6}{1} = 24.6{:}1$

(1:220,228), (2:64–67,83)

12. A. This patient showed no signs of respiratory disease. His history indicated none as well. The patient was overdiuresed and developed iatrogenic metabolic alkalosis as a consequence.

Although, quantitatively, chronic ventilatory failure and compensated respiratory acidosis are feasible, the scenario gives no indication that any respiratory condition exists.

Furthermore, if the patient were experiencing a primary respiratory problem consistent with respiratory acidosis, the HCO_3^-/CO_2 ratio would not have exceeded 20:1 because that would have represented overcompensation. A ratio of 24.6:1 would have represented overcompensation.

(1:602), (6:535),

13. E. $\dfrac{FEV_3}{FVC} \times 100 = FEV_{3\%}$

$$\dfrac{7.29 \text{ liters}}{7.60 \text{ liters}} \times 100 = 95.9\%$$

(3:43), (17:29–30)

14. A. The FEV_1 is often presented as a percentage of the FVC obtained by the following calculation:

$$\dfrac{FEV_1}{FVC} \times 100 = FEV_{1\%}$$

Normally, greater than 75% of one's FVC can be exhaled in the first second.

(3:43), (6:232–233), (10:87), (17:29–30), (26:21)

15. B. The subject is instructed to perform an FVC, after which he is told to maximally and rapidly inspire to TLC.

Both inspiratory and expiratory measurements of volumes and flows can be obtained from a flow-volume loop. A flow-volume loop will provide the same data obtained from an FVC recording plus inspiratory and expiratory flows at 75%, 50%, and 25% of the vital capacity.

Parameters such as V_T, IRV, and ERV are obtained only by superimposing a V_T loop on a flow-volume loop.

(6:244), (10:98), (17:35)

16. A. As the oxyhemoglobin curve shifts to the right, the oxygen-hemoglobin affinity decreases. This mechanism facilitates oxygen uptake by the tissues. Factors causing the Hb-O_2 dissociation curve to shift right are (1) hypercapnia, (2) hyperther-

mia, (3) increased 2,3-DPG, and (4) acidemia. The pH 7.31 represents the greatest drop in Hb-O_2 affinity, consequently, the greatest arterial-venous oxygen tension difference.
(1:208), (6:263), (8:68–71), (12:186), (27:206)

17. B. After the patient breathes 100% oxygen for 7 minutes during the 7-minute nitrogen washout test, his alveolar nitrogen should be less than 2.5%. This test assesses the degree of unevenness of ventilation.

The slope of the tracing (log %N_2 versus volume) is influenced by the patient's ventilatory rate, V_T and FRC.

A %N_2 greater than 2.5% at the end of the maneuver is indicative of maldistribution of ventilation. It should be noted that most young, healthy adults will wash out their nitrogen to 1% or less in 7 minutes.
(6:242–244), (17:53)

18. E. The Severinghaus electrode measures the potential difference across the pH-sensitive glass that separates two electrolyte solutions, one of known pH and the other of unknown pH. CO_2 diffuses across a Teflon or silicone membrane into the unknown solution and alters its pH according to the following reaction:

$$CO_2 + H_2O \rightleftharpoons H_2CO_3 \rightleftharpoons H^+ + HCO_3^-$$

The potential difference is measured on a voltmeter and is read out as P_{CO_2}. The Severinghaus electrode potentiometrically measures the P_{CO_2}.
(6:983), (12:10), (17:136), (25:180), (27:31–33)

19. B. Carbon monoxide is used to measure lung diffusion capacity ($D_{L_{CO}}$) because it has an affinity for Hb 210 times greater than that of oxygen. Also, the blood CO level is assumed to be near zero. However, smokers tend to have CO levels greater than normal, depending on how heavily they smoke. The gas mixture used in the single-breath study is 0.3% CO, 10% He, and air.
(10:150), (17:61), (25:173), (26:28)

20. C. Ventilator patients can have fiberoptic bronchoscopy performed with relatively little interference with their mechanical ventilation. This procedure may be performed under either local or general anesthesia. Anaerobic cultures can be readily obtained via this technique.
(1:567), (3:399), (6:892)

21. C. STEP 1: Convert the volume in the Tissot spirometer from milliliters to liters.

$$1 \text{ cc} = 10^{-3} \text{ liter}$$
$$(27{,}000 \text{ cc})(10^{-3} \text{ liter/cc}) = 27 \text{ liters}$$

STEP 2: Use the formula for calculating the FRC via the open-circuit technique.

$$FRC = \frac{\left(\begin{array}{c}\text{final \%N}_2 \text{ in}\\ \text{Tissot spirometer}\end{array}\right)\left(\begin{array}{c}\text{exhaled volume}\\ \text{collected in Tissot}\\ \text{spirometer}\end{array}\right)^*}{\text{alveolar \%N}_2}$$

$$= \frac{(9\%)(27 \text{ liters})}{75\%}$$

$$= 3.24 \text{ liters}$$

STEP 3: Calculate the residual volume (RV) from the formula below.

$$RV = FRC - ERV$$
$$= 3.24 \text{ liters} - 1.22 \text{ liters}$$
$$= 2.02 \text{ liters}$$

The formula shown here does not include the following corrective factors: (1) test duration (ordinarily, 7 minutes), (2) blood and tissue N_2 removal factor, (3) V_D spirometer circuitry, and (4) spirometer (ambient) temperature. (Refer to Ruppel, G., *Manual of Pulmonary Function Testing*, 4th ed., C. V. Mosby, St. Louis, 1987 for specific computations.)

(6:243,966), (10:103), (12:15), (17:3,187), (25:134), (26:8)

22. C. The RV/TLC ratio can be determined as follows.

STEP 1: $\dfrac{RV}{TLC} \times 100 = RV/TLC\%$

STEP 2: $\dfrac{2.02 \text{ liters}}{9.56 \text{ liters}} \times 100 = 21.1\%$

(17:14), (25:197)

23. C. This person exhibits higher than predicted flowrates, which can also occur in a restrictive lung disease. However, the large TLC and normal RV/TLC ratio (along with the good flowrates) rule out either obstruction or restriction. This person displays normal lung mechanics.

(6:235), (8:130), (10:93), (12:134), (17:17–38), (25:201), (26:21)

24. B. The Sanz (pH) electrode incorporates glass that is pH sensitive. As a consequence, a potential difference is established between the H^+ ion concentration in the constant pH solution and the H^+ ion concentration in the blood sample. The Ag/AgCl measuring electrode is in contact with the buffer solution, while the $Hg/HgCl_2$ calomel reference electrode communicates with the Ag/AgCl electrode. The Sanz electrode measures the potential difference between the H^+ ion concentration in the solution and the H^+ ion concentration in the blood sample.

(6:983), (17:136), (27:31,32,37)

---

*This formula is actually derived from the relationship $C_1V_1 = C_2V_2$, where C_1 = initial concentration; V_1 = initial volume; C_2 = final concentration; and V_2 = final volume.

25. D. The alveolar air equation should be used.

$$PA_{O_2} = (P_B - P_{H_2O})F_{I_{O_2}} - PA_{CO_2}\left(F_{I_{O_2}} + \frac{1 - F_{I_{O_2}}}{R}\right)$$

where

PA_{O_2} = alveolar oxygen tension
P_B = barometric pressure
P_{H_2O} = water vapor pressure
$F_{I_{O_2}}$ = fraction of inspired oxygen
PA_{CO_2} = alveolar oxygen tension (Because it is assumed that there is complete equilibration between the alveoli and the blood, the Pa_{CO_2} can substitute for the PA_{CO_2}.)
R = respiratory quotient ($\dot{V}_{CO_2}/\dot{V}_{O_2}$)

$$PA_{O_2} = (760 \text{ torr} - 47 \text{ torr})0.31 - 49 \text{ torr}\left(0.31 + \frac{1 - 0.31}{0.8}\right)$$

$$= (713 \text{ torr})0.31 - 49 \text{ torr}(1.17)$$

$$= 221 \text{ torr} - 57.33 \text{ torr}$$

$$= 163.67 \text{ torr}$$

A shorter form of the alveolar air equation is often used in clinical situations for expediency. For example,

$$PA_{O_2} = (P_B - P_{H_2O})F_{I_{O_2}} - \left(\frac{Pa_{CO_2}}{R}\right)$$

$$= (760 \text{ torr} - 47 \text{ torr})0.31 - \left(\frac{49 \text{ torr}}{0.8}\right)$$

$$= 221 \text{ torr} - 61.25 \text{ torr}$$

$$= 159.75 \text{ torr}$$

(1:717), (2:19,22,131–132), (3:65), (12:11), (17:182)

26. E. Restrictive lung disorders, for example, obesity, kyphoscoliosis, and pectus excavatum, are generally characterized by decreased lung volumes and capacities. Flowrates can be normal or increased because lung recoil properties are ordinarily normal in these conditions. However, severe restrictive decreases will show decreased lung volumes and capacities, as well as decreased flowrates.
(3:337), (8:126), (10:92), (17:33), (25:200), (26:21)

27. C. Generally, four forced expiratory time volumes are reported after a subject performs a forced vital capacity. These forced expiratory volumes are $FEV_{0.5}$, $FEV_{1.0}$, $FEV_{2.0}$, and $FEV_{3.0}$.

The normal values for each of these FEVT parameters expressed as a percentage of normal FVC are as follows:

$$FEV_{0.5\%} = 50\% \text{ to } 60\%$$
$$FEV_{1\%} = 75\% \text{ to } 85\%$$

$$FEV_{2\%} = 94\%$$
$$FEV_{3\%} = 97\%$$
$$FEV_{2\%} = \frac{FEV_{2.0}\ (actual)}{FVC\ (actual)} \times 100$$
$$= \frac{7.03\ liters}{7.48\ liters} \times 100$$
$$= 94\%$$

(8:128), (10:28–30), (17:30), (25:137–139)

28. E. Inspection of the Hb-O_2 dissociation curve shows that as the curve shifts to the left ($\downarrow$ [H^+]; $\uparrow$ pH; $\downarrow$ Pa_{CO_2}; $\downarrow$ temperature; $\downarrow$ 2,3-DPG), the release of oxygen to the tissues is hindered ($\uparrow$ Hb-O_2 affinity). At the same time, the P_{50} value decreases. When the curve shifts to the left, a lower partial pressure of oxygen is needed to saturate 50% of the hemoglobin in circulation.

(1:205), (3:91,92,141), (6:261), (8:78)

29. D. COPD characteristically presents the flow-volume curve for an FVC, as shown in the question. This configuration results from the reduced expiratory flowrates associated with diseases, such as pulmonary emphysema and chronic bronchitis.

Restrictive diseases, on the other hand, present a flow-volume curve similar to a normal one; however, the tracing is usually much shorter because of the reduced volumes and capacities associated with such diseases. Expiratory flows generally appear normal.

(3:128–134), (10:94), (17:33–36), (26:21)

30. D. The normal, average adult male has an FRC of approximately 2,400 cc. This value represents approximately 40% of the TLC (6,000 ml).

(1:164), (12:16), (17:8)

31. C. The Wright respirometer is a useful portable device for measuring tidal volume, minute volume, and slow (nonforced) vital capacity at the patient's bedside. The rotating vanes of the Wright respirometer spin as gas flows through the device. The volume exhaled is indicated on the dial (face) of the device, which is calibrated in liters and fractions of liters. Because the device is rather delicate, high flowrates (greater than 300 liters/minute) may damage the device. It is for this reason that measuring a forced vital capacity with the Wright respirometer is discouraged. Low flowrates (less than 3 liters/minute) may produce inaccurate measurements.

(1:639), (5:219–221), (17:128)

32. C. Like the ^{133}Xe elimination study, the single-breath CO_2 elimination procedure provides an index of ventilation and pulmonary perfusion uniformity.

(6:966), (12:180), (17:61–69)

33. C. Normal, average adults should be able to exhale at least 83% of their FVC in 1 second ($FEV_{1\%}$ = 83%).

(10:95), (17:27–30), (30:328)

34. D. The maximum voluntary ventilation (MVV), formerly the maximum breathing capacity (MBC), is performed by the patient as he takes in rapid, deep, successive breaths for 15 seconds. The RV can be calculated from data obtained from the open-circuit N_2 washout and the closed-circuit He equilibration techniques, or from body plethysmography.

(6:232–234), (10:78,89,102), (17:3–8,27,39), (30:331)

35. B. A person having an acute asthmatic episode typically exhibits hypoxemia and has a respiratory alkalosis (hypocapnia). The hypoxemia probably results from the maldistribution of ventilation caused by the diffuse bronchospasm. Because of the increased airway resistance throughout the tracheobronchial tree, some lung regions experience high $\dot{V}A/\dot{Q}C$ ratios, and others low $\dot{V}A/\dot{Q}C$ ratios. The low $\dot{V}A/\dot{Q}C$ ratios produce venous admixtures resulting in hypoxemia. During an asthmatic attack, the person's ventilatory rate is ordinarily high (30 to 40 breaths/min). The rapid ventilatory rate produces a low Pa_{CO_2} and a respiratory alkalosis.

If the asthmatic episode is refractory to medical treatment, the hypoxemia worsens and the patient begins presenting with a higher Pa_{CO_2}. The acid-base abnormality at this point is a mixed acidosis—metabolic (lactic acid) and respiratory (alveolar hypoventilation).

(6:750), (10:174–175), (11:53–54), (13:87,90), (24:171), (27:250–251)

36. C. The TLC is composed of all the lung volumes and capacities (Figure 155). The IC plus the RV contains all the lung volumes and capacities except the ERV. Therefore,

$$TLC - (IC + RV) = ERV$$

LUNG VOLUMES AND CAPACITIES

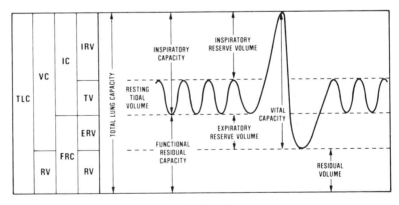

FIGURE 155

(6:232), (8:12), (10:85), (12:15), (17:2)

37. C. The ability to generate a sufficient forced vital capacity is essential to producing an effective cough. The inhalation of an adequate volume is necessary along with the ability to rapidly exhale.

(3:42–43,75,146,149), (8:226,382), (10:228)

38. B. The compression of the airways during the exhalation phase of the single-breath nitrogen elimination test causes airways to close as the lungs empty to the residual volume. The closing capacity represents the volume at which airway closure (small airways) occurs. It is expressed as a percentage of the total lung capacity, that is, (CC ÷ TLC)100.
(6:251), (17:50–52), (25:160,208), (26:38), (30:332)

39. E. Bronchiolar collapse during exhalation contributes to air trapping in pulmonary emphysema, and elastic lung recoil is lost because of connective tissue destruction. These factors contribute to the hyperinflated condition (↑ TLC) that exists with pulmonary emphysema.
(6:237), (8:126–128), (10:76), (17:13–15), (25:196–197), (26:21,37)

40. D. The RV/TLC ratio for normal young adults ranges between 20% and 35%.
(6:237–238), (8:11–13,127), (12:16), (17:14)

41. A. Small-airway characteristics are represented by the $FEF_{25\%-75\%}$ measurement, which reflects the flowrate during the middle 50% of the FVC maneuver. A reduction in the FVC is nonspecific for obstructive diseases or restrictive abnormalities. The $FEV_{1\%}$ is normal or increased in restrictive diseases. The $FEF_{200-1200}$ reflects the status of the large airways also.
(6:233), (8:128–134), (10:86–88), (17:31–32)

42. C. After performing a VC maneuver, the subject inspires 100% O_2 to TLC. At that point, he begins to exhale as slowly and as evenly as possible. When exhalation proceeds in that manner, the tracing shown in Figure 145 appears.
The tracing presents four phases: phase I, the first part of the exhaled volume containing only 100% O_2 (anatomic dead space gas); phase II, increasing amounts of N_2 exhaled as alveolar gas mixes with anatomic dead space gas; phase III, gas from alveolar units of the basal and middle lung zones; and phase IV, alveolar gas from the apices.
(6:242), (12:137), (17:50–53), (30:332)

43. E. The $\Delta\%N_2$ can be obtained from the single-breath N_2 elimination curve (Figure 145). The first 750 cc of the exhaled volume essentially represent dead space gas (phases I and II). Alveolar gas is obtained from phase III. The normal $\Delta\%N_2$ value for healthy young adults is $\leq 1.5\%$. Obstructive lung diseases cause the $\Delta\%N_2$ value to exceed 1.5%, which reflects uneven distribution of gas throughout the lungs. The $\Delta\%N_2$ will increase, reflecting the degree of unevenness of ventilation and varying expiratory flowrates.
(6:242), (17:50–53)

44. E. The closed-circuit helium dilution and the open-circuit N_2 washout tests are limited in the degree of accuracy when performed on patients with blebs or bullae (i.e., obstructive pulmonary disease). The pathologic conditions result in poor ventilation; consequently, these lung areas, where ventilation is poor, do not participate (or only to a very limited degree) in the gas distribution methods.
Body plethysmography, based on pressure-volume relationships, takes these poorly ventilated areas into consideration. Hence, the body plethysmograph will

render a higher (more accurate) FRC value in pulmonary emphysema, for example, than the gas distribution tests.
(10:104), (17:3–10)

45. D. One complete breath of 100% O_2 is inspired from the RV level to the TLC level. The subject then exhales slowly and evenly to the RV level.
(6:242), (10:49), (17:50), (25:156), (26:22)

46. C. Mass spectrometry monitoring is based on the ability of gases to be ionized and separated as a result of the molecular mass of their ions. In an ionization chamber, the sample gas molecules, including those of oxygen, are converted to positive ions by the loss of electrons. The gases are then separated according to the molecular mass of their ions. For example, oxygen ions have a larger mass than nitrogen ions. The percentage of the gas or gases in the sample is determined by the number of ions present of each gas within the sample. Continuous analysis of the gases is possible. The response time of spectrometers is rapid.
(5:210), (6:395), (17:134)

47. A. Letter E in Figure 156 designates the ERV. The letter designations for the other lung volumes and capacities are as follows:

LUNG VOLUMES AND CAPACITIES

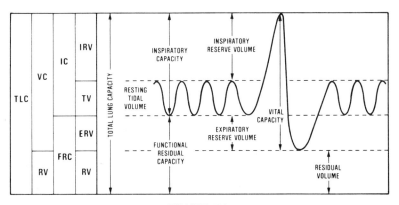

FIGURE 156

A = TLC
B = V_T
C = IC
D = FRC
E = ERV
F = VC
G = RV
(6:232), (10:185), (12:15), (17:2), (25:196), (26:5)

48. D. The methacholine challenge test is a bronchial provocation test used to determine the extent of airway reactivity, especially in individuals who are symptomatic, but

have normal pulmonary function studies or equivocal bronchodilator studies. Challenge testing may be performed in conjunction with before and after bronchodilator studies, and is often done as a preliminary to an exercise-induced asthma evaluation. The hyperactive airway bronchoconstricts when challenged with very low concentrations of some of the actual mediators of immune response, such as methacholine. The objective of the test is to determine the minimum exposure of methacholine that can precipitate a 20% decrease in the FEV_1. Methacholine increases parasympathetic tone in bronchial smooth muscle, resulting in bronchoconstriction.

(6:795), (8:261–262), (17:107)

49. C. The $FEF_{25\%-75\%}$ (Figure 157) is the forced expiratory flowrate during the middle 50% of the FVC maneuver. It represents the flowrate through medium and small airways.

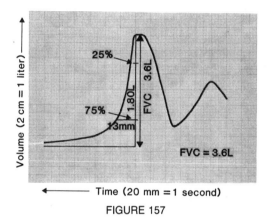

FIGURE 157

STEP 1: Determine the FVC.

The FVC is obtained by measuring the vertical distance from peak inspiration (TLC) to the point of maximum exhalation. Because 2 cm equal one liter, 7.2 cm is equal to 3.60 liters.

STEP 2: Locate the 25% and 75% points of the FVC on a vertical line representing the volume of the FVC.

$$3.60 \text{ liters} \times 25\% = 0.90 \text{ liter}$$
$$3.60 \text{ liters} \times 75\% = 2.70 \text{ liters}$$

STEP 3: Determine the volume by measuring the vertical distance between these two points. The volume is 1.80 liters.

STEP 4: Measure the horizontal distance from the 75% mark to the volume-time tracing. It measures 13 mm.

STEP 5: Calculate the time factor by dividing the horizontal distance 13 mm by the pen speed 20 mm/sec.

$$\frac{13 \text{ mm}}{20 \text{ mm/sec}} = 0.65 \text{ sec}$$

STEP 6: Calculate the $FEF_{25\%-75\%}$ by dividing the volume obtained in Step 3 by the time factor from Step 5.

$$\frac{1.80 \text{ liters}}{0.65 \text{ second}} = 2.77 \text{ liters/sec}$$

(1:175–178),   (4:210–211),   (6:233,961),   (8:129),   (17:31–32),   (24:72), (26:20–21), (30:325–326)

50. E. Spinal deformity conditions, such as kyphoscoliosis, present with reduced compliance of both the lungs and chest wall. Consequently, the vital capacity and TLC are reduced. Flow resistance is only moderately increased. The FEV_1/FVC ratio ($FEV_{1\%}$) is usual within normal limits because the FEV_1 and FVC are often proportionally reduced. Minute ventilation is often increased via lowered tidal volumes accompanied by higher ventilatory rates to produce the least expenditure of muscle energy.
(1:296–298), (3:337), (8:354)

51. B. Ventricular tachycardia is the dysrhythmia shown in Figure 148. The other dysrhythmias listed are shown in Figures 158 to 161.

A.

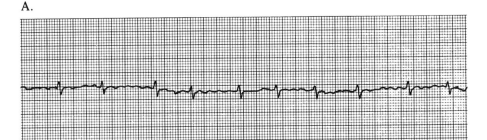

atrial flutter

FIGURE 158

C.

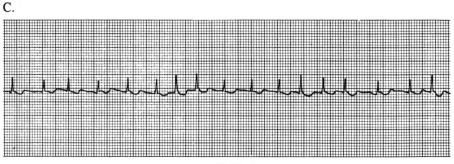

atrial fibrillation

FIGURE 159

D.

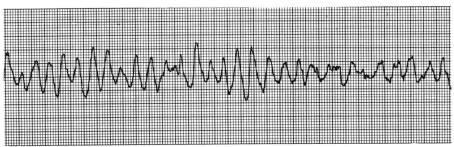

ventricular fibrillation

FIGURE 160

E.

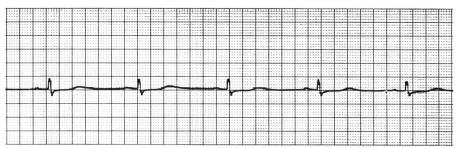

sinus bradycardia

FIGURE 161

(30:368,371,377)

52. A. Figure 149 illustrates the characteristic waveforms that are ordinarily observed during the insertion of a Swan-Ganz catheter in a patient.

> waveform A = right atrial pressure
> waveform B = right ventricular pressure
> waveform C = pulmonary artery pressure
> waveform D = pulmonary capillary wedge pressure

(9:98), (*Pressure Monitoring Instruments for Critical Care*, Spacelabs, Figure 35, p 5-2), (47:128)

53. D. Thrombosis is a likely complication associated with arterial cannulation. However, with proper care techniques the benefits far outweigh any potential complications of the procedure.
(6:941), (27:150), (34:240–241,318)

54. B. Ventricular depolarization on an ECG is represented by the QRS complex. The normal time interval for the QRS complex is 0.03 to 0.12 second. Figure 162 de-

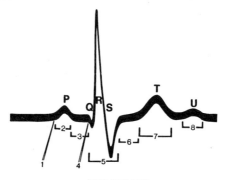

FIGURE 162

picts a normal lead II ECG. The sequential electrophysiologic events of a normal cardiac cycle are labeled and keyed to Table 15 at the bottom of the page. (1:249–250), (4:261), (30:360,367), (47:117–118)

55. D. When airway resistance is being determined via body plethysmography, the patient breathes through an unobstructed airway (shutter opened) as the flowrate ($\dot{V}$) and plethysmograph pressure (PB) are being obtained. The shutter closes then for the alveolar pressure (PA) and plethysmograph pressure (PB) measurements. Airway resistance is then calculated as follows:

$$R_{aw} = \frac{\text{shutter closed}}{\text{shutter open}} = \frac{P_A/P_B}{\dot{V}/P_B} = \frac{P_A}{\dot{V}}$$

(1:181–182), (6:249–251,964), (8:30–31), (17:44–46)

56. E. The common sites used for the insertion of indwelling arterial catheters used during exercise testing are the radial and brachial arteries.
(17:95)

TABLE 15

Sequential electrical events of the cardiac cycle	Electrocardiographic representation
1. Impulse from the sinus node	Not visible
2. Depolarization of the atria	P wave
3. Depolarization of the AV node	Isoelectric
4. Repolarization of the atria	Usually obscured by the QRS complex

5. Depolarization of the ventricles
  a. intraventricular septum
  b. right and left ventricles
	QRS complex
	  a. initial portion
	  b. central and terminal portions

6. Activated state of the ventricles immediately after depolarization	ST segment; isoelectric
7. Repolarization of the ventricles	T wave
8. After-potentials following repolarization of the ventricles	U wave

57. A. These arterial blood gas data are consistent with someone experiencing diabetic ketoacidosis. The acute increase in blood [H$^+$] has stimulated the peripheral chemoreceptors (carotid and aortic bodies) to reflexly signal the lungs to increase minute ventilation, hence, the decreased Pa$_{CO_2}$. The fact that the respiratory apparatus has made attempts to eliminate acid via hyperventilation signifies a compensatory effort. However, because the pH has not returned to the normal range (7.35 to 7.45), the compensatory effort is termed partial. Finally, the increased metabolically produced hydrogen ions have depleted the bicarbonate/carbonic acid buffer system.

(1:228–238), (4:203,205), (6:1010–1015), (8:89–92), (27:245,261)

58. D. Three physiologic factors influence the D$_{L_{CO}}$: (1) the diffusion capacity of the alveolar-capillary membrane (D$_{M_{CO}}$), (2) the pulmonary capillary blood volume (Vc), and (3) the rate of the reaction time between carbon monoxide (CO) and hemoglobin (θ). Quantitatively, the relationship is as follows:

$$\frac{1}{D_{L_{CO}}} = \frac{1}{D_M} + \frac{1}{V_C \times \theta}$$

The factor D$_M$ is considered the membrane component, while the factor (Vc $\times$ θ) is called the blood component.

Notice that the D$_{L_{CO}}$ is a conductance, or a reciprocal of resistance. The clinical applications of these considerations are shown in Table 16. In the case of anemia and decreased hematocrit, the D$_{L_{CO}}$ is reduced because of the reduced rate of reaction between CO and hemoglobin (θ). In the situations involving supine body position and exercise, the D$_{L_{CO}}$ is increased because of an increased pulmonary capillary blood volume (Vc). Lastly, diffuse pulmonary fibrosis and granulomatosis both decrease the D$_{L_{CO}}$ because of impeding the movement (diffusion) of CO across the alveolar-capillary membrane (D$_{M_{CO}}$).

TABLE 16

Clinical Conditions	D$_{L_{CO}}$	Equation Component Influenced
Anemia	↓	θ
Decreased hematocrit	↓	θ
Supine body position	↑	Vc
Exercise	↑	Vc
Diffuse pulmonary fibrosis	↓	D$_{M_{CO}}$
Granulomatosis	↓	D$_{M_{CO}}$

(6:968), (8:72–75), (12:114–117), (32:127–129)

59. C. Response to bronchodilator administration is considered significant when certain pulmonary function parameters increase by more than 15% to 20%. In this instance, the FVC improved by only 1.5%. The FEV$_1$ improved only 4.0%; the FEF$_{25\%-75\%}$ increased 4.2%.

Bronchodilator improvement is calculated according to the following formula.

$$\frac{\left(\begin{array}{c}\text{post-bronchodilator}\\ \text{value}\end{array}\right) - \left(\begin{array}{c}\text{pre-bronchodilator}\\ \text{value}\end{array}\right)}{\text{pre-bronchodilator value}} \times 100 = \%\ \text{improvement}$$

(12:11–12), (17:106), (30:339–341)

60. C. Persons having kyphoscoliosis and chronic obstructive pulmonary disease (COPD) characteristically have arterial blood gas data that indicate hypercapnia, hypoxemia, and acidemia. Because of the chronic nature of these pulmonary diseases, the renal system has had time to compensate (increased HCO_3^-) for the respiratory acidemia. The interpretation for such a blood gas and acid-base status is compensated respiratory acidosis.
(1:231–232), (4:203,205), (6:278,845,1014), (8:371), (17:73), (27:101,106, 257–258)

61. B. Letter D in the arterial pressure tracing shown in Figure 150 indicates the pulse pressure. The pulse pressure is the quantitive difference between the systolic pressure and the diastolic pressure. For example, if the blood pressure is 120/80 mm Hg, the pulse pressure is 40 mm Hg.

$$120\ \text{mm Hg} - 80\ \text{mm Hg} = 40\ \text{mm Hg}$$

The other components of the arterial pressure tracing shown are

A = diastolic pressure
B = mean arterial pressure
C = systolic pressure

(4:230)

62. A. The central venous pressue (CVP) represents the mean right atrial pressure. The value of measuring the CVP lies in the fact that it effectively monitors (1) blood volume, (2) venous return, and (3) right ventricular function. Because venous tone determines the venous vascular space, it directly influences the CVP. For example, vasodilatation of the venous circulation results in decreased venous return and decreased right atrial filling pressures; consequently, the CVP decreases. Venous vasoconstriction produces the opposite effect. When the CVP is measured as the right ventricular end-diastolic pressure (RVEDP), it is a good indicator of right ventricular preload.
An infarction of the right ventricle causes a decreased compliance of that cardiac chamber and results in an increased CVP value. The normal adult CVP range is 0 to 8 cm H_2O.
(4:231–232), (9:55-56)

63. B. The Allen test is performed to assess the adequacy of collateral circulation through the hand. The patency of the ulnar artery is determined by compressing both arteries simultaneously, and then releasing pressure from the ulnar artery while the radial remains compressed.
(6:258), (9:104), (27:145–147), (30:348)

64. D. Before-and-after bronchodilator pulmonary function studies are performed to ascertain the degree of reversibility of airway obstruction. Improvement in lung dynamics is deemed significant if certain pulmonary function parameters increase 15% to 20%.

Among factors required to optimize test results is the need to provide an adequate amount of time between test trials after the administration of the bronchodilator. A time interval of 5 to 10 minutes is generally considered sufficient to allow the medication to produce its desired effect. However, the time interval will differ depending on which bronchodilator is used.

(6:960), (17:180), (*American Review of Respiratory Disease*, 119:836, 1979)

65. A. STEP 1: Use the formula for calculating pulmonary vascular resistance (PVR).

$$PVR = \frac{\overline{PAP} - PCWP}{\dot{Q}_T}$$

where

$$PVR = \text{pulmonary vascular resistance}$$
$$\overline{PAP} = \text{mean pulmonary artery pressure}$$
$$PCWP = \text{pulmonary capillary wedge pressure}$$
$$\dot{Q}_T = \text{cardiac output}$$

STEP 2: Insert the known values and solve for PVR.

$$PVR = \frac{15 \text{ mm Hg} - 5 \text{ mm Hg}}{5 \text{ liters/min}}$$
$$= \frac{10 \text{ mm Hg}}{5 \text{ liters/min}}$$
$$= 2 \text{ mm Hg/liter/min}$$

(4:235)

66. E. The two factors that influence the pH of arterial blood are the Pa_{CO_2} (respiratory acid-base component) and the HCO_3^- (metabolic acid-base component). Table 17 illustrates the relationship between these two acid-base components and their effect on arterial blood pH.

For example, in an uncompensated respiratory alkalosis hyperventilation causes the Pa_{CO_2} to decrease (< 35 mm Hg) and the pH to increase (> 7.45). The HCO_3^- value will remain in the normal range (22 to 26 mEq/liter) until the renal mechanism begins to compensate. Therefore, a Pa_{CO_2} of 30 mm Hg is compatible with an uncompensated respiratory acidosis.

(1:229), (4:203,205), (6:278), (8:87–88,90–91), (24:88–91), (27:135,Table 13-3)

67. C. Pulmonary artery catheter ballon rupture can be prevented by any one of the following four measures: (1) slow balloon inflation with a minimum amount of air to obtain a pulmonary wedge pressure measurement; (2) monitor the pulmonary artery diastolic pressure as an indicator of pulmonary artery wedge pressure and left ventricular end-diastolic pressure; (3) allow passive balloon deflation through

TABLE 17

Acid base abnormality	Pa_{CO_2} (mm Hg)	HCO_3^- (mEq/liter)	pH[a]
1. Uncompensated (acute) respiratory acidosis	> 45	22–26	< 7.35
2. Compensated (chronic) respiratory acidosis	> 45	> 26	Just under 7.35
3. Uncompensated (acute) respiratory alkalosis	< 35	22–26	> 7.45
4. Compensated (chronic) respiratory alkalosis	< 35	< 22	Just above 7.45
5. Uncompensated (acute) metabolic acidosis	35–45	< 22	< 7.35
6. Compensated (chronic) metabolic acidosis	< 35	< 22	Just below 7.35
7. Uncompensated (acute) metabolic alkalosis	35–45	> 26	> 7.45
8. Compensated (chronic) metabolic alkalosis	> 45[b]	> 26	> 7.45[b]

[a] Compensatory mechanisms ordinarily do *not* return the pH value to within normal limits. When compensation has occurred, the pH will generally be just below the lower limit of normal (compensated acidois), or just above the upper limit of normal (compensated alkalosis), depending on the primary acid-base disturbance.

[b] The Pa_{CO_2} rarely exceeds 50 mm Hg during a compensated metabolic alkalosis. Therefore, the pH in this situation will generally be somewhat higher than the upper limit of normal.

the stopcock after obtaining a pulmonary artery wedge pressue reading; and (4) remove the syringe from the stopcock after balloon inflation. (9:73,88)

68. A. The following arterial parameters can be *directly* measured during arterial blood gas analysis via a blood gas analyzer.

1. P_{O_2}
2. P_{CO_2}
3. pH

The following parameters are calculated during arterial blood gas analysis via a blood gas analyzer.

1. HCO_3^-
2. S_{O_2}
3. [Hb]

(34:223,226,250,253)

69. C. The following pulmonary measurements are made during the performance of exercise testing.

1. respiratory exchange ratio (R)
2. minute ventilation ($\dot{V}E$)
3. ventilatory frequency (f)
4. oxygen consumption ($\dot{V}_{O_2}$)
5. carbon dioxide production ($\dot{V}_{CO_2}$)

The forced expiratory volume in 1 second (FEV₁) is obtained along with other spirometric data during pulmonary function studies usually conducted before the exercise test. Spirometric data also may be obtained after exercise testing to ascertain the presence of exercise-induced obstruction to flow.

Frequency dependence of compliance, considered by some pulmonary physiologists to be a sensitive indicator of early small airways (diameter, < 2 mm) disease, is measured via the use of an intra-esophageal balloon and a body plethysmograph. A decreasing dynamic compliance (CL_{dyn}) associated with increasing ventilatory frequency (f) is said to be indicative of airway obstruction.

(6:968), (12:136), (17:18), (24:47), (32:23,45)

70. E. Two humoral factors influence arterial blood pH. One is the level of dissolved carbon dioxide (Pa_{CO_2}), which is controlled by the ventilatory apparatus. If hyperventilation predominates, while the metabolic component of the acid-base status remains normal ([HCO₃⁻] = 22 to 26 mEq/liter), the arterial pH will be alkalotic (> 7.45). Conversely, if hypoventilation prevails, while the metabolic acid-base component is normal, arterial pH will be acidotic (< 7.35).

The other factor influencing arterial blood pH is the plasma bicarbonate concentration (metabolic component of the acid-base status). When the [HCO₃⁻] rises, while the ventilatory apparatus remains normal (Pa_{CO_2} = 35 to 45 mm Hg), the arterial blood pH also rises (alkalemia; > 7.45). On the other hand, when the [HCO₃⁻] falls, while the Pa_{CO_2} remains normal, the pH of arterial blood likewise falls (acidemia; < 7.35).

In the presence of an uncompensated metabolic alkalosis, the ventilatory apparatus remains normal (Pa_{CO_2} = 35 mm Hg to 45 mm Hg) while the [HCO₃⁻] increases (> 26 mEq/liter). An arterial pH of 7.50 would be consistent with an uncompensated metabolic alkalosis.

(1:229), (4:203,205), (6:277,278), (8:87–88,90–91), (17:73), (24:89–92), (27:123)

71. C. The mean pulmonary capillary wedge pressure (PCWP) in a normal adult ranges from 2 to 12 mm Hg.

The inability of the left ventricle to accept or receive a normal stroke volume (60 cc to 130 cc) will create back pressure from the left atrium and into the pulmonary vasculature. The back pressure will be reflected as an elevated pulmonary capillary wedge pressure. In the case of mitral valve stenosis, blood flow from the left atrium into the left ventricle is restricted because of the narrowing between these two chambers. Because the left ventricle receives an insufficient blood volume, the increased volume in the left atrium is reflected as an increased pressure toward the pulmonary vasculature, and elevates the PCWP.

When the left ventricle itself becomes an inadequate pump (e.g., left ventricular myocardial infarction), blood volume also accumulates in the pulmonary vasculature and causes an increased PCWP.

Right ventricular failure or tricuspid valve stenosis will cause less blood to enter the pulmonary vasculature, and will *not* elevate the PCWP.
(1:270–273), (4:234–235), (9:9–12,73–76)

72. B. During the steady-state carbon monoxide lung diffusion capacity study, the subject is instructed to tidally breathe an air-carbon monoxide (0.1% to 0.2% CO) mixture for about 6 minutes. During the last 2 minutes of the study the subject's expirate is collected and an arterial blood sample is obtained. The collected exhaled gas is analyzed for the P_{O_2}, P_{CO_2}, and P_{CO}; the arterial blood sample is analyzed for the Pa_{CO_2}.

The Pa_{CO_2} sustitutes for the PA_{CO_2} in the modified Bohr equation shown below.

$$V_D = V_T \left(\frac{PA_{CO_2} - P\bar{E}_{CO_2}}{PA_{CO_2}} \right) = V_T \left(\frac{P\bar{E}_{CO} - PA_{CO}}{PI_{CO} - PA_{CO}} \right)$$

where

V_D = the dead space volume
V_T = the tidal volume
PA_{CO_2} = the alveolar CO_2 tension; equal to the Pa_{CO_2} value
$P\bar{E}_{CO_2}$ = the mixed exhaled CO_2 tension
$P\bar{E}_{CO}$ = the mixed exhaled CO tension
PA_{CO} = the alveolar CO tension
PI_{CO} = the inspired CO tension

Rearranging,

$$PA_{CO} = PI_{CO} - \frac{PA_{CO_2}}{P\bar{E}_{CO_2}} (PI_{CO} - P\bar{E}_{CO})$$

The calculated PA_{CO} is then used to compute the DL_{CO} (liters/min/mm Hg) as follows:

$$DL_{CO} = \frac{\dot{V}_{CO}}{PA_{CO}}$$

The $\dot{V}_{CO}$ is the carbon monoxide consumption expressed in liters/min.
(17:63), (22:352–353)

73. C. STEP 1: Determine the initial volume in the spirometer system according to the following formula.

$$V = \frac{\text{helium added (liters)}}{\text{initial helium concentration}}$$

$$V = \frac{0.70 \text{ liter}}{0.10}$$

$$V = 7.0 \text{ liters}$$

STEP 2: Calculate the FRC using the following formula.

$$FRC = \left[\frac{(\text{initial He\%} - \text{final He\%})}{\text{final He\%}} \times \text{initial volume} \right] - \left(\begin{array}{c} \text{He} \\ \text{absorption} \\ \text{factor} \end{array} \right)$$

$$FRC = \left[\frac{(0.10 - 0.075)}{0.075} \times 7.0 \text{ liters} \right] - 0.10 \text{ liter}$$

FRC = 2.23 liters (ATPS)

(1:168), (4:275–276), (6:960), (14:14–15), (17:5,187), (22:17), (26:8), (30:321), (32:59)

74. B. The combined gas law is used for volume corrections.

$$\frac{P_1 V_1}{T_1} = \frac{P_2 V_2}{T_2}$$

STEP 1: Convert °C to °K.

T_1:   25°C

T_2:   37°C

$T_1 = °K = 25°C + 273$

$= 298°K$

$T_2 = °K = 37°C + 273$

$= 310°K$

STEP 2: Correct the pressure at their respective temperatures for the presence of P_{H_2O}. (See Appendix III.)

P_1:   760 mm Hg

P_2:   760 mm Hg

At 25°C, the P_{H_2O} is 23.8 mm Hg. Therefore,

P_1 (corrected) = 760 mm Hg − 23.8 mm Hg

P_1 (corrected) = 736 mm Hg

At 37°C, the P_{H_2O} is 47 mm Hg. Therefore,

P_2 (corrected) = 760 mm Hg − 47 mm Hg

P_2 (corrected) = 713 mm Hg

STEP 3: Convert the FRC measured at ATPS to BTPS using the combined gas law.

$P_1 = 760$ mm Hg $P_2 = 713$ mm Hg

$V_1 = 2.23$ liters $V_2 = ?$

$T_1 = 298°K$ $T_2 = 310°K$

$P_{H_2O} = 23.8$ mm Hg $P_{H_2O} = 47$ mm Hg

$P_1 = $ (corrected) 736 mm Hg $P_2 = $ (corrected) 713 mm Hg

$$\frac{(P_1 - P_{H_2O})V_1}{T_1} = \frac{(P_2 - P_{H_2O})V_2}{T_2}$$

$$V_2 = \frac{(P_1 - P_{H_2O})V_1T_2}{(P_2 - P_{H_2O})T_1}$$

$$V_2 = \frac{(736 \text{ mm Hg})(2.23 \text{ liters})(310°\text{K})}{(713 \text{ mm Hg})(298°\text{K})}$$

$$V_2 = 2.39 \text{ liters}$$

(1:26), (2:126–127), (6:960), (17:117), (30:341–342)

75. A. Stroke volume is influenced by (1) ventricular preload, or ventricular end-diastolic volume, (2) ventricular afterload, and (3) the state of myocardial contractility.

Ventricular preload, or ventricular end-diastolic volume, refers to the volume of blood that enters the ventricle during diastole. The volume of blood occupying the ventricle at ventricular end-diastole directly influences myocardial fiber length, which, in turn (up to a sarcomere length of 2.2 μ), increases the contractile force (Frank-Starling relationship).

Ventricular afterload represents the stress on the ventricular walls during ventricular systole. Factors, such as aortic valve stenosis and arterial hypertension, cause an increased resistance to the outflow of blood from the left ventricle. Such factors increase the strain on the ventricular walls and increase afterload.

Myocardial contractility is influenced by a number of factors. The sympathetic nervous system greatly influences the force of myocardial contractility. Myocardial infarction reduces myocardial contractility because some degree of myocardial tissue becomes necrotic and no longer participates in contraction. Certain pharmacologic agents have negative inotropic influences. These include propranolol and procainamide. Examples of positive inotropic medications are dopamine, dobutamine, and epinephrine.

(4:130–137), (9:9–11)

76. B. The patient performing the before-and-after bronchodilator study most likely has bronchial asthma, which is a reversible airway disease. Pulmonary emphysema is a chronic obstructive lung disease which is ordinarily not responsive to bronchodilator therapy. Pickwickian syndrome, pneumoconioses, and pneumonias (bacterial and viral) are restrictive lung diseases which do not respond to the administration of a bronchodilator.

(4:311), (6:791), (8:131,278), (17:106), (30:340), (34:215)

77. E. The measurement $\Delta N_{2_{750-1,250}}$ represents the nitrogen concentration difference between the 750-ml point and the 1,250-ml point on the single-breath nitrogen elimination curve. This measurement serves as an index (along with the phase III portion of the curve) of the uniformity of ventilation. The $\Delta N_{2_{750-1,250}}$ is normally less than 1.5%. It can be as high as 3.0% in healthy elderly adults. The $\Delta N_{2_{750-1,250}}$ for the tracing shown in Figure 163 is less than 3.0%. The $\%N_2$ at 750 ml is 20% and the $\%N_2$ at 1,250 ml is 22%. Therefore, the ΔN_2 is determined as follows

$$\begin{array}{r} 22\% \text{ N}_2 \text{ at } 1{,}250 \text{ ml} \\ - 20\% \text{ N}_2 \text{ at } 750 \text{ ml} \\ \hline 2\% \ \Delta\text{N}_2 \end{array}$$

(1:184–185), (4:279–281), (6:242–243), (8:135–136), (13:14–15,17–18), (17:50–53), (24:106–107), (30:332), (34:105–106,109)

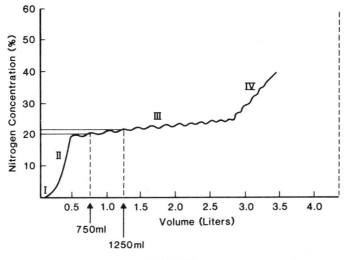

FIGURE 163

78. B. The formula for calculating the P_{O_2} calibration factor for a blood gas analyzer is as follows:

$$P_{O_2} = F_{O_2}(P_B - P_{H_2O})$$

Insert the known values and calculate the P_{O_2} calibration factor.

$$P_{O_2} = 0.12(760 \text{ torr} - 47 \text{ torr})$$
$$= 0.12(713 \text{ torr})$$
$$= 85.6 \text{ torr}$$

(2:127–130), (6:986), (27:161)

79. B. If a pH (Sanz) electrode shown in Figure 164 is calibrated and is introduced with a blood sample (in the sampling chamber) having a pH of 6.840, the potential dif-

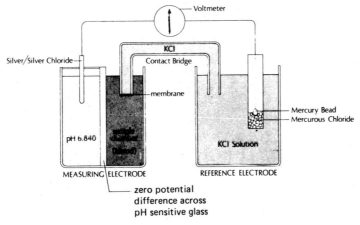

FIGURE 164

ference measured by the instrument should be 0.00 millivolt. The reason for the absence of a potential difference across the pH-sensitive glass in the measuring electrode is that, in this instance, both half-cells contain solutions having a pH of 6.840.

(4:418–420), (5:211–213), (6:980,982), (17:136), (27:29–31)

80. D. The frequency distribution curve shown in Figure 165 illustrates a normal (gaussian) distribution of data points for a series of P_{CO_2} measurements made by a Severinghaus electrode. The standard deviation (SD) provides information concerning the accuracy and reliability of any P_{CO_2} value. For example, 68% of all the values fall within 1 SD of the mean; 95% of all values reside within 2 SDs, whereas 99% of all values are included within 3 SDs.

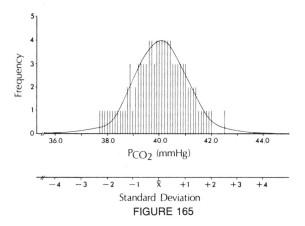

FIGURE 165

(6:988–989), (27:162–166), (34:53–56)

REFERENCES

1. Spearman, C., and Sheldon, R., *Egan's Fundamentals of Respiratory Therapy,* 4th ed., C.V. Mosby, St. Louis, 1982.
2. Wojciechowski, W., *Respiratory Care Sciences: An Integrated Approach,* John Wiley & Sons, New York, 1985.
3. Shapiro, B., Harrison R., Kacmarek, R., and Cane, R., *Clinical Application of Respiratory Care,* 3rd ed., Year Book Medical Publishers, Chicago, 1985.
4. Kacmarek, R., Mack, C., and Dimas, S., *The Essentials of Respiratory Therapy,* 2nd ed., Year Book Medical Publishers, Chicago, 1985.
5. McPherson, S., *Respiratory Therapy Equipment,* 3rd ed., C.V. Mosby, St. Louis, 1985.
6. Burton, G., and Hodgkin, J., *Respiratory Care: A Guide to Clinical Practice,* 2nd ed. J.B. Lippincott, Philadelphia, 1985.
7. Frownfelter, D., *Chest Physical Therapy and Cardiopulmonary Rehabilitation, An Interdisciplinary Approach,* Year Book Medical Publishers, Chicago, 1978.
8. Cherniack, R., and Cherniack, L., *Respiration in Health and Disease,* 3rd ed., W.B. Saunders, Philadelphia, 1983.
9. Daily, E., and Schroeder, G., *Techniques in Bedside Hemodynamic Monitoring,* 3rd ed., C.V. Mosby, St. Louis, 1985.

10. Des Jardins, R., *Clinical Manifestations of Respiratory Disease,* Year Book Medical Publishers, Chicago, 1984.
11. Mitchell, R., *Synopsis of Clinical Pulmonary Disease,* 3rd ed., C.V. Mosby, St. Louis, 1982.
12. Comroe, J., *Physiology of Respiration,* 3rd ed., Year Book Medical Publishers, Chicago, 1974.
13. West, J., *Pulmonary Pathophysiology—The Essentials,* 2nd ed., Williams & Wilkins, Baltimore, 1982.
14. West, J., *Respiratory Physiology—The Essentials,* 3rd ed., Williams & Wilkins, Baltimore, 1985.
15. Martz, K., et al., *Management of the Patient-Ventilator System: A Team Approach,* 2nd ed., C.V. Mosby, St. Louis, 1984.
16. Shoup, C., and McHenry, R., *Laboratory Exercises in Respiratory Therapy,* 2nd ed., C.V. Mosby, St. Louis, 1983.
17. Ruppel, G., *Manual of Pulmonary Function Testing,* 3rd ed., C.V. Mosby, St. Louis, 1982.
18. Appelbaum, E., and Bruce, D., *Tracheal Intubation,* W.B. Saunders, Philadelphia, 1976.
19. Rau, J., *Respiratory Therapy Pharmacology,* 2nd ed., Year Book Medical Publishers, Chicago, 1984.
20. United States Department of Health, Education, and Welfare, Public Health Service, *Isolation Techniques for Use in Hospitals,* 2nd ed., Washington, D.C., 1975.
21. Brooks, S., *Integrated Basic Science,* 4th ed., C.V. Mosby, St. Louis, 1979.
22. Comroe, J., *The Lung,* Year Book Medical Publishers, Chicago, 1962.
23. Shibel, E., and Moser, K., *Respiratory Emergencies,* 2nd ed., C.V. Mosby, St. Louis, 1982.
24. Tisi, G., *Pulmonary Physiology in Clinical Medicine,* 2nd ed., Williams & Wilkins, Baltimore, 1985.
25. Cherniack, R., *Pulmonary Function Testing,* W.B. Saunders, Philadelphia, 1977.
26. Altose M., *The Physiological Basis of Pulmonary Function Testing,* Clinical Symposia-CIBA, Vol. 31, No. 2, Summit, New Jersey, 1979.
27. Shapiro, B., Harrison, R., and Walton, J., *Clinical Application of Arterial Blood Gases,* 3rd ed., Year Book Medical Publishers, Chicago, 1982.
28. West, J., *Ventilation/Blood Flow and Gas Exchange,* 3rd ed., Blackwell Scientific Publications, 1979.
29. Slonim, N., and Hamilton, K., *Respiratory Physiology,* 4th ed., C.V. Mosby, St. Louis, 1981.
30. Rarey, K., and Youtsey, J., *Respiratory Patient Care,* Prentice-Hall, Englewood Cliffs, 1981.
31. Berne, R., and Levy, M., *Physiology,* C.V. Mosby, St. Louis, 1983.
32. Levitzky, M., *Pulmonary Physiology,* 2nd ed., McGraw-Hill, New York, 1986.
33. Wilson, P., Bell, C., and Norton, A., *Rehabilitation of the Heart and Lungs,* SensorMedics, 1980.
34. Clausen, J., and Zarins, L., *Pulmonary Function Testing Guidelines and Controversies,* Academic Press, New York, 1982.
35. Klaus, M., and Fanaroff, A., *Care of the High-Risk Neonate,* 2nd ed., W.B. Saunders, Philadelphia, 1979.
36. Lough, M., et al., *Pediatric Respiratory Therapy,* 3rd ed., Year Book Medical Publishers, Chicago, 1985.
37. Levin, D., et al., *A Practical Guide to Pediatric Intensive Care,* 2nd ed., C.V. Mosby, St. Louis, 1984.
38. O'Ryan, J., and Burns, D., *Pulmonary Rehabilitation from Hospital to Home,* Year Book Medical Publishers, Chicago, 1984.
39. Bell, C., et al., *Home Care and Rehabilitation in Respiratory Medicine,* J.B. Lippincott, Philadelphia, 1984.
40. Wilkins, R., et al., *Clinical Assessment in Respiratory Care,* C.V. Mosby, St. Louis, 1985.

41. Jones, N., and Campbell, E., *Clinical Exercise Testing,* 2nd ed., W.B. Saunders, Philadelphia, 1982.
42. Goldsmith, J., and Karotkin, E., *Assisted Ventilation of the Neonate,* W.B. Saunders, Philadelphia, 1981.
43. Blowers, M., and Sims, R., *How to Read an ECG,* 3rd ed., Medical Economics, New Jersey, 1983.
44. Eubanks, D., and Bone, R., *Comprehensive Respiratory Care,* C.V. Mosby, St. Louis, 1985.
45. Rattenborg, C., *Clinical Use of Mechanical Ventilation,* Year Book Medical Publishers, Chicago, 1981.
46. Witkowski, A. S., *Pulmonary Assessment: A Clinical Guide,* J.B. Lippincott, Philadelphia, 1985.
47. Op't Holt, T. B., *Assessment Based Respiratory Care,* John Wiley & Sons, New York, 1986.

PEDIATRICS AND PERINATOLOGY ASSESSMENT

PURPOSE: The purpose of this 50-item section is to evaluate your knowledge and understanding of the clinical application of respiratory care principles and practices as they pertain to pediatric and neonatal patients. Included in this section will be oxygen and medical gas therapy, aerosol/humidity therapy, intermittent therapy, mechanical ventilation, airway management, pharmacology, and diagnostic procedures.

DIRECTIONS: Each of the questions or incomplete statements is followed by five suggested answers. Select the one which is the best in each case and then blacken the corresponding space on the answer sheet.

1. When the red flag on an incubator is horizontal and the oxygen flowrate is 8 liters/min, approximately, what oxygen concentration can be expected inside the incubator?

   A. 28%   D. 45%
   B. 32%   E. 60%
   C. 39%

2. What may be the consequences of applying continuous positive airway pressure (CPAP) to an infant who has a normal lung compliance.

   I. pulmonary hypertension
   II. reduced venous return
   III. air trapping
   IV. pulmonary oxygen toxicity

   A. II, III only   D. I, II, III only
   B. III, IV only   E. I, II, III, IV
   C. I, II, IV only

3. Which of the following statements accurately describe mist tents?

   I. Mist tents tend to be cooler than the ambient air.
   II. An ultrasonic nebulizer may be used in conjunction with a mist tent.

III. The maximum oxygen concentration ranges from 40% to 60%.

IV. Patients with cystic fibrosis or pneumonia may find this mode of therapy useful.

A. I, III only

B. II, IV only

C. I, II, III only

D. II, III, IV only

E. I, II, III, IV

4. Which of the following factors affect the mean airway pressure ($\overline{P}_{aw}$) during mechanical ventilation of an infant?

   I. peak inspiratory pressure

   II. inspiratory time

   III. shape of the airway pressure waveform

   IV. positive end-expiratory pressure

A. I, II, III, IV

B. I, IV only

C. I, II, III only

D. I, III, IV only

E. I, III only

5. What would be the most likely consequence to a neonate receiving 40% oxygen at ambient temperature and humidity via an oxygen hood?

A. decreased Pa_{CO_2}

B. hyperthermia

C. decreased mean pulmonary artery pressure

D. increased oxygen consumption

E. polycythemia

6. Which of the following statements are true concerning the use of IPPB therapy on children?

   I. A surgical candidate should be introduced to this mode of therapy in the presurgical stage.

   II. The treatment should be of at least 30 minutes duration.

   III. The pressure during the treatment should range between 30 cm H_2O to 40 cm H_2O.

   IV. The patient should be instructed to breathe deeply and slowly during the treatment.

A. I, II, IV only

B. II, III only

C. I, III only

D. I, IV only

E. I, III, IV only

7. Which infant ventilator(s) is(are) fluidically controlled?

   I. Sechrist IV-100B

   II. Bear Cub BP 2001

   III. Healthdyne 105

   IV. Bio-Med MVP-10

A. II only   D. II, III only
B. III, IV only   E. IV only
C. I, IV only

8. Which of the following statements is true concerning the measurement of an infant's body temperature?

   A. The axillary temperature is about 2°F less than the rectal temperature.
   B. The rectal temperature is approximately 1°F less than the oral temperature.
   C. The oral temperature is about 2°F greater than the axillary temperature.
   D. The rectal temperature is approximately 1°F greater than the axillary temperature.
   E. The oral temperature is about 1°F greater than the rectal temperature.

9. Which of the following statements accurately describe the transcutaneous oxygen monitor?

   I. The temperature of the electrode must be increased to maintain identity between the Pa_{O_2} and the TcP_{O_2} during conditions of hypoperfusion.
   II. A decreased TcP_{O_2} value may be indicative of a low cardiac output.
   III. The position of the electrode is important if the infant has a patent ductus arteriosus.
   IV. As the cardiac output falls, the heat output of the electrode decreases.

   A. II, IV only   D. II, III only
   B. I, II, IV only   E. I, II, III, IV
   C. I, III only

10. What is the primary problem for blood gas analysis associated with squeezing the puncture site when performing a heel stick on an infant?

    A. It causes the rupture of red blood cells.
    B. It causes venous blood to mix with arterial blood.
    C. The direct compression of the area actually reduces the blood flow.
    D. Interstitial fluid contaminates the sample.
    E. It increases the blood flow to the area, thereby causing an erroneously high P_{O_2}.

11. Which of the following conditions is considered to be a common complication of rigid bronchoscopy in infants?

    A. subglottic croup   D. hemoptysis
    B. bronchospasm   E. rhinorrhea
    C. vocal cord paralysis

12. Which letter on the diagram shown in Figure 166 indicates the preferred site of insertion of a central venous pressure catheter in an infant?

    A. A   D. D
    B. B   E. E
    C. C

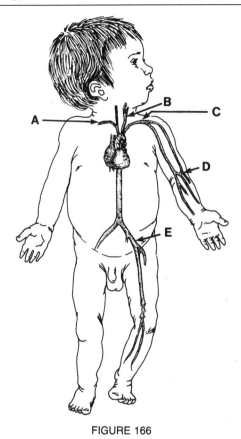

FIGURE 166

13. What gas should be used to partially inflate the balloon of a Swan-Ganz catheter once a venous waveform is observed?

A. oxygen   D. air
B. carbon dioxide   E. nitrogen
C. helium

14. Which of the following statements are true concerning the Penlon infant resuscitator bag?

 I. It can deliver oxygen concentrations up to 100%.
 II. It generally does *not* require oxygen flowrates greater than 8 liters/min.
 III. The patient valve is a one-way leaf valve.
 IV. A small hole is incorporated in the cupped disk at the bag outlet and functions as a pressure relief.

A. I, II, III, IV   D. II, IV only
B. II, III only   E. I, II, IV only
C. I, III, IV only

15. What type of humidification system is provided for Bear Cub BP 2001 by the manufacturer?

    A. heated blow-by humidifier
    B. cascade humidifier
    C. wick humidifier
    D. bubble humidifier
    E. 500-cc micronebulizer

16. Which of the following statements are true concerning umbilical artery catheters (UACs)?

    I. The waveform display will be devoid of a dicrotic notch.
    II. Blood obtained from a UAC in an infant with a patent ductus arteriosus may reveal a low Sa_{O_2}.
    III. UACs sometimes have a tendency to dislodge and migrate spontaneously.
    IV. UAC waveforms have the same characteristics as a peripheral artery waveform.

    A. II, III, IV only
    B. II, III only
    C. I, IV only
    D. I, II, III only
    E. III, IV only

17. Which of the following guidelines is appropriate for determining the proper size oral endotracheal tube for a small child about to be placed on a mechanical ventilator?

    A. The outer diameter of the tube should be about the same size as the infant's small finger.
    B. The tube should be just wide enough to allow the passage of a suction catheter.
    C. The size tube that creates a complete seal with the subglottic area should be used.
    D. The tube should be large enough to support the mechanical ventilator tubing.
    E. The outer diameter should allow for a small air leak at an inflation pressure of 25 cm H_2O.

18. Which of the following neonatal clinical conditions may sometimes be effectively treated with CPAP?

    I. persistent fetal circulation
    II. respiratory distress syndrome
    III. retrolental fibroplasia
    IV. acute ventilatory failure

    A. II, III only
    B. I, III only
    C. I, II only
    D. I, II, III only
    E. II, III, IV only

19. What determines the direction of blood flow across a patent ductus arteriosus in extrauterine life?

    A. whether the foramen ovale is patent or closed
    B. systemic vascular resistance
    C. polycythemia

D. pulmonary vascular resistance

E. the presence of central and peripheral cyanosis

20. What is the purpose of the oxygen challenge test?

A. to determine the percentage of shunt

B. to determine an infant's risk of oxygen toxicity

C. to determine the influence a high F_{IO_2} has on an infant's ventilation

D. to determine the amount of dead space ventilation an infant has

E. to determine if an infant has a pulmonary disease or a cardiac disease

21. Which infant ventilator(s) allow(s) for the inspiratory time to be directly selected?

   I. Sechrist IV-100B

  II. Healthdyne 105

 III. Bear Cub BP 2001

 IV. Bourns BP 200

A. II only

B. III, IV only

C. IV only

D. I, II, III only

E. I, II, III, IV

22. Which physiologic changes may be caused in a neonate by the delivery of an air-oxygen mixture that is too warm?

   I. hyperventilation

  II. apnea

 III. hyperthermia

 IV. tetany

A. II, IV only

B. II, III only

C. II, III, IV only

D. I, IV only

E. I, III, IV only

23. Which aerosolized medication may be useful for a child with allergic asthma about to take an aerosol treatment of nebulized cromolyn sodium?

A. Mucomyst

B. 0.45% normal saline

C. normal saline

D. hypertonic saline

E. bronchodilator

24. A 9-year-old boy aspirated a peanut while standing and watching a Mardi Gras parade in downtown Mobile. He was rushed immediately to the University of South Alabama Medical Center where a chest radiograph was taken. Where in the tracheobronchial tree is the peanut *most* likely to have lodged?

A. in the posterior basal segment of the right lower lobe

B. in the lingula

C. in the right middle lobe

D. in the anterior basal segment of the left lower lobe

E. in the anterior segment of the left lower lobe

Questions 25 and 26 refer to the same patient.

A 4-year-old girl is admitted to the Emergency Room presenting the following clinical manifestations: fever, aphonia, and inspiratory stridor. On physical examination she presented with severe dyspnea and severe retractions. The girl assumed a sitting position, leaning forward with her chin projected outward. She was also drooling.

25. What is this girl's probable diagnosis?

A. epiglottitis

B. laryngotracheobronchitis

C. bronchiolitis

D. pneumonia

E. pneumothorax

26. What is the appropriate therapeutic intervention at this time?

A. an aerosol mask with an F_{IO_2} of 0.40

B. endotracheal intubation and mechanical ventilation

C. endotracheal intubation and humidified oxygen

D. IPPB with alupent

E. a bronchodilator administered via a hand-held nebulizer

27. Why is it important to maintain an adequate volume of water in the reservoir of the humidifier on an infant mechanical ventilator?

   I. to prevent the compliance of the delivery tubing from decreasing

   II. to avoid a decrease in the tidal volume

   III. to prevent the flowrate from decreasing

   IV. to avoid the loss of humidification

A. I, II, IV only

B. II, III, IV only

C. II, IV only

D. I, III only

E. I, II, III, IV

28. What is the *most* common site of post-extubation edema in infants?

A. supraglottic region

B. subglottic region

C. retroarytenoid region

D. vestibular region

E. aryepiglottic region

29. What is the accepted sequence of therapeutic interventions in treating an infant in respiratory distress syndrome?

A. oxygenate, mechanically ventilate, apply CPAP

B. institute IMV, apply CPAP

C. mechanically ventilate, apply CPAP, oxygenate

D. institute controlled mechanical ventilation, institute IMV or CPAP, oxygenate

E. oxygenate, apply CPAP, mechanically ventilate

Questions 30 and 31 refer to the same patient.

A 12-month-old boy in mild respiratory distress was brought to the Emergency Room by his mother. The mother stated that her son had a frequent, dry cough and a slight fever (38.5°C) for a few days. A lateral roentgenogram of the neck revealed slight subglottic edema.

30. What is the probable diagnosis?

   A. acute bronchitis   D. bronchiolitis

   B. epiglottitis   E. laryngotracheobronchitis

   C. transient pulmonary hypertension

31. What is the appropriate therapeutic intervention at this time?

   A. endotracheal intubation and mechanical ventilation

   B. aerosolized antibiotics

   C. IPPB with normal saline

   D. endotracheal intubation with humidification and oxygenation

   E. unheated aerosol with racemic epinephrine

32. Which of the following expressions represent forms of high-frequency ventilation?

   I. high-frequency oscillation

   II. high-frequency impulse ventilations

   III. high-frequency jet ventilation

   IV. high-frequency positive pressure ventilation

   A. I, II only   D. III, IV only

   B. II, III, IV only   E. I, II, III, IV

   C. I, III, IV only

33. Which of the following therapeutic modalities may be beneficial in the treatment of cystic fibrosis in a nonhospitalized patient?

   I. intermittent positive pressure breathing treatments

   II. aerosol therapy

   III. chest physiotherapy

   IV. oxygen administration

   A. I, II, III, IV   D. II, IV only

   B. I, II, III only   E. II, III, IV only

   C. III, IV only

34. An infant being born at a gestational age of 36 weeks presents in the perineum with meconium staining. The infant's naso- and oropharynx have been thoroughly suctioned. Once delivered, the infant appears to be in mild respiratory distress. What therapeutic action would be appropriate at this time?

   A. Place the infant on nasal CPAP of 5 cm H_2O with an $F_{I_{O_2}}$ of 0.50.

   B. Place the infant in an oxyhood with an $F_{I_{O_2}}$ of 0.40.

C. Intubate the infant and place her on controlled mechanical ventilation with a PEEP of 5 cm H_2O and an FI_{O_2} of 0.50.

D. Intubate the infant and place her on IMV with an FI_{O_2} of 0.40.

E. The infant should have a tracheotomy performed, and then be placed on controlled mechanical ventilation with a PEEP of 5 cm H_2O and an FI_{O_2} of 0.40.

35. What is the major problem associated with the use of an oxygen hood?

A. It increases the infant's oxygen consumption.

B. The high temperatures that develop inside tend to cause the infant to become febrile.

C. The oxygen environment must be disturbed to feed the infant.

D. The oxygen concentration tends to increase inside the hood because of the small enclosure.

E. Carbon dioxide retention is sometimes a problem because of the small enclosure.

Questions 36, 37, and 38 refer to the information below.

36. While you are setting up the Bear Cub to ventilate a 2,000-g neonate, the neonatologist asks you to determine the inspiratory flowrate necessary to maintain an inspiratory/expiratory (I/E) ratio of 1:3 while delivering a tidal volume of 36 ml at a ventilatory rate of 30 breaths/min. Assume that a peak inspiratory pressure of 20 cm H_2O will be achieved.

A. 5.40 liters/min   D. 2.16 liters/min

B. 4.32 liters/min   E. 1.08 liters/min

C. 3.24 liters/min

37. What is the patient's actual V_T if the tubing compliance is 1.0 cc/cm H_2O?

A. 36 cc   D. 16 cc

B. 30 cc   E. 10 cc

C. 20 cc

38. If the patient's tidal volume was found to be too large, what would be the appropriate adjustment?

A. Decrease the inspiratory flowrate.

B. Add positive end-expiratory pressure.

C. Increase the ventilatory frequency.

D. Decrease the FI_{O_2}.

E. Decrease the pressure limit.

39. What pathophysiologic condition may result from the delivery of high oxygen concentrations and prolonged mechanical ventilation to a neonate?

A. persistent fetal circulation   D. retrolental fibroplasia

B. hyaline membrane disease   E. necrotizing enterocolitis

C. bronchopulmonary dysplasia

40. You receive an order to administer an ultrasonic nebulization treatment to a pediatric burn patient who is burned over 40% of his body and has a *Staphylococcus aureus* wound infection. The child's wounds do not have dressings on them. What form of isolation technique should you follow as you prepare to enter the patient's room?

    A. enteric precautions   D. strict isolation
    B. wound and skin precautions   E. respiratory isolation
    C. protective isolation

41. An infant in the neonatal intensive care unit is being mechanically ventilated in the control mode via a Bourns LS 104-150 Infant Ventilator. The infant is receiving a rate of 40 breaths/min and a minute ventilation of 600 cc/min.

    The neonatologist prescribes that the mode of ventilation be switched to assist/control. The control rate is now set at 25 breaths/min. The infant was initially noted to have a ventilatory rate of 30 breaths/min. However, after approximately 10 minutes of observation, the respiratory care practitioner perceives *no* assisted ventilations.

    What is the infant's minute ventilation at this time? Assume that tubing compliance is negligible.

    A. 0 cc/min   D. 375 cc/min
    B. 150 cc/min   E. 450 cc/min
    C. 180 cc/min

42. When the Bear Cub is used for neonatal mechanical ventilation, how is it generally operated?

    A. as a time-cycled, pressure-limited ventilator
    B. as a time-cycled, time-limited ventilator
    C. as a volume-cycled, pressure-limited ventilator
    D. as a volume-cycled, time-limited ventilator
    E. as a pressure-cycled, time-limited ventilator

43. Which of the following statements are true concerning the Cole pediatric endotracheal tube?

    I. The distal end (tip) is narrower than the proximal end.
    II. It increases the mechanical dead space.
    III. The resistance through the Cole tube is less than the resistance through a tube with the same caliber as the tip.
    IV. It is sometimes associated with laryngeal dilatation.

    A. I, II, III, IV   D. I, III only
    B. II, III, IV only   E. I, II, IV only
    C. I, II, III only

44. Which of the following statements correctly refer to the technique of performing a heel stick on a neonate for an arterial blood gas sample?

    I. A scalpel blade is generally used.

II. The depth of the puncture is determined by the amount of the bleeding produced.

III. The heel and surrounding area should be warmed for about 3 minutes at an approximate temperature of 38°C to 40°C.

IV. It is acceptable to make the puncture on the lateral aspect of the plantar surface.

A. I, II, III, IV   D. III, IV only

B. I, IV only   E. I, II, III only

C. II, III only

45. Which of the following statements describe the proper technique of oral endotracheal intubation of the neonate?

   I. The tip of a MacIntosh blade exposes the vocal cords by directly lifting up the epiglottis.

  II. The laryngoscope blade is inserted into the left side of the mouth to move the tongue out of the way.

 III. A Miller blade tip is placed in the vallecula to expose the vocal cords.

 IV. The endotracheal tube is inserted from the right side of the mouth and advanced through the glottis under direct visualization.

A. II, III, IV only   D. II, III only

B. III, IV only   E. I, II, IV only

C. I, II only

46. A 3-year-old boy is brought into the Emergency Room intubated and manually resuscitated after being in a house fire. When you arrive on the scene, he is breathing spontaneously. The arterial puncture that you perform reveals a Pa_{O_2} of 95 mm Hg; a Pa_{CO_2} of 43 mm Hg; and a carboxyhemoglobin (COHb) level of 12.0%. Which therapeutic intervention would be most appropriate at this time.

A. Place him on a Sechrist IV-100B ventilator in the control mode with an F_{IO_2} of 1.0.

B. Place him on a BP 200 ventilator in the IMV mode with an F_{IO_2} of 0.60.

C. Place the boy on a Siemens Servo 900 C ventilator in the control mode with an F_{IO_2} of 0.40.

D. Place the boy on a Brigg's adaptor at 100% oxygen.

E. Place him on a Babybird with a CPAP of 10 cm H_2O and an F_{IO_2} of 0.60.

47. What is the minimum liter flow of oxygen required to prevent carbon dioxide accumulation inside an oxygen hood?

A. 3 liters/min   D. 10 liters/min

B. 5 liters/min   E. 15 liters/min

C. 7 liters/min

48. What size endotracheal tube would be appropriate for a 5-year-old girl who is of normal size for her age?

A. 4.0 to 4.5 mm (I.D.)

B. 4.5 to 5.0 mm (I.D.)

C. 5.0 to 5.5 mm (I.D.)

D. 5.5 to 6.0 mm (I.D.)

E. 6.0 to 6.5 mm (I.D.)

49. What is the appropriate pressure range for routine tracheobronchial suctioning of neonatal patients?

A. -20 to -50 mm Hg

B. -50 to -90 mm Hg

C. -90 to -115 mm Hg

D. -110 to -125 mm Hg

E. -120 to -150 mm Hg

50. Which of the following procedures constitute recommended steps for weaning an infant from CPAP?

   I. The F_{IO_2} should be lowered by 0.03 to 0.05 each time the Pa_{O_2} exceeds 70 mm Hg.

   II. Once the inspired oxygen concentration reaches 40%, the pressure should be decreased 5 cm H_2O each hour.

   III. When a CPAP of 2 to 3 cm H_2O is attained, the patient should be placed in an oxygen hood at 60% oxygen.

   IV. Low birth weight infants may need a CPAP lowered to about 4 cm H_2O with the F_{IO_2} gradually lowered to 0.21.

A. I, IV only

B. II, III only

C. I, II, III only

D. III, IV only

E. I, II, IV only

ASSESSMENT ANSWER SHEET

DIRECTIONS: Darken the space under the selected answer.

	A	B	C	D	E		A	B	C	D	E
1.	[ ]	[ ]	[ ]	[ ]	[ ]	26.	[ ]	[ ]	[ ]	[ ]	[ ]
2.	[ ]	[ ]	[ ]	[ ]	[ ]	27.	[ ]	[ ]	[ ]	[ ]	[ ]
3.	[ ]	[ ]	[ ]	[ ]	[ ]	28.	[ ]	[ ]	[ ]	[ ]	[ ]
4.	[ ]	[ ]	[ ]	[ ]	[ ]	29.	[ ]	[ ]	[ ]	[ ]	[ ]
5.	[ ]	[ ]	[ ]	[ ]	[ ]	30.	[ ]	[ ]	[ ]	[ ]	[ ]
6.	[ ]	[ ]	[ ]	[ ]	[ ]	31.	[ ]	[ ]	[ ]	[ ]	[ ]
7.	[ ]	[ ]	[ ]	[ ]	[ ]	32.	[ ]	[ ]	[ ]	[ ]	[ ]
8.	[ ]	[ ]	[ ]	[ ]	[ ]	33.	[ ]	[ ]	[ ]	[ ]	[ ]
9.	[ ]	[ ]	[ ]	[ ]	[ ]	34.	[ ]	[ ]	[ ]	[ ]	[ ]
10.	[ ]	[ ]	[ ]	[ ]	[ ]	35.	[ ]	[ ]	[ ]	[ ]	[ ]
11.	[ ]	[ ]	[ ]	[ ]	[ ]	36.	[ ]	[ ]	[ ]	[ ]	[ ]
12.	[ ]	[ ]	[ ]	[ ]	[ ]	37.	[ ]	[ ]	[ ]	[ ]	[ ]
13.	[ ]	[ ]	[ ]	[ ]	[ ]	38.	[ ]	[ ]	[ ]	[ ]	[ ]
14.	[ ]	[ ]	[ ]	[ ]	[ ]	39.	[ ]	[ ]	[ ]	[ ]	[ ]
15.	[ ]	[ ]	[ ]	[ ]	[ ]	40.	[ ]	[ ]	[ ]	[ ]	[ ]
16.	[ ]	[ ]	[ ]	[ ]	[ ]	41.	[ ]	[ ]	[ ]	[ ]	[ ]
17.	[ ]	[ ]	[ ]	[ ]	[ ]	42.	[ ]	[ ]	[ ]	[ ]	[ ]
18.	[ ]	[ ]	[ ]	[ ]	[ ]	43.	[ ]	[ ]	[ ]	[ ]	[ ]
19.	[ ]	[ ]	[ ]	[ ]	[ ]	44.	[ ]	[ ]	[ ]	[ ]	[ ]
20.	[ ]	[ ]	[ ]	[ ]	[ ]	45.	[ ]	[ ]	[ ]	[ ]	[ ]
21.	[ ]	[ ]	[ ]	[ ]	[ ]	46.	[ ]	[ ]	[ ]	[ ]	[ ]
22.	[ ]	[ ]	[ ]	[ ]	[ ]	47.	[ ]	[ ]	[ ]	[ ]	[ ]
23.	[ ]	[ ]	[ ]	[ ]	[ ]	48.	[ ]	[ ]	[ ]	[ ]	[ ]
24.	[ ]	[ ]	[ ]	[ ]	[ ]	49	[ ]	[ ]	[ ]	[ ]	[ ]
25.	[ ]	[ ]	[ ]	[ ]	[ ]	50.	[ ]	[ ]	[ ]	[ ]	[ ]

PEDIATRICS AND PERINATOLOGY ANALYSES

Note: The references listed after each analysis are numbered and keyed to the reference list located at the end of this section. The first number indicates the text. The second number indicates the page where information about the question can be found. For example, (1:219,384) means that reference number 1 is to be used and that on pages 219 and 384 information about the question will be found. Frequently, it will be necessary to read beyond the page number indicated to obtain complete information. Therefore, reference to the question will be found either on the page indicated or on subsequent pages.

1. C. When the red flag is horizontal and the oxygen liter flow is set at 8 liters/min, the approximate oxygen concentration in the incubator will be 36% to 40%. Note Tables 18A and 18B.

   TABLE 18A Horizontal Flag

Oxygen Flowrate	Oxygen Concentration
4 lpm	28% to 31%
6 lpm	32% to 36%
8 lpm	36% to 40%

   TABLE 18B Vertical Flag

Oxygen Flowrate	Oxygen Concentration
8 lpm	70% to 75%
10 lpm	75% to 80%
12 lpm	80% to 85%

   (5:103), (6:701), (36:128–129), (37:552), (42:83–84)

2. A. When continuous positive airway pressure (CPAP) is applied to an infant with normally compliant lungs (0.2 liter/cm H_2O), the positive pressure is transmitted throughout the thorax. Consequently, such complications as (1) decreased venous return, (2) reduced cardiac output, (3) air leaks, and (4) air trapping may occur. When CPAP is applied to lungs of decreased compliance, less pressure is transmitted throughout the thorax.

   Therapeutically, CPAP is generally intended to increase the FRC, improve ventilation-perfusion ($\dot{V}_A/\dot{Q}_C$) ratios, and reduce right-to-left shunting produced by atelectasis or low $\dot{V}_A/\dot{Q}_C$ units.

   (3:435–438,439), (4:500), (6:557,850), (36:56,131)

3. D. Mist tents are used therapeutically for a variety of clinical conditions. These include cystic fibrosis, pneumonia, bronchitis, etc. The device provides an enclosed environment of oxygen, high humidity, and aerosol particles. The temperature of

the tents is somewhat higher than the ambient temperature. Therefore, to remove the patient's body heat, the devices are cooled either with refrigeration coils or ice. Aerosols can be provided to the enclosure by either an ultrasonic nebulizer or a pneumatic nebulizer. The maximum oxygen concentration that can be achieved with this unit ranges between 40% to 60%.
(5:97–102), (36:142–143), (37:552)

4. A. Mean airway pressure ($\overline{P}_{aw}$) is the average pressure at the airway opening during a ventilatory cycle. One ventilatory cycle is the sum of the inspiratory time and the expiratory time (I_T + E_T = length of ventilatory cycle). Ventilator changes that cause the $\overline{P}_{aw}$ to increase without reducing the cardiac output usually improve oxygenation. The following factors influence the mean airway pressure (1) positive end-expiratory pressure (PEEP), (2) peak inspiratory pressure (PIP), (3) the shape of the airway pressure waveform, and (4) the inspiratory time (I_T).
(36:161–162)

5. D. Oxygen hoods are clear, plastic enclosures that are placed over an infant's or neonate's head. Heated, humidified oxygen is delivered to the patient via this device. It is imperative that the delivered gas be appropriately warmed to maintain the infant's or neonate's neutral thermal environment. If the delivered gas is too cool, it will cause the infant's oxygen consumption to increase. Cooling can lead to decreased peripheral circulation, a mixed (metabolic and respiratory) acidosis, pulmonary vasoconstriction, hypoxemia, hypoxia, and apnea. Therefore, frequent temperature monitoring is necessary.
(5:102–104), (6:700,701), (35:94–106), (36:130), (37:551)

6. D. Intermittent positive pressure breathing (IPPB) may be useful in treating bronchospasm, impaired ventilatory mechanics, and postoperative patients. Presurgically, the patient should be instructed on the therapeutic modality that will be administered postoperatively. Doing so will enhance the efficacy of the therapy, and allay patient fear and anxiety when the therapy is acutally administered. An IPPB treatment generally is 10 to 15 minutes in duration. The pressure settings ordinarily range between 10 cm H_2O to 20 cm H_2O. The optimum breathing pattern includes having the patient breathe slowly and deeply to improve the distribution of the inhaled gas.
(4:406–411), (6:527–554), (36:143–144)

7. E. The Bio-Med MVP-10 is fluidically controlled. The Bear Cub 2001, the Sechrist IV-100, the Sechrist IV-100 B, and the Healthdyne 105 are electronically controlled. Even though the Sechrist ventilators incorporate fluidic components, the controls are operated electronically. The only mode available without the electronics is CPAP.
(5:558,563,572,575), (36:177,179–180)

8. A. The following relationship generally occurs among the three methods of obtaining infant body temperatures. The rectal temperature is about 1°F greater than the oral temperature. The axillary temperature is approximately 1°F lower than the oral temperature. Therefore, the axillary temperature is about 2°F less than the rectal temperature.

For example, the three sites might indicate the following temperatures on the same infant:

> Rectal: 97°F
> Oral: 96°F
> Axillary: 95°F

Body temperatures of infants are measured by either the rectal or axillary method. (36:37)

9. E. The relationship betwen the dissolved arterial oxygen tension (Pa_{O_2}) and the transcutaneous partial pressure of oxygen (TcP_{O_2}) is high when the Pa_{O_2} ranges between 30 mm Hg and 100 mm Hg. However, the relationship diminishes in hypoperfused states during which time the heat output of the electrode must be increased. There are limits as to how high the temperature can be advanced to promote a high TcP_{O_2} in the face of hypoperfusion because of the danger of skin burns. Theoretically, increasing the electrode temperature can increase the TcP_{O_2}, but the increase is limited by practical concerns.

Some evidence has indicated that when the TcP_{O_2} falls below the mixed venous partial pressure of oxygen ($P\overline{v}_{O_2}$), the infant's cardiac output is about 30% of normal. It has been observed that cardiac arrest can occur within 30 to 75 minutes after the time when the $P\overline{v}_{O_2}$ exceeded the TcP_{O_2}. When a right-to-left shunt exists across a patent ductus arteriosus, the transcutaneous electrode should be placed on the right upper portion of the chest to reflect preductal blood.

(9:143–144), (17:138), (36:137–139), (Respiratory Therapy, "Practical, Noninvasive Monitoring of Oxygenation," Vol. 16, No. 1, Jan/Feb 1986)

10. B. The respiratory care practitioner should not squeeze the puncture site when performing a heel stick because the blood sample will likely become contaminated with venous blood from the area. As a result, the P_{O_2} will tend to be lower than actual, whereas the P_{CO_2} will be higher than actual.

(34:323), (42:226–227)

11. A. The most common complication associated with rigid bronchoscopy is subglottic edema. This condition develops anywhere from a few minutes to hours after the procedure. Aerosolized epinephrine, Micronephrin or Vaponefrin are useful in treating this postbronchoscopy complication.

(36:217)

12. B. Letter B in Figure 166 indicates the location of the external jugular vein which is usually the preferred site for CVP catheter insertion because it generally is the most accessible.

> A = right subclavian vein
> B = external jugular vein
> C = left subclavian vein
> D = basilic vein
> E = femoral vein

These other sites are also locations where a CVP catheter may be inserted. (6:943), (9:146–147)

13. B. It is recommended that carbon dioxide gas be used to partially (about one-half of the recommended volume) inflate the balloon of a Swan-Ganz catheter, as the catheter enters the superior vena cava. This practice is suggested for neonates because of the increased risk of right-to-left shunts. If the balloon bursts, the potential for an air embolism lessens.

(9:153)

14. E. The Penlon infant resuscitator (Figure 167) uses a cupped-disk valve at the bag outlet (patient valve). Manual compression of the bag causes the cupped disk to open the bag outlet and close the exhalation port. A small opening in the cupped-disk valve acts as a pressure relief valve, preventing excessive pressure from building up on inspiration. During exhalation the negative (subatmospheric) pressure inside the resuscitator causes the cupped-disk valve to close the bag outlet and open the exhalation port.

The presence of an oxygen inlet and a reservoir provides the means for administering up to 100% oxygen. Ordinarily, the resuscitator does not require flowrates greater than 8 liters/min.

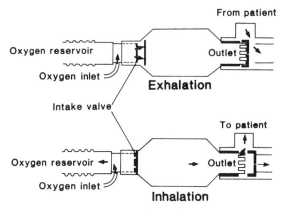

FIGURE 167

(5:185–186)

15. A. The Bear Cub BP 2001 is provided with a heated blow-by humidifier by the manufacturer.

(5:562)

16. A. An umbilical artery catheter (UAC) waveform has the same characteristics as that of a peripheral artery, including a prominent dicrotic notch which is located higher on the monitor because of its proximity to the heart. Umbilical artery catheters may spontaneously dislodge and migrate. Therefore, they require frequent monitoring. Neonates who have a patent ductus arteriosus (PDA) may display a low Sa_{O_2} because right-to-left shunting may exist across the PDA.

(9:159–161)

17. E. A reasonable guideline to use when selecting an oral endotracheal tube for an infant about to be mechanically ventilated is to insert a tube that will allow for a rel-

atively small leak around the tube at an inflation pressure of 25 cm H₂O. Based on this guideline, it is suggested that if no leak occurs at this pressure the tube be removed and replaced by one somewhat smaller.

(36:211)

18. C. Continuous positive airway pressure (CPAP) is defined as the application of positive end-expiratory pressure (PEEP) to a spontaneously breathing patient during the entire ventilatory cycle (inspiration and exhalation). Although no standards exist dictating the point of CPAP implementation, one guideline suggests its use when an F_{IO_2} greater than 0.70 is required to maintain a Pa_{O_2} greater than 50 mm Hg to 60 mm Hg in spontaneously breathing patients who have no carbon dioxide retention. CPAP is frequently used for neonates who have infant respiratory distress syndrome. It sometimes improves the oxygenation status of neonates having persistent fetal circulation. CPAP is also commonly used to help wean infants from mechanical ventilation.

(6:568,718–723), (36:56–58,66), (37:542–544), (42:172–177)

19. D. Blood will flow across a patent ductus arteriosus (PDA) from right to left when the pulmonary vascular resistance is high. In clinical conditions where this exists, e.g., RDS, blood flows from the pulmonary artery to the aorta. When normal vascular pressures exist, i.e., systemic vascular resistance greater than pulmonary vascular resistance, blood will flow from left to right, or from the aorta, across the PDA, to the pulmonary artery. Right-to-left shunting is associated with hypoxemia, whereas left-to-right shunting is *not*. Figure 167A depicts a patent ductus arteriosus.

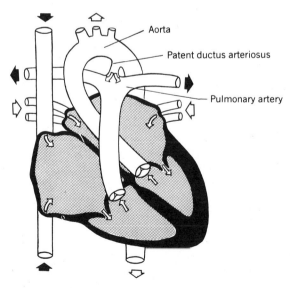

FIGURE 167A

(4:337,339–340), (6:741), (36:21–22,111,117)

20. E. The purpose of the oxygen challenge test is to determine if an infant has a pulmonary disease or a cardiac disease. An F_{IO_2} of 1.0 is administered to determine the extent the Pa_{O_2} rises. If the infant has an anatomic shunt from a cardiac anomaly, the Pa_{O_2} may only slightly increase. If the Pa_{O_2} increases, the infant likely has a pulmonary disease. A severe pulmonary disease may produce little improvement in the Pa_{O_2}. In such cases further clinical evaluation is necessary.
(6:741–742), (36:43–44)

21. E. The Sechrist IV-100 and IV-100B, the Healthdyne 105, the Bourns BP 200, and the Bear Cub BP 2001 possess the capability of having the inspiratory time directly set.
(5:553,558,563,575), (36:156,176,177,179–180)

22. B. When oxygen is delivered it should be humidified and warmed. Unheated gas mixtures delivered to infants increase their oxygen consumption ($\dot{V}_{O_2}$). Gas that is too warm can cause hyperthermia and apnea. The ideal temperature to which the air-oxygen mixture should be heated is to the infant's neutral thermal temperature.
(6:700,701), (36:130)

23. E. For children who have allergic asthma and take aerosolized cromolyn sodium treatments, an aerosolized bronchodilator before the cromolyn treatment may be useful to enhance the penetration and deposition of the cromolyn.
(6:796)

24. A. Because of the anatomic arrangement of the tracheobronchial tree at the bifurcation of the trachea into the left and right mainstem bronchi, the peanut will tend to follow the path of least resistance and enter the right mainstem bronchus. The right mainstem bronchus branches 40° to 60° of the midline, whereas the left mainstem bronchus comes off at a more acute angle, i.e., 20° to 30° of the midline. Because the child was positioned in an upright manner, chances are the peanut would make its way into the right lower lobe. At this point, there is probably an equal chance for it to enter either the anterior basal, lateral basal, medial basal (cardiac), or the posterior basal segment because each of these segments branches at about 45° to the vertical.
(1:94–96), (4:54,398–399), (6:651)

25. A. Epiglottitis, usually caused by the bacterium *Hemophilus influenzae* type B, is a ventilatory emergency. The clinical presentation of this disease is quite dramatic. The child is usually in respiratory distress and displays retractions varying in degree. The child may be hoarse or aphonic and may have inspiratory stridor. As the airway obstruction worsens, the patient sits up and leans forward with his chin jutting outward to facilitate ventilations. Drooling is usually present.
The definitive diagnosis is made when direct visualization of the epiglottis reveals that it is swollen and inflamed (Figure 168).
(4:354–355), (6:776), (8:274), (36:84–85), (37:202–207,545)

26. C. Oral or nasal tracheal intubation is generally performed. If an airway cannot be established via either of these routes, a tracheotomy is done. Once an airway is

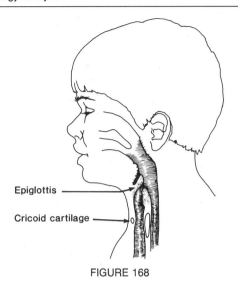

Epiglottis

Cricoid cartilage

FIGURE 168

established, humidified oxygen is required. These patients require the airway for less than 5 days.

(4:354–355), (6:776), (8:274), (36:84–85), (37:202–207,545)

27. C. Maintaining an adequate supply of water in the humidification reservoir is important for a number of reasons. For example, a decreased water level will (1) impair the humidification process, (2) increase the compliance of the ventilator delivery tubing, and (3) decrease the delivered tidal volume to the infant.

(36:183), (42:130)

28. B. Subglottic edema is the most common cause of reintubation of infants who have been extubated. The cricoid cartilage, which is the only laryngeal cartilage that entirely circumscribes the larynx, resides in the most narrow portion of the larynx in infants. It is this area that creates the "seal" for the noncuffed pediatric endotracheal tubes.

(3:268), (36:211), (37:191)

29. E. For the treatment of infant respiratory distress syndrome (IRDS), initially the clinician attempts to oxygenate. If the infant's Pa_{O_2} cannot be maintained at greater than 50 mm Hg on an F_{IO_2} of 0.8, the infant should be intubated and placed on CPAP. Low pressures (approximately 5 cm H_2O) are used along with a high F_{IO_2}. If the Pa_{O_2} still remains below 50 mm Hg, the CPAP should be increased gradually up to 10 cm H_2O. If at a CPAP of 10 cm H_2O the oxygenation is not improved, mechanical ventilation with IMV is instituted.

Note: The reader should keep in mind that clinical philosophies, as well as early indications, such as x-ray findings, gestational age, etc., result in deviations from these guidelines.

(36:48–49,56–58), (37:228), (42:118)

30. E. Laryngotracheobronchitis, or croup (Figure 169), is commonly caused by the parainfluenza virus, the respiratory syncytial virus (RSV), and the adenovirus. The clinical manifestations include a low-grade fever and nonproductive cough both of which precede the onset of croup by a few days. As the subglottic edema develops and worsens, respiratory distress becomes apparent. Unlike epiglottitis, a lateral x-ray view of the neck reveals a normal epiglottis; however, edema can be seen below the glottis.

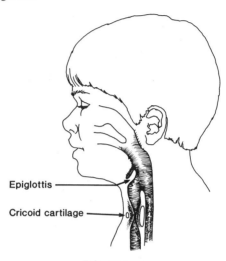

Epiglottis

Cricoid cartilage

FIGURE 169

(4:354), (6:776–777), (36:86–88), (37:197)

31. E. The subglottic edema frequently responds well to a cool air mist or an air-oxygen mixture. Because of this favorable response, many children never become admitted to the hospital. Not uncommonly, sitting with the child in a bathroom with a hot shower running to create steam relieves the symptoms. Once in the hospital, the method of treatment generally includes the use of unheated aerosols and racemic epinephrine (an alpha-adrenergic agonist) to reduce the subglottic edema. (4:354), (6:776–777), (36:86–88), (37:197)

32. C. Ventilatory rates greater than or equal to 60 breaths/min (1 Hertz = 1 cycle/sec = 60 cycles/min) are referred to as high-frequency ventilation. High-frequency ventilation is usually divided into three categories. High-frequency oscillation (HFO) actively transports gas to the lungs, cycling anywhere from 5 Hertz to 30 Hertz (300 cycles/min to 1,800 cycles/min). High-frequency jet ventilation (HFJV) operates between 100 cycles/min and 150 cycles/min. High-frequency jet ventilation creates in the lungs a jet mixing effect which theoretically accounts for gas delivery to the alveoli. High-frequency positive pressure ventilation (HFPPV) involves the use of a conventional positive pressure ventilator. However, the amount of internal compressible volume is negligible. This variety of high-frequency ventilation can deliver frequencies between 60 cycles/min and 100 cycles/min.

The gas movement mechanism hypothesized to account for most of the gas delivery to the peripheral airways during high-frequency ventilation is termed *augmented diffusion*. It is postulated that rapidly delivered tidal volume boluses delivered by these ventilators produce eddy currents and vortices (turbulent flow) that progressively advance gas molecules to the alveoli where molecular diffusion occurs. The high velocity of the gas molecules purportedly enhances the diffusion of the gas molecules by a factor of several thousand compared with that associated with molecular diffusion. Figure 170 presents a schematic of the proposed gas movement mechanisms occurring during high-frequency ventilation. During high-frequency ventilation augmented diffusion is considered to account for most of the gas transport from generation 0 (trachea) through generation 15 (bronchioles), and molecular diffusion is responsible for most of the gas movement from generation 16 (terminal bronchioles) through generation 23 (alveoli).

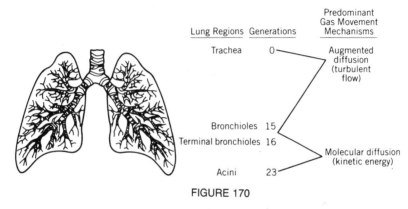

FIGURE 170

Figure 171 illustrates the proposed gas movement mechanisms associated with conventional ventilation. During conventional ventilation generations 0 through 15 (trachea to bronchioles) experience bulk flow or convective gas movement; generations 16 through 23 (terminal bronchioles to alveoli) are characterized by molecular diffusion.

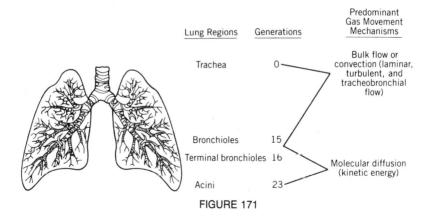

FIGURE 171

(1:525–527), (2:149–152), (3:442–448), (36:63–64,186–190)

33. E. Intermittent positive pressure breathing (IPPB) ordinarily is not prescribed for cystic fibrosis patients because of the increased risk of producing a pneumothorax. Cystic fibrosis patients often have blebs and bullae which are susceptible to rupture in the presence of high mean intrathoracic pressures.

Aerosol therapy is indicated in cystic fibrosis because it enhances the liquefaction of the thick tracheobronchial secretions, and is a convenient mode of medication delivery. Chest physiotherapy (postural drainage, percussion, and vibration) further assists in the regimen of treatment of this disease.

Nonhospitalized cystic fibrosis patients generally do not require oxygen at home. Despite the presence of some degree of hypoxemia, these patients can adequately ventilate and gas exchange while breathing room air. During a hospitalization the administration of oxygen is not uncommon.

(3:137,153,504), (4:352–353), (6:771–775), (36:100–102)

34. B. Meconium is the fluid normally located in the intestinal tract of a fetus. Some form of intrauterine stress, e.g., fetal asphyxia, is thought to be responsible for the presence of meconium in the amniotic fluid. Infants less than 34 weeks' gestation are rarely meconium stained at birth. This condition is usually confined to term infants.

An infant presenting meconium staining at birth should receive thorough naso- and oropharyngeal suctioning immediately when its head appears at the perineum. After the meconium-stained infant is delivered, it is highly desirable to visualize the cords with a laryngoscope before the infant draws its first breath. If any meconium is noted, an endotracheal tube should be immediately inserted and suction applied through the endotracheal tube to clear any meconium that may have entered the trachea. All of this should be accomplished quickly and before the infant draws its first breath.

Meconium aspiration causes maldistribution of the infant's first ventilations of extrauterine life. The maldistribution of ventilation impairs gas exchange, causes respiratory distress (dependent primarily on the amount of meconium aspirated), and decreases lung compliance. In a situation where the amount of meconium aspirated produces mild respiratory distress, the infant can be placed in an oxygen-enriched environment, e.g., an oxyhood. Additionally, the infant will require chest physiotherapy, further suctioning, and observation.

Intubation followed by the institution of CPAP of mechanical ventilation is indicated when the infant is in severe respiratory distress.

(4:337), (6:733–734), (36:33,44,65–67), (37:233–235)

35. C. The major problem or disadvantage common to the use of an oxygen hood is the disruption of the oxygen-enriched environment of the enclosure for feeding or any other patient care about the head and/or face.

(5:102–104), (6:701), (36:130), (37:551–552)

36. C. STEP 1: Determine the number of time segments comprising a complete ventilatory cycle.

$$I + E = \text{time segments in a ventilatory cycle}$$
$$1 + 3 = 4$$

STEP 2: Obtain the minute ventilation ($\dot{V}_E$) from the following relationship. $(V_T)(f) = \dot{V}_E$

1. 36 cc = 0.036 liter
2. 0.036 liter $\times$ 30 breaths/min = 1.08 liters/min

STEP 3: Calculate the inspiratory flowrate according to the following expression.

$$\text{inspiratory flowrate} = \dot{V}_E \left(\begin{array}{c} \text{time segments in} \\ \text{a ventilatory} \\ \text{cycle} \end{array} \right)$$

$$= (1.08 \text{ liters/min})(4)$$
$$= 3.24 \text{ liters/min}$$

(36:159–162), (42:130–131,137)

37. D. STEP 1: Multiply the compliance factor (1.0 cc/cm H_2O) by the peak inspiratory pressure (20 cm H_2O).

$$\text{(compliance factor)(PIP)} = \text{compressible volume}$$
$$(1.0 \text{ cc/}\cancel{\text{cm } H_2O})(20 \text{ } \cancel{\text{cm } H_2O}) = 20 \text{ cc}$$

STEP 2: Determine the patient's V_T.

$$\text{(delivered volume)} - \text{(compressible volume)} = V_T$$
$$36 \text{ cc} - 20 \text{ cc} = 16 \text{ cc}$$

(42:137–138), (45:58–59)

38. A. By decreasing the inspiratory flowrate, less volume/time ($\dot{V}$) would enter the lungs. Consequently, the tidal volume would be lessened and the peak inspiratory pressure (PIP) would, likewise, be reduced. Lowering the inspiratory flowrate on time-cycled infant ventilators will not affect the I/E ratio.
(42:43–44, 116)

39. C. Bronchopulmonary dysplasia (BPD) has no precise etiology. It is associated with the application of high oxygen concentrations and prolonged mechanical ventilation. The destructive activity of oxygen radicals on lung tissues is implicated along with the high mean airway pressures affecting airway linings. BPD usually develops in preterm, low birth weight infants who are treated for infant respiratory distress syndrome (IRDS).
(1:456), (2:247–254), (3:456), (4:336–337), (6:397–398,725–727), (36:54–55, 138), (42:188–189) *

40. D. Strict isolation is suggested for burn patients who have wound infections caused by *Staphylococcus aureus*. Burn patients experiencing gram-negative nosocomial bacterial wound infections generally require wound and skin precautions.
(20:31)

41. E. The minute ventilation ($\dot{V}_E$) is a function of the tidal volume (V_T) and the ventilatory rate (f).

$$\dot{V}_E = V_T \times f$$

Therefore, the infant's $\dot{V}T$ while in the control mode can be obtained as follows:

$$VT = \frac{\dot{V}E}{f}$$

$$= \frac{600 \text{ cc/min}}{40 \text{ breaths/min}}$$

$$= 15 \text{ cc}$$

Consequently, when the ventilator rate was changed to 30 breaths/min in the pressure control mode, the infant's $\dot{V}E$ became approximately:

$$(15 \text{ cc/breath})(30 \text{ breaths/min}) = 450 \text{ cc/min}$$

(1:118–119), (5:536,537,541), (8:50–51), (36:155)

42. A. The Bourns Bear Cub (BP 2001) is classified as a pneumatically powered, electronically controlled, continuous flow, time-cycled, pressure-limited ventilator. (5:558–563), (36:177–178)

43. A. The Cole tube unlike the Murphy tube is tapered toward the tip. It has a larger proximal diameter and a smaller distal diameter. The narrowed tip passes into the larynx, while the wider portion of the tube rests at the site of the cricoid cartilage (the larynx's narrowest aspect). The advantages of the Cole tube include (1) reduced resistance through the lumen as compared with a tube with the same diameter as the Cole's distal end, and (2) reduced risk of inadvertent entry into right mainstem bronchus. The wider, proximal end increases the mechanical dead space. Because this tube rests in the larynx, prolonged intubation is sometimes associated with laryngeal dilatation.

Figure 172 illustrates features of the Cole and Murphy pediatric endotracheal tubes.

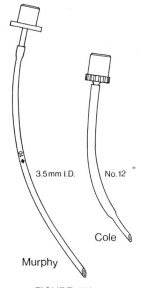

3.5 mm I.D.   No. 12

Cole

Murphy

FIGURE 172

(5:175), (42:68–69)

44. D. The heel should be warmed in a water bath or wrapped in a warm towel for about 3 minutes at an approximate temperature range of 38°C to 40°C. After the site is aseptically prepared, the respiratory care practitioner should use a 3-mm lancet to puncture either the medial or lateral aspect of the plantar surface. Ideally, the puncture made with the lancet should not exceed a depth of 2.4 mm. However, the "cleanest" cut and best bleeding are generally accomplished by a swift jab of the lancet into the puncture site. Therefore, the suggested depth may be exceeded. The point of the matter is that the puncture should *not* be inordinately deep.
(34:323), (42:226)

45. B. When oral endotracheal intubation is performed on a neonate, a Miller (straight) blade is inserted into the mouth midline, and directed forward and leftward to move the tongue away from the right side (Figure 173). The tip of the laryngo-scope (Miller) blade is placed in the vallecula to allow for visualization of the vo-cal cords and glottis. At this point, the endotracheal tube is inserted from the right side of the mouth and advanced through the glottis (Figure 174, page 600).

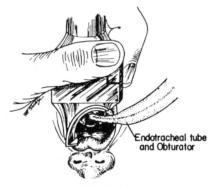

Endotracheal tube and Obturator

FIGURE 173

(35:31–34), (36:210–211), (42:68–71), (44:508–509)

46. D. Carbon monoxide has an affinity for hemoglobin 210 times greater than that of oxygen. Carbon monoxide poisoning does not influence the Pa_{O_2}; consequently, the peripheral chemoreceptors are not stimulated to send hyperventilatory signals to the medulla oblongata. However, the Sa_{O_2} is affected by CO poisoning.
The situation here presents a child who has not had severe CO poisoning, as re-vealed by the 12.0% COHb level. The appropriate treatment for this patient is to maintain the patent airway and administer 100% oxygen via a Briggs adapter. The 100% oxygen is to be given until the COHb level drops to 10% or less. At that time the $F_{I_{O_2}}$ can be reduced. Severe cases of CO poisoning often require mechan-ical ventilation.
(37:177–178)

47. B. A minimum liter flow of 5 liters/min of oxygen is necessary to prevent carbon dioxide accumulation inside an oxygen hood. Other considerations that are neces-sary for this modality of oxygen administration include (1) temperature, (2) hu-midification, and (3) oxygen concentration.
(6:700–701), (36:130–131), (35:179), (37:551–552), (42:79)

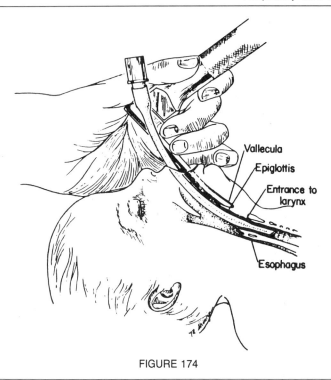

Vallecula

Epiglottis

Entrance to larynx

Esophagus

FIGURE 174

48. D. Use the following formula to determine the appropriate size endotracheal tube for a pediatric patient.

$$\text{tube size (I.D.)} = \left(\frac{\text{age in years}}{4}\right) + 4.5$$

$$= \left(\frac{5}{4}\right) + 4.5$$

$$= 1.25 + 4.5$$

$$= 5.65 \text{ mm (I.D.)}$$

The formula is *not* applicable to patients less than 2 years old.
(37:536)

49. B. The suction pressure that is ordinarily set for routine infant tracheobronchial suctioning ranges between −50 mm Hg to −90 mm Hg. The accepted range for children is −90 mm Hg to −115 mm Hg.
(37:567)

50. A. The following steps are *recommended* for the purpose of weaning an infant from CPAP.

STEP 1: Each time the infant's Pa_{O_2} exceeds 70 mm Hg, the $F_{I_{O_2}}$ should be decreased from 0.03 to 0.05 (3% to 5%).

STEP 2: When an F_{IO_2} of 0.40 is attained, the CPAP pressure should be reduced 2 cm H_2O every 2 to 4 hours, until a CPAP of 2 to 3 cm H_2O is achieved.

STEP 3: At that point, the patient should be placed in an oxygen hood and the F_{IO_2} increased to 0.45 to 0.50.

Low birth weight patients may require a CPAP level of 4 cm H_2O, until the F_{IO_2} is brought to room air level.

(35:210), (37:177)

REFERENCES

1. Spearman, C., and Sheldon, R., *Egan's Fundamentals of Respiratory Therapy*, 4th ed., C.V. Mosby, St. Louis, 1982.
2. Wojciechowski, W., *Respiratory Care Sciences: An Integrated Approach*, John Wiley & Sons, New York, 1985.
3. Shapiro, B., Harrison, R., Kacmarek, R., and Cane, R., *Clinical Application of Respiratory Care*, 3rd ed., Year Book Medical Publishers, Chicago, 1985.
4. Kacmarek, R., Mack, C., and Dimas, S., *The Essentials of Respiratory Therapy*, 2nd ed., Year Book Medical Publishers, Chicago, 1985.
5. McPherson, S., *Respiratory Therapy Equipment*, 3rd ed., C.V. Mosby, St. Louis, 1985.
6. Burton, G., and Hodgkin, J., *Respiratory Care: A Guide to Clinical Practice*, 2nd ed., J.B. Lippincott, Philadelphia, 1985.
7. Frownfelter, D., *Chest Physical Therapy and Cardiopulmonary Rehabilitation, An Interdisciplinary Approach*, Year Book Medical Publishers, Chicago, 1978.
8. Cherniack, R., and Cherniack, L., *Respiration in Health and Disease*, 3rd ed., W. B. Saunders, Philadelphia, 1983.
9. Daily, E., and Schroeder, G., *Techniques in Bedside Hemodynamic Monitoring*, 3rd ed., C.V. Mosby, St. Louis, 1985.
10. Des Jardins, R., *Clinical Manifestations of Respiratory Disease*, Year Book Medical Publishers, Chicago, 1984.
11. Mitchell, R., *Synopsis of Clinical Pulmonary Disease*, 3rd ed., C.V. Mosby, St. Louis, 1982.
12. Comroe, J., *Physiology of Respiration*, 3rd ed., Year Book Medical Publishers, Chicago, 1974.
13. West, J., *Pulmonary Pathophysiology—The Essentials*, 2nd ed., Williams & Wilkins, Baltimore, 1982.
14. West, J., *Respiratory Physiology—The Essentials*, 3rd ed., Williams & Wilkins, Baltimore, 1985.
15. Martz, K., et al., *Management of the Patient-Ventilator System: A Team Approach*, 2nd ed., C.V. Mosby, St. Louis, 1984.
16. Shoup, C., and McHenry, R., *Laboratory Exercises in Respiratory Therapy*, 2nd ed., C.V. Mosby, St. Louis, 1983.
17. Ruppel, G., *Manual of Pulmonary Function Testing*, 3rd ed., C.V. Mosby, St. Louis, 1982.
18. Appelbaum, E., and Brucc, D., *Tracheal Intubation*, W.B. Saunders, Philadelphia, 1976.
19. Rau, J., *Respiratory Therapy Pharmacology*, 2nd ed., Year Book Medical Publishers, Chicago, 1984.
20. United States Department of Health, Education, and Welfare, Public Health Service, *Isolation Techniques for Use in Hospitals*, 2nd ed., Washington, D.C., 1975.
21. Brooks, S., *Integrated Basic Science*, 4th ed., C.V. Mosby, St. Louis, 1979.
22. Comroe, J., *The Lung*, Year Book Medical Publishers, Chicago, 1962.

23. Shibel, E., and Moser, K., *Respiratory Emergencies,* 2nd ed., C.V. Mosby, St. Louis, 1982.

24. Tisi, G., *Pulmonary Physiology in Clinical Medicine,* 2nd ed., Williams & Wilkins, Baltimore, 1985.

25. Cherniack, R., *Pulmonary Function Testing,* W.B. Saunders, Philadelphia, 1977.

26. Altose, M., *The Physiological Basis of Pulmonary Function Testing,* Clinical Symposia-CIBA, Vol. 31, No. 2, Summit, New Jersey, 1979.

27. Shapiro, B., Harrison, R., and Walton, J., *Clinical Application of Arterial Blood Gases,* 3rd ed., Year Book Medical Publishers, Chicago, 1982.

28. West, J., *Ventilation/Blood Flow and Gas Exchange,* 3rd ed., Blackwell Scientific Publications, 1979.

29. Slonim, N., and Hamilton, K., *Respiratory Physiology,* 4th ed., C.V. Mosby, St. Louis, 1981.

30. Rarey, K., and Youtsey, J., *Respiratory Patient Care,* Prentice-Hall, Englewood Cliffs, 1981.

31. Berne, R., and Levy, M., *Physiology,* C.V. Mosby, St. Louis, 1983.

32. Levitzky, M., *Pulmonary Physiology,* 2nd ed., McGraw-Hill, New York, 1986.

33. Wilson, P., Bell, C., and Norton, A., *Rehabilitation of the Heart and Lungs,* SensorMedics, 1980.

34. Clausen, J., and Zarins, L., *Pulmonary Function Testing Guidelines and Controversies,* Academic Press, New York, 1982.

35. Klaus, M., and Fanaroff, A., *Care of the High-Risk Neonate,* 2nd ed., W.B. Saunders, Philadelphia, 1979.

36. Lough, M., et al., *Pediatric Respiratory Therapy,* 3rd ed., Year Book Medical Publishers, Chicago, 1985.

37. Levin, D., et al., *A Practical Guide to Pediatric Intensive Care,* 2nd ed., C.V. Mosby, St. Louis, 1984.

38. O'Ryan, J., and Burns, D., *Pulmonary Rehabilitation from Hospital to Home,* Year Book Medical Publishers, Chicago, 1984.

39. Bell, C., et al., *Home Care and Rehabilitation in Respiratory Medicine,* J.B. Lippincott, Philadelphia, 1984.

40. Wilkins, R., et al., *Clinical Assessment in Respiratory Care,* C.V. Mosby, St. Louis, 1985.

41. Jones, N., and Campbell, E., *Clinical Exercise Testing,* 2nd ed., W.B. Saunders, Philadelphia, 1982.

42. Goldsmith, J., and Karotkin, E., *Assisted Ventilation of the Neonate,* W.B. Saunders, Philadelphia, 1981.

43. Blowers, M., and Sims, R., *How to Read an ECG,* 3rd ed., Medical Economics, New Jersey, 1983.

44. Eubanks, D., and Bone, R., *Comprehensive Respiratory Care,* C.V. Mosby, St. Louis, 1985.

45. Rattenborg, C., *Clinical Use of Mechanical Ventilation,* Year Book Medical Publishers, Chicago, 1981.

46. Witkowski, A.S., *Pulmonary Assessment: A Clinical Guide,* J.B. Lippincott, Philadelphia, 1985.

47. Op't Holt, T.B., *Assessment Based Respiratory Care,* John Wiley & Sons, New York, 1986.

CARDIOPULMONARY REHABILITATION AND HOME CARE ASSESSMENT

PURPOSE: The purpose of this 50-item section is to help you evaluate your knowledge and understanding of the content area of cardiopulmonary rehabilitation and home respiratory care. Included in this assessment are patient evaluation, components of a cardiopulmonary rehabilitation program, interviewing techniques, exercise testing, home oxygen therapy, and home mechanical ventilation.

DIRECTIONS: Each of the questions or incomplete statements is followed by five suggested answers. Select the one which is the best in each case and then blacken the corresponding space on the answer sheet.

1. Which of the following statements accurately describe an oxygen concentrator?

    I. The oxygen delivered by concentrators operating according to the molecular sieve principle do *not* require humidification because the moisture in the air is also concentrated and delivered with the oxygen.

    II. Most oxygen concentrators can deliver oxygen at flowrates ranging from 1 liter/min to 15 liters/min.

    III. Most oxygen concentrators are capable of an oxygen percentage ranging from 85% to 90+%.

    IV. With oxygen concentrators, the flowrate on the flowmeter is inversely proportional to the oxygen percentage delivered.

    A. II, IV only   D. III, IV only

    B. I, III only   E. I, III, IV only

    C. II, III only

2. While you are conducting an interview with a patient, she states that she has smoked three packs of cigarettes a day for 15 years. How many pack-years would you record in the patient's history?

    A. 3 pack-years   D. 30 pack-years

    B. 5 pack-years   E. 45 pack-years

    C. 15 pack-years

3. Which of the following pulmonary abnormalities is likely to have the characteristics listed below?

    1. increased vocal and tactile fremitus

    2. bronchial breath sounds

    3. dull percussion note over the affected area

    A. chronic airways obstruction   D. fibrosis

    B. consolidation   E. pneumothorax

    C. pleural effusion

4. When should either sterile water or sterile normal saline prepared in the home for therapeutic use be discarded?

    A. 1 day   D. 4 days

    B. 2 days   E. 5 days

    C. 3 days

5. What is the appropriate sequence of care used in a pulmonary rehabilitation program?

    I. assess patient progress

  II. determine goals

  III. outline rehabilitation program components

  IV. patient selection

  V. initial patient evaluation

  VI. long-term follow-up

  A. III, II, V, IV, I, VI   D. V, III, IV, I, II, VI

  B. V, IV, II, III, VI, I   E. II, IV, III, V, I, VI

  C. IV, V, II, III, I, VI

6. Which of the following clinical conditions represent contraindications for exercise testing?

  I. uncontrolled asthma

  II. unstable angina

  III. hypertension

  IV. symptomatic congestive heart failure

  A. I, II, III, IV   D. I, II only

  B. I, III only   E. II, IV only

  C. II, III, IV only

7. Marasmus develops from inadequate _____ and _____ intake.

  A. protein; calorie   D. glucose; carbohydrate

  B. carbohydrate; fat   E. calorie; carbohydrate

  C. fat; calorie

8. How should the exterior surfaces of a mechanical ventilator used in the home be kept clean?

  A. A damp cloth can be used to remove accumulated dust.

  B. Soap and water should be applied.

  C. A vinegar-water solution should be used to clean the exterior.

  D. A 70% ethyl alcohol solution can be used.

  E. A lint-free dust cloth can be applied.

9. An increased or unchanged V_D/V_T ratio with exercise may be indicative of which physiologic alteration(s) or condition(s)?

  I. chronic bronchitis

  II. ventilation/perfusion mismatching

  III. pulmonary emphysema

  IV. such a response is normal with exercise

  A. IV only   D. I, II, III only

  B. I, III only   E. II, III only

  C. II only

10. Which of the following physiologic events would cause the value of the ventilation-perfusion ratio to differ from the respiratory quotient?

    I. hyperventilation
    II. exercise
    III. sleep
    IV. anaerobic metabolism

    A. II, IV only   D. I, II, IV only
    B. I, II only   E. I, II, III, IV
    C. I, II, III only

11. Which of the following clinical conditions cause mediastinal shift?

    I. consolidation
    II. atelectasis
    III. fibrosis
    IV. pleural effusion

    A. II, III, IV only   D. II, IV only
    B. I, III only   E. I, II, III, IV
    C. I, II, III only

12. Which of the following oxygen appliances would be inappropriate to use with an oxygen concentrator?

    I. Venturi mask
    II. aerosol mask
    III. nasal cannula
    IV. partial re-breathing mask

    A. II, IV only   D. II, III, IV only
    B. I, II, IV only   E. I, II only
    C. III, IV only

13. The delivery of oxygen to the lungs is best represented by which equation?

    A. $\dfrac{V_D}{V_T} = \dfrac{Pa_{CO_2} - P\overline{E}_{CO_2}}{Pa_{CO_2}}$

    B. $\dot{V}_{O_2} = \dot{Q}_T(Ca_{O_2} - C\overline{v}_{O_2})$

    C. $\dot{V}_A = \dot{V}_E - \dot{V}_D$

    D. $\dfrac{\dot{Q}_S}{\dot{Q}_T} = \dfrac{Cc_{O_2} - Ca_{O_2}}{Cc_{O_2} - C\overline{v}_{O_2}}$

    E. $P(A\text{-}a)O_2 = P_{A_{O_2}} - Pa_{O_2}$

14. What is the primary objective of oxygen therapy for a chronic obstructive pulmonary disease (COPD) patient?

    A. to maintain the patient's Pa_{O_2} between 55 mm Hg to 60 mm Hg
    B. to eliminate the hypoxic drive

C. to elevate the patient's Pa_{O_2} between 80 mm Hg to 100 mm Hg

D. to normalize the oxygen saturation

E. to alleviate the hypercapnia

15. Which of the following factors comprise the exercise components of an exercise prescription?

   I. intensity
   II. duration
   III. frequency
   IV. mode

   A. I, III only   D. I, III only
   B. II, III, IV only   E. I, II, III, IV
   C. II, IV only

16. What will be the numerical value of the respiratory quotient if carbohydrates are solely metabolized?

   A. 1.0   D. 0.7
   B. 0.9   E. 0.6
   C. 0.8

17. Which of the following protocols are used in a cardiopulmonary rehabilitation program?

   I. Balke
   II. Sigaard-Anderson
   III. Naughton
   IV. Astrup
   V. Bruce

   A. II, III, V only   D. II, IV only
   B. I, III only   E. II, III only
   C. I, III, V only

18. Which of the following metabolic changes are often associated with chronic obstructive pulmonary disease?

   I. lean body mass depletion
   II. anorexia
   III. protein deficiency
   IV. impaired vitamin absorption

   A. I, II, III, IV   D. I, III only
   B. I, III, IV only   E. II, III only
   C. II, IV only

19. Which of the following clinical conditions are associated with only a slight increase in the steady-state diffusing capacity during exercise testing?

    I. diffusion defect

    II. pulmonary emphysema

    III. primary pulmonary hypertension

    IV. chronic bronchitis

A. I, II, III, IV   D. I, III only

B. II, IV only   E. II, III, IV only

C. I, II, IV only

20. If a COPD patient has a body temperature of 39°C, by what percentage has her energy requirements been increased?

A. 12%   D. 44%

B. 24%   E. 50%

C. 30%

21. Which of the following terms are synonyms for oxygen consumption?

    I. oxygen uptake

    II. oxygen pulse

    III. oxygen intake

    IV. oxygen debt

A. I, III only   D. I, IV only

B. I, II, III only   E. III, IV only

C. II, III only

22. Which of the following evaluation procedures or maneuvers are performed via auscultation?

    I. tactile fremitus

    II. whispering pectoriloquy

    III. egophony

    IV. vocal fremitus

A. I, II, III, IV   D. I, IV only

B. II, III only   E. I, II, III only

C. II, III, IV only

23. Which relationship represents the oxygen pulse?

A. $\dot{V}_{O_2}$/heartbeat

B. $\dfrac{Sa_{O_2}}{C.O.}$

C. Pa_{O_2}/Sa_{O_2}

D. $\dfrac{Sa_{O_2}/[Hb]}{heartbeat}$

E. $\dot{V}_{O_2}/Pa_{O_2} \times Sa_{O_2}$

24. When conducting exercise testing associated with pulmonary rehabilitation, how is the dyspnea index (DI) calculated?

A. $\dfrac{\dot{V}_{O_2}}{FVC} \times 100$

D. $\dfrac{V_D/V_T}{FVC} \times 100$

B. $\dfrac{\dot{V}_E}{MVV} \times 100$

E. $\dfrac{V_T \times f}{FEV_1} \times 100$

C. $\dfrac{FVC}{\dot{V}_{O_2}/\dot{V}_{CO_2}} \times 100$

25. Which of the following safety precautions must be taken by the patient when using a liquid oxygen system at home?

   I. The patient must always wear protective clothing when using the liquid oxygen system.

   II. The patient must vent the reservoir unit when it is being filled with liquid oxygen.

   III. When filling the reservoir, the patient must always wear protective glasses and gloves.

   IV. The patient must change the cannula each day if the liquid oxygen is in use more than 15 hours per day.

   A. II, IV only   D. I, III only

   B. II, III, IV only   E. I, II, III, IV

   C. I, II, III only

26. What is the relationship between heart rate and oxygen consumption during exercise testing?

   A. linear   D. hyperbolic

   B. sigmoid   E. curvilinear

   C. parabolic

27. Which of the following clinical conditions cause a mediastinal shift toward the affected side?

   I. consolidation

   II. fibrosis

   III. pleural effusion

   IV. atelectasis

   V. pneumothorax

   A. III, V only   D. I, II only

   B. I, II, IV only   E. I, II, III, IV only

   C. II, IV only

28. Palpation can help determine which of the following physical findings?

   I. the patient's use of accessory muscles

   II. chest wall movement

   III. malformation of the bony thorax and spine

   IV. tracheal deviation

A. II, IV only   D. I, II only

B. I, III, IV only   E. II, III, IV only

C. III, IV only

29. Supplemental oxygen for at least 15 hours per day purportedly delays the onset of which of the following pathophysiologic changes in a COPD patient?

   I. pneumonia

  II. pulmonary hypertension

 III. cor pulmonale

 IV. syncope

A. II, III only   D. II, III, IV only

B. I, IV only   E. I, II, III only

C. III, IV only

30. In a pulmonary rehabilitation program who is generally responsible for evaluating a patient's activities of daily living?

   I. respiratory care practitioners

  II. physical therapists

 III. nutritionists

 IV. occupational therapists

A. II, IV only   D. I, II, IV only

B. I, II only   E. II, III, IV only

C. I, III only

31. Which of the following precautions should be used by patients who experience respiratory difficulty from cold weather?

   I. They should breathe through their mouths to help reduce the airway resistance and work of breathing.

  II. They should cover their mouths with a mask or a scarf.

 III. They should face the wind to supplement the flow of air into their lungs.

 IV. They should walk slower to reduce their energy expenditure and their work of breathing.

A. I, II, IV only   D. II, IV only

B. II, III only   E. I, II, III, IV

C. I, IV only

32. Which of the following statements describes the least exertional method for a COPD patient to lift an object off the floor?

A. The patient should bend over to pick up the object.

B. The patient should kneel on one knee and bend the other, then lift the object.

C. The patient should squat, then lift the object with arms outwardly extended.

D. The patient should bend at the knees keeping the back straight, and lift the object.

    E. The patient should lift the object onto a nearby chair, then lift it from the seat of the chair.

33. What are the anticipated physiologic changes from pursed-lip breathing used by a resting COPD patient?

    I. decreased ventilatory rate
    II. increased $\dot{V}_{O_2}$
    III. increased Pa_{O_2}
    IV. increased V_T

    A. I, II, III, IV   D. I, II, III only
    B. II, III only   E. I, III, IV only
    C. I, IV only

34. Dyspnea is classified as severe if the dyspnea index (DI) exceeds _____ .

    A. 80%   D. 50%
    B. 70%   E. 40%
    C. 60%

36. If a patient needs supplemental oxygen during exercise testing, what is the minimum Sa_{O_2} and Pa_{O_2} that is generally accepted before terminating the procedure?

    A. Sa_{O_2} 85%; Pa_{O_2} 55 torr   D. Sa_{O_2} 60%; Pa_{O_2} 50 torr
    B. Sa_{O_2} 70%; Pa_{O_2} 60 torr   E. Sa_{O_2} 95%; Pa_{O_2} 100 torr
    C. Sa_{O_2} 90%; Pa_{O_2} 80 torr

36. Which of the following types of diet metabolically produces the greatest amount of carbon dioxide, thereby requiring a higher energy expenditure for CO_2 removal via ventilation?

    A. carbohydrates only   D. fats and carbohydrates
    B. fats only   E. fats, carbohydrates, and proteins
    C. proteins only

37. Which of the following methods of oxygen delivery at 3 liters/min is the *least* expensive for continuous use in the home?

    A. piped-in oxygen   D. a compressed gas cylinder
    B. an oxygen concentrator   E. fractional distillation
    C. a liquid oxygen system

38. What is the approximate $\dot{V}_{O_2}$ for a resting healthy adult who has an ideal body weight of 75 kg?

    A. 241 ml/min   D. 274 ml/min
    B. 250 ml/min   E. 289 ml/min
    C. 263 ml/min

39. What is the approximate caloric requirement at rest per day for the person in question 38?

    A. 1,374 kcal/day
    B. 1,800 kcal/day
    C. 1,894 kcal/day
    D. 1,973 kcal/day
    E. 2,081 kcal/day

40. How frequently should a nebulizer be cleaned when used by a home care patient?

    A. daily
    B. every 3 days
    C. weekly
    D. monthly
    E. when it show signs of being dirty

41. How should a patient who suctions herself be instructed to enhance the removal of secretions from the left lung?

    A. The patient should be instructed to lie on her left side and advance the catheter into the tracheobronchial tree.
    B. The patient should be instructed to lie on her right side and advance the catheter into the tracheobronchial tree.
    C. The patient should be instructed to sit up and turn her head to the left while advancing the catheter into the tracheobronchial tree.
    D. The patient should be instructed to sit up and turn her head to the right while advancing the catheter into the tracheobronchial tree.
    E. The patient should be instructed to sit up and face forward while advancing the catheter into the tracheobronchial tree.

42. What is the proper sequence of activities for performing a physical assessment of the chest?

    A. inspection, percussion, palpation, and auscultation
    B. palpation, inspection, percussion, and auscultation
    C. percussion, inspection, palpation, and auscultation
    D. inspection, palpation, percussion, and auscultation
    E. inspection, percussion, auscultation, and palpation

43. Which of the following skeletal characteristics of the thorax are associated with pulmonary emphysema?

    I. increased convexity (posteriorly) of the thoracic spine
    II. increased anteroposterior diameter
    III. clavicular lift during inspiration
    IV. increased transverse diameter

    A. I, II, III, IV
    B. I, III only
    C. II, IV only
    D. II, III, IV only
    E. I, II, IV only

44. Which value(s) and/or expression(s) represent(s) one MET.

I. 3.5 ml O_2/kg · min

II. 250 ml O_2/min

III. $\dfrac{\text{resting } \dot{V}_{O_2}}{\text{exercising } \dot{V}_{O_2}}$

IV. $\left(\dfrac{\dot{V}_{CO_2}}{\dot{V}_{O_2}}\right)_{\text{resting}} \left(\dfrac{\dot{V}_{CO_2}}{\dot{V}_{O_2}}\right)_{\text{exercising}}$

A. II only

B. III, IV only

C. I, IV only

D. I only

E. I, II only

45. Which of the following modes of oxygen delivery would be *most* cost effective for a home care patient using a cannula operating at 1 liter/min only at night?

   I. oxygen concentrator

   II. compressed gas cylinder

   III. liquid oxygen system

   IV. any one of these modes, because the oxygen usage is so small

A. IV only

B. II, III only

C. II only

D. I only

E. I, III only

46. How should a pulmonary emphysema patient be instructed to cough?

   A. She should be instructed to inhale to total lung capacity, breathhold for one second, then forcefully exhale.

   B. She should be instructed to inhale a moderate volume of air slowly through the nose, then rapidly and forcefully exhale.

   C. She should be instructed to inhale rapidly to mid-inspiration, then rapidly and forcefully exhale.

   D. She should be instructed to inhale a moderate tidal volume, then perform a series of short expiratory efforts.

   E. She should be instructed to use only a throat-clearing maneuver.

47. Which of the following statements are proper components of stair climbing instructions for a COPD patient?

   I. The patient should inhale while stepping up and exhale when his foot rests on the stair.

   II. The patient should rest between each step.

   III. The patient should incorporate pursed-lip breathing during this activity.

   IV. The patient should be breathing with a normal ventilatory pattern before beginning to ascend the stairs.

A. II, III, IV only

B. I, III, IV only

C. I, II, III only

D. I, II, IV only

E. I, II, III, IV

48. Why should COPD patients avoid using tranquilizers to induce sleep?

    I. They stimulate mucus production.
    II. They tend to suppress the cough mechanism.
    III. They produce a rebound effect and the patient may awaken anxious the next morning.
    IV. They may depress ventilations.

    A. I, II, IV only
    B. III, IV only
    C. I, III, IV only
    D. II, III only
    E. II, IV only

49. Which of the following maneuvers constitute breathing exercises or breathing retraining techniques?

    I. clavicular elevation
    II. diaphragmatic breathing
    III. sternocleidomastoid breathing
    IV. glossopharyngeal breathing
    V. lateral costal expansion

    A. I, III, IV only
    B. II, V only
    C. I, II, IV, V only
    D. II, III, V only
    E. I, III, IV, V only

50. Which of the following outcomes represent objectives of a rehabilitation program?

    I. improve patient self-image
    II. decrease work of breathing
    III. eliminate the need for bronchial hygiene
    IV. increase muscle efficiency

    A. I, III, IV only
    B. II, IV only
    C. I, III only
    D. I, II, IV only
    E. II, III, IV only

ASSESSMENT ANSWER SHEET

DIRECTIONS: Darken the space under the selected answer.

	A	B	C	D	E		A	B	C	D	E
1.	[ ]	[ ]	[ ]	[ ]	[ ]	26.	[ ]	[ ]	[ ]	[ ]	[ ]
2.	[ ]	[ ]	[ ]	[ ]	[ ]	27.	[ ]	[ ]	[ ]	[ ]	[ ]
3.	[ ]	[ ]	[ ]	[ ]	[ ]	28.	[ ]	[ ]	[ ]	[ ]	[ ]
4.	[ ]	[ ]	[ ]	[ ]	[ ]	29.	[ ]	[ ]	[ ]	[ ]	[ ]
5.	[ ]	[ ]	[ ]	[ ]	[ ]	30.	[ ]	[ ]	[ ]	[ ]	[ ]
6.	[ ]	[ ]	[ ]	[ ]	[ ]	31.	[ ]	[ ]	[ ]	[ ]	[ ]
7.	[ ]	[ ]	[ ]	[ ]	[ ]	32.	[ ]	[ ]	[ ]	[ ]	[ ]
8.	[ ]	[ ]	[ ]	[ ]	[ ]	33.	[ ]	[ ]	[ ]	[ ]	[ ]
9.	[ ]	[ ]	[ ]	[ ]	[ ]	34.	[ ]	[ ]	[ ]	[ ]	[ ]
10.	[ ]	[ ]	[ ]	[ ]	[ ]	35.	[ ]	[ ]	[ ]	[ ]	[ ]
11.	[ ]	[ ]	[ ]	[ ]	[ ]	36.	[ ]	[ ]	[ ]	[ ]	[ ]
12.	[ ]	[ ]	[ ]	[ ]	[ ]	37.	[ ]	[ ]	[ ]	[ ]	[ ]
13.	[ ]	[ ]	[ ]	[ ]	[ ]	38.	[ ]	[ ]	[ ]	[ ]	[ ]
14.	[ ]	[ ]	[ ]	[ ]	[ ]	39.	[ ]	[ ]	[ ]	[ ]	[ ]
15.	[ ]	[ ]	[ ]	[ ]	[ ]	40.	[ ]	[ ]	[ ]	[ ]	[ ]
16.	[ ]	[ ]	[ ]	[ ]	[ ]	41.	[ ]	[ ]	[ ]	[ ]	[ ]
17.	[ ]	[ ]	[ ]	[ ]	[ ]	42.	[ ]	[ ]	[ ]	[ ]	[ ]
18.	[ ]	[ ]	[ ]	[ ]	[ ]	43.	[ ]	[ ]	[ ]	[ ]	[ ]
19.	[ ]	[ ]	[ ]	[ ]	[ ]	44.	[ ]	[ ]	[ ]	[ ]	[ ]
20.	[ ]	[ ]	[ ]	[ ]	[ ]	45.	[ ]	[ ]	[ ]	[ ]	[ ]
21.	[ ]	[ ]	[ ]	[ ]	[ ]	46.	[ ]	[ ]	[ ]	[ ]	[ ]
22.	[ ]	[ ]	[ ]	[ ]	[ ]	47.	[ ]	[ ]	[ ]	[ ]	[ ]
23.	[ ]	[ ]	[ ]	[ ]	[ ]	48.	[ ]	[ ]	[ ]	[ ]	[ ]
24.	[ ]	[ ]	[ ]	[ ]	[ ]	49.	[ ]	[ ]	[ ]	[ ]	[ ]
25.	[ ]	[ ]	[ ]	[ ]	[ ]	50.	[ ]	[ ]	[ ]	[ ]	[ ]

CARDIOPULMONARY REHABILITATION AND HOME CARE ANALYSES

Note: The references listed after each analysis are numbered and keyed to the reference list located at the end of this section. The first number indicates the text. The second number indicates the page where information about the question can be found. For example, (1:219,384) means that reference number 1 is to be used and that on pages 219 and 384 information about the question will be found. Frequently, it will be necesary to read beyond the page number indicated to obtain complete information. Therefore, reference to the question will be found either on the page indicated or on subsequent pages.

1. D. Two types of oxygen concentrators are available. One type uses molecular sieves, and the other uses permeable plastic membranes. The molecular sieve variety incorporates an air compressor that forces room air to a set of sieves where nitrogen is separated from the air.

    Permeable plastic membrane concentrators have plastic membranes that are permeable to room air. The solubility and diffusivity of each gas component of room air determine the rate of diffusion across this membrane. Oxygen diffuses across faster than nitrogen. A compressor maintains a constant vacuum across the plastic membranes to enhance oxygen diffusion.

    Some oxygen concentrators can provide liter flows of less than 1 and up to 6 liters/min. The oxygen delivered usually has to be humidified. The oxygen concentration delivered varies inversely with the flowrate setting on the flowmeter. For example, the Mountain Medical Mini O_2 delivers 93% O_2 at 1 to 2 liters/min and 85% O_2 at 3 liters/min.
    (5:71–73), (38:123), 39:190–193)

2. E. Because of the direct relationship between cigarette smoking and cardiopulmonary disease, it is imperative to note the smoking history of every patient being evaluated. The standard method of documenting a person's cigarette consumption over the years is to use the pack-year measure. A pack-year is defined as the number of packs of cigarettes smoked each day times the number of years the person has smoked. For example, a person who has smoked three packs of cigarettes a day for 15 years has a 45 pack-year smoking history (i.e., 3 packs/day × 15 years = 45 pack-years).
    (40:15)

3. B. Lung consolidation is usually associated with bacterial and viral pneumonias, and is characterized by (1) increased vocal and tactile fremitus, (2) bronchial breath sounds, and (3) dull percussion notes over the area of consolidation. Chest movement on the affected side is sometimes reduced.

    In severe chronic airway obstruction breath sounds are either reduced or absent. Tactile and vocal fremitus are reduced and percussion produces resonant sounds.

    In a pleural effusion tactile fremitus is usually absent, and breath sounds are absent or reduced. Percussion produces a dull or flat sound.

    A fibrotic process produces reduced percussion sounds and inspiratory rales.
    (8:307–308), (40:82–85)

4. C. Sterile water or sterile normal saline prepared in the home for therapeutic use should be discarded after 3 days if the preparation is not entirely consumed by that time.

(40:220–221)

5. C. According to the American Thoracic Society (ATS), a pulmonary rehabilitation program should follow the sequence of care outlined below.

1. Patient selection: Consideration should be given to (a) the severity of the patient's disease, (b) the patient's psychosocial status, and (c) the personal factors.

2. Initial patient evaluation: Diagnostic data from pulmonary function studies, electrocardiography, chest radiography, etc., are needed to tailor the program to the patient.

3. Determine goals: Long-term and short-term goals must be established to ultimately provide a basis for program evaluation.

4. Outline program components: Pulmonary rehabilitation program components should include (a) physical therapy, (b) respiratory therapy, (c) education, (d) exercise conditioning, and (e) general considerations (environmental factors, pharmacologic intervention, etc.)

5. Assess patient progress: Evaluation of patient progress allows for program changes to be implemented if necessary.

6. Long-term follow-up: This helps to objectively evaluate the patient's progress and provides for educational reinforcement.

(6:680–681), (American Review of Respiratory Disease, *American Thoracic Society—Pulmonary Rehabilitation: An Official Statement of the ATS Executive Committee,* 124:663, 1981)

6. A. A number of diseases or clinical conditions are considered absolute contraindications for exercise testing. These include (1) uncontrolled asthma, (2) unstable angina, (3) hypertension, (4) symptomatic congestive heart failure, (5) acute myocarditis, (6) myocardial disease associated with ischemic changes on an ECG, and (7) febrile state.

(38:39)

7. A. Marasmus is the term that describes the condition resulting from a calorie deficit accompanied by a protein deficiency. Kwashiorkor malnutrition is characterized by a depletion of protein stores when the caloric supply is devoid of, or inadequate in, protein.

Nutritional assessment of the patient may reveal one of these two types of malnutrition. A combination of the two may also be present.

(38:87), (39:87–89)

8. D. The exterior aspects of a mechanical ventilator used in the home can be cleaned effectively with either 70% ethyl alcohol or a broad-spectrum germicide.

(38:229)

9. D. The dead space-tidal volume ratio (V_D/V_T) in a normal person ranges between

0.25 to 0.35 at rest. It usually decreases with progressive exercise to values ranging between 0.05 to 0.20.

The Bohr equation is used to calculate the V_D/V_T.

$$\frac{V_D}{V_T} = \frac{Pa_{CO_2} - P\bar{E}_{CO_2}}{Pa_{CO_2}}$$

where

V_D = the dead space volume

V_T = the tidal volume

Pa_{CO_2} = the arterial carbon dioxide tension

$P\bar{E}_{CO_2}$ = the mean exhaled carbon dioxide tension

Normally, during exercise the $P\bar{E}_{CO_2}$ increases as the tidal volume increases and approaches the Pa_{CO_2} value; consequently, the V_D/V_T ratio decreases. An increased or unchanged V_D/V_T ratio during exercise testing can be caused by high $\dot{V}_A/\dot{Q}_C$ ratios or small tidal volume increases. The V_D/V_T will increase or remain unchanged in COPD (chronic bronchitis and pulmonary emphysema), diseases associated with high ventilation-perfusion ratios, and diffuse pulmonary fibrosis. (1:119–120), (33:48), 41:29–30)

10. D. The ventilation-perfusion ratio represents the minute alveolar ventilation per pulmonary capillary perfusion, i.e., $\dot{V}_A/\dot{Q}_C$. The respiratory quotient refers to the carbon dioxide production over the oxygen consumption—$\dot{V}_{CO_2}/\dot{V}_{O_2}$. In a normal, resting adult person the $\dot{V}_A/\dot{Q}_C$ is ordinarily equal to the $\dot{V}_{CO_2}/\dot{V}_{O_2}$. The $\dot{V}_A/\dot{Q}_C$ is usually 4 liters/min over 5 liters/min; hence,

$$\text{ventilation-perfusion ratio} = \frac{\dot{V}_A}{\dot{Q}_C} = \frac{4 \text{ liters/min}}{5 \text{ liters/min}} = 0.8$$

In a normal, resting adult person the carbon dioxide production is about 200 ml/min and the oxygen consumption is 250 ml/min, therefore

$$\text{respiratory quotient} = \frac{\dot{V}_{CO_2}}{\dot{V}_{O_2}} = \frac{200 \text{ ml/min}}{250 \text{ ml/min}} = 0.8$$

During hyperventilation and exercise, anaerobic metabolism will increase the carbon dioxide production without proportionately increasing the oxygen consumption. (17:93), (33:45–46), (41:15)

11. A. Lobar atelectasis shown in Figure 175 causes the mediastinum to shift to the affected side. For example, if the right lower lobe is atelectatic, the mediastinum will shift to the right side.

Fibrosis of the lung parenchyma will result in a shift of the mediastinum to the affected side. Figure 176 illustrates this situation. A pleural effusion can cause the mediastinum to shift toward the unaffected lung. If, in the presence of a pleural effusion, the mediastinum is normally positioned, adhesions or an underlying atelectasis is suspected. Figure 177 depicts a right-sided pleural effusion. A consolidation, as seen in a lobar pneumonia, produces no mediastinal shift. A consolidation is demonstrated in Figure 178. (8:276,308,315,347), (40:82–85)

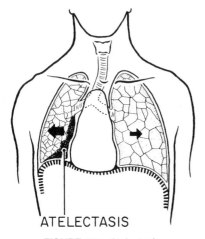

ATELECTASIS

FIGURE 175. Atelectasis.

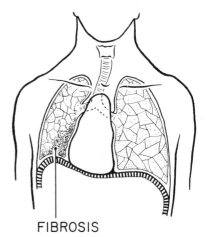

FIBROSIS

FIGURE 176. Fibrosis.

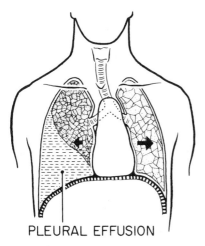

PLEURAL EFFUSION

FIGURE 177. Pleural effusion.

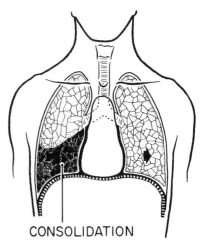

CONSOLIDATION

FIGURE 178. Consolidation.

12. B. Oxygen concentrators provide inadequate flowrates and oxygen concentrations to properly serve as the source for the operation of a Venturi mask, an aerosol mask, and a partial re-breathing mask. Increased flowrates from a concentrator produce lower oxygen concentrations. The two are inversely related.

A nasal cannula attached to a bubble humidifier can appropriately provide oxygenation needs for a variety of home care patients.

(5:71–73), (38:123), (39:192–195)

13. C. The delivery of oxygen to the lungs is best represented by the relationship

$$\dot{V}_A = \dot{V}_E - \dot{V}_D$$

where

$$\dot{V}_A = \text{minute alveolar ventilation}$$
$$\dot{V}_E = \text{minute ventilation}$$
$$\dot{V}_D = \text{minute dead space ventilation}$$

The amount of oxygen that is delivered to the lungs is dependent upon minute ventilation and minute dead space ventilation. For example, if the amount of dead space increases, the tidal volume (V_T) and/or ventilatory rate (f) must increase to provide an adequate amount of oxygen to the lungs for the tissue demands. If the minute ventilation is not sufficient to overcome the increased dead space volume, alveolar ventilation falls and oxygen delivery to the lungs decreases.
(1:118–120), (33:44), (41:28–29)

14. A. The primary objective of oxygen therapy for a COPD patient is to maintain that person's Pa_{O_2} at approximately 55 mm Hg to 60 mm Hg. Elevating the Pa_{O_2} beyond 60 mm Hg may eliminate the person's hypoxic drive. For some COPD patient's the hypoxic drive is the only stimulus for breathing.

Another consequence of oxygen therapy for a COPD patient may be a lessening or elimination of pulmonary hypertension, which is usually caused by (1) a decreased alveolar oxygen tension, (2) a decreased arterial oxygen tension, and (3) acidemia.
(3:172–173,176–177,512), (38:115,119)

15. E. When designing an exercise prescription for a patient, the practitioner must consider four components—intensity, duration, frequency, and mode. Intensity refers to the work phase of the exercise. The patient works to achieve a target heart rate. The duration of the exercise sessions will be determined by the severity of the disease. As the patient progresses through an exercise program, the duration can be increased. The frequency relates to the number of exercise sessions per day or per week. Initially, a patient may exercise for shorter periods, but two or three times per day. As the duration of the sessions increases, the number of sessions each day may decrease. The mode refers to the type of exercise conducted, e.g., walking and exercycling.
(33:23–24,31), (38:78–80)

16. A. The respiratory quotient (RQ) is defined as the carbon dioxide production ($\dot{V}_{CO_2}$) divided by the oxygen consumption ($\dot{V}_{O_2}$). The respiratory quotient is related to metabolism, i.e., the foodstuffs used for energy production.

When carbohydrates only are metabolized, the $\dot{V}_{CO_2}$ equals the $\dot{V}_{O_2}$, and the respiratory quotient will be 1.00. The following biochemical reaction shows the oxidation of glucose.

$$C_6H_{12}O_6 + 6\ O_2 \longrightarrow 6\ CO_2 + 6\ H_2O$$
$$R = \frac{6\ CO_2}{6\ O_2} = \frac{1}{1} = 1.0$$

When fats only are metabolized, the $\dot{V}_{CO_2}$ is less than the $\dot{V}_{O_2}$. The oxidation of palmitic acid (a fat) is shown below.

$$C_{15}H_{31}COOH + 23\ O_2 \longrightarrow 16\ CO_2 + 16\ H_2O$$

$$R = \frac{16\ CO_2}{23\ O_2} = 0.7$$

The respiratory quotient for proteins only reflects the average of the individual respiratory quotients of the amino acids. It generally averages 0.80. Proteins are not major sources of energy.

A mixed diet produces a respiratory quotient between 0.80 and 0.90.

(31:917), (33:7,45–46), (38:137–138), (40:333,337), (41:20)

17. C. A protocol is used in conjunction with exercise testing in cardiopulmonary rehabilitation programs to help evaluate a patient's performance. It provides standards for comparison of patient responses to stepwise, progressively increasing workloads. Examples of protocols commonly used include (1) Balke, (2) Naughton, and (3) Bruce.

(33:22–23), (39:38–39)

18. A. Chronic obstructive pulmonary disease (COPD) is associated with several metabolic changes. Weight loss occurs in proportion to the severity of the COPD. The weight loss appears to produce general malaise which, in turn, leads to anorexia contributing to further weight loss. If protein malnutrition occurs, lean body mass depletion follows. Lean body mass depletion produces respiratory muscle inefficiency. This condition places constraints on the patient's physical activity, as well as predisposing him to ventilatory failure. The protein malnutrition, accompanying the weight loss when an infection is present, may interfere with vitamin and mineral absorption.

(38:135–136)

19. A. The physiologic measurements that are made during an exercise will vary according to the testing protocol used. However, certain measurements are quite common. These include (1) ventilatory rate, (2) minute ventilation, (3) oxygen consumption, (4) carbon dioxide production, (5) respiratory exchange ratio, (6) metabolic equivalents, (7) arterial blood analysis, and (8) ventilatory equivalent for oxygen and carbon dioxide. Sometimes the V_D/V_T ratio and the steady-state carbon monoxide lung diffusion capacity study are obtained.

It has been found that in healthy persons the diffusion capacity increases substantially during exercise testing. The pulmonary capillary lung volume (V_C) and the membrane diffusing capacity (D_M) increase, thereby increasing the $D_{L_{CO}}$. In certain cardiopulmonary diseases the $D_{L_{CO}}$ is below normal at rest, and increases slightly during exercise testing. Such diseases include pulmonary emphysema, severe diffusion impairments, primary pulmonary hypertension, and chronic bronchitis.

(17:68), (32:127–129), (33:49–50)

20. B. For each degree Celsius rise in body temperature, the energy requirements increase by approximately 11% to 13%. Therefore, if a patient's temperature rises 2°C above normal, the energy requirements of that person will increase between 22% and 26%. The person's diet should be high in calories, protein, carbohydrates, salt, and fluids at that time.

(39:115)

21. A. Oxygen consumption, symbolized as $\dot{V}_{O_2}$, is synonymous with the terms oxygen uptake and oxygen intake. The normal value for the $\dot{V}_{O_2}$ in a resting person is about 250 ml/min.

    (33:23,26)

22. C. In addition to perceiving normal and abnormal (adventitious) breath sounds, auscultation is used to perform whispering pectoriloquy and egophony, and to detect vocal fremitus.

    High-frequency vibrations produced during whispering are ordinarily filtered by normal lung tissue. When lung consolidation is present, the ability of the lung tissue to continue filtering these high-frequency vibrations is lost. Instead these vibrations are transmitted to the chest wall. When whispering pectoriloquy is performed, the patient is instructed to whisper the words *ninety-nine,* or *one, two, three,* while the practitioner listens with the stethoscope against the patient's chest.

    Egophony is present over lung parenchyma compressed by a pleural effusion. A stethoscope is placed over the chest and the patient is told to say, "e-e-e-e." Egophony is present if the sound heard through the stethoscope is that of "a-a-a-a." This is described as e-to-a changes.

    Vocal fremitus refers to the vibrations that are perceived via auscultation when the patient phonates. Tactile fremitus refers to feeling these vibrations when the practitioner's hand is placed on the patient's chest wall.

    (8:214–222), (38:59,61), (39:20–23), (40:72–73)

23. A. The oxygen pulse is the oxygen consumption per heartbeat, i.e.

    $$O_2 \text{ pulse} = \frac{\dot{V}_{O_2}}{\text{heartbeat}}$$

    Normally, the O_2 pulse ranges between 2.54 and 4.00 ml O_2/beat at rest. The oxygen pulse rises normally during exercise to as high as 10 to 15 ml O_2/beat. Cardiac patients may have a normal or below normal oxygen pulse at rest. However, during exercise it does not increase to expected values.

    (17:93–94), (33:41), (41:158)

24. B. The dyspnea index (DI) relates the minute ventilation ($\dot{V}_E$), achieved during the last minute of an exercise test (at a submaximal level), to the maximum voluntary ventilation (MVV).

    The MVV is usually approximated by multiplying the FEV_1 by 35, i.e.,

    $$MVV = FEV_1 \times 35$$

    The degree of dyspnea, as derived from the dyspnea index, is shown in Table 19 shown on page 624.

    (17:87–89), (33:39), (41:64)

25. C. A number of safety precautions must be followed when using a home liquid oxygen delivery system. For example, the patient must always wear clothing that protects her skin because oxygen liquifies at $-297°F$ and can burn the skin. Also, the reservoir and the portable unit must be vented periodically to prevent pressure buildup from vaporized oxygen. Additionally, to prevent against splashing of liq-

TABLE 19

DI	Classification
< 35%	Normal for walking at 2 mph and 0% grade
35% to 50%	Mild to moderate
> 50%	Severe

uid oxygen, protective eyewear and gloves must be worn by the patient when filling the portable unit.
(39:198–200)

26. A. The relationship between oxygen consumption ($\dot{V}_{O_2}$) and heart rate (HR) during exercise testing is linear. An exercise prescription is developed according to this relationship.
(33:28)

27. C. Both lobar atelectasis and fibrosis of lung tissue will cause the mediastinum to shift toward the side where the pathophysiology is located, i.e., affected lung. A pulmonary consolidation produces no mediastinal shift. A pneumothorax and a pleural effusion can cause the mediastinum to shift toward the unaffected lung. See Figures 175-178 on page 620.
(8:216,276,308,315,347), (40:82–85)

28. A. Palpation is performed by the practitioner as she places her hands on the patient's thorax and observes the degree and symmetry of chest wall movement. Via palpation, the clinician can evaluate thoracic expansion, tactile fremitus, tracheal (mediastinal) deviation, and chest pain.

Thoracic expansion or chest wall movement can be evaluated when the practitioner places her hands on the patient's chest wall and instructs the patient to breathe. Figure 179 illustrates chest wall movement of the upper lobes. Movement of the right middle lobe, lingula, and the lower lobes can be evaluated in a similar

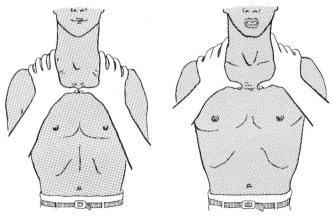

FIGURE 179

manner. The diagram on the left represents end-exhalation, and the diagram on the right shows end-inspiration. Note how the hands have moved equally.

Tactile fremitus refers to perceiving vibrations created by the vocal cords through the chest wall during phonation. The patient is ordinarily instructed to say *one, two, three,* or *ninety-nine.* Lung consolidation increases tactile fremitus—there are more vibrations transmitted to the hands.

Mediastinal shift is assessed by placing a fully extended finger medial to the sternoclavicular joint. If equal resistance is felt on both sides, the trachea is midline. The apex of the heart can also be felt to assess the presence of mediastinal shift.

(3:64), (8:215–219), (38:57–60), (40:59–62)

29. A. It has been said that supplemental oxygen delivered to COPD patients for at least 15 hours per day delays the onset of pulmonary hypertension and cor pulmonale.

    The factors primarily responsible for the development of pulmonary hypertension include (1) a decreased alveolar oxygen tension, (2) a decreased arterial oxygen tension, and (3) acidemia.

    The decreased $P_{A_{O_2}}$ and Pa_{O_2} cause pulmonary vasoconstriction and contribute to the development of pulmonary hypertension. Oxygen administration will improve the $P_{A_{O_2}}$ and Pa_{O_2} and thereby tend to diminish the tendency to develop pulmonary hypertension.

    (6:683), (38:115), (Daily Requirement of Oxygen to Reverse Pulmonary Hypertension in Patients with Chronic Bronchitis, Br Med J 3:724, 1972)

30. A. Physical therapists and/or occupational therapists are generally responsible for evaluating a patient's activities of daily living.

    (6:692)

31. D. Environmental conditions frequently have an adverse influence on a pulmonary patient's breathing. For example, cold weather can cause shortness of breath, coughing, or bronchospasm. Such patients should adhere to the following precautions:

    1. dress warmly
    2. walk slowly
    3. avoid the wind
    4. cover the mouth with a mask or scarf

    (40:137)

32. D. Proper body mechanics and breath control are important points to implement for a COPD patient, as they tend to reduce the work of breathing. For example, when lifting an object from the floor the patient should bend at the knees, maintain a straight back, then lift the object while exhaling slowly through pursed lips.

    (40:132)

33. E. By performing pursed-lip breathing, a COPD patient is expected to increase her tidal volume, lower her ventilatory rate, and raise her Pa_{O_2}. Some investigators found that the Sa_{O_2} also increased, while the Pa_{CO_2} decreased.

    (6:691), (38:68), (The Effects of Slow Deep Breathing on the Blood Gas Exchange in Emphysema, Am Rev Respir Dis 88:485–492, 1963), (Ventilation and

Arterial Blood Gas Exchange Induced by Pursed-Lips Breathing, J Appl Physiol 28:784–789, 1970)

34. D. The dyspnea index (DI) is a parameter that is used to assess the degree of ventilatory limitations to exercise. It is obtained by dividing the minute ventilation ($\dot{V}_E$) in the last minute of the exercise test by the maximum voluntary ventilation (MVV) and expressing it as a percent. The equation is

$$DI = \left(\frac{\dot{V}_E}{MVV}\right)100$$

A DI > 50% usually indicates severe dyspnea. Moderate dyspnea is classified as a DI between 35% to 50%. Dyspnea is absent when the DI is < 35%.
(17:87–78), (33:39), (41:64)

35. A. Patients who require supplemental oxygen at rest do so because of some mechanical or pathophysiologic defect. During exercise testing this ventilatory defect becomes accentuated; the lungs are incapable of performing gas exchange adequately. As a consequence, any hypoxemic condition worsens. Therefore, supplemental oxygenation may need to be increased during exercise testing. Generally, an oxygen saturation (Sa_{O_2}) greater than 85%, and a dissolved arterial oxygen tension (Pa_{O_2}) greater than 55 mm Hg, are minimally acceptable during the procedure. If the oxygenation status falls below this level, the exercise test is usually terminated. Inadequate oxygenation is potentially hazardous to patients, especially for organ tissues sensitive to oxygen deprivation, e.g., the myocardium.
(33:43,51–52,54)

36. A. Alveolar ventilation ($\dot{V}_A$) is the minute ventilation ($\dot{V}_E$) minus the dead space ventilation ($\dot{V}_D$).

$$\dot{V}_A = \dot{V}_E - \dot{V}_D$$

The following equation indicates the relationship between the alveolar carbon dioxide tension (P_{ACO_2}) and the alveolar ventilation ($\dot{V}_A$) for any given level of metabolism.

$$P_{ACO_2} = K\left(\frac{\dot{V}_{CO_2}}{\dot{V}_A}\right)$$

where

$$
\begin{aligned}
P_{ACO_2} &= \text{alveolar carbon dioxide tension} \\
K &= \text{proportionality constant} \\
\dot{V}_{CO_2} &= \text{carbon dioxide production} \\
\dot{V}_A &= \text{alveolar ventilation}
\end{aligned}
$$

Increased metabolic activity, e.g., increased carbon dioxide production, will cause the level of alveolar ventilation to increase. The increased CO_2 production associated with a high carbohydrate intake may have an adverse effect on cardiopulmonary patients in terms of their work of breathing.
(8:366–367), (31:685), (33:45–46), (38:138–139), (41:20)

37. B. The least expensive or most cost effective method of providing 3 liters/min of continuous supplemental oxygen to a patient at home is an oxygen concentrator.

    There are instances when compressed gas cylinders are more cost-effective. For example, a patient requiring a liter/minute of nocturnal oxygen would find the liquid system and the concentrator more expensive.

    (6:690), (38:123–126), (39:179)

38. C. A healthy resting adult demands approximately 3.5 ml of oxygen per kilogram of ideal body weight per minute. Therefore, to determine a person's oxygen consumption ($\dot{V}_{O_2}$), multiply the ideal body weight by 3.5 ml O_2/kg/min. For example,

$$75 \text{ kg} \times 3.5 \text{ ml } O_2/\text{kg}/\text{min} = 262.5 \text{ ml } O_2/\text{min}$$

    (33:28,68), (38:137), (41:122)

39. C. One liter of oxygen produces about 5 kcal of heat. The amount of oxygen in liters consumed per day times 5 kcal will provide the approximate daily caloric requirement for a person at rest. For example,

    STEP 1: Use the relationship below to determine the caloric requirements per minute.

    1. 263 ml/min = 0.263 liter/min
    2. (estimated $\dot{V}_{O_2}$ at rest)(5 kcal/liter) = kcal/min
       (0.263 liter/min)(5 kcal/liter) = 1.315 kcal/min

    STEP 2: The daily caloric requirements at rest can be calculated as follows:

    1. 1 day = 24 hours = 1,440 min
    2. (1.315 kcal/min)(1,440 min/day) = 1,894 kcal/day

    (33:67), (38:136–137)

40. A. It is recommended that patients who receive aerosol therapy at home clean their equipment (nebulizer, mouthpiece, etc.) daily, preferably after the last treatment of the day.

    (6:452–453), (39:209–211)

41. D. At the carina, the right mainstem bronchus arises from the trachea at an angle ranging from 20° to 30° from the midline. The left mainstem bronchus arises from the same point, but at an angle ranging from 45° to 60° from the midline.

    Based on this anatomic arrangement, a suction catheter, for example, will tend to follow the direction of the right mainstem bronchus. Therefore, to increase the possibility of inserting a suction catheter into the left mainstem bronchus, the patient should be instructed to turn her head to the right while advancing the suction catheter into the tracheobronchial tree. Similarly, the suction catheter supposedly will enter the right mainstem bronchus more easily if the patient is instructed to turn her head to the left while advancing the catheter into the tracheobronchial tree.

    (4:54), (3:253), (6:515), (39:52,236,239)

42. D. When performing a physical examination of the chest, the clinician should adhere to the following order: (1) inspection, (2) palpation, (3) percussion, and (4) auscultation.

    (6:286–295), (38:51–62), (39:13–23), (40:51–73)

43. A. A patient having pulmonary emphysema will sometimes display the following skeletal thoracic deformities:

    1. a kyphotic posture—increased convexity of the thoracic spine directed posteriorly
    2. increased anteroposterior diameter—consistent with the air trapping caused by the pathophysiology of the disease
    3. clavicular lift on inspiration—an attempt to gain a mechanical advantage to facilitate inspiration and to reduce the work of breathing
    4. increased transverse diameter—consistent with the air trapping (increased RV and TLC) caused by the pathophysiology of the disease.

    (4:305–306), (6:797), (8:286–292,659), (40:361)

44. D. One MET is equal to the resting oxygen consumption. During activity METS are calculated by dividing the metabolic oxygen consumption during exercise by the oxygen consumption at rest. One MET is equivalent to 1.0 kcal/kg · hr, or 3.5 ml O_2/kg · min.

    (41:11,230)

45. C. A compressed gas cylinder would be the most cost-effective mode of oxygen delivery for a home care patient receiving only nocturnal oxygen at a liter flow of 1 liter/min.

    (6:690), (38:123–125)

46. D. Pulmonary emphysema patients have difficulty with air trapping when coughing improperly. This loss of lung tissue reduces the normal elastic recoil properties of the lungs. Rapid air compression (rapid ascent of the diaphragm) generates supra-atmospheric intrapleural pressures. These high pressures can cause the airways to collapse. Therefore, forceful expiratory maneuvers should generally be avoided for these patients. Because the cough is associated with a rapid elevation of the diaphragm and supra-atmospheric intrapleural pressures, emphysematous patients should be taught a cough technique that can avoid these deleterious consequences, yet still assist in their bronchial hygiene. For example, the person should be instructed to inhale a moderate tidal volume (slightly more than the tidal volume), and exhale using a series of short compressions (not maximally forceful).

    (6:667–670), (39:164–166)

47. A. A COPD patient should be breathing in a comfortable ventilatory pattern before the stair climb is attempted. As he begins his ascent, he should exhale through pursed lips as he steps up and inhale when his foot comes to rest on each stair. He should be instructed to stop at each step to maintain a controlled and comfortable breathing pattern.

    (38:73,76–75)

48. E. COPD patients should avoid using tranquilizers or sleeping pills to induce sleep because these agents have a tendency to depress the cough mechanism and the ventilatory center.

(39:140)

49. B. Breathing exercises and breathing retraining techniques include

1. diaphragmatic breathing
2. lateral costal expansion
3. localized expansion
4. pursed-lip breathing

(4:403–404), (6:659–664), (38:66), (39:158)

50. D. A number of outcomes are sought in a rehabilitation program. These include (1) decreasing the work of breathing; (2) improving ventilation; (3) improving exercise tolerance; (4) reducing the use of accessory muscles of ventilation; (5) improving bronchial hygiene; (6) reducing stress and anxiety caused by the disease process; and (7) providing emotional, social, and psychologic support.

(38:6–7), (39:46–47), (41:1–9)

REFERENCES

1. Spearman, C., and Sheldon, R., *Egan's Fundamentals of Respiratory Therapy,* 4th ed., C.V. Mosby, St. Louis, 1982.
2. Wojciechowski, W., *Respiratory Care Sciences: An Integrated Approach,* John Wiley & Sons, New York, 1985.
3. Shapiro, B., Harrison, R., Kacmarek, R., and Cane, R., *Clinical Application of Respiratory Care,* 3rd ed., Year Book Medical Publishers, Chicago, 1985.
4. Kacmarek, R., Mack, C., and Dimas, S., *The Essentials of Respiratory Therapy,* 2nd ed., Year Book Medical Publishers, Chicago, 1985.
5. McPherson, S., *Respiratory Therapy Equipment,* 3rd ed., C.V. Mosby, St. Louis, 1985.
6. Burton, G., and Hodgkin, J., *Respiratory Care: A Guide to Clinical Practice,* 2nd ed., J.B. Lippincott, Philadelphia, 1985.
7. Frownfelter, D., *Chest Physical Therapy and Cardiopulmonary Rehabilitation, An Interdisciplinary Approach,* Year Book Medical Publishers, Chicago, 1978.
8. Cherniack, R., and Cherniack, L., *Respiration in Health and Disease,* 3rd ed., W.B. Saunders, Philadelphia, 1983.
9. Daily, E., and Schroeder, G., *Techniques in Bedside Hemodynamic Monitoring,* 3rd ed., C.V. Mosby, St. Louis, 1985.
10. Des Jardins, R., *Clinical Manifestations of Respiratory Disease,* Year Book Medical Publishers, Chicago, 1984.
11. Mitchell, R., *Synopsis of Clinical Pulmonary Disease,* 3rd ed., C.V. Mosby, St. Louis, 1982.
12. Comroe, J., *Physiology of Respiration,* 3rd ed., Year Book Medical Publishers, Chicago, 1974.
13. West, J., *Pulmonary Pathophysiology—The Essentials,* 2nd ed., Williams & Wilkins, Baltimore, 1982.
14. West, J., *Respiratory Physiology—The Essentials,* 3rd ed., Williams & Wilkins, Baltimore, 1985.
15. Martz, K., et al., *Management of the Patient-Ventilator System: A Team Approach,* 2nd ed., C.V. Mosby, St. Louis, 1984.

16. Shoup, C., and McHenry, R., *Laboratory Exercises in Respiratory Therapy*, 2nd ed., C.V. Mosby, St. Louis, 1983.

17. Ruppel, G., *Manual of Pulmonary Function Testing*, 3rd ed., C.V. Mosby, St. Louis, 1982.

18. Appelbaum, E., and Bruce, D., *Tracheal Intubation*, W.B. Saunders, Philadelphia, 1976.

19. Rau, J., *Respiratory Therapy Pharmacology*, 2nd ed., Year Book Medical Publishers, Chicago, 1984.

20. United States Department of Health, Education, and Welfare, Public Health Service, *Isolation Techniques for Use in Hospitals*, 2nd ed., Washington, D.C., 1975.

21. Brooks, S., *Integrated Basic Science*, 4th ed., C.V. Mosby, St. Louis, 1979.

22. Comroe, J., *The Lung*, Year Book Medical Publishers, Chicago, 1962.

23. Shibel, E., and Moser, K., *Respiratory Emergencies*, 2nd ed., C.V. Mosby, St. Louis, 1982.

24. Tisi, G., *Pulmonary Physiology in Clinical Medicine*, 2nd ed., Williams & Wilkins, Baltimore, 1985.

25. Cherniack, R., *Pulmonary Function Testing*, W.B. Saunders, Philadelphia, 1977.

26. Altose, M., *The Physiological Basis of Pulmonary Function Testing*, Clinical Symposia-CIBA, Vol. 31, No. 2, Summit, New Jersey, 1979.

27. Shapiro, B., Harrison, R., and Walton, J., *Clinical Application of Arterial Blood Gases*, 3rd ed., Year Book Medical Publishers, Chicago, 1982.

28. West, J., *Ventilation/Blood Flow and Gas Exchange*, 3rd ed., Blackwell Scientific Publications, 1979.

29. Slonim, N., and Hamilton, K., *Respiratory Physiology*, 4th ed., C. V. Mosby, St. Louis, 1981.

30. Rarey, K., and Youtsey, J., *Respiratory Patient Care*, Prentice-Hall, Englewood Cliffs, 1981.

31. Berne, R., and Levy, M., *Physiology*, C. V. Mosby, St. Louis, 1983.

32. Levitzky, M., *Pulmonary Physiology*, 2nd ed., McGraw-Hill, New York, 1986.

33. Wilson, P., Bell, C., and Norton, A., *Rehabilitation of the Heart and Lungs*, SensorMedics, 1980.

34. Clausen, J., and Zarins, L. *Pulmonary Function Testing Guidelines and Controversies*, Academic Press, New York, 1982.

35. Klaus, M., and Fanaroff, A., *Care of the High-Risk Neonate*, 2nd ed., W. B. Saunders, Philadelphia, 1979.

36. Lough, M., et al., *Pediatric Respiratory Therapy*, 3rd ed., Year Book Medical Publishers, Chicago, 1985.

37. Levin, D., et al., *A Practical Guide to Pediatric Intensive Care*, 2nd ed., C. V. Mosby, St. Louis, 1984.

38. O'Ryan, J., and Burns, D., *Pulmonary Rehabilitation from Hospital to Home*, Year Book Medical Publishers, Chicago, 1984.

39. Bell, C., et al., *Home Care and Rehabilitation in Respiratory Medicine*, J. B. Lippincott, Philadelphia, 1984.

40. Wilkins, R., et al., *Clinical Assessment in Respiratory Care*, C. V. Mosby, St. Louis, 1985.

41. Jones, N., and Campbell, E., *Clinical Exercise Testing*, 2nd ed., W. B. Saunders, Philadelphia, 1982.

42. Goldsmith, J., and Karotkin, E., *Assisted Ventilation of the Neonate*, W. B. Saunders, Philadelphia, 1981.

43. Blowers, M., and Sims, R., *How to Read an ECG*, 3rd ed., Medical Economics, New Jersey, 1983.

44. Eubanks, D., and Bone, R., *Comprehensive Respiratory Care*, C. V. Mosby, St. Louis, 1985.

45. Rattenborg, C., *Clinical Use of Mechanical Ventilation*, Year Book Medical Publishers, Chicago, 1981.

46. Witkowksi, A. S., *Pulmonary Assessment: A Clinical Guide*, J. B. Lippincott, Philadelphia, 1985.

47. Op't Holt, T. B., *Assessment Based Respiratory Care*, John Wiley & Sons, New York, 1986.

SECTION 5

APPENDIXES

APPENDIX I

MATHEMATICS ASSESSMENT EQUATIONS

The information contained here is required for the calculations in the Mathematics Assessment in the Basic Sciences Section. Persons using the Mathematics Assessment to solely
evaluate their mathematic skills should refer to the conversion factors, formulae, etc.,
listed here before performing the computations. Persons who are using this assessment to
evaluate their recall of such information should attempt the calculations before referring to
this appendix.

The answers and solutions to these calculations are located in the Mathematics Answers
and Analyses Section.

1. One kilogram (kg) equals 2.2 pounds (lb).
2. Use the formula

$$°F = \left[\left(\frac{9}{5} \right) (°C) + 32 \right]$$

4. Use the following rule governing the division of exponential numbers.

$$\frac{10^x}{10^y} = 10^x \div 10^y = 10^{x-y}$$

5. Use the factor 1.36 cm H_2O/mm Hg, or 1.36 cm H_2O/torr.
6. The capacity for water at 37°C is 43.8 g/m³ or 43.8 mg/liter. Use the relationship

$$\text{percent relative humidity} = \frac{\text{content}}{\text{capacity}} \times 100$$

7. Use the expression

$$FEV_{1\%} = \frac{FEV_1}{FVC} \times 100$$

8. Use the formula

$$\% \text{ oxygen saturation} = \frac{\text{content}}{\text{capacity}} \times 100$$

9. The expression for MAP is

$$MAP = \frac{\text{systolic pressure} + 2(\text{diastolic pressure})}{3}$$

10. The units of each factor in Reynold's equation are shown below.

$$R_N = \frac{\left(\frac{cm}{sec} \right) \left(\frac{kg}{cm^3} \right) (cm)}{\frac{kg \times cm \times sec}{sec^2 \times cm^2}}$$

11. Use the relationship

$$\frac{1}{C_L} + \frac{1}{C_{CW}} = \frac{1}{C_{L-CW}}$$

12. Use the equation

$$R = \frac{\Delta P}{\dot{V}}$$

13. Use the relationship

$$\frac{\text{air liter flow}}{\text{oxygen liter flow}}$$

14. Use the formula

$$°C = (°F - 32)\frac{5}{9}$$

15. Use the rule that governs the division of numbers having exponents.

$$\frac{A \times 10^x}{B \times 10^y} = (A \div B)10^{x-y}$$

16. Use the relationship

$$\frac{\text{inspiratory time}}{\text{expiratory time}} = I/E \text{ ratio}$$

17. Use the expression (Bohr equation)

$$\frac{V_D}{V_T} = \frac{Pa_{CO_2} - P\bar{E}_{CO_2}}{Pa_{CO_2}}$$

18. Use the formula (classic shunt equation)

$$\frac{\dot{Q}s}{\dot{Q}_T} = \frac{Cc_{O_2} - Ca_{O_2}}{Cc_{O_2} - C\bar{v}_{O_2}} \times 100$$

The end-pulmonary capillary O_2 content (Cc_{O_2}) = 24.78 vol%
The arterial O_2 content (Ca_{O_2}) = 24.36 vol%
The venous O_2 content ($C\bar{v}_{O_2}$) = 20.86 vol%

20. Use the equation

$$\text{humidity deficit} = \text{capacity} - \text{content}$$

21. Use the formula

$$C.I. = \frac{C.O.}{BSA}$$

22. One cubic foot of oxygen has a volume of 28.3 liters. The formula to use is

$$\frac{\text{conversion}}{\text{factor}} = \frac{\left(\begin{array}{c}\text{cubic feet of gas}\\\text{in a full cylinder}\end{array}\right) \times \left(\begin{array}{c}\text{number of liters/cubic}\\\text{foot of gas}\end{array}\right)}{\text{pressure in a full cylinder}}$$

23. The formula for flow duration is

$$\text{flow duration} = \frac{(\text{gauge pressure})(\text{conversion factor})}{\text{flowrate}}$$

25. Use the proportion

$$V_1 C_1 = V_2 C_2$$

APPENDIX II

COMMON LOGARITHMS OF NUMBERS[a]

N	0	1	2	3	4	5	6	7	8	9
10	0000	0043	0086	0128	0170	0212	0253	0294	0334	0374
11	0414	0453	0492	0531	0569	0607	0645	0682	0719	0755
12	0792	0828	0864	0899	0934	0969	1004	1038	1072	1106
13	1139	1173	1206	1239	1271	1303	1335	1367	1399	1430
14	1461	1492	1523	1553	1584	1614	1644	1673	1703	1732
15	1761	1790	1818	1847	1875	1903	1931	1959	1987	2014
16	2041	2068	2095	2122	2148	2175	2201	2227	2253	2279
17	2304	2330	2335	2380	2405	2430	2455	2480	2504	2529
18	2553	2577	2601	2625	2648	2672	2695	2718	2742	2765
19	2788	2810	2833	2856	2878	2900	2923	2945	2967	2989
20	3010	3032	3054	3075	3096	3118	3139	3160	3181	3201
21	3222	3243	3263	3284	3304	3324	3345	3365	3385	3404
22	3424	3444	3464	3483	3502	3522	3541	3560	3579	3598
23	3617	3636	3655	3674	3692	3711	3729	3747	3766	3784
24	3802	3820	3838	3856	3874	3892	3909	3927	3945	3962
25	3979	3997	4014	4031	4048	4065	4082	4099	4116	4133
26	4150	4166	4183	4200	4216	4232	4249	4265	4281	4298
27	4314	4330	4346	4362	4378	4393	4409	4425	4440	4456
28	4472	4487	4502	4518	4533	4548	4564	4579	4594	4609
29	4624	4639	4654	4669	4683	4698	4713	4728	4742	4757
30	4771	4786	4800	4814	4829	4843	4857	4871	4886	4900
31	4914	4928	4942	4955	4969	4983	4997	5011	5024	5038
32	5051	5065	5079	5092	5105	5119	5132	5145	5159	5172
33	5185	5198	5211	5224	5237	5250	5263	5276	5289	5302
34	5315	5328	5340	5353	5366	5378	5391	5403	5416	5428
35	5441	5453	5465	5478	5490	5502	5514	5527	5539	5551
36	5563	5575	5587	5599	5611	5623	5635	5647	5658	5670
37	5682	5694	5705	5717	5729	5740	5752	5763	5775	5786
38	5798	5809	5821	5832	5843	5855	5866	5877	5888	5899
39	5911	5922	5933	5944	5955	5966	5977	5988	5999	6010
40	6021	6031	6042	6053	6064	6075	6085	6096	6107	6117
41	6128	6138	6149	6160	6170	6180	6191	6201	6212	6222
42	6232	6243	6253	6263	6274	6284	6294	6304	6314	6325
43	6335	6345	6355	6365	6375	6385	6395	6405	6415	6425
44	6435	6444	6454	6464	6474	6484	6493	6503	6513	6522
45	6532	6542	6551	6561	6571	6580	6590	6599	6609	6618
46	6628	6637	6646	6656	6665	6675	6684	6693	6702	6712
47	6721	6730	6739	6749	6758	6767	6776	6785	6794	6803
48	6812	6821	6830	6839	6848	6857	6866	6875	6884	6893
49	6902	6911	6920	6928	6937	6946	6955	6964	6972	6981
N	0	1	2	3	4	5	6	7	8	9

[a]This table gives the mantissas of numbers with the decimal point omitted in each case. Characteristics are determined by inspection from the numbers.

COMMON LOGARITHMS OF NUMBERS[a] (continued)

N	0	1	2	3	4	5	6	7	8	9
50	6990	6998	7007	7016	7024	7033	7042	7050	7059	7067
51	7076	7084	7093	7101	7110	7118	7126	7135	7143	7152
52	7160	7168	7177	7185	7193	7202	7210	7218	7226	7235
53	7243	7251	7259	7267	7275	7284	7292	7300	7308	7316
54	7324	7332	7340	7348	7356	7364	7372	7380	7388	7396
55	7404	7412	7419	7427	7435	7443	7451	7459	7466	7474
56	7482	7490	7497	7505	7513	7520	7528	7536	7543	7551
57	7559	7566	7574	7582	7589	7597	7604	7612	7619	7627
58	7634	7642	7649	7657	7664	7672	7679	7686	7694	7701
59	7709	7716	7723	7731	7738	7745	7752	7760	7767	7774
60	7782	7789	7796	7803	7810	7818	7825	7832	7839	7846
61	7853	7860	7868	7875	7892	7889	7896	7903	7910	7917
62	7924	7931	7938	7945	7952	7959	7966	7973	7980	7987
63	7993	8000	8007	8014	8021	8028	8035	8041	8048	8055
64	8062	8069	8075	8082	8089	8096	8102	8109	8116	8122
65	8129	8136	8142	8149	8156	8162	8169	8176	8182	8189
66	8195	8202	8209	8215	8222	8228	8235	8241	8248	8254
67	8261	8267	8274	8280	8287	8293	8299	8306	8312	8319
68	8325	8331	8338	8344	8351	8357	8363	8370	8376	8382
69	8388	8395	8401	8407	8414	8420	8426	8432	8439	8445
70	8451	8457	8463	8470	8476	8482	8488	8494	8500	8506
71	8513	8519	8525	8531	8537	8543	8549	8555	8561	8567
72	8573	8579	8585	8591	8597	8603	8609	8615	8621	8627
73	8633	8639	8645	8651	8657	8663	8669	8675	8681	8686
74	8692	8698	8704	8710	8716	8722	8727	8733	8739	8745
75	8751	8756	8762	8768	8774	8779	8785	8791	8797	8802
76	8808	8814	8820	8825	8831	8837	8842	8848	8854	8859
77	8865	8871	8876	8882	8887	8893	8899	8904	8910	8915
78	8921	8927	8932	8938	8943	8949	8954	8960	8965	8971
79	8976	8982	8987	8993	8998	9004	9009	9015	9020	9025
80	9031	9036	9042	9047	9053	9058	9063	9069	9074	9079
81	9085	9090	9096	9101	9106	9112	9117	9122	9128	9133
82	9138	9143	9149	9154	9159	9165	9170	9175	9180	9186
83	9191	9196	9201	9206	9212	9217	9222	9227	9232	9238
84	9243	9248	9253	9258	9263	9269	9274	9279	9284	9289
85	9294	9299	9304	9309	9315	9320	9325	9330	9335	9340
86	9345	9350	9355	9360	9365	9370	9375	9380	9385	9390
87	9395	9400	9405	9410	9415	9420	9425	9430	9435	9440
88	9445	9450	9455	9460	9465	9469	9474	9479	9484	9489
89	9494	9499	9504	9509	9513	9518	9523	9528	9533	9538
N	0	1	2	3	4	5	6	7	8	9

[a]This table gives the mantissas of numbers with the decimal point omitted in each case.
Characteristics are determined by inspection from the numbers.

COMMON LOGARITHMS OF NUMBERS[a] (continued)

N	0	1	2	3	4	5	6	7	8	9
90	9542	9547	9552	9557	9562	9566	9571	9576	9581	9586
81	9590	9595	9600	9605	9609	9614	9619	9624	9628	9633
92	9638	9643	9647	9652	9657	9661	9666	9671	9675	9680
93	9685	9689	9694	9699	9703	9708	9713	9717	9722	9727
94	9731	9736	9741	9745	9750	9754	9759	9763	9768	9773
95	9777	9782	9786	9791	9795	9800	9805	9809	9814	9818
96	9823	9827	9832	9836	9841	9845	9850	9854	9859	9863
97	9868	9872	9877	9881	9886	9890	9894	9899	9903	9908
98	9912	9917	9921	9926	9930	9934	9939	9943	9948	9952
99	9956	9961	9965	9969	9974	9978	9983	9987	9991	9996
N	0	1	2	3	4	5	6	7	8	9

[a]This table gives the mantissas of numbers with the decimal point omitted in each case.
Characteristics are determined by inspection from the numbers.

APPENDIX III

VAPOR PRESSURE OF WATER

Temperature (°C)	Vapor Pressure (mm Hg)
20	17.5
21	18.7
22	19.8
23	21.1
24	22.4
25	23.8
26	25.2
27	26.7
28	28.3
29	30.0
30	31.8
31	33.7
32	35.7
33	37.8
34	39.9
35	42.2
36	44.6
37	47.0
38	49.7
39	52.4
40	55.3

APPENDIX IV

PERIODIC TABLE OF THE ELEMENTS

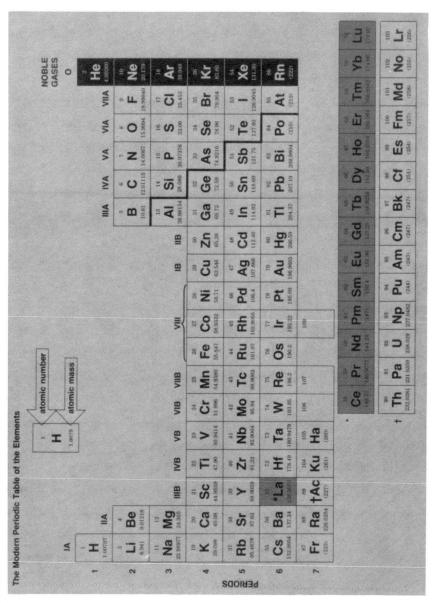

The Modern Periodic Table of the Elements

APPENDIX V

OXIDATION POTENTIALS

Anode	Anode reaction	Oxidation potential (standard hydrogen electrode = 0)
$Zn;Zn^{+2}$	$Zn \rightarrow Zn^{+2} + 2e^-$	+0.76 volt
$Pb;Pb^{+2}$	$Pb \rightarrow Pb^{+2} + 2e^-$	+0.13 volt
$H_2;H^{+1}$	$H_2 \rightarrow 2H^{+1} + 2e^-$	0.00 volt
$Cu;Cu^{+2}$	$Cu \rightarrow Cu^{+2} + 2e^-$	−0.34 volt
$Hg;Hg^{+2}$	$Hg \rightarrow Hg^{+2} + 2e^-$	−0.79 volt
$Ag;Ag^{+1}$	$Ag \rightarrow Ag^{+1} + 1e^-$	−0.80 volt
$Pt;Pt^{+2}$	$Pt \rightarrow Pt^{+2} + 2e^-$	−1.20 volts
$Au;Au^{+3}$	$Au \rightarrow Au^{+3} + 3e^-$	−1.50 volts

ILLUSTRATION CREDITS

1. Figures 1, 27: Reprinted with permission from Dubois, E.F., *Basal Metabolism in Health and Disease*, 3rd ed., Lea & Febiger, Philadelphia, 1936.

2. Figures 9, 26, 32, 33, 34: Reprinted with permission from Shapiro, B.A., Harrison, R.A., and Walton, J.R., *Clinical Application of Blood Gases*, 3rd ed., Year Book Medical Publishers, Chicago, 1982.

3. Figure 18: Reprinted with permission from Dripps, R.D., Comroe, J.D., Jr., American Journal of Physiology, 143:43, 1947.

4. Figure 19: Reprinted with permission from "Understanding Hemodynamic Measurements Made With the Swan-Ganz® Catherer" American Edwards Laboratories.

5. Figures 24, 84: Reprinted with permission from Spearman, C., et al., *Egan's Fundamentals of Respiratory Therapy*, 4th ed., St. Louis, C.V. Mosby, 1982.

6. Figure 38: Reprinted with permission from Wilson, R.F., *Principles and Techniques of Critical Care*, Vol. 1, F. A. Davis Company (Renal Physiology, Figure 6, page 10).

7. Figures 49, 115–120, 128: Reprinted with permission from Kacmarek, R.M., Mack, C.W., and Dimas, S., *The Essentials of Respiratory Therapy*, 2nd ed., Year Book Medical Publishers, Chicago, 1985.

8. Figure 150: Modified and reprinted with permission from Little, R.C., *Physiology of the Heart and Circulation*, 2nd ed., Year Book Medical Publishers, Chicago, 1981.

9. Figures 71, 76: Reprinted with permission from Radford, E.P., et al., Clinical Use of a Nomogram to Estimate Proper Ventilation During Artificial Respiration, The New England Journal of Medicine, 251:877–884, 1954.

10. Figures 73, 74, 75: Reprinted with permission from *Clinical Educational Aids* #1, and 7, G157, G163, Ross Laboratories, Columbus, OH 43216, 1978.

11. Figures 71C, 77: Reprinted with permission from Avery, M.E., *The Lung and Its Disorders in the Newborn Infant*, 2nd ed., W.B. Saunders, Philadelphia, 1964.

12. Figure 86: Reprinted with permission from Physical Principles of Respiratory Therapy Equipment, Ohmeda, Division of the BOC Group, Inc. Madison, Wisconsin, 1978.

13. Figure 114: Reprinted with permission from American Medical Association, Journal of the American Medical Association, August 1, Vol. 244, Number 5, page 264, Figure 1, 1980.

14. Figures 132, 141: Reprinted with permission from Wilkins, R., et al., *Clinical Assessment in Respiratory Care*, C.V. Mosby, St. Louis, 1985.

641

15. Figures 134–138: Reprinted with permission from Op't Holt, T., *Assessment Based Respiratory Care*, John Wiley & Sons, New York, 1986.

16. Figure 140: Reprinted with permission from Garrett, A., and Adams, V., *Pocket Handbook of Common Cardiac Arrhythmias: Recognition and Treatment*, J.B. Lippincott, Philadelphia, 1986.

17. Figure 172: Reprinted with permission from Goldsmith, J., and Karotkin, E., *Assisted Ventilation of the Neonate*, W.B. Saunders, Philadelphia, 1981.

18. Figures 173, 174: Reprinted with permission from Klaus, M.H., and Fanaroff, A.A., *Care of the High Risk Neonate*, 2nd ed., W.B. Saunders, Philadelphia, 1979.

19. Figures 175–179: Reprinted with permission from Cherniack, R., and Cherniack, L., *Respiration in Health and Disease*, 3rd ed., W.B. Saunders, Philadelphia, 1983.

20. Figures 2–5, 17, 25, 28, 29, 30, 42, 78–82, 89, 90, 99, 100, 101, 107–112, 131, 143, 146: Reprinted with permission from Wojciechowski, W., *Comprehensive Review of Respiratory Therapy*, 1st ed., John Wiley & Sons, New York, 1981.

21. Figures 22, 39, 43–48, 51–57, 60, 62–64, 66, 67, 170, 171: Reprinted with permission from Wojciechowski, W., *Respiratory Care Sciences: An Integrated Approach*, John Wiley & Sons, New York, 1985.

22. Figures 145, 147, 151–153, 157–161, 163–165: Reprinted with permission from Wojciechowski, W., *Comprehensive Review of Pulmonary Function*, John Wiley & Sons, New York, 1986.

23. Figure 162: Reprinted with permission from Phillip, R., and Feeney, M., *The Cardiac Rhythm; a Systematic Approach to Interpretation*, 2nd ed., W.B. Saunders, Philadelphia, 1980.

24. Figure 61: Reprinted with permission from Ruch, T.C., and Patton, H.D., *Physiology and Biophysics*, W.B. Saunders, Philadelphia, 1974.